Clear Cell Renal Cell Carcinoma 2021–2022

Clear Cell Renal Cell Carcinoma 2021–2022

Editors

Claudia Manini
José I. López

MDPI • Basel • Beijing • Wuhan • Barcelona • Belgrade • Manchester • Tokyo • Cluj • Tianjin

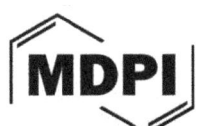

Editors
Claudia Manini
San Giovanni Bosco Hospital
Turin, Italy

José I. López
Biocruces-Bizkaia Health
Research Institute
Spain

Editorial Office
MDPI
St. Alban-Anlage 66
4052 Basel, Switzerland

This is a reprint of articles from the Special Issue published online in the open access journal *Cancers* (ISSN 2072-6694) (available at: https://www.mdpi.com/journal/cancers/special_issues/Clear_Cell_Renal_Cell_Carcinoma).

For citation purposes, cite each article independently as indicated on the article page online and as indicated below:

LastName, A.A.; LastName, B.B.; LastName, C.C. Article Title. *Journal Name* **Year**, *Volume Number*, Page Range.

ISBN 978-3-0365-5517-1 (Hbk)
ISBN 978-3-0365-5518-8 (PDF)

Cover image courtesy of José I. López

© 2022 by the authors. Articles in this book are Open Access and distributed under the Creative Commons Attribution (CC BY) license, which allows users to download, copy and build upon published articles, as long as the author and publisher are properly credited, which ensures maximum dissemination and a wider impact of our publications.

The book as a whole is distributed by MDPI under the terms and conditions of the Creative Commons license CC BY-NC-ND.

Contents

About the Editors ix

Claudia Manini and José I. López
Updating Clear Cell Renal Cell Carcinoma (a Tribute to Prof. Ondrej Hes)
Reprinted from: *Cancers* **2022**, *14*, 3990, doi:10.3390/cancers14163990 1

Kristyna Prochazkova, Nikola Ptakova, Reza Alaghehbandan, Sean R. Williamson, Tomáš Vaněček, Josef Vodicka, Vladislav Treska, Joanna Rogala, Kristyna Pivovarcikova, Kvetoslava Michalova, Maryna Slisarenko, Milan Hora, Michal Michal and Ondrej Hes
Mutation Profile Variability in the Primary Tumor and Multiple Pulmonary Metastases of Clear Cell Renal Cell Carcinoma. A Review of the Literature and Analysis of Four Metastatic Cases
Reprinted from: *Cancers* **2021**, *13*, 5906, doi:10.3390/cancers13235906 7

Tomas Pitra, Kristyna Pivovarcikova, Reza Alaghehbandan, Adriena Bartos Vesela, Radek Tupy, Milan Hora and Ondrej Hes
A Comprehensive Commentary on the Multilocular Cystic Renal Neoplasm of Low Malignant Potential: A Urologist's Perspective
Reprinted from: *Cancers* **2022**, *14*, 831, doi:10.3390/cancers14030831 21

Claudia Manini, Estíbaliz López-Fernández and José I. López
Towards Personalized Sampling in Clear Cell Renal Cell Carcinomas
Reprinted from: *Cancers* **2022**, *14*, 3381, doi:10.3390/cancers14143381 33

José Pedro Sequeira, Vera Constâncio, Sofia Salta, João Lobo, Daniela Barros-Silva, Carina Carvalho-Maia, Jéssica Rodrigues, Isaac Braga, Rui Henrique and Carmen Jerónimo
LiKidMiRs: A ddPCR-Based Panel of 4 Circulating miRNAs for Detection of Renal Cell Carcinoma
Reprinted from: *Cancers* **2022**, *14*, 858, doi:10.3390/cancers14040858 41

Nikhil Gopal, Pouria Yazdian Anari, Evrim Turkbey, Elizabeth C. Jones and Ashkan A. Malayeri
The Next Paradigm Shift in the Management of Clear Cell Renal Cancer: Radiogenomics—Definition, Current Advances, and Future Directions
Reprinted from: *Cancers* **2022**, *14*, 793, doi:10.3390/cancers14030793 57

Yann-Alexandre Vano, Sylvain Ladoire, Réza Elaidi, Slimane Dermeche, Jean-Christophe Eymard, Sabrina Falkowski, Marine Gross-Goupil, Gabriel Malouf, Bérangère Narciso, Christophe Sajous, Sophie Tartas, Eric Voog and Alain Ravaud
First-Line Treatment of Metastatic Clear Cell Renal Cell Carcinoma: What Are the Most Appropriate Combination Therapies?
Reprinted from: *Cancers* **2021**, *13*, 5548, doi:10.3390/cancers13215548 77

Gorka Larrinaga, Jon Danel Solano-Iturri, Peio Errarte, Miguel Unda, Ana Loizaga-Iriarte, Amparo Pérez-Fernández, Enrique Echevarría, Aintzane Asumendi, Claudia Manini, Javier C. Angulo and José I. López
Soluble PD-L1 Is an Independent Prognostic Factor in Clear Cell Renal Cell Carcinoma
Reprinted from: *Cancers* **2021**, *13*, 667, doi:10.3390/cancers13040667 91

Pablo Álvarez Ballesteros, Jesús Chamorro, María San Román-Gil, Javier Pozas, Victoria Gómez Dos Santos, Álvaro Ruiz Granados, Enrique Grande, Teresa Alonso-Gordoa and Javier Molina-Cerrillo
Molecular Mechanisms of Resistance to Immunotherapy and Antiangiogenic Treatments in Clear Cell Renal Cell Carcinoma
Reprinted from: *Cancers* **2021**, *13*, 5981, doi:10.3390/cancers13235981 . . . . **109**

Javier C. Angulo, Claudia Manini, Jose I. López, Angel Pueyo, Begoña Colás and Santiago Ropero
The Role of Epigenetics in the Progression of Clear Cell Renal Cell Carcinoma and the Basis for Future Epigenetic Treatments
Reprinted from: *Cancers* **2021**, *13*, 2071, doi:10.3390/cancers13092071 . . . . **133**

Myung-Chul Kim, Zeng Jin, Ryan Kolb, Nicholas Borcherding, Jonathan Alexander Chatzkel, Sara Moscovita Falzarano and Weizhou Zhang
Updates on Immunotherapy and Immune Landscape in Renal Clear Cell Carcinoma
Reprinted from: *Cancers* **2021**, *13*, 5856, doi:10.3390/cancers13225856 . . . . **163**

María Armesto, Maitane Marquez, María Arestin, Peio Errarte, Ane Rubio, Lorea Manterola, Jose I. López and Charles H. Lawrie
Integrated mRNA and miRNA Transcriptomic Analyses Reveals Divergent Mechanisms of Sunitinib Resistance in Clear Cell Renal Cell Carcinoma (ccRCC)
Reprinted from: *Cancers* **2021**, *13*, 4401, doi:10.3390/cancers13174401 . . . . **189**

Agnese Paderi, Roberta Giorgione, Elisa Giommoni, Marinella Micol Mela, Virginia Rossi, Laura Doni, Andrea Minervini, Marco Carini, Serena Pillozzi and Lorenzo Antonuzzo
Association between Immune Related Adverse Events and Outcome in Patients with Metastatic Renal Cell Carcinoma Treated with Immune Checkpoint Inhibitors
Reprinted from: *Cancers* **2021**, *13*, 860, doi:10.3390/cancers13040860 . . . . **211**

Philipp J. Stenzel, Nina Hörner, Sebastian Foersch, Daniel-Christoph Wagner, Igor Tsaur, Anita Thomas, Axel Haferkamp, Stephan Macher-Goeppinger, Wilfried Roth, Stefan Porubsky and Katrin E. Tagscherer
Nivolumab Reduces PD1 Expression and Alters Density and Proliferation of Tumor Infiltrating Immune Cells in a Tissue Slice Culture Model of Renal Cell Carcinoma
Reprinted from: *Cancers* **2021**, *13*, 4511, doi:10.3390/cancers13184511 . . . . **223**

ByulA Jee, Eunjeong Seo, Kyunghee Park, Yi Rang Kim, Sun-ju Byeon, Sang Min Lee, Jae Hoon Chung, Wan Song, Hyun Hwan Sung, Hwang Gyun Jeon, Byong Chang Jeong, Seong Il Seo, Seong Soo Jeon, Hyun Moo Lee, Se Hoon Park, Woong-Yang Park and Minyong Kang
Molecular Subtypes Based on Genomic and Transcriptomic Features Correlate with the Responsiveness to Immune Checkpoint Inhibitors in Metastatic Clear Cell Renal Cell Carcinoma
Reprinted from: *Cancers* **2022**, *14*, 2354, doi:10.3390/cancers14102354 . . . . **237**

Kalle E. Mattila, Paula Vainio and Panu M. Jaakkola
Prognostic Factors for Localized Clear Cell Renal Cell Carcinoma and Their Application in Adjuvant Therapy
Reprinted from: *Cancers* **2022**, *14*, 239, doi:10.3390/cancers14010239 . . . . **257**

Juan Pablo Melana, Francesco Mignolli, Tania Stoyanoff, María V. Aguirre, María A. Balboa, Jesús Balsinde and Juan Pablo Rodríguez
The Hypoxic Microenvironment Induces Stearoyl-CoA Desaturase-1 Overexpression and Lipidomic Profile Changes in Clear Cell Renal Cell Carcinoma
Reprinted from: *Cancers* **2021**, *13*, 2962, doi:10.3390/cancers13122962 . . . . **271**

Kazuho Saiga, Chisato Ohe, Takashi Yoshida, Haruyuki Ohsugi, Junichi Ikeda,
Naho Atsumi, Yuri Noda, Yoshiki Yasukochi, Koichiro Higasa, Hisanori Taniguchi,
Hidefumi Kinoshita and Koji Tsuta
PBRM1 Immunohistochemical Expression Profile Correlates with Histomorphological Features
and Endothelial Expression of Tumor Vasculature for Clear Cell Renal Cell Carcinoma
Reprinted from: *Cancers* **2022**, *14*, 1062, doi:10.3390/cancers14041062 . . . . **287**

Sari Khaleel, Andrew Katims, Shivaram Cumarasamy, Shoshana Rosenzweig,
Kyrollis Attalla, A Ari Hakimi and Reza Mehrazin
Radiogenomics in Clear Cell Renal Cell Carcinoma: A Review of the Current Status and Future
Directions
Reprinted from: *Cancers* **2022**, *14*, 2085, doi:10.3390/cancers14092085 . . . . **299**

Fiorella L. Roldán, Laura Izquierdo, Mercedes Ingelmo-Torres, Juan José Lozano,
Raquel Carrasco, Alexandra Cuñado, Oscar Reig, Lourdes Mengual and Antonio Alcaraz
Prognostic Gene Expression-Based Signature in Clear-Cell Renal Cell Carcinoma
Reprinted from: *Cancers* **2022**, *14*, 3754, doi:10.3390/cancers14153754 . . . . **317**

About the Editors

Claudia Manini

Claudia Manini is head of the Department of Pathology at San Giovanni Bosco Hospital in Turin, Italy. She graduated from the Faculty of Medicine and Surgery and post-graduated in Surgical Pathology at the University of Turin, Turin, Italy. Dr. Manini has served as pathologist for more than 25 years in several hospitals in Italy, developing an expertise in diagnostic uropathology, neuropathology and gynecopathology. She is also affiliated with the Department of Public Health and Pediatric Sciences at the University of Turin. Her main interest is translational pathology.

Jose I. López

Jose I. López is Advisor Researcher of the Biomarkers in Cancer Unit at the Biocruces-Bizkaia Health Research Institute. He graduated at the Faculty of Medicine, University of the Basque Country, Leioa, Spain, and trained in Pathology at the Hospital Universitario 12 de Octubre, Madrid, Spain. He received his PhD degree at the Universidad Complutense of Madrid, Spain. Dr. Lopez has served as a pathologist for more than 30 years in several hospitals in Spain, and subspecializes in Uropathology, where he has published more than 200 peer-reviewed articles and reviews. Dr. Lopez is interested in translational uropathology in general and in renal cancer in particular and has collaborated with several international research groups unveiling the genomic landscape of urological cancer. Intratumor heterogeneity, tumor sampling, tumor microenvironment, tumor ecology, immunotherapy, and basic mechanisms of carcinogenesis are his main topics of interest.

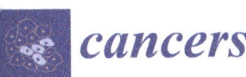

Editorial

Updating Clear Cell Renal Cell Carcinoma (a Tribute to Prof. Ondrej Hes)

Claudia Manini [1,2] and José I. López [3,*]

1. Department of Pathology, San Giovanni Bosco Hospital, 10154 Turin, Italy
2. Department of Sciences of Public Health and Pediatrics, University of Turin, 10124 Turin, Italy
3. Unit of Biomarkers, Biocruces-Bizkaia Health Research Institute, 48903 Barakaldo, Spain
* Correspondence: joseignacio.lopez@osakidetza.eus or jilpath@gmail.com

This Special Issue provides an insight into critical issues concerning clear cell renal cell carcinomas (CCRCCs), reflecting the recent level of intricacy reached by renal oncology. The collection includes nineteen papers (nine articles, eight reviews, one perspective, and one commentary) which deal with contemporary diagnostic, prognostic, and therapeutic aspects of this tumor. Moreover, this Special Issue aims to provide a humble and sincere homage to the memory of Prof. Ondrej Hes, a worldwide referential Czech pathologist in renal cancer, who passed away unexpectedly on 2 July 2022 at the age of 54. We are honored to have two contributions co-authored by him (refs. [1,2]) in this collection.

Manini et al. [3] focus on tumor sampling as a cornerstone to scrutinize the complexity of intratumor heterogeneity (ITH) in CCRCC. Based on the recent molecular findings of tumor regionalization [4], the authors propose focalizing tumor sampling on peripheral zones, where ITH is expected to be the highest. Conversely, the tumor interior, where metastasizing subclones develop, is more homogeneous.

Sequeira et al. [5] show that a specific pattern of miRNA expression characterizes CCRCC with a sensitivity of 74.78%. This pattern includes hsa-miR-126-3p and hsa-miR-200b-3p levels. The authors conclude that this minimally invasive test may be useful to detect CCRCC in the early stages of tumor development.

Gopal et al. [6] review the current advances and future directions of the use of radiogenomics in the management of CCRCC. The authors update the issue and stress the promising correlation found between imaging features and gene expression patterns in several neoplasms, particularly in CCRCC.

Vano et al. [7] review the first-line treatment options in metastatic CCRCC. They state that a strategy based on the International Metastatic Database Consortium is currently recommended with either pembrolizumab and axitinib, cabozantinib and nivolumab, or levantinib and pembrolizumab given as the first-line treatment for all patients. Additionally, patients with an intermediate or poor risk should be treated with nivolumab and ipilimumab. They indicate that several issues, such as PD-L1 status, are unresolved and deserve further analyses. Thus, making therapeutic decisions based on a reliable immunohistochemical detection of the PD-L1 is still a matter of controversy [8].

Larrinaga et al. [9] compare the plasma and tissue expression of PD-1 and PD-L1 in a series of 89 CCRCCs. This unprecedented analysis yielded some significant results, for example, the plasmatic levels of both proteins were lower in CCRCC patients than in the controls. The study also confirms that the high expression of PD-1 and PD-L1 in tumor tissue was associated with tumor grade, size, and tumor necrosis. While PD-1 was associated with tumor stage (pT), PD-L1 was associated with metastases. The combination of plasmatic and tissue positivity increased the level of significance to predict the prognosis of these patients.

Several contributions deal with the ever-changing landscape of therapies and resistances to therapies occurring in these tumors. Three clinical reviews [10–12] and one article analyzing sunitinib resistance in CCRCC cell lines [13] revisit this particularly important issue.

Ballesteros et al. [10] focus on the molecular mechanisms of resistance to immunotherapy and antiangiogenic drugs. Resistance associated with tyrosine-kinase inhibitors include molecular mechanisms related to hypoxia, the angiogenic switch, epithelial-to-mesenchymal transition, the activation of bypass pathways, the lysosomal sequestration of tyrosine kinase inhibitors, non-coding RNAs and single-nucleotide polymorphism, and the tumor microenvironment. Among the pathways associated with resistance to immune checkpoint inhibitors, the authors analyze interferon gamma signaling, Wnt/β-catenin, MAPK, PI3K/AKT/mTOR, cell cycle checkpoint, the loss of major histocompatibility complexes I and II, and the tumor microenvironment.

Angulo et al. [11] analyze the epigenetic landscape of CCRCCs. Thus, abnormal DNA methylation, methyl-binding proteins, post-translational histone modifications, miRNAs, long non-coding RNAs, and RNA methylation are thoroughly reviewed. Furthermore, the authors revise the epigenetic-based therapeutic opportunities for CCRCCs and the caveats and limitations of these treatments.

Kim et al. [12] update the immune landscape and the immunotherapy opportunities of CCRCCs, i.e., cytokine-based immunotherapy, tyrosine kinase and mTOR inhibitors, and immune checkpoint inhibitors. The authors also focus on single-cell genomics to analyze the tumor microenvironment.

Sunitinib is a standard first-line treatment for metastatic CCRCCs [14]. Armesto et al. [13] have identified miRNA:target interactions involved in sunitinib resistance using three CCRCC cell lines (786-O, A498, and Caki-1). They have demonstrated that the use of in vitro models of sunitinib resistance, combined with an integrated approach of miRNA and gene expression, can identify divergent mechanisms of resistance with potential benefit for patients.

Paderi et al. [15] retrospectively evaluate the immune-related adverse effect of nivolumab and ipilimumab in 43 patients with metastatic renal cell carcinomas, 36 of them being CCRCCs. They conclude that adverse effects, such as thyroid dysfunction and cutaneous reactions, were associated with longer progression-free survivals and that patients that experienced more than one adverse effect presented a better response to treatment. Endocrine disorders, notably thyroid toxicities, must be taken into account since they present clinically with vague symptoms and unclear clinical pictures. The effect of nivolumab on the PD-1 expression in a culture model of CCRCC has been analyzed by Stenzel et al. [16]. They conclude that data obtained from ex vivo tissue slice culture may predict patient response to nivolumab. The influence of molecular subtypes based on genomic and transcriptomic features in the responsiveness of metastatic CCRCCs to immune checkpoint inhibitors has been reviewed by Jee et al. [17].

Mattila et al. [18] analyze the existing prognostic features and prediction models for localized CCRCCs, a growing group of tumors with an unpredictable clinical course. They conclude that prognostic factors and prediction models may help evaluate the risk of recurrence after surgical resection in localized CCRCCs, which would reduce follow-up imaging in low-risk cases. Additionally, better prediction models would help select patients for adjuvant trial therapies.

Lipidomic analysis adds interesting information in normal and neoplastic kidneys. Molecular histology has recently been profiled in non-tumor kidney tissue using the mass spectrometry of lipids [19]. Data obtained in this study demonstrate that up to seven lipidic patterns correlate with different parts of the nephron, allowing one to distinguish characteristic lipidic fingerprints in different individuals. The lipidomic analysis performed in samples from 12 CCRCCs has demonstrated the overexpression of stearoyl-CoA desaturase-1 (SCD-1) induced by the hypoxic microenvironment [20] which is characteristic of this neoplasm. The authors have detected a particular lipidomic composition involving SCD-1 in the center of CCRCC which in turns depends on the high hypoxic status found at this level. They conclude that SCD-1 may be a potential target in future treatments of these tumors. Other authors have detected that metastasizing clones of CCRCCs are located in the tumor's center [4], where hypoxia is high and the struggle for survival is fierce.

The molecular heterogeneity in paired primary and metastatic samples of CCRCCs has previously been analyzed [21,22]. Prochazkova et al. [1] have studied the mutational variability between primary CCRCCs (four cases) and their multiple pulmonary metastases (nine metastases in total). The authors conclude that all the cases studied displayed high mutational variability not only when comparing the primary tumors, but also among the metastases themselves. These findings confirm the previous analyses which stress the high inter- and intratumor variability in most CCRCCs, a feature of critical importance when making therapeutic decisions for patients.

Recent studies have shown that the angiogenic type of CCRCC is linked to *PBRM1* gene loss [23]. In this Special Issue, Saiga et al. [24] correlate the immunohistochemical expression of PBRM1 with specific architectural and vascular patterns in CCRCCs. The authors found that endothelial expression tends to be lost in cases with low PBRM1 expression. Previous studies of the same research group have demonstrated that a vascularity-based architectural classification of CCRCC has prognostic implications [25].

Khaleel et al. [26] analyze the translation between the radiologic phenotype and the underlying genotype available in the current radiogenomics literature of CCRCCs, reviewing PubMed, Medline, Cochrane Library, Google Scholar, and the Web of Science databases. Most studies use computed tomography images and the most common genomic mutations of CCRCC (VHL, PBRM1, BAP1, SETD2, and KDM5C) for such translation. They conclude that the field is promising but further studies are needed to implement this approach in clinical practice.

Roldán et al. [27] define a gene-expression-based signature in CCRCCs with prognostic implications based on a whole-transcriptome profiling of 26 cases. They found a total of 132 genes related to prognosis; however, following a Cox analysis, a nomogram including *CERCAM, MIA2, HS6ST2, ONE-CUT2, SOX12,* and *TMEM132A* genes, together with pT stage, tumor size, and ISUP grade, has been generated. The authors conclude that this nomogram discriminates between two different groups of CCRCCs with different probabilities of recurrence and predicts cancer-specific survival.

A commentary in this CCRCC Special Issue refers to the urologist's perspective of the so-called multilocular cystic renal neoplasm of low malignant potential [2]. The clinical, radiological, and pathological findings as well as the therapeutic management are reviewed. They conclude that this entity is a lesion with excellent prognosis in which a conservative nephron-sparing treatment, if technically possible from the surgeon's perspective, should be performed.

Author Contributions: C.M. and J.I.L. designed and wrote the manuscript. All authors have read and agreed to the published version of the manuscript.

Funding: This research received no external funding.

Conflicts of Interest: The authors declare no conflict of interest.

References

1. Prochazkova, K.; Ptakova, N.; Alaghehbandan, R.; Williamson, S.R.; Vaněček, T.; Vodicka, J.; Treska, V.; Rogala, J.; Pivovarcikova, K.; Michalova, K.; et al. Mutation Profile Variability in the Primary Tumor and Multiple Pulmonary Metastases of Clear Cell Renal Cell Carcinoma. A Review of the Literature and Analysis of Four Metastatic Cases. *Cancers* **2021**, *13*, 5906. [CrossRef] [PubMed]
2. Pitra, T.; Pivovarcikova, K.; Alaghehbandan, R.; Vesela, A.B.; Tupy, R.; Hora, M.; Hes, O. A Comprehensive Commentary on the Multilocular Cystic Renal Neoplasm of Low Malignant Potential: A Urologist's Perspective. *Cancers* **2022**, *14*, 831. [CrossRef] [PubMed]
3. Manini, C.; López-Fernández, E.; López, J.I. Towards Personalized Sampling in Clear Cell Renal Cell Carcinomas. *Cancers* **2022**, *14*, 3381. [CrossRef]
4. Zhao, Y.; Fu, X.; López, J.I.; Rowan, A.; Au, L.; Fendler, A.; Hazell, S.; Xu, H.; Horswell, S.; Shepherd, S.T.C.; et al. Selection of metastasis competent subclones in the tumour interior. *Nat. Ecol. Evol.* **2021**, *5*, 1033–1045. [CrossRef]

5. Sequeira, J.P.; Constâncio, V.; Salta, S.; Lobo, J.; Barros-Silva, D.; Carvalho-Maia, C.; Rodrigues, J.; Braga, I.; Henrique, R.; Jerónimo, C. LiKidMiRs: A ddPCR-Based Panel of 4 Circulating miRNAs for Detection of Renal Cell Carcinoma. *Cancers* 2022, *14*, 858. [CrossRef]
6. Gopal, N.; Anari, P.Y.; Turkbey, E.; Jones, E.C.; Malayeri, A.A. The Next Paradigm Shift in the Management of Clear Cell Renal Cancer: Radiogenomics—Definition, Current Advances, and Future Directions. *Cancers* 2022, *14*, 793. [CrossRef] [PubMed]
7. Vano, Y.-A.; Ladoire, S.; Elaidi, R.; Dermeche, S.; Eymard, J.-C.; Falkowski, S.; Gross-Goupil, M.; Malouf, G.; Narciso, B.; Sajous, C.; et al. First-Line Treatment of Metastatic Clear Cell Renal Cell Carcinoma: What Are the Most Appropriate Combination Therapies? *Cancers* 2021, *13*, 5548. [CrossRef]
8. Nunes-Xavier, C.E.; Angulo, J.C.; Pulido, R.; López, J.I. A Critical Insight into the Clinical Translation of PD-1/PD-L1 Blockade Therapy in Clear Cell Renal Cell Carcinoma. *Curr. Urol. Rep.* 2019, *20*, 1. [CrossRef]
9. Larrinaga, G.; Solano-Iturri, J.D.; Errarte, P.; Unda, M.; Loizaga-Iriarte, A.; Pérez-Fernández, A.; Echevarría, E.; Asumendi, A.; Manini, C.; Angulo, J.C.; et al. Soluble PD-L1 Is an Independent Prognostic Factor in Clear Cell Renal Cell Carcinoma. *Cancers* 2021, *13*, 667. [CrossRef]
10. Alvarez Ballesteros, P.; Chamorro, J.; San Román-Gil, M.; Pozas, J.; Gómez Dos Santos, V.; Ruiz Granados, A.; Grande, E.; Alonso-Gordoa, T.; Molina-Cerrillo, J. Molecular mechanisms of resistance to immunotherapy and antiangiogenic treatments in clear cell renal cell carcinoma. *Cancers* 2021, *13*, 5981. [CrossRef]
11. Angulo, J.; Manini, C.; López, J.; Pueyo, A.; Colás, B.; Ropero, S. The Role of Epigenetics in the Progression of Clear Cell Renal Cell Carcinoma and the Basis for Future Epigenetic Treatments. *Cancers* 2021, *13*, 2071. [CrossRef] [PubMed]
12. Kim, M.-C.; Jin, Z.; Kolb, R.; Borcherding, N.; Chatzkel, J.A.; Falzarano, S.M.; Zhang, W. Updates on Immunotherapy and Immune Landscape in Renal Clear Cell Carcinoma. *Cancers* 2021, *13*, 5856. [CrossRef] [PubMed]
13. Armesto, M.; Marquez, M.; Arestín, M.; Errarte, P.; Rubio, A.; Manterola, L.; López, J.I.; Lawrie, C.H. Integrated mRNA and miRNA transcriptomic analyses reveals divergent mechanisms of sunitinib resistance in clear cell renal cell carcinoma (ccRCC). *Cancers* 2021, *13*, 4401. [CrossRef] [PubMed]
14. Motzer, R.J.; Hutson, T.E.; Tomczak, P.; Michaelson, M.D.; Bukowski, R.M.; Rixe, O.; Oudard, S.; Negrier, S.; Szczylik, C.; Kim, S.T.; et al. Sunitinib versus Interferon Alfa in Metastatic Renal-Cell Carcinoma. *N. Engl. J. Med.* 2007, *356*, 115–124. [CrossRef] [PubMed]
15. Paderi, A.; Giorgione, R.; Giommoni, E.; Micol Mela, M.; Rossi, V.; Doni, L.; Minervini, A.; Carini, M.; Pillozzi, S.; Antonuzzo, L. Association between Immune Related Adverse Events and Outcome in Patients with Metastatic Renal Cell Carcinoma Treated with Immune Checkpoint Inhibitors. *Cancers* 2021, *13*, 860. [CrossRef] [PubMed]
16. Stenzel, P.J.; Hörner, N.; Foersch, S.; Wagner, D.-C.; Tsaur, I.; Thomas, A.; Haferkamp, A.; Macher-Goeppinger, S.; Roth, W.; Porubsky, S.; et al. Nivolumab Reduces PD1 Expression and Alters Density and Proliferation of Tumor Infiltrating Immune Cells in a Tissue Slice Culture Model of Renal Cell Carcinoma. *Cancers* 2021, *13*, 4511. [CrossRef]
17. Jee, B.; Seo, E.; Park, K.; Kim, Y.R.; Byeon, S.-J.; Lee, S.M.; Chung, J.H.; Song, W.; Sung, H.H.; Jeon, H.G.; et al. Molecular Subtypes Based on Genomic and Transcriptomic Features Correlate with the Responsiveness to Immune Checkpoint Inhibitors in Metastatic Clear Cell Renal Cell Carcinoma. *Cancers* 2022, *14*, 2354. [CrossRef]
18. Mattila, K.E.; Vainio, P.; Jaakkola, P.M. Prognostic Factors for Localized Clear Cell Renal Cell Carcinoma and Their Application in Adjuvant Therapy. *Cancers* 2022, *14*, 239. [CrossRef]
19. Martín-Saiz, L.; Mosteiro, L.; Solano-Iturri, J.D.; Rueda, Y.; Martín-Allende, J.; Imaz, I.; Olano, I.; Ochoa, B.; Fresnedo, O.; Fernández, J.A.; et al. High-Resolution Human Kidney Molecular Histology by Imaging Mass Spectrometry of Lipids. *Anal. Chem.* 2021, *93*, 9364–9372. [CrossRef]
20. Melana, J.; Mignolli, F.; Stoyanoff, T.; Aguirre, M.; Balboa, M.; Balsinde, J.; Rodríguez, J. The Hypoxic Microenvironment Induces Stearoyl-CoA Desaturase-1 Overexpression and Lipidomic Profile Changes in Clear Cell Renal Cell Carcinoma. *Cancers* 2021, *13*, 2962. [CrossRef]
21. Eckel-Passow, J.E.; Serie, D.J.; Cheville, J.C.; Ho, T.H.; Kapur, P.; Brugarolas, J.; Thompson, R.H.; Leibovich, B.C.; Kwon, E.D.; Joseph, R.W.; et al. BAP1 and PBRM1 in metastatic clear cell renal cell carcinoma: Tumor heterogeneity and concordance with paired primary tumor. *BMC Urol.* 2017, *17*, 19. [CrossRef] [PubMed]
22. Turajlic, S.; Xu, H.; Litchfield, K.; Rowan, A.; Chambers, T.; Lopez, J.I.; Nicol, D.; O'Brien, T.; Larkin, J.; Horswell, S.; et al. Tracking Cancer Evolution Reveals Constrained Routes to Metastases: TRACERx Renal. *Cell* 2018, *173*, 581–594. [CrossRef] [PubMed]
23. Brugarolas, J.; Rajaram, S.; Christie, A.; Kapur, P. The Evolution of Angiogenic and Inflamed Tumors: The Renal Cancer Paradigm. *Cancer Cell* 2020, *38*, 771–773. [CrossRef] [PubMed]
24. Saiga, K.; Ohe, C.; Yoshida, T.; Ohsugi, H.; Ikeda, J.; Atsumi, N.; Noda, Y.; Yasukochi, Y.; Higasa, K.; Taniguchi, H.; et al. PBRM1 Immunohistochemical Expression Profile Correlates with Histomorphological Features and Endothelial Expression of Tumor Vasculature for Clear Cell Renal Cell Carcinoma. *Cancers* 2022, *14*, 1062. [CrossRef]
25. Ohe, C.; Yoshida, T.; Amin, M.B.; Atsumi, N.; Ikeda, J.; Saiga, K.; Noda, Y.; Yasukochi, Y.; Ohashi, R.; Ohsugi, H.; et al. Development and validation of a vascularity-based architectural classification for clear cell renal cell carcinoma: Correlation with conventional pathological prognostic factors, gene expression patterns, and clinical outcomes. *Mod. Pathol.* 2022, *35*, 816–824. [CrossRef]

26. Khaleel, S.; Katims, A.; Cumarasamy, S.; Rosenzweig, S.; Attalla, K.; Hakimi, A.A.; Mehrazin, R. Radiogenomics in Clear Cell Renal Cell Carcinoma: A Review of the Current Status and Future Directions. *Cancers* **2022**, *14*, 2085. [CrossRef]
27. Roldán, F.L.; Izquierdo, L.; Ingelmo-Torres, M.; Lozano, J.J.; Carrasco, R.; Cuñado, A.; Reig, O.; Mengual, L.; Alcaraz, A. Prognostic Gene Expression-Based Signature in Clear-Cell Renal Cell Carcinoma. *Cancers* **2022**, *14*, 3754. [CrossRef]

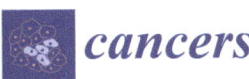

Review

Mutation Profile Variability in the Primary Tumor and Multiple Pulmonary Metastases of Clear Cell Renal Cell Carcinoma. A Review of the Literature and Analysis of Four Metastatic Cases

Kristyna Prochazkova [1], Nikola Ptakova [2], Reza Alaghehbandan [3], Sean R. Williamson [4], Tomáš Vaněček [5], Josef Vodicka [1], Vladislav Treska [1], Joanna Rogala [5], Kristyna Pivovarcikova [5], Kvetoslava Michalova [5], Maryna Slisarenko [5], Milan Hora [6], Michal Michal [5] and Ondrej Hes [5,*]

Citation: Prochazkova, K.; Ptakova, N.; Alaghehbandan, R.; Williamson, S.R.; Vaněček, T.; Vodicka, J.; Treska, V.; Rogala, J.; Pivovarcikova, K.; Michalova, K.; et al. Mutation Profile Variability in the Primary Tumor and Multiple Pulmonary Metastases of Clear Cell Renal Cell Carcinoma. A Review of the Literature and Analysis of Four Metastatic Cases. *Cancers* **2021**, *13*, 5906. https://doi.org/10.3390/cancers13235906

Academic Editors: José I. López and Claudia Manini

Received: 21 September 2021
Accepted: 22 November 2021
Published: 24 November 2021

Publisher's Note: MDPI stays neutral with regard to jurisdictional claims in published maps and institutional affiliations.

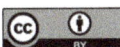

Copyright: © 2021 by the authors. Licensee MDPI, Basel, Switzerland. This article is an open access article distributed under the terms and conditions of the Creative Commons Attribution (CC BY) license (https://creativecommons.org/licenses/by/4.0/).

1. Department of Surgery, Faculty of Medicine in Pilsen and University Hospital Pilsen, Charles University, 304 60 Pilsen, Czech Republic; Prochazkovak@fnplzen.cz (K.P.); vodicka@fnplzen.cz (J.V.); treska@fnplzen.cz (V.T.)
2. Second Faculty of Medicine, Charles University, 150 06 Prague, Czech Republic; ptakova@biopticka.cz
3. Department of Pathology, University of British Columbia, Vancouver, BC 2329, Canada; Reza.Alaghehbandan@fraserhealth.ca
4. Robert J. Tomsich Pathology and Laboratory Medicine Institute and Glickman Urological Institute, Cleveland Clinic, Cleveland, OH 44195, USA; williamson.sean@outlook.com
5. Department of Pathology, Faculty of Medicine in Pilsen and University Hospital Pilsen, Charles University, 305 99 Pilsen, Czech Republic; vanecek@bioptica.cz (T.V.); superrrogalik7@gmail.com (J.R.); Pivovarcikova@fnplzen.cz (K.P.); Kvetoslava.Michalova@biopticka.cz (K.M.); MarynaSlisarenko@gmail.com (M.S.); Michal@biopticka.cz (M.M.)
6. Department of Urology, Faculty of Medicine in Pilsen and University Hospital Pilsen, Charles University, 305 99 Pilsen, Czech Republic; horam@biopticka.cz
* Correspondence: hes@biopticka.cz

Simple Summary: Clear cell renal cell carcinoma (CCRCC) is well known for intra-tumoral heterogeneity. However, there are limited data focusing on the inter-tumoral and inter-metastatic heterogeneity of CCRCC. In one study, primary and metastatic tumors were classified as clear cell type A or B subtypes, using nanostring expression technology. It was found that primary and metastatic tumors of CCRCC differed in nearly one half of patients. Approximately one quarter of metastatic tumors display inter-metastatic heterogeneity. Another study, using an immunohistochemical assay, found inter-metastatic tumor heterogeneity of BAP1 in only 1 of 32 patients (3%). Comparing gene expression across patient-matched primary-metastatic tumor pairs, 98% had concordant BAP1 status. We aimed to review published data and to examine mutation profile variability in primary and multiple pulmonary metastases (PMs) in our cohort of four patients with metastatic CCRCC.

Abstract: (1) Background: There are limited data concerning inter-tumoral and inter-metastatic heterogeneity in clear cell renal cell carcinoma (CCRCC). The aim of our study was to review published data and to examine mutation profile variability in primary and multiple pulmonary metastases (PMs) in our cohort of four patients with metastatic CCRCC. (2) Methods: Four patients were enrolled in this study. The clinical characteristics, types of surgeries, histopathologic results, immunohistochemical and genetic evaluations of corresponding primary tumor and PMs, and follow-up data were recorded. (3) Results: In our series, the most commonly mutated genes were those in the canonically dysregulated VHL pathway, which were detected in both primary tumors and corresponding metastasis. There were genetic profile differences between primary and metastatic tumors, as well as among particular metastases in one patient. (4) Conclusions: CCRCC shows heterogeneity between the primary tumor and its metastasis. Such mutational changes may be responsible for suboptimal treatment outcomes in targeted therapy settings.

Keywords: clear cell renal cell carcinoma; intra-tumoral heterogeneity; inter-tumoral heterogeneity; inter-metastatic heterogeneity

1. Introduction

Clear cell renal cell carcinoma (CCRCC) is the most common renal carcinoma, accounting for more than 70% of adult renal cancer [1,2]. Nonsurgical therapy for metastatic RCC (mRCC) has limited efficacy, with a median overall survival (OS) of 26.4–32.0 months [2]. The lung is one of the most affected metastatic sites in patients with CCRCC. If clinically feasible, metastasectomy is preferable for metastatic disease [3]. The 5 year survival rates after a complete pulmonary metastasectomy range from 36 to 83% [4].

CCRCC is well known for intra-tumoral heterogeneity [2,5–10] and morphologic, immunohistochemical and genetic differences also exist between the primary tumor and its metastases (inter-tumoral heterogeneity) [11–14]. Furthermore, heterogeneity among multiple metastases in a single patient (inter-metastatic heterogeneity) has been reported [11,14].

VHL, *BAP1*, *PBRM1*, and *SETD2* are the most frequently mutated genes, all located on chromosome 3p. Chromosome arm 3p loss is a common event in primary CCRCC, and in difficult diagnostic pathology cases, molecular evaluation can be used to support a diagnosis of CCRCC, such as chromosome 3p loss (FISH, cytogenetics, or copy number analysis) or VHL mutational analysis. However, 3p loss may not be entirely specific for clear cell RCC in all contexts [15]. For example, chromosome 3p loss has been recognized in subsets of papillary RCC, unclassified RCC, and RCC with the amplification of the 6p21/*TFEB* gene region, including in tumors with non-clear cell morphology and without *VHL* alterations [16–18]. Although the majority of CCRCCs show mutation in the *VHL* gene, LOH3p, or the hypermethylation status of *VHL* gene, 25–30% of CCRCCs show other molecular genetic changes [2]. The molecular study of the Cancer Genome Atlas Research Network identified 19 significantly mutated genes, with alterations of *VHL*, *PBRM1*, *SETD2*, *KDMC*, *PTEN*, *BAP1*, *MTOR* and *TP53*, being the eight most frequent [2,19].

CCRCC is ideal for studying intra-tumoral heterogeneity, since adjuvant therapy is not standard practice [3]. Therefore, the effect of therapy on the development of resistance or tumor changes can be excluded. The aim of this review was to summarize the current knowledge on intra-tumoral, inter-tumoral, and inter-metastatic heterogeneity in CCRCC at the morphologic, immunohistochemical, and molecular-genetic levels.

1.1. Morphology and Immunohistochemistry
1.1.1. Intra-Tumoral Heterogeneity

López et al. [5] drew attention to the problem of tumor sampling, particularly in CCRCC where some large tumors may display areas with different colors and/or textures on gross sections. It is worth noting that even neoplastic cell populations in CCRCC, which may seem homogenous microscopically, indeed may be very heterogeneous at the molecular level with different mutation profiles in different parts of the tumor [6]. In routine clinical practice, more than 95% of the tissue of a given 10 cm tumor is not analyzed, when following typical sampling protocols (i.e., one block per 1–2 cm of the tumor). In these cases, the histo-molecular data that might be derived from non-sampled areas of the tumor are lost. Therefore, some authors suggest that a multisite tumor sampling approach would be more informative than routine sampling [6,7].

CCRCC is typically immunoreactive for PAX8, PAX2, pankeratin (AE1–AE3), CAM5.2, and epithelial membrane antigens. Carbonic anhydrase 9 (CA9) is positive in a diffuse membranous pattern in 75–100% of CCRCC; however, high-grade tumors may exhibit a reduced immunohistochemical expression [2]. According to the latest edition of the WHO classification of genitourinary tumors, keratin 7 positivity in CCRCC is only seen in isolated cells, in rare high-grade tumors, and is often used to distinguish CCRCC from chromophobe RCC [2]. However, in a recent study by Gonzalez et al. examining keratin 7 reactivity in a spectrum of 75 CCRCC tumors, it was shown that low-grade CCRCCs were more frequently positive than high-grade tumors [8].

1.1.2. Inter-Tumoral Heterogeneity

Eckel-Passow and colleagues analyzed the immunohistochemical expression of BAP1 and PBRM1 in primary and metastatic tumors from 97 patients. In their cohort, 20% of primary tumors showed the loss of BAP1 staining and 57% showed the loss of PBRM1. They demonstrated subtle molecular heterogeneity in the metastatic tumors with similar morphology. Comparing expression across patient-matched primary-metastatic tumor pairs, the authors reported that 98% had concordant BAP1 status (90% PBRM1). Only two patients demonstrated discordant BAP1 immunohistochemical expression, with the loss of BAP1 during the progression to metastatic disease [11].

1.1.3. Inter-Metastatic Heterogeneity

Eckel-Passow et al. [11] also determined the inter-metastatic tumor heterogeneity of BAP1 using immunohistochemical examination. However, they found heterogeneity of BAP1 in only 1 patient in a cohort of 32 patients (3%). The primary tumor for this patient was BAP1 positive, whereas the first bone metastasis was IHC negative, and the second bone metastasis) was IHC positive. In this study, the authors also examined intra-metastatic tumor heterogeneity, and found a 100% concordance in BAP1 between 12 patients. The limitation of this study was that the expression was determined using an immunohistochemical assay only, with no further molecular genetic validation.

1.2. Molecular Genetic Analysis

1.2.1. Intra-Tumoral Heterogeneity

Gerlinger et al. analyzed material from four tumors (core biopsy) in four patients with metastatic CCRCC. They demonstrated intra-tumoral heterogeneity for a mutation within an auto-inhibitory domain of the mTOR kinase. Mutational intratumoral heterogeneity was found for multiple tumor suppressor genes resulting in a loss of function. Multiple distinct mutations of *SETD2*, *PTEN*, and *KDM5C* genes were found within a single tumor [9].

In their subsequent study, the authors showed that ultra-deep sequencing identified intra-tumoral heterogeneity in all cases. Using multiregional exome sequencing, the authors reported the following as the most prevalent mutations: *PBRM1* 60%, *SETD2* 30%, *BAP1* 40%, *KDM5C* 10%, *TP53* 40%, *ATM* 10%, *ARID1A* 10%, *PTEN* 20%, *MTOR* 10%, *PIK3CA* 20%, and *TSC2* 10%. The combined prevalence of the indicated PI3K-mTOR pathway genes (*PTEN*, *PIK3CA*, *TSC2*, *MTOR*) was up to 60% [10].

1.2.2. Inter-Tumoral Heterogeneity

According to Serie et al. [14], heterogeneity between primary and distant simultaneous metastases affects half of the patients with metastatic CCRCC. The authors analyzed primary CCRCC and their metastases using nanostring technology. Nanostring assays were successful in 91 primary tumors and 123 metastases from different organs, most frequently from the lung. ClearCode 34 genes were also analyzed for all tumors. They divided primary and secondary tumors into so-called ccA and ccB subtypes, based on the proposed stratification by Brooks et al. [12]. They further compared ccA/ccB subtypes across patient-matched primary and metastatic CCRCC tumors and documented discordance in 43% of patients.

1.2.3. Inter-Metastatic Heterogeneity

Serie et al. [14] also evaluated inter-metastatic tumor heterogeneity. Thirty patients in their cohort had more than one metastatic tumor. Seven of the 30 (23%) had metastatic tumors with discordant ccA/ccB subtypes.

2. Materials and Methods

Pulmonary metastasectomy for metastatic CCRCC (single or multiple metastases) was performed in 35 patients (without evidence of local residual disease, recurrence, or any disease other than pulmonary metastases) in a single academic institution (Department of

Surgery, University Hospital in Pilsen) from January 2001 to January 2019. From this cohort, 13 patients had undergone multifocal surgical treatments for their pulmonary metastases of CCRCC. Four patients were excluded from our study since the primary tumor was not available. Five patients were later excluded from the study because of low DNA quality. Finally, four cases were selected and enrolled into the study.

The following clinical and pathologic characteristics were obtained: gender, age at diagnosis, tumor size, pathologic stage [20], histologic grade (ISUP/WHO) [2], progression-free interval (PFI is defined as the time period between curative primary kidney surgery and the first detection of metastatic disease), pulmonary metastases details (site, size of the largest metastasis, synchronous or metachronous, number, and laterality), the type of pulmonary surgery, histopathology results, the type of adjuvant therapies, and follow-up data.

The primary tumor was diagnosed based on morphology and the immunohistochemical (IHC) profile. The tissues were processed as published previously [21]. The following primary antibodies were used: keratin 7 (OV-TL12/30, monoclonal, DakoCytomation, 1:200), vimentin (D9, monoclonal, NeoMarkers, Westinghouse, CA, USA, 1:1000), carbonic anhydrase 9 (rhCA9, monoclonal, R&D Systems, Abingdon, GB, USA, 1:100), PD-L1 (22C3, monoclonal, Cell Signaling, Danvers, MA, USA, 1:25), and Ki67 (MIB1, monoclonal, Dako, Glostrup, Denmark, 1:1000). The primary antibodies were visualized using a supersensitive streptavidin–biotin–peroxidase complex (BioGenex, Fremont, CA, USA). Internal biotin was blocked by the standard protocol used by the Ventana BenchMark XT automated stainer (hydrogen peroxide-based). Appropriate positive and negative controls were applied. The immunohistochemical evaluation was based on the staining percentage of cells: focal positive < 50%, diffuse positive > 50%, and negative (−) 0%. For the PD-L1 antibody, a total % of positive neoplastic cells and % of intervening stromal cells and lymphocytes was recorded.

2.1. Mutation Analysis

A mutation analysis detection of tumor and non-tumor tissue was performed using a TruSight Oncology 500 (TSO500) panel (Illumina, San Diego, CA, USA) [22]. In two cases, data from the TruSight Tumor 170 panel (TS170) (Illumina) were used for samples with low DNA quality. The gene list was previously published [23]. Total nucleic acid was extracted using an FFPE DNA kit (automated on an RSC 48 Instrument, Promega, Madison, WI, USA). Purified DNA was quantified using a Qubit Broad Range DNA assay (Thermo Fisher Scientific, Waltham, MA, USA). The quality of DNA was assessed using the FFPE QC kit (Illumina). DNA samples with Cq < 5 were used for further analysis. After DNA enzymatic fragmentation with a KAPA Frag Kit (Kapa Biosystems, Washington, MA, USA), DNA libraries were prepared with the TSO500/TS170 (Illumina) according to the manufacturer's protocol. Sequencing was performed on the NextSeq 500 sequencer (Illumina) following the manufacturer's recommendations. A data analysis was performed using the TSO500/TS170 application on the BaseSpace Sequence Hub (Illumina). DNA variant filtering and annotation were performed using the cloud-based tool Variant Interpreter (Illumina). A custom variant filter was set up including only variants with coding consequences at an allelic frequency of 5% and higher. The cut-off was set at 1% only in the case of mutations known in related tumor tissue. Comparing tumor and non-tumor data, germline alterations were excluded. The remaining subset of variants was checked visually, and suspected artefactual variants were excluded.

2.2. Analysis of VHL Promoter Methylation

The detection of promoter methylation was carried out via methylation-specific PCR as previously described [24].

2.3. LOH Analysis

For an LOH analysis of neoplastic tissue DNA, ten STR (short tandem repeats) markers D3S666, D3S1270, D3S1300, D3S1581, D3S1597, D3S1600, D3S1603, D3S1768, D3S2338 and D3S3630 located on the short arm of chromosome 3 (3p) were chosen from the database (Gene Bank UniSTS) [25].

3. Results

Four patients were enrolled in the study. Clinicopathologic data are summarized in Table 1. The patients were two men and two women, with ages ranging from 53.6 to 67.4 years (mean 61.5, median 62.5 years) at the time of renal surgery. Radical nephrectomy was performed in three cases. In one case, nephron sparing surgery was performed, but during the follow-up period, radical nephrectomy was completed due to recurrence (after a period of 72.6 months). Tumor size ranged from 30 mm to 75 mm (mean 53.5, median 54.5). The pathologic stage included 1× pT2a, 1× pT3a, and 2× pT1a. At the time of diagnosis, one patient had synchronous pulmonary lesions. The median progression-free interval (PFI) of the other cases was 40.5 months.

The mean age at the time of pulmonary metastasectomy was 65.5 years. Two patients had bilateral lung metastases, which were resected in a multistage fashion in independent surgeries. Overall, nine metastases were removed (in three patients, there were two metastases; in one patient, there were three metastases).

Signs of aggressive behavior were found approximately 2 to 35 months after pulmonary metastasectomy (metastatic progression to bones, lung, mediastinum, lymph nodes, and brain; median PFI was 18.7). Follow-up data were available for all patients, ranging approximately from 88 to 123 months (mean 104.4, median 103.4 months). For brain metastasis, surgical treatment using a gamma knife was performed. However, this patient died of peritonitis 3 months after the brain surgery. One patient died from the progression of the disease to the lung and bone 6 years after pulmonary surgery. To date, one patient with a progression of disease after 2 months (lymphatic tissue, bones, kidney) and one patient with a progression of disease 35 months (lymph nodes) after pulmonary surgery are alive.

Table 1. Primary tumors: clinicopathological features.

	Patient 1	Patient 2	Patient 3	Patient 4
Sex	F	M	M	F
Age (years)	61.6	67.4	63.4	53.6
Size (mm)	39	75	30	70
pT (UICC 2017)	pT1a	pT2a	pT1a	pT3b
Grade (WHO/ISUP)	3	2	2	2
TTP meta 1	40.5	M1	59.6	38.1
TTP meta 2	40.5	M1	81.1	38.1
TTP meta 3	-	-	81.1	

F, female; M, male; M1, M1 stage (pulmonary metastases at the time of the renal cancer diagnosis); TTP, time to pulmonary progression (months).

3.1. Morphology

All cases showed morphologic features typical of CCRCC. Primary tumors were arranged in a solid alveolar pattern, and occasionally with smaller cystic areas. The rich vasculature characteristic of CCRCC was noted in all primary tumors. Only small foci of necrosis or regressive changes were recorded. Neoplastic cells were mostly voluminous with clear to pale eosinophilic cytoplasm. The histologic grade was 2 in three tumors and 3 in one tumor. Metastases showed relatively uniform morphology, arranged mostly in solid architecture and composed of predominantly clear cells. The histologic grade was 2 in 8/9 metastatic foci and 3 in 1/9 metastases (Table 2).

Table 2. Grade of the primary tumors and metastases.

	Patient 1	Patient 2	Patient 3	Patient 4
Primary tumor grade	3	2	2	2
Met 1 grade	2	2	3	2
Met 2 grade	2	2	2	2
Met 3 grade			2	

Met, metastasis.

3.2. Immunohistochemical Analysis

All primary tumors and metastases were positive for CA9 (diffuse strong positivity) and vimentin. The Ki-67 proliferation index ranged from 3–12 positive cells/high-power field (under 10%). Primary tumors and metastases were negative for keratin 7.

The primary tumor and metastases were immunohistochemically examined using BAP1 antibody. Except for one tumor (patient 4), all primary tumors were BAP1 negative. In patient 3, negative BAP1 in the primary tumor and positive BAP1 in two of three PMs were documented.

PD-L1 reactivity was evaluated in all available samples. Only one primary tumor showed significant positivity (up to 30% of neoplastic cells); however, no positivity was documented in the available tissue from pulmonary metastasis (Table 3).

Table 3. PD-L1 reactivity in the primary tumor and metastases.

PD-L1	Case 1	Case 2	Case 3	Case 4
Primary tumor	* 0% ** 0%	* 0% ** 0%	* up to 5% ** 0%	* 30% ** 0%
Met 1	NA	* 0% ** 0%	* 0% ** up to 5%	* 0% ** 0%
Met 2	* up to 5% ** 0%	* 0% ** 0%	NA	NA
Met 3			NA	

Met, metastasis; * PD-L1 in neoplastic cells; ** PD-L1 in tumor infiltrating lymphocytes and stroma; NA, not available.

3.3. Molecular Genetic Analysis

Results of the molecular genetic analysis are summarized in Table 4. Typical *VHL* gene alterations were found in three primary tumors and their PMs (75%). In the patient without *VHL* mutation, we found alterations in *CUL3*, *DOT1L*, *SETD2* and *TSC1* in the primary tumor, with the addition of *BAP1* gene mutation in its analyzable PMs.

The comparison of mutation pattern among primary tumors and their PMs showed heterogeneity in three (75%) cases. In one case (patient 1), inter-metastatic differences were also found. In one metastasis, the mutation of *GNAQ* and loss of LOH3p were detected; however, in the second metastasis those changes were not confirmed. The comparison is displayed in Table 5.

Table 4. Mutational profile of primary tumors and their PMs using TSO500/TS170 panels.

	Gene	Protein ID:Protein Alteration	Transcript ID: Mutation	Allele Frequency
Patient 1—primary tumor TMB—6.5	MSH6	NP_000170.1:p.(Ala780Ser)	NM_000179.2:c.2338G>T	0.2586
	MYOD1	NP_002469.2:p.(Glu158Lys)	NM_002478.4:c.472G>A	0.2071
	PBRM1	NP_060783.3:p.(Tyr893Ter)	NM_018313.4:c.2679T>A	0.2885
	SETD2	NP_054878.5:p.(Lys2471Ile)	NM_014159.6:c.7412A>T	0.3654
	TFE3	NP_006512.2:p.(Pro374Ala)	NM_006521.5:c.1120C>G	0.2237
	VHL	NP_000542.1:p.(Ser65Ter)	NM_000551.3:c.194C>A	0.3855

Table 4. Cont.

	Gene	Protein ID:Protein Alteration	Transcript ID: Mutation	Allele Frequency
Patient 1—metastasis 1 TMB—5.5	BCORL1	NP_001171701.1:p.(Pro787Thr)	NM_001184772.2:c.2359C>A	0.2074
	MSH6	NP_000170.1:p.(Ala780Ser)	NM_000179.2:c.2338G>T	0.256
	MYOD1	NP_002469.2:p.(Glu158Lys)	NM_002478.4:c.472G>A	0.256
	PBRM1	NP_060783.3:p.(Tyr893Ter)	NM_018313.4:c.2679T>A	0.2657
	SETD2	NP_054878.5:p.(Lys2471Ile)	NM_014159.6:c.7412A>T	0.2372
	TSC1	NP_000359.1:p.(Glu839Ter)	NM_000368.4:c.2515G>T	0.3039
	VHL	NP_000542.1:p.(Ser65Ter)	NM_000551.3:c.194C>A	0.2896
Patient 1—metastasis 2	MSH6	NP_000170.1:p.(Ala780Ser)	NM_000179.2:c.2338G>T	0.30
	TSC1	NP_000359.1:p.(Glu839Ter)	NM_000368.4:c.2515G>T	0.39
	VHL	NP_000542.1:p.(Ser65Ter)	NM_000551.3:c.194C>A	0.40
	GNAQ	NP_002063.2:p.(Tyr101Ter)	NM_002072.4:c.303C>A	0.08
Patient 2—primary tumor TMB—4.7	CDK12	NP_057591.2:p.(Leu529PhefsTer81)	NM_016507.2:c.1585del	0.1264
	PTEN		NM_000314.6:c.492+1del	0.2
	REL	NP_002899.1:p.(Ser274Cys)	NM_002908.3:c.821C>G	0.0685
	SETD2	NP_054878.5:p.(Gly1467ArgfsTer8)	NM_014159.6:c.4398dup	0.105
	TGFBR2	NP_001020018.1:p.(Glu510Asp)	NM_001024847.2:c.1530A>C	0.0857
	VHL		NM_000551.3:c.463+2T>A	0.1091
Patient 2—metastasis 1 TMB—6.3	CDK12	NP_057591.2:p.(Leu529PhefsTer81)	NM_016507.2:c.1585del	0.0993
	PTEN		NM_000314.6:c.492+1del	0.2207
	REL	NP_002899.1:p.(Ser274Cys)	NM_002908.3:c.821C>G	0.1138
	SETD2	NP_054878.5:p.(Gly1467ArgfsTer8)	NM_014159.6:c.4398dup	0.1229
	TGFBR2	NP_001020018.1:p.(Glu510Asp)	NM_001024847.2:c.1530A>C	0.15
	VHL		NM_000551.3:c.463+2T>A	0.1044
Patient 2—metastasis 2 TMB—7.1	CDK12	NP_057591.2:p.(Leu529PhefsTer81)	NM_016507.2:c.1585del	0.0989
	PTEN		NM_000314.6:c.492+1del	0.2308
	REL	NP_002899.1:p.(Ser274Cys)	NM_002908.3:c.821C>G	0.1059
	SETD2	NP_054878.5:p.(Gly1467ArgfsTer8)	NM_014159.6:c.4398dup	0.1365
	TGFBR2	NP_001020018.1:p.(Glu510Asp)	NM_001024847.2:c.1530A>C	0.0856
	VHL		NM_000551.3:c.463+2T>A	0.0828
Patient 3—primary tumor TMB—4.7	CUL3	NP_001244127.1:p.(Val452PhefsTer9)	NM_001257198.1:c.1354del	0.1523
	DOT1L	NP_115871.1:p.(Met147Ile)	NM_032482.2:c.441G>T	0.1664
	SETD2	NP_054878.5:p.(Gln2070Ter)	NM_014159.6:c.6208C>T	0.1696
	TSC1	NP_000359.1:p.(Asn364LysfsTer5)	NM_000368.4:c.1091dup	0.195
Patient 3—metastasis 1 TMB—4.7	BAP1	NP_004647.1:p.(Arg385Ter)	NM_004656.3:c.1153C>T	0.1193
	CUL3	NP_001244127.1:p.(Val452PhefsTer9)	NM_001257198.1:c.1354del	0.1127
	DOT1L	NP_115871.1:p.(Met147Ile)	NM_032482.2:c.441G>T	0.1032
	SETD2	NP_054878.5:p.(Gln2070Ter)	NM_014159.6:c.6208C>T	0.1191
	TSC1	NP_000359.1:p.(Asn364LysfsTer5)	NM_000368.4:c.1091dup	0.0714
Patient 3—metastasis 2 TMB—4	BAP1	NP_004647.1:p.(Arg385Ter)	NM_004656.3:c.1153C>T	0.1026
	CUL3	NP_001244127.1:p.(Val452PhefsTer9)	NM_001257198.1:c.1354del	0.1076
	DOT1L	NP_115871.1:p.(Met147Ile)	NM_032482.2:c.441G>T	0.0642
	SETD2	NP_054878.5:p.(Gln2070Ter)	NM_014159.6:c.6208C>T	0.1177
	TSC1	NP_000359.1:p.(Asn364LysfsTer5)	NM_000368.4:c.1091dup	0.0559
Patient 4—primary tumor TMB—3.1	ARID5B	NP_115575.1:p.(Ala954Asp)	NM_032199.2:c.2861C>A	0.0835
	BAP1	NP_004647.1:p.(Gly703SerfsTer30)	NM_004656.3:c.2107_2116del	0.1046
	VHL	NP_000542.1:p.(Arg69AlafsTer82)	NM_000551.3:c.201_225del	0.0917
	XIAP	NP_001158.2:p.(Ser169Tyr)	NM_001167.3:c.506C>A	0.0583
Patient 4—metastasis 1 TMB—1.6	ARID5B	NP_115575.1:p.(Ala954Asp)	NM_032199.2:c.2861C>A	0.0835
	BAP1		NM_004656.3:c.122+1G>T	0.0806
	VHL	NP_000542.1:p.(Arg69AlafsTer82)	NM_000551.3:c.201_225del	0.0718
Patient 4—metastasis 2	BAP1		NM_004656.3:c.122+1G>T	0.03
	VHL	NP_000542.1:p.(Arg69AlafsTer82)	NM_000551.3:c.201_225del	0.06

Tumor/metastasis differences highlighted by red color. TMB, Tumor Mutation Burden; TS170 data in gray.

Table 5. The genetic profile of primary tumors and their PMs.

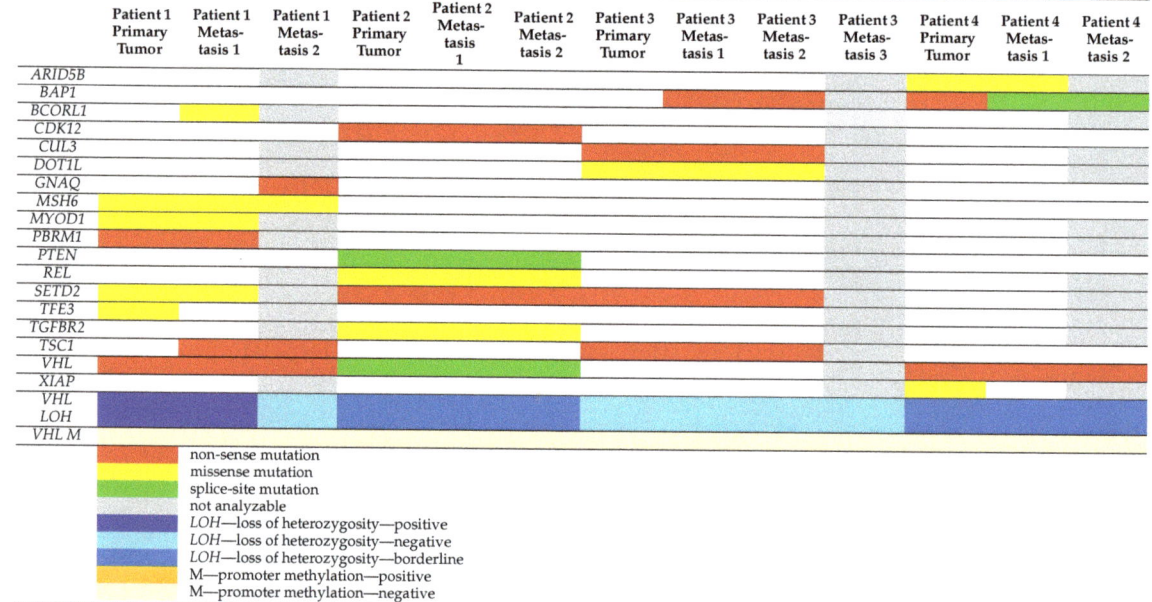

4. Discussion

The loss of the short arm of chromosome 3 in CCRCC is a ubiquitous somatic event, accompanied by the inactivation of the remaining *VHL* gene through mutation or methylation (in >90%) [26–29].

The *VHL* gene product (pVHL) is a component of E3 ubiquitin ligase complex, a key regulator of the cellular response to hypoxia. The E3 ubiquitin ligase complex promotes the degradation of its substrates including the alpha subunit of the hypoxia inducible factor (HIFα). The loss of *VHL* results in the accumulation of HIF-α, leading to the constitutive expression of HIF target genes. These genes are involved in angiogenesis (e.g., *VEGF*), glycolysis and glucose transport (e.g., *GLUT1*), and erythropoiesis (e.g., *EPO*), which molecularly characterize CCRCC [30,31]. Mutations in other members of the E3 ubiquitin ligase complex such as elongin C (*ELOC/TCEB1*) and cullin 2 (*CUL2*) occur rarely and are mutually exclusive to *VHL*. Although there are differences between tumors with mutations in *TCEB1* and *VHL*, the dysregulation of the VHL pathway may explain the overlapping morphology and immunohistochemical profile [32].

Chromosome 3p loss may be identified using different molecular genetic methods. This and the mutation or promoter hypermethylation of *VHL* are so common in CCRCC that a subset of tumors without such alterations may be misclassified [33]; however, the usage of extensive molecular testing is rare in current clinical practice. Varying driver gene alterations underpin CCRCC evolution and biology [34,35]. CCRCCs with *VHL* loss as the only driver event are indolent and rarely metastasize.

The loss of 3p results in the simultaneous loss of three other tumor suppressor genes that are frequently mutated in CCRCC: *Polybromo 1* (*PBRM1*) (~50%), *SET domain containing 2* (*SETD2*) (~20%), and *BRCA1-associated protein 1* (*BAP1*) (~15%) [26,32,36]. It should be noted that tumorigenesis in CCRCC follows a trunk-branch evolution [37], in which the trunk mutation (*VHL*) is responsible for tumorigenesis and sub-clonal mutations (i.e., *PBRM1*, *SETD2*, *BAP1*) are developed during disease progression.

Similar to *VHL*, *PBRM1* is often mutated early during tumor development [38]. *PBRM1*-mutated tumors with subsequent *SETD2* mutations, driver somatic copy number alterations, or P13K pathway alterations have a more attenuated disease course [36,37,39]. In contrast, CCRCCs with *BAP1* mutations or multiple driver mutations are associated with aggressive clinical behavior and early metastatic disease. Additional driver mutations and somatic copy number alterations include (i) inactivating mutations in histone modifying genes (*KDM5C* and *KDM6A*), (ii) mutations in the mTOR pathway genes (*TSC1*, *TSC2*, *MTOR*, *PIK3CA*, *PTEN*), (iii) the loss of TP53, and (iv) losses of chromosomes 14 and 9 [26,34,40].

Recent large scale gene expression analyses of metastatic CCRCC identified unique molecular subsets with distinct drug response characteristics [38,41]. CCRCC with high angiogenic gene signatures had a favorable response to anti-angiogenic therapies and were enriched with PBRM1 loss [35,41]. In contrast, CCRCCs with an inflamed microenvironment were associated with the highest PD-L1 expression, preferential responsiveness to regimes containing immune checkpoint inhibitors and the highest rates of sarcomatoid change and *BAP1* mutations [38,39,41].

Passow et al. [11] also showed inter-metastatic tumor heterogeneity in BAP1 immunohistochemical reactivity in their study. The primary tumor in their study was BAP1 IHC positive, the first bone metastasis (synchronous) was IHC negative, and the second bone metastasis (diagnosed approximately 9 months later) was BAP1 IHC positive. In our study, we also observed variability in BAP1 immunohistochemical reactivity. In one of our cases (no. 3), the primary tumor and one of its metastases (PM3) were both BAP1 negative, whereas its two other distant metastases (PM1, PM2) were BAP1 positive. Of note, these IHC findings were consistent with the mutation analysis. BAP1 IHC expression also perfectly matched with the mutation profile in our fourth case, although two different *BAP1* mutations were unexpectedly found in the primary tumor and its PM. We assume that this phenomenon could be a result of genetic drift during tumor progression

There are two genetic "supergroups" in RCCs: the Krebs cycle group and the mTOR/TSC group. CCRCC is by far the most common example of the Krebs cycle group, whereas the mTOR/TSC group includes a number of newly recognized novel tumors such as eosinophilic solid and cystic RCC (ESC-RCC), eosinophilic vacuolated tumor (EVT), low-grade oncocytic tumor (LOT), and RCC with prominent fibromyomatous stroma (RCC FMS), for which the mutation of *TSC1*, *TSC2* and/or *MTOR* is typical [42].

The mTOR pathway is an intracellular signaling pathway important for regulating the cell cycle. The most common genes involved in the tumorigenesis of the mTOR pathway group are *TSC1*, *TSC2*, and *MTOR*.

The mutation of the *TSC* genes in CCRCC is unusual but has been documented. Pang et al. [43] reported a rare case of CCRCC with novel biallelic somatic mutations in *TSC2*. This was a case of a 14-year-old female with VHL syndrome, where histologic findings were typical of CCRCC morphology. In addition, immunohistochemical findings also showed immunohistochemical expression for keratin, vimentin, CD10, and RCC, with negative results for CA9, keratin 7 and TFE3 staining. In our series, one of our patients (patient 1) demonstrated an interesting combination of mutations of *VHL* and *TSC1* in the PM, whereas we did not observe this phenomenon in the primary tumor. In the second patient, we verified a combination of *VHL* and *PTEN* mutations in the primary tumor and both metastases. In our third patient, the primary tumor showed a combination of *TSC1*, *CUL3*, *DOT1L* and *SETD2* gene mutations (but not *BAP1*), whereas the PM had the same genetic mutations plus *BAP1* mutation. This patient had metastatic disease at multiple sites post-surgery with disease progression. These molecular genetic findings indicate that in metastatic lesions, subclonal driver mutations are potentially responsible for spread and possible treatment failure. Such driver mutations were potentially missed due to sampling error or a lower number in samples analyzed by bulk sequencing. Another explanation might be the development of driver mutations over the course of the treatment. Current evidence suggests that treatment resistance and/or failure is caused by the resistant subclones, which were not targeted by the initial treatment [37]. We believe that optimizing the sampling approach in the metastatic setting, including the biopsy of newly developed metastatic CCRCC lesions, is important and can aid in effective therapeutic regimens due to the possible continued propagation of subclones.

One of the important novel renal entities in the differential diagnosis of CCRCC is RCC FMS [42]. Recognizing RCC FMS not only has academic value, but it also carries potential clinical implications and therapeutic management. Based on limited clinical data, these tumors tend to behave in an indolent fashion in most cases. In the largest cohort study of RCC FMS published to date [44], no evidence of recurrence or progression after surgical removal was documented. RCC FMS was included in the 2016 WHO classification of renal tumors as an emerging/provisional entity as "RCC with (angio) leiomyomatous stroma" [2]. However, distinct diagnostic criteria were not defined by the WHO classification. In the Genitourinary Pathology Society (GUPS) update review paper, the diagnostic histologic criteria for this distinct subtype of RCC have recently been established [42]. Tumors are composed of invariably voluminous epithelial clear cell components, which are typically diffusely positive for keratin 7 and of fibroleiomyomatous stroma. In this type of RCC, recurrent mutations involving the genes of the TSC/MTOR pathway were found. A subset of tumors with almost identical morphologic features showed mutations involving *ELOC* (also referred to as *TCEB1*), typically associated with the monosomy of chromosome 8 [44]. Both tumor subtypes lack *VHL* or chromosome 3p abnormalities [42,44]. In fact, it is not clear whether *TSC/MTOR* and *ELOC* mutated RCC with fibromyomatous stroma are two different tumor types, or just part of the molecular genetic variability within one tumor entity. Recently, one tumor with confirmed monosomy 8 and *ELOC* deletion as well as a *TSC1* mutation was documented [32,44].

RCC FMS are suggested to be more frequently sporadic; however, identical tumors were documented in patients with TSC. However, although the duration of the follow-up period is limited, most RCC FMS with *TSC/MTOR* mutations have demonstrated an indolent biological behavior [44]. However, lymph node metastases have been reported in rare cases associated with TSC recently. Although the initial report on *ELOC* (*TCEB1*)-associated RCC FMS suggested indolent behavior, an aggressive clinical course was recently described [45].

5. Conclusions

CCRCC are highly heterogeneous tumors, with complex molecular profiles both in the primary and metastatic settings. Tumor mutational profiles can be different not only between primary and metastatic tumors but also among multiple metastatic lesions themselves. It is evident that a one-size-fits-all approach is not optimal for treating advanced CCRCC and treatments need to be personalized. In this regard, optimizing tumor sampling and clinical management approaches in metastatic settings is crucial in order to identify subclonal mutations, which can ultimately lead to effective targeted therapies. The future of the successful personalized treatment and management of CCRCC is contingent upon a good understanding and accurate accounting for tumor heterogeneity.

The results of previously published studies and our own results show that CCRCC is a genetically heterogeneous tumor. The genetic background and mutation profile are highly variable within the primary tumor. However, data about the molecular genetic profile of the primary tumor and multiple metastases are very limited. It is apparent that the mutation profile can be different not only between the primary tumor and metastasis, but also among multiple metastases. Such important findings raise the question of the direct testing of each metastasis before the potential targeted therapy. Current clinical practice largely reflects genetic changes in primary tumors only. Because current oncologic treatment is reserved mostly for unresectable primary tumors and metastatic disease, we believe that such findings may become of critical importance.

Author Contributions: Methodology, K.P. (Kristyna Prochazkova), O.H., T.V., J.V. and V.T.; validation, T.V., O.H., K.M. and K.P. (Kristyna Prochazkova); formal analysis, O.H., K.P. (Kristyna Prochazkova) and T.V.; investigation, K.P. (Kristyna Prochazkova), O.H., T.V., J.V., N.P., J.R., K.P. (Kristyna Pivovarcikova), K.M. and M.S.; resources, K.P. (Kristyna Prochazkova), O.H., T.V., J.V. and V.T.; writing—original draft preparation, K.P. (Kristyna Prochazkova), O.H., T.V. and J.V.; writing—review and editing, K.P. (Kristyna Prochazkova), O.H., T.V., J.V. and V.T.; visualization, K.P. (Kristyna Prochazkova), O.H. and T.V.; supervision, O.H., S.R.W., M.M., R.A., M.H. and V.T.; project administration, K.P. (Kristyna Prochazkova), O.H., T.V., J.V. and V.T. All authors have read and agreed to the published version of the manuscript.

Funding: This research was funded by the grant SVV-2020-2022 No 260539, by the Charles University Research Fund (Progres Q39), the grant of Ministry of Health of the Czech Republic – Conceptual Development of Research Organization (Faculty Hospital in Pilsen—FNPI 00669806).

Institutional Review Board Statement: All procedures performed in studies involving human participants were in accordance with the ethical standards of the institutional and/or national research committee and with the 1964 Helsinki declaration and its later amendments or comparable ethical standards.

Informed Consent Statement: Informed consent was obtained from all subjects involved in the study.

Data Availability Statement: Data is contained within the article.

Acknowledgments: The work was supported by the grant SVV-2020-2022 No 260539, by the Charles University Research Fund (Progres Q39), the grant of Ministry of Health of the Czech Republic—Conceptual Development of Research Organization (Faculty Hospital in Pilsen—FNPI 00669806).

Conflicts of Interest: The authors declare no conflict of interest.

References

1. López, J.I. Renal Tumors with Clear Cells. A Review. *Pathol. Res. Pract.* **2013**, *209*, 137–146. [CrossRef] [PubMed]
2. Moch, H.; Humphrey, P.H.; Ulbright, T.M.; Reuter, V.E. (Eds.) *WHO Classification of Tumours of the Urinary System and Male Genital Organs*, 4th ed.; IARC: Lyon, France, 2016; 356p.
3. Ljungberg, B.; Bensalah, K.; Canfield, S.; Dabestani, S.; Hofmann, F.; Hora, M.; Kuczyk, M.A.; Lam, T.; Marconi, L.; Merseburger, A.S.; et al. EAU Guidelines on Renal Cell Carcinoma: 2014 Update. *Eur. Urol.* **2015**, *67*, 913–924. [CrossRef] [PubMed]
4. Procházková, K.; Vodička, J.; Fichtl, J.; Krákorová, G.; Šebek, J.; Roušarová, M.; Hošek, P.; Brookman May, S.D.; Hes, O.; Hora, M.; et al. Outcomes for Patients after Resection of Pulmonary Metastases from Clear Cell Renal Cell Carcinoma: 18 Years of Experience. *Urol. Int.* **2019**, *103*, 297–302. [CrossRef] [PubMed]
5. López, J.I.; Angulo, J.C. Pathological Bases and Clinical Impact of Intratumor Heterogeneity in Clear Cell Renal Cell Carcinoma. *Curr. Urol. Rep.* **2018**, *19*, 3. [CrossRef]
6. López, J.I.; Cortés, J.M. Multisite Tumor Sampling: A New Tumor Selection Method to Enhance Intratumor Heterogeneity Detection. *Hum. Pathol.* **2017**, *64*, 1–6. [CrossRef] [PubMed]
7. Cortés, J.M.; de Petris, G.; López, J.I. Detection of Intratumor Heterogeneity in Modern Pathology: A Multisite Tumor Sampling Perspective. *Front. Med.* **2017**, *4*, 25. [CrossRef]
8. Gonzalez, M.L.; Alagehbandan, R.; Pivovarcikova, K.; Michalova, K.; Rogala, J.; Martinek, P.; Foix, M.P.; Mundo, E.C.; Comperat, E.; Ulamec, M.; et al. Reactivity of CK7 across the Spectrum of Renal Cell Carcinomas with Clear Cells. *Histopathology* **2019**, *74*, 608–617. [CrossRef]
9. Gerlinger, M.; Rowan, A.J.; Horswell, S.; Math, M.; Larkin, J.; Endesfelder, D.; Gronroos, E.; Martinez, P.; Matthews, N.; Stewart, A.; et al. Intratumor Heterogeneity and Branched Evolution Revealed by Multiregion Sequencing. *N. Engl. J. Med.* **2012**, *366*, 883–892. [CrossRef]
10. Marco Gerlinger, Stuart Horswell, James Larkin, Andrew J Rowan, Max P Salm, Ignacio Varela, Rosalie Fisher, Nicholas McGranahan, Nicholas Matthews, Claudio R Santos, Pierre Martinez, Benjamin Phillimore, Sharmin Begum, Adam Rabinowitz, Bradley Spencer-Dene, Sakshi Gulati, Paul A Bates, Gordon Stamp, Lisa Pickering, Martin Gore, David L Nicol, Steven Hazell, P Andrew Futreal, Aengus Stewart, Charles Swanton Genomic Architecture and Evolution of Clear Cell Renal Cell Carcinomas Defined by Multiregion Sequencing. *Nat. Genet.* **2014**, *46*, 225–233. [CrossRef]
11. Eckel-Passow, J.E.; Serie, D.J.; Cheville, J.C.; Ho, T.H.; Kapur, P.; Brugarolas, J.; Thompson, R.H.; Leibovich, B.C.; Kwon, E.D.; Joseph, R.W.; et al. BAP1 and PBRM1 in Metastatic Clear Cell Renal Cell Carcinoma: Tumor Heterogeneity and Concordance with Paired Primary Tumor. *BMC Urol.* **2017**, *17*, 19. [CrossRef]

12. Brooks, S.A.; Brannon, A.R.; Parker, J.S.; Fisher, J.C.; Sen, O.; Kattan, M.W.; Hakimi, A.A.; Hsieh, J.J.; Choueiri, T.K.; Tamboli, P.; et al. ClearCode34: A Prognostic Risk Predictor for Localized Clear Cell Renal Cell Carcinoma. *Eur. Urol.* **2014**, *66*, 77–84. [CrossRef] [PubMed]
13. A Rose Brannon, Anupama Reddy, Michael Seiler, Alexandra Arreola, Dominic T Moore, Raj S Pruthi, Eric M Wallen, Matthew E Nielsen, Huiqing Liu, Katherine L Nathanson, Börje Ljungberg, Hongjuan Zhao, James D Brooks, Shridar Ganesan, Gyan Bhanot, W Kimryn Rathmell Molecular Stratification of Clear Cell Renal Cell Carcinoma by Consensus Clustering Reveals Distinct Subtypes and Survival Patterns. *Genes Cancer* **2010**, *1*, 152–163. [CrossRef]
14. Serie, D.J.; Joseph, R.W.; Cheville, J.C.; Ho, T.H.; Parasramka, M.; Hilton, T.; Thompson, R.H.; Leibovich, B.C.; Parker, A.S.; Eckel-Passow, J.E. Clear Cell Type A and B Molecular Subtypes in Metastatic Clear Cell Renal Cell Carcinoma: Tumor Heterogeneity and Aggressiveness. *Eur. Urol.* **2017**, *71*, 979–985. [CrossRef] [PubMed]
15. Williamson, S.R.; Halat, S.; Eble, J.N.; Grignon, D.J.; Lopez-Beltran, A.; Montironi, R.; Tan, P.-H.; Wang, M.; Zhang, S.; MacLennan, G.T.; et al. Multilocular Cystic Renal Cell Carcinoma: Similarities and Differences in Immunoprofile Compared With Clear Cell Renal Cell Carcinoma. *Am. J. Surg. Pathol.* **2012**, *36*, 1425–1433. [CrossRef]
16. Chen, Y.-B.; Xu, J.; Skanderup, A.J.; Dong, Y.; Brannon, A.R.; Wang, L.; Won, H.H.; Wang, P.I.; Nanjangud, G.J.; Jungbluth, A.A.; et al. Molecular Analysis of Aggressive Renal Cell Carcinoma with Unclassified Histology Reveals Distinct Subsets. *Nat. Commun.* **2016**, *7*, 13131. [CrossRef]
17. Williamson, S.R.; Grignon, D.J.; Cheng, L.; Favazza, L.; Gondim, D.D.; Carskadon, S.; Gupta, N.S.; Chitale, D.A.; Kalyana-Sundaram, S.; Palanisamy, N. Renal Cell Carcinoma With Chromosome 6p Amplification Including the TFEB Gene: A Novel Mechanism of Tumor Pathogenesis? *Am. J. Surg. Pathol.* **2017**, *41*, 287–298. [CrossRef]
18. Klatte, T.; Said, J.W.; Seligson, D.B.; Rao, P.N.; de Martino, M.; Shuch, B.; Zomorodian, N.; Kabbinavar, F.F.; Belldegrun, A.S.; Pantuck, A.J. Pathological, Immunohistochemical and Cytogenetic Features of Papillary Renal Cell Carcinoma with Clear Cell Features. *J. Urol.* **2011**, *185*, 30–36. [CrossRef]
19. Cancer Genome Atlas Research Network Comprehensive Molecular Characterization of Clear Cell Renal Cell Carcinoma. *Nature* **2013**, *499*, 43–49. [CrossRef]
20. Brierley, J.D.; Gospodarowicz, M.K. Wittekind Christian. In *TNM Classification of Malignant Tumours*, 8th ed.; Wiley-Blackwell: Hoboken, NJ, USA, 2016; ISBN 978-1-119-26357-9.
21. Farcaş, M.; Gatalica, Z.; Trpkov, K.; Swensen, J.; Zhou, M.; Alaghehbandan, R.; Williamson, S.R.; Magi-Galluzzi, C.; Gill, A.J.; Tretiakova, M.; et al. Eosinophilic Vacuolated Tumor (EVT) of Kidney Demonstrates Sporadic TSC/MTOR Mutations: Next-Generation Sequencing Multi-Institutional Study of 19 Cases. *Mod. Pathol.* **2021**. [CrossRef]
22. Pestinger, V.; Smith, M.; Sillo, T.; Findlay, J.M.; Laes, J.-F.; Martin, G.; Middleton, G.; Taniere, P.; Beggs, A.D. Use of an Integrated Pan-Cancer Oncology Enrichment Next-Generation Sequencing Assay to Measure Tumour Mutational Burden and Detect Clinically Actionable Variants. *Mol. Diagn. Ther.* **2020**, *24*, 339–349. [CrossRef]
23. Na, K.; Kim, H.-S.; Shim, H.S.; Chang, J.H.; Kang, S.-G.; Kim, S.H. Targeted Next-Generation Sequencing Panel (TruSight Tumor 170) in Diffuse Glioma: A Single Institutional Experience of 135 Cases. *J. Neuro-Oncol.* **2019**, *142*, 445–454. [CrossRef] [PubMed]
24. Petersson, F.; Martinek, P.; Vanecek, T.; Pivovarcikova, K.; Peckova, K.; Ondic, O.; Perez-Montiel, D.; Skenderi, F.; Ulamec, M.; Nenutil, R.; et al. Renal Cell Carcinoma With Leiomyomatous Stroma: A Group of Tumors With Indistinguishable Histopathologic Features, But 2 Distinct Genetic Profiles: Next-Generation Sequencing Analysis of 6 Cases Negative for Aberrations Related to the VHL Gene. *Appl. Immunohistochem. Mol. Morphol.* **2018**, *26*, 192–197. [CrossRef] [PubMed]
25. Kojima, F.; Bulimbasic, S.; Alaghehbandan, R.; Martinek, P.; Vanecek, T.; Michalova, K.; Pivovarcikova, K.; Michal, M.; Hora, M.; Murata, S.; et al. Clear Cell Renal Cell Carcinoma with Paneth-like Cells: Clinicopathologic, Morphologic, Immunohistochemical, Ultrastructural, and Molecular Analysis of 13 Cases. *Ann. Diagn. Pathol.* **2019**, *41*, 96–101. [CrossRef]
26. Ricketts, C.J.; De Cubas, A.A.; Fan, H.; Smith, C.C.; Lang, M.; Reznik, E.; Bowlby, R.; Gibb, E.A.; Akbani, R.; Beroukhim, R.; et al. The Cancer Genome Atlas Comprehensive Molecular Characterization of Renal Cell Carcinoma. *Cell Rep.* **2018**, *23*, 313–326.e5. [CrossRef]
27. Nickerson, M.L.; Jaeger, E.; Shi, Y.; Durocher, J.A.; Mahurkar, S.; Zaridze, D.; Matveev, V.; Janout, V.; Kollarova, H.; Bencko, V.; et al. Improved Identification of von Hippel-Lindau Gene Alterations in Clear Cell Renal Tumors. *Clin. Cancer Res.* **2008**, *14*, 4726–4734. [CrossRef]
28. Zbar, B.; Brauch, H.; Talmadge, C.; Linehan, M. Loss of Alleles of Loci on the Short Arm of Chromosome 3 in Renal Cell Carcinoma. *Nature* **1987**, *327*, 721–724. [CrossRef] [PubMed]
29. Mitchell, T.J.; Turajlic, S.; Rowan, A.; Nicol, D.; Farmery, J.H.R.; O'Brien, T.; Martincorena, I.; Tarpey, P.; Angelopoulos, N.; Yates, L.R.; et al. Timing the Landmark Events in the Evolution of Clear Cell Renal Cell Cancer: TRACERx Renal. *Cell* **2018**, *173*, 611–623.e17. [CrossRef]
30. Choueiri, T.K.; Kaelin, W.G. Targeting the HIF2–VEGF Axis in Renal Cell Carcinoma. *Nat. Med.* **2020**, *26*, 1519–1530. [CrossRef]
31. Brugarolas, J. Molecular Genetics of Clear-Cell Renal Cell Carcinoma. *J. Clin. Oncol.* **2014**, *32*, 1968–1976. [CrossRef]
32. Hakimi, A.A.; Tickoo, S.K.; Jacobsen, A.; Sarungbam, J.; Sfakianos, J.P.; Sato, Y.; Morikawa, T.; Kume, H.; Fukayama, M.; Homma, Y.; et al. TCEB1-Mutated Renal Cell Carcinoma: A Distinct Genomic and Morphological Subtype. *Mod. Pathol.* **2015**, *28*, 845–853. [CrossRef]

33. Favazza, L.; Chitale, D.A.; Barod, R.; Rogers, C.G.; Kalyana-Sundaram, S.; Palanisamy, N.; Gupta, N.S.; Williamson, S.R. Renal Cell Tumors with Clear Cell Histology and Intact VHL and Chromosome 3p: A Histological Review of Tumors from the Cancer Genome Atlas Database. *Mod. Pathol.* **2017**, *30*, 1603–1612. [CrossRef]
34. Turajlic, S.; Xu, H.; Litchfield, K.; Rowan, A.; Horswell, S.; Chambers, T.; O'Brien, T.; Lopez, J.I.; Watkins, T.B.K.; Nicol, D.; et al. Deterministic Evolutionary Trajectories Influence Primary Tumor Growth: TRACERx Renal. *Cell* **2018**, *173*, 595–610.e11. [CrossRef]
35. Cai, Q.; Christie, A.; Rajaram, S.; Zhou, Q.; Araj, E.; Chintalapati, S.; Singla, N.; Cadeddu, J.; Margulis, V.; Pedrosa, I.; et al. Corrigendum to "Ontological Analyses Reveal Clinically-Significant Clear Cell Renal Cell Carcinoma Subtypes with Convergent Evolutionary Trajectories into an Aggressive Type" [EBioMedicine 51 (2020) 102526]. *EBioMedicine* **2020**, *55*, 102707. [CrossRef] [PubMed]
36. Peña-Llopis, S.; Christie, A.; Xie, X.-J.; Brugarolas, J. Cooperation and Antagonism among Cancer Genes: The Renal Cancer Paradigm. *Cancer Res.* **2013**, *73*, 4173–4179. [CrossRef] [PubMed]
37. Beksac, A.T.; Paulucci, D.J.; Blum, K.A.; Yadav, S.S.; Sfakianos, J.P.; Badani, K.K. Heterogeneity in Renal Cell Carcinoma. *Urol. Oncol. Semin. Orig. Investig.* **2017**, *35*, 507–515. [CrossRef]
38. Brugarolas, J.; Rajaram, S.; Christie, A.; Kapur, P. The Evolution of Angiogenic and Inflamed Tumors: The Renal Cancer Paradigm. *Cancer Cell* **2020**, *38*, 771–773. [CrossRef]
39. Wang, T.; Lu, R.; Kapur, P.; Jaiswal, B.S.; Hannan, R.; Zhang, Z.; Pedrosa, I.; Luke, J.J.; Zhang, H.; Goldstein, L.D.; et al. An Empirical Approach Leveraging Tumorgrafts to Dissect the Tumor Microenvironment in Renal Cell Carcinoma Identifies Missing Link to Prognostic Inflammatory Factors. *Cancer Discov.* **2018**, *8*, 1142–1155. [CrossRef] [PubMed]
40. Turajlic, S.; Xu, H.; Litchfield, K.; Rowan, A.; Chambers, T.; Lopez, J.I.; Nicol, D.; O'Brien, T.; Larkin, J.; Horswell, S.; et al. Tracking Cancer Evolution Reveals Constrained Routes to Metastases: TRACERx Renal. *Cell* **2018**, *173*, 581–594.e12. [CrossRef] [PubMed]
41. Motzer, R.J.; Banchereau, R.; Hamidi, H.; Powles, T.; McDermott, D.; Atkins, M.B.; Escudier, B.; Liu, L.-F.; Leng, N.; Abbas, A.R.; et al. Molecular Subsets in Renal Cancer Determine Outcome to Checkpoint and Angiogenesis Blockade. *Cancer Cell* **2020**, *38*, 803–817.e4. [CrossRef]
42. Trpkov, K.; Williamson, S.R.; Gill, A.J.; Adeniran, A.J.; Agaimy, A.; Alaghehbandan, R.; Amin, M.B.; Argani, P.; Chen, Y.-B.; Cheng, L.; et al. Novel, Emerging and Provisional Renal Entities: The Genitourinary Pathology Society (GUPS) Update on Renal Neoplasia. *Mod. Pathol.* **2021**, *34*, 1167–1184. [CrossRef]
43. Pang, J.; Wang, L.; Xu, J.; Xie, Q.; Liu, Q.; Tong, D.; Liu, G.; Huang, Y.; Yang, X.; Pan, J.; et al. A Renal Cell Carcinoma with Biallelic Somatic TSC2 Mutation: Clinical Study and Literature Review. *Urology* **2019**, *133*, 96–102. [CrossRef] [PubMed]
44. Shah, R.B.; Stohr, B.A.; Tu, Z.J.; Gao, Y.; Przybycin, C.G.; Nguyen, J.; Cox, R.M.; Rashid-Kolvear, F.; Weindel, M.D.; Farkas, D.H.; et al. "Renal Cell Carcinoma With Leiomyomatous Stroma" Harbor Somatic Mutations of TSC1, TSC2, MTOR, and/or ELOC (TCEB1): Clinicopathologic and Molecular Characterization of 18 Sporadic Tumors Supports a Distinct Entity. *Am. J. Surg. Pathol.* **2020**, *44*, 571–581. [CrossRef] [PubMed]
45. DiNatale, R.G.; Gorelick, A.N.; Makarov, V.; Blum, K.A.; Silagy, A.W.; Freeman, B.; Chowell, D.; Marcon, J.; Mano, R.; Sanchez, A.; et al. Putative Drivers of Aggressiveness in TCEB1-Mutant Renal Cell Carcinoma: An Emerging Entity with Variable Clinical Course. *Eur. Urol. Focus* **2021**, *7*, 381–389. [CrossRef] [PubMed]

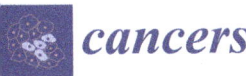

Commentary

A Comprehensive Commentary on the Multilocular Cystic Renal Neoplasm of Low Malignant Potential: A Urologist's Perspective

Tomas Pitra [1,*], Kristyna Pivovarcikova [2], Reza Alaghehbandan [3], Adriena Bartos Vesela [1], Radek Tupy [4], Milan Hora [1] and Ondrej Hes [2]

1. Department of Urology, Faculty Hospital in Pilsen, Charles University in Prague, 30599 Pilsen, Czech Republic; veselaad@fnplzen.cz (A.B.V.); horam@fnplzen.cz (M.H.)
2. Sikl's Department of Pathology, Faculty Hospital in Pilsen, Charles University in Prague, 30599 Pilsen, Czech Republic; pivovarcikovak@fnplzen.cz (K.P.); hes@fnplzen.cz (O.H.)
3. Department of Pathology, Faculty of Medicine, University of British Columbia, Royal Columbian Hospital, Vancouver, BC V6T 1Z4, Canada; reza.alagh@gmail.com
4. Department of Radiology, Faculty Hospital in Pilsen, Charles University in Prague, 30599 Pilsen, Czech Republic; tupyr@fnplzen.cz
* Correspondence: pitrat@fnplzen.cz

Citation: Pitra, T.; Pivovarcikova, K.; Alaghehbandan, R.; Bartos Vesela, A.; Tupy, R.; Hora, M.; Hes, O. A Comprehensive Commentary on the Multilocular Cystic Renal Neoplasm of Low Malignant Potential: A Urologist's Perspective. *Cancers* **2022**, *14*, 831. https://doi.org/10.3390/cancers14030831

Academic Editors: Claudia Manini and José I. López

Received: 30 November 2021
Accepted: 3 February 2022
Published: 6 February 2022

Publisher's Note: MDPI stays neutral with regard to jurisdictional claims in published maps and institutional affiliations.

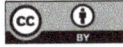

Copyright: © 2022 by the authors. Licensee MDPI, Basel, Switzerland. This article is an open access article distributed under the terms and conditions of the Creative Commons Attribution (CC BY) license (https://creativecommons.org/licenses/by/4.0/).

Simple Summary: Multilocular cystic renal neoplasm of low malignant potential (MCRNLMP) is a cystic renal neoplasm with an excellent prognosis. This neoplasm was previously named as "multilocular cystic renal cell carcinoma", which is now considered obsolete. In 2016, the WHO distinguished this neoplasm of low malignant potential from cystic renal cell carcinomas, which have some overlapping morphologic features.

Abstract: Multilocular cystic renal neoplasm of low malignant potential (MCRNLMP) is a cystic renal tumor with indolent clinical behavior. In most of cases, it is an incidental finding during the examination of other health issues. The true incidence rate is estimated to be between 1.5% and 4% of all RCCs. These lesions are classified according to the Bosniak classification as Bosniak category III. There is a wide spectrum of diagnostic tools that can be utilized in the identification of this tumor, such as computed tomography (CT), magnetic resonance (MRI) or contrast-enhanced ultrasonography (CEUS). Management choices of these lesions range from conservative approaches, such as clinical follow-up, to surgery. Minimally invasive techniques (i.e., robotic surgery and laparoscopy) are preferred, with an emphasis on nephron sparing surgery, if clinically feasible.

Keywords: kidney; cystic tumor; imaging; magnetic resonance; surgery

1. Introduction

Multilocular cystic renal neoplasm of low malignant potential (MCRNLMP) is a benign cystic lesion of the kidney, which was previously known as multilocular cystic renal cell carcinoma (MCRCC). This entity was initially described in 1982 by Lewis et al. [1]. Over time, the diagnostic criteria have changed from initially being defined as a tumor in which solid typical renal cell carcinoma exhibit less than 10% of the total mass [2]. A subsequent proposal suggested a cutoff point of 25% [3]. Finally, the 2012 International Society of Urological Pathology (ISUP) Vancouver Modification of the 2004 World Health Organization (WHO) Histologic Classification of Kidney Tumors recommended the re-designation of MCRCC as a multilocular cystic renal neoplasm of low malignant potential (MCRNLMP) [4,5]. MCRNLMP has a similar genetic profile and histopathological characteristics to that of clear cell renal cell carcinoma (CCRCC), but with a completely different prognostic feature with no progression or metastatic potential, because there are no reports of disease progression or metastases to date [6–11]. The 2016 WHO classification defined

MCRNLMP as a tumor entirely composed of multiple cysts, of which the septa contain small groups of clear cells without expansive growth, and is morphologically indistinguishable from low-grade CCRCC [12]. It should be noted that MCRNLMP follows strict histologic criteria that would allow any expansive growth, the presence of which qualifies the tumor as a cystic CCRCC [5,12].

2. Clinical Characteristics

MCRNLMP is a relatively rare entity, representing approximately less than 1% of all renal tumors, affecting middle-aged adults with a slight male predominance [2,13–15]. Most cases are asymptomatic and found incidentally. However, in the setting of large tumors, patients may present with gross hematuria, flank pain, palpable mass and abdominal discomfort, and sometimes digestive symptoms [3,16].

3. Imaging Studies

MCRNLMP is often initially identified on B-mode ultrasound as a well-defined multilocular cystic lesion with numerous septa, filled with serous or complicated fluid. Given the cystic nature of the lesion, further investigation by computed tomography (CT) using contrast agent is still the gold standard in classification and subsequent decision making in the field of cystic tumors of the kidney. The Bosniak classification with five groups (I, II, IIF, III and IV) is used as standard for defining cystic tumors of the kidney on CT. Results of CT scans and strict definitions of the Bosniak category of the cystic lesion are crucial for the further management of these lesions [17–21]. According to Bosniak, great parts of MCRNLMPs are defined/described as Bosniak category II, IIF or III [22,23]. In indeterminate cases where the CT imagining shows Bosniak category IIF–III, other imaging modalities (i.e., MRI), with greater precision and better visualization of the inner architecture of the septa, can be utilized [24,25] (Figure 1). In patients who cannot undergo CT or MRI, the preferred modality choice would be contrast-enhanced ultrasound (CEUS) [26–30]. This modality is now recognized as a diagnostic tool with at least the same effectiveness and imaging precision of cystic lesion as contrast-enhanced magnetic resonance or contrast-enhanced computed tomography [21,31–33].

3.1. Bosniak Classification

The first time the Bosniak classification was proposed and published was in 1986 [18]. In the following years and decades, this classification underwent several updates. Originally, four groups were expanded into five groups, adding a new unit—Bosniak IIF. The latest update of the Bosniak classification came in 2019 [34–36].

Each Bosniak group is evaluated according to the structure of the cystic lesion, the number of septa, the thickness and regularity/irregularity of the septa and wall, the presence of contrast enhancement in the septa, and the presence of calcifications or soft-tissue nodules.

Bosniak I group—simple cyst, uncomplicated. Defined by a thin wall, no septa, and no contrast enhancement.

Bosniak II group—minimally complex cyst, minimally complicated. Defined by a thin wall and septa, calcifications can be present, and no contrast enhancement.

Bosniak IIF group—slightly thickened wall, thin septa with visible, but not measurable enhancement, and the presence of calcifications.

Bosniak III group—indeterminate cystic tumor, thickened, irregular wall and septa, and measurable contrast enhancement.

Bosniak IV group—cystic tumor, soft-tissue nodules with measurable enhancement.

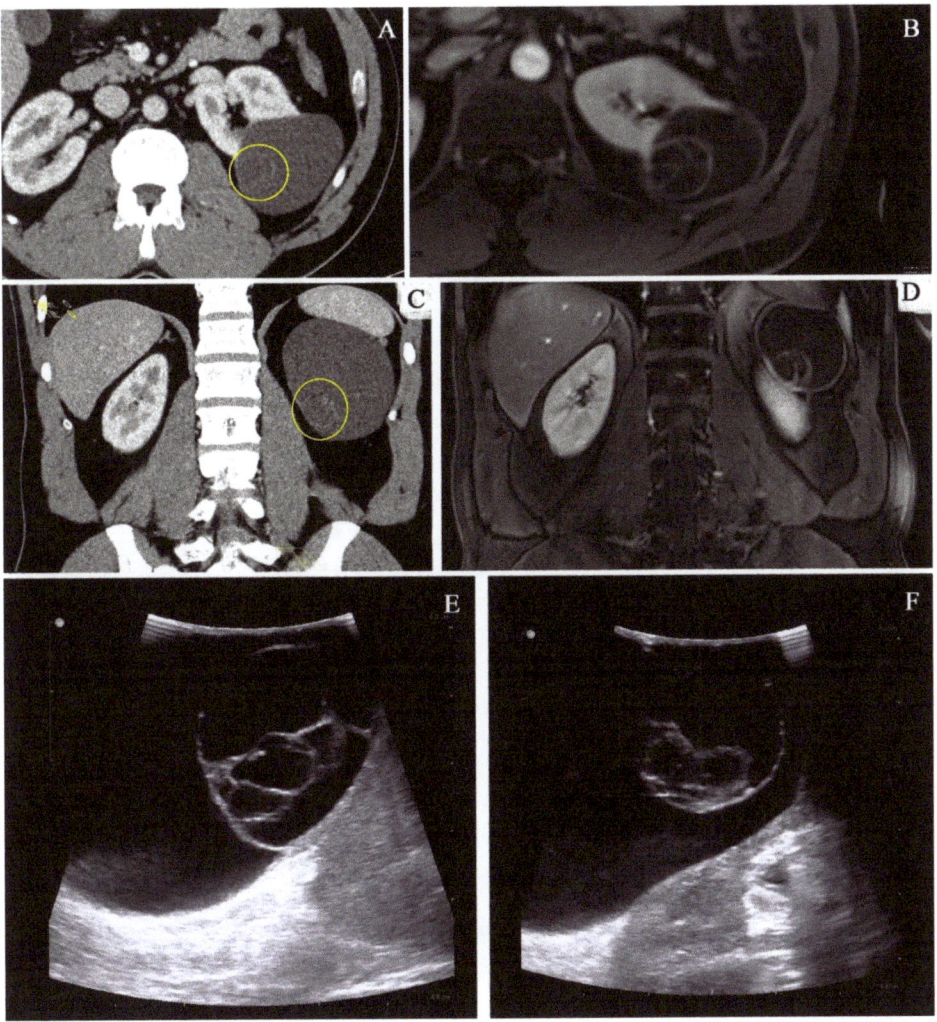

Figure 1. Imaging methods: comparison of CT imaging (**A,C**) and MRI (**B,D**) of the same lesion. There is a clearly visible benefit of MRI in imaging of the inner architecture with more precise imaging of the septa. (**E,F**) Intraoperative ultrasound image of MCRNLMP.

3.2. Differential Diagnostics

Due to its cystic nature, MCRNLMP could be misdiagnosed as another cystic tumor of the kidney, according to imaging studies. In differential diagnostics, it could be diagnosed as a hemorrhagic or inflamed cyst, or mixed epithelial and stromal tumor of the kidney (MESTK) [22]. A recent study from Song et al. [33] described a series of six cases of Xp11 translocation renal cell carcinoma, which have some morphological features mimicking MCRNLMP. Entities in the differential diagnosis are summarized in Table 1.

Table 1. Differential diagnosis.

Entity in Differential Diagnosis	Clinical Characteristics	Imaging Studies	Macroscopic Findings	Microscopic Findings	Immunoprofile	Molecular Genetic Findings
MCRNLMP	Indolent behavior, frequently incidental finding, no clinical symptoms.	Mostly Bosniak III on CT/MRI	Variably large non-communicating cysts, no solid component	Cystic spaces lined by clear cells lining, low grade nuclei (WHO/ISUP grade 1–2), no expansile/solid nodular growth, no necrosis, no vascular invasion, no sarcomatoid changes	PAX8 +, CANH +, CK7 +, AMACR −, ER −, PR −	Chromosome 3p deletion, VHL mutation
Renal cortical cyst	Benign, symptoms only in big size lesion	Bosniak I or II on CT	Usually unilocular, thin-walled cortical cyst	Cystic space lined by single layer of cuboidal/flattened cells/atrophic epithelium	PAX8 −	No specific changes
CCRCC with cystic changes (or regressive changes)	Malignant lesion with favorable behavior compared with CCRCC	Bosniak III or IV on CT/MRI	Solid component, necrosis, hemorrhage may be present	Composed of cells with clear cytoplasm and distinct membrane, solid nodule present at least focally; necrosis, vascular invasion, and sarcomatoid changes may be present, even high-grade feature	PAX8 +, CANH +, CD10 +, AE1/3 +, Vimentin +, CK7 +/− (usually −/focally), AMACR −(usually), TFE3 −, HMB45 −, Melan A −	Chromosome 3p deletion, VHL mutation, VHL promoter methylation
MEST	Usually perimenopausal women, benign with possible rare malignant transformation	Bosniak III or IV on CT/MRI	Solitary, well circumscribed (unencapsulated), mixture of solid and cystic areas	Stromal (collagenous/edematous/spindle/ovarian-like) and epithelial (cysts of various size with flat/cuboidal/columnar/hobnail epithelial lining) component	PAX8 + (epithelium), ER + (stroma), PR + (stroma), inhibin + (stroma), HMB45 −, Melan A −	No specific changes
MiT family RCC (some variant of Xp11 translocation RCC [33]	Malignant, rare entity	Mostly Bosniak III or IV on CT/MRI	Multicystic mass, with a circumscribed appearance	Well-delimited, multilocular cystic lesion with thin membranous and fibrous septa, lined by a single layer of cell with clear to eosinophilic cytoplasm, WHO/ISUP grade 1/2 nuclei, no solid nodule	Cytokeratins +/−, TFE3 +, PAX8 +, CANH −	TFE3 gene rearrangements (MED15-TFE3 gene fusion)

MCRNLMP, multilocular cystic renal neoplasm of low malignant potential; CCRCC, clear cell renal cell carcinoma; MEST, mixed epithelial and stromal tumor; CANH, carbonic anhydrase; AMACR, alpha methyacyl CoA racemase; ER, estrogen receptors; PR, progesterone receptors; + positive; − negative; +/− variable.

4. Therapeutic Management

The therapeutic management of cystic lesions of the kidney (including MCRNLMP) is still based on the results of imaging studies and precise categorization according to the Bosniak classification system. Each Bosniak category is associated with the individual risk of malignancy and the malignancy rate. The malignancy rate is based on typical signs of each group-complexity of the lesion and the characteristics mentioned above (Section 3.1). The malignancy rates in Bosniak I and II, based on recent cohorts in the literature, are given as 3.2% and 6%, respectively [37]. The Bosniak IIF malignancy rate is reported as 6.7% [37] or 18% [38]. The Bosniak III malignancy rate is 55.1% [37]. In Bosniak IV, the malignancy rate is reported as 91% [37].

There is no need for intervention or regular follow-up in Bosniak I and II category, except for large lesions with clinical symptoms. Bosniak IIF is a cystic lesion, where regular follow-up is recommended. However, no strict consensus protocol has been provided, and the follow-up protocols or eventual surgical intervention are still controversial. Follow-up is the preferred choice of management. There are multiple proposed recommendations in the literature on how to manage these lesions. Bosniak et al. proposed a follow-up regimen based on CT scans 6 months after diagnosis. In cases of no progression, another imaging study should be performed once per year [39]. Another study from Weibl et al. suggested follow-up CT scans every 6 months in the first 2 years, and then continuing with the imaging study once every year. The authors incorporated MRI in the follow-up regimen, which should be performed minimally in the first 4 years of follow-up [40,41]. For Bosniak III category lesions, there are two options available: (1) surgical treatment, possibly with minimally invasive nephron sparing surgery with regard to the oncological radicality of the procedure; and (2) strict clinical follow-up, as per the recent guidelines of the European Association of Urology [42]. Bosniak IV is treated as a solid tumor of the kidney, with the surgical interventions described above.

5. Pathological Findings

5.1. Macroscopic Findings

MCRNLMP exclusively consists of variably large non-communicating cysts (0.4–14 cm) [9,10], which are separated by thin septa and filled with serous, gelatinous, hemorrhagic, or mixed fluid (Figures 2 and 3). There are no solid components in these lesions, and, in fact, the presence of such solid nodules would not be compatible with the diagnosis of this entity [9,10,12,43]. Most patients have unilateral lesions with no laterality predominance [3,9,44].

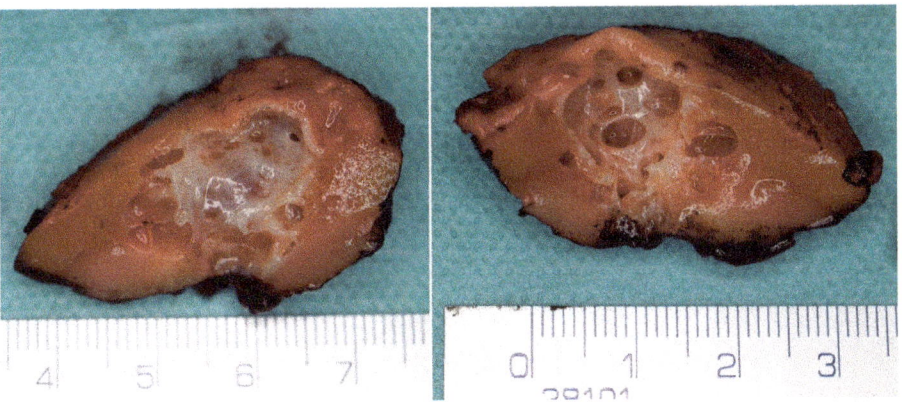

Figure 2. Macroscopic appearance of the MCRNLMP specimen from nephron sparing surgery. There is a multicystic lesion with a thin septa and variable sized cystic spaces without solid expansion.

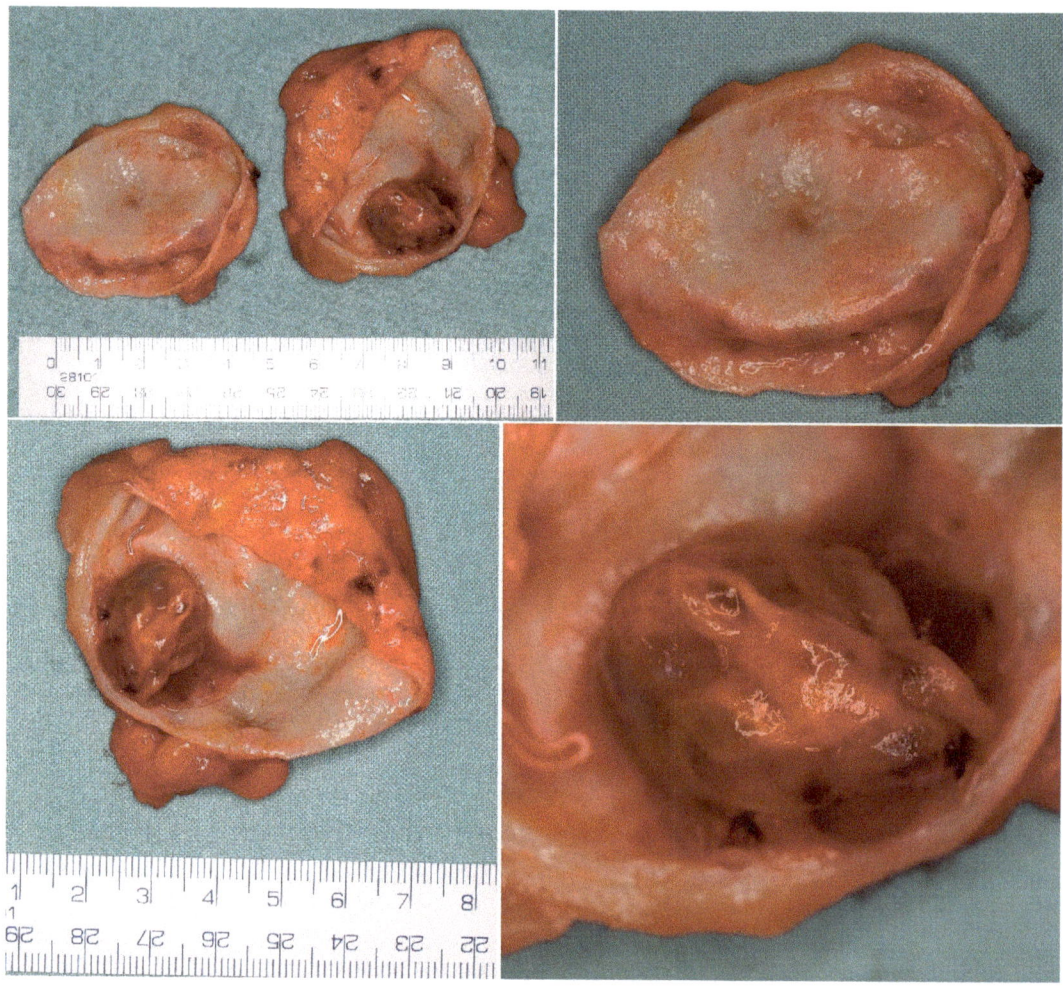

Figure 3. Macroscopic appearance of an MCRNLMP specimen from nephron sparing surgery. The dominant cystic space contains smaller cystic expansion. The absence of solid mass is crucial for the diagnosis of MCRNLMP, and must be proved by microscopic examination of the specimen.

5.2. Microscopic Findings

The neoplasm is composed of the cystic spaces lined by clear cells, exhibiting low-grade nuclei without nucleoli (WHO/ISUP grade 1–2). No expansive/solid nodular growth of clear tumor cells, necrosis, vascular invasion or sarcomatoid changes have been noted in MCRNLMP. In rare cases, the linings of cysts may show multilayering, granular cytoplasm of cells and the formation of small intracystic papillae. Furthermore, the septa may exhibit calcification or ossification [12,45] (Figure 4).

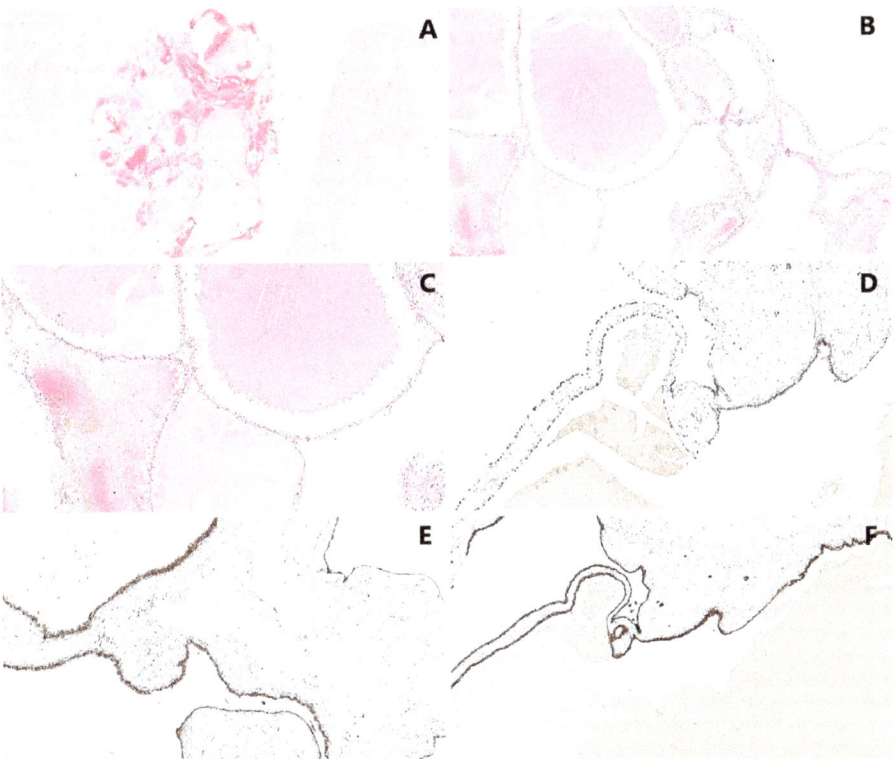

Figure 4. Histological appearance of MCRNLMP: (**A,B**) The lesion is characterized by the formation of cystic spaces—various sized cysts are separated by thin, fibrous septa (magnification 10×, resp. 60×). (**C**) The epithelial lining is composed by neoplastic cells with clear cytoplasm arranged in a single layer (magnification 160×). (**D**) The epithelial lining is positive in PAX8 (magnification 10×). (**E**) Equally, carbonic anhydrase IX (CAIX) shows positivity in neoplastic cells (magnification 10×). (**F**) Strong immunoreactivity was proved in CK7 (magnification 10×).

5.3. Immunohistochemical Findings

Neoplastic cells are typically PAX2-, PAX8-, and carbonic anhydrase IX (CAIX)-positive [46–48]. In wider immunohistochemical panels, MCRNLMP is usually negative in α-methylacyl-CoA-racemase, progesterone and estrogen receptor. Strong immunoreactivity was proven in EMA, CAM5.2 and CK7 [44,49].

Some authors used less common immunohistochemical staining techniques in their immunohistochemical studies—Kuroda et al. demonstrated the immunoreactivity of the cytoplasm of tumor cells in adipophilin which corresponded to lipid droplets [44]. Adipophilin expression in CCRCC has previously been reported, which may reflect a close relationship between MCRNLMP and CCRCC [50]. Kim et al. recently examined a number of immunostains between MCRNLMP and CCRCC. According to their study, the expressions of TGAse-2 and Ki-67 were significantly different between these two groups [12,51].

5.4. Molecular Genetic Findings

VHL gene mutations were found in 25% of MCRNLMP [47], and deletions of chromosome 3p in 74% of cases in comparison with 89% of CCRCC. These findings can support the concept of MCRNLMP being genetically related to CCRCC [52]. Kuroda et al. also reported a loss of heterozygosity (LOH) in chromosome 3p in one MCRNLMP case [44]. Tretiakova et al. found a high rate of chromosome 3 abnormalities with chromosome 3 monosomy in 3/3 MCRNLMP cases [10]. Raspollini et al. conducted a comparison study between CCRCC and MCRNLMP using a genetic mutational analysis. There were no significant genetic differences between these two groups, except for *KRAS* mutation. According to their results, the *KRAS* mutation may be helpful for distinguishing between CCRCC and MCRNLP, despite their histologic similarities [53]. Kim et al. identified six novel genetic alterations, including *SET domain-containing 2* (*SETD2*), *lysine methyltransferase 2C* (*KMT2C*), *tuberous sclerosis complex 2* (*TSC2*), *GRB10 interacting GYF protein 2* (*GIGYF2*), *fibroblast growth factor receptor 3* (*FGFR3*) and *breakpoint cluster region protein* (*BCR*), also known as *renal carcinoma antigen NY-REN-26* (*BCR*), which could be potential candidate genes for differentiating between MCRNLMP and MCRCC [54].

6. Prognosis

The prognosis of MCRNLMP is excellent, with no cases of progression or metastatic spread [55]. This fact is based on multiple publications including more than 200 patients with clinical follow-ups longer than 5 years [1,5,6,9].

7. Discussion

Since the first report of MCRNLMP (then MCRCC) in 1982 [1], this entity has evolved, frequently being characterized, specified, named/re-named, and classified [2,3]. Firstly, it was characterized as a cystic neoplasm with less than 10% [2] and then less than 25% solid area [3]. Finally, MCRNLMP is described as a tumor entirely composed of cystic spaces with no expansive/solid nodules [56,57]. The original classification as multilocular cystic renal cell carcinoma (MCRCC) was re-designated as MCRNLMP, according to the ISUP recommendation, and became a part of the current WHO classification of renal tumors (2016) [5,12]. The nuclear grade (WHO/ISUP) of MCRNLMP is typically 1 (in two thirds of cases), or grade 2 (in one-third of MCRNLMP). WHO/ISUP grade 3 is not compatible with the diagnosis of MCRNLMP [10].

Chromosomal abnormalities were described in various studies, and chromosome 3p deletion was proved in 74% of MCRNLMP [52]. The *von Hippel-Lindau* (*VHL*) gene mutations were described in 25% of cases of MCRNLMP [47]. Furthermore, one case of loss of heterozygosity (LOH) in chromosome 3p in MCRNLMP was presented by Kuroda et al. [44].

The accurate incidence of MCRNLMP is not known, because of its rarity and variable diagnostic criteria used in various studies. However, it is estimated that MCRNLMP accounts for fewer than 1% of all renal neoplasms [16,23,58–60].

As with other cystic lesions of the kidney, MCRNLMP should be precisely diagnosed using proper imaging methods prior to treatment planning. The gold standard in imaging of the cystic tumors of the kidney is contrast-enhanced CT. The Bosniak classification is currently utilized to stratify the lesion accordingly [18–21,36]. In indeterminate cases where the initial CT imaging is not conclusive enough, a second imaging choice, such as MRI, needs to be utilized; some studies have demonstrated its benefit in diagnostics of cystic lesions of the kidney [24,25]. Other potential imaging modalities which can be used include contrast-enhanced ultrasound (CEUS) [26–29,61,62]. Typically, MCRNLMP is categorized as a cystic lesion, category Bosniak IIF or III [22,23]. Imaging studies cannot precisely distinguish MCRNLMP from other cystic lesions preoperatively [16,44,58,59,63].

The therapeutic management of MCRNLMP consists of strict clinical follow-ups or surgical interventions. There is still no strict protocol as to how and when to follow up Bosniak IIF category lesions. Weibl et al. suggested a CT scan in the follow-up every 6 months in the first 2 years, and then continuing with imaging studies once every year. The authors incorporated MRI into the follow-up regimen, which should be performed minimally in the first 4 years of follow-up [40]. In the past, Bosniak III lesions were strictly associated with surgical intervention. However, according to the recent EAU guidelines [42], it is possible to strictly follow-up such cases. The current preferred surgical approach is minimally invasive nephron-sparing surgery, which may allow the laparoscopic or robotic resection of such lesion, if technically feasible and oncological radicality is achievable.

In summary, MCRNLMP is a cystic lesion of the kidney with excellent prognosis. In 2016, the WHO separated this neoplasm of low malignant potential from cystic renal cell carcinomas, which have some overlapping morphologic features. Minimally invasive procedures (i.e., robotic surgery and laparoscopy) are preferred, with emphasis on nephron sparing surgery, if clinically feasible.

Author Contributions: Conceptualization, T.P. and K.P.; resources—A.B.V.; writing—original draft preparation, T.P.; writing—review and editing, R.A., O.H. and R.T.; supervision O.H. and M.H. All authors have read and agreed to the published version of the manuscript.

Funding: This study was funded by the grant SVV-2020-2022 No 260539, by the Charles University Research Fund (Progres Q39), the grant of Ministry of Health of the Czech Republic – Conceptual Development of Research Organization (Faculty Hospital in Pilsen—FNPI 00669806).

Conflicts of Interest: The authors declare no conflict of interest.

References

1. Lewis, R.H.; Clark, M.A.; Dobson, C.L.; O'Connell, K.J. Multilocular cystic renal adenocarcinoma arising in a solitary kidney. *J Urol.* **1982**, *127*, 314–316. [CrossRef]
2. Murad, T.; Komaiko, W.; Oyasu, R.; Bauer, K. Multilocular cystic renal cell carcinoma. *Am. J. Clin. Pathol.* **1991**, *95*, 633–637. [CrossRef] [PubMed]
3. Corica, F.A.; Iczkowski, K.A.; Cheng, L.; Zincke, H.; Blute, M.L.; Wendel, A.; Sebo, T.J.; Neumann, R.; Botswick, D.G. Cystic renal cell carcinoma is cured by resection: A study of 24 cases with long-term followup. *J. Urol.* **1999**, *161*, 408–411. [CrossRef]
4. Kristiansen, G.; Delahunt, B.; Srigley, J.R.; Lüders, C.; Lunkenheimer, J.M.; Gevensleben, H.; Thiesler, T.; Montironi, R.; Egevad, L. Vancouver classification of renal tumors: Recommendations of the 2012 consensus conference of the International Society of Urological Pathology (ISUP). *Der Pathol.* **2015**, *36*, 310–316.
5. Srigley, J.R.; Delahunt, B.; Eble, J.N.; Egevad, L.; Epstein, J.I.; Grignon, D.; Hes, O.; Moch, H.; Montironi, R.; Tickoo, S.T.; et al. The International Society of Urological Pathology (ISUP) Vancouver Classification of Renal Neoplasia. *Am. J. Surg. Pathol.* **2013**, *37*, 1469–1489. [CrossRef]
6. Bhatt, J.R.; Jewett, M.A.; Richard, P.O.; Kawaguchi, S.; Timilshina, N.; Evans, A.; Alibhai, S.; Finelli, A. Multilocular Cystic Renal Cell Carcinoma: Pathological T Staging Makes No Difference to Favorable Outcomes and Should be Reclassified. *J. Urol.* **2016**, *196*, 1350–1355. [CrossRef]
7. Chen, S.; Jin, B.; Xu, L.; Fu, G.; Meng, H.; Liu, B.; Li, J.; Xia, D. Cystic renal cell carcinoma: A report of 67 cases including 4 cases with concurrent renal cell carcinoma. *BMC Urol.* **2014**, *14*, 87. [CrossRef]
8. Li, T.; Chen, J.; Jiang, Y.; Ning, X.; Peng, S.; Wang, J.; He, Q.; Yang, X.; Gong, K. Multilocular Cystic Renal Cell Neoplasm of Low Malignant Potential: A Series of 76 Cases. *Clin Genitourin. Cancer* **2016**, *14*, e553–e557. [CrossRef]
9. Suzigan, S.; López-Beltrán, A.; Montironi, R.; Drut, R.; Romero, A.; Hayashi, T.; Gentili, A.L.C.; Fonseca, P.S.P.; deTorres, I.; Billis, A.; et al. Multilocular cystic renal cell carcinoma: A report of 45 cases of a kidney tumor of low malignant potential. *Am. J. Clin. Pathol.* **2006**, *125*, 217–222. [CrossRef]
10. Tretiakova, M.; Mehta, V.; Kocherginsky, M.; Minor, A.; Shen, S.S.; Sirintrapun, S.J.; Yao, J.L.; Alvarado-Cabrero, I.; Antic, T.; Eggener, S.; et al. Predominantly cystic clear cell renal cell carcinoma and multilocular cystic renal neoplasm of low malignant potential form a low-grade spectrum. *Virchows Arch.* **2018**, *473*, 85–93. [CrossRef]
11. Westerman, M.E.; Cheville, J.C.; Lohse, C.M.; Sharma, V.; Boorjian, S.A.; Leibovich, B.C.; Thompson, R.H. Long-Term Outcomes of Patients with Low Grade Cystic Renal Epithelial Neoplasms. *Urology* **2019**, *133*, 145–150. [CrossRef]
12. Moch, H.; Cubilla, A.L.; Humphrey, P.A.; Reuter, V.E.; Ulbright, T.M. The 2016 WHO Classification of Tumours of the Urinary System and Male Genital Organs-Part A: Renal, Penile, and Testicular Tumours. *Eur. Urol.* **2016**, *70*, 93–105. [CrossRef] [PubMed]
13. Nassir, A.; Jollimore, J.; Gupta, R.; Bell, D.; Norman, R. Multilocular cystic renal cell carcinoma: A series of 12 cases and review of the literature. *Urology* **2002**, *60*, 421–427. [CrossRef]
14. Agarwal, S.; Agrawal, U.; Mohanty, N.K.; Saxena, S. Multilocular cystic renal cell carcinoma: A case report of a rare entity. *Arch. Pathol. Lab. Med.* **2011**, *135*, 290–292. [CrossRef] [PubMed]
15. Sabhiki, A.; Abrari, A.; Sachdev, R.; Chawla, A.; Vaidya, A. Multilocular cystic renal cell carcinoma: A diagnostic rarity. *Indian J. Pathol. Microbiol.* **2008**, *51*, 457–458. [PubMed]
16. Gong, K.; Zhang, N.; He, Z.; Zhou, L.; Lin, G.; Na, Y. Multilocular cystic renal cell carcinoma: An experience of clinical management for 31 cases. *J. Cancer Res. Clin. Oncol.* **2008**, *134*, 433–437. [CrossRef] [PubMed]
17. Curry, N.S.; Cochran, S.T.; Bissada, N.K. Cystic renal masses: Accurate Bosniak classification requires adequate renal CT. *AJR Am. J. Roentgenol.* **2000**, *175*, 339–342. [CrossRef] [PubMed]
18. Bosniak, M.A. The current radiological approach to renal cysts. *Radiology* **1986**, *158*, 1–10. [CrossRef]

19. Bosniak, M.A. Diagnosis and management of patients with complicated cystic lesions of the kidney. *AJR Am. J. Roentgenol.* **1997**, *169*, 819–821. [CrossRef]
20. Bosniak, M.A. The use of the Bosniak classification system for renal cysts and cystic tumors. *J. Urol.* **1997**, *157*, 1852–1853. [CrossRef]
21. Israel, G.M.; Bosniak, M.A. An update of the Bosniak renal cyst classification system. *Urology* **2005**, *66*, 484–488. [CrossRef] [PubMed]
22. Hora, M.; Hes, O.; Michal, M.; Boudova, L.; Chudacek, Z.; Kreuzberg, B.; Klecka, J. Extensively cystic renal neoplasms in adults (Bosniak classification II or III)-possible common histological diagnoses: Multilocular cystic renal cell carcinoma, cystic nephroma, and mixed epithelial and stromal tumor of the kidney. *Int. Urol. Nephrol.* **2005**, *37*, 743–750. [CrossRef] [PubMed]
23. You, D.; Shim, M.; Jeong, I.G.; Song, C.; Kim, J.K.; Ro, J.Y.; Hong, J.H.; Ahn, H.; Kim, C.S. Multilocular cystic renal cell carcinoma: Clinicopathological features and preoperative prediction using multiphase computed tomography. *BJU Int.* **2011**, *108*, 1444–1449. [CrossRef] [PubMed]
24. Pitra, T.; Pivovarcikova, K.; Tupy, R.; Alaghehbandan, R.; Barakova, T.; Travnicek, I.; Prochazkova, K.; Klatte, T.; Chlosta, P.; Hes, O.; et al. Magnetic resonance imaging as an adjunct diagnostic tool in computed tomography defined Bosniak IIF-III renal cysts: A multicenter study. *World J. Urol.* **2018**, *36*, 905–911. [CrossRef]
25. Ferreira, A.M.; Reis, R.B.; Kajiwara, P.P.; Silva, G.E.; Elias, J.; Muglia, V.F. MRI evaluation of complex renal cysts using the Bosniak classification: A comparison to CT. *Abdom Radiol.* **2016**, *41*, 2011–2019. [CrossRef]
26. Clevert, D.A.; Minaifar, N.; Weckbach, S.; Jung, E.M.; Stock, K.; Reiser, M.; Staehler, M. Multislice computed tomography versus contrast-enhanced ultrasound in evaluation of complex cystic renal masses using the Bosniak classification system. *Clin. Hemorheol. Microcirc.* **2008**, *39*, 171–178. [CrossRef]
27. Graumann, O.; Osther, S.S.; Karstoft, J.; Hørlyck, A.; Osther, P.J. Bosniak classification system: A prospective comparison of CT, contrast-enhanced US, and MR for categorizing complex renal cystic masses. *Acta Radiol.* **2015**, *57*, 1409–1417. [CrossRef]
28. Ignee, A.; Straub, B.; Brix, D.; Schuessler, G.; Ott, M.; Dietrich, C.F. The value of contrast enhanced ultrasound (CEUS) in the characterisation of patients with renal masses. *Clin. Hemorheol. Microcirc.* **2010**, *46*, 275–290. [CrossRef]
29. Rübenthaler, J.; Bogner, F.; Reiser, M.; Clevert, D.A. Contrast-Enhanced Ultrasound (CEUS) of the Kidneys by Using the Bosniak Classification. *Ultraschall Med.* **2016**, *37*, 234–251. [CrossRef]
30. Shan, K.; Fu, A.B.D.L.; Liu, N.; Cai, Q.; Fu, Q.; Liu, L.; Sun, X.; Zhang, Z. Contrast-enhanced Ultrasound (CEUS) vs contrast-enhanced computed tomography for multilocular cystic renal neoplasm of low malignant potential: A retrospective analysis for diagnostic performance study. *Medicine* **2020**, *99*, e23110. [CrossRef]
31. Hindman, N.M. Imaging of Cystic Renal Masses. *Radiol. Clin. N. Am.* **2017**, *55*, 259–277. [CrossRef] [PubMed]
32. Robbin, M.L.; Lockhart, M.E.; Barr, R.G. Renal imaging with ultrasound contrast: Current status. *Radiol. Clin. N. Am.* **2003**, *41*, 963–978. [CrossRef]
33. Cantisani, V.; Bertolotto, M.; Clevert, D.A.; Correas, J.M.; Drudi, F.M.; Fischer, T.; Gilja, O.H.; Granata, A.; Graumann, O.; Harvey, C.J.; et al. EFSUMB 2020 Proposal for a Contrast-Enhanced Ultrasound-Adapted Bosniak Cyst Categorization-Position Statement. *Ultraschall Med.* **2021**, *42*, 154–166. [CrossRef] [PubMed]
34. Edney, E.; Davenport, M.S.; Curci, N.; Schieda, N.; Krishna, S.; Hindman, N.; Silverman, S.G.; Pedrosa, I. Bosniak classification of cystic renal masses, version 2019: Interpretation pitfalls and recommendations to avoid misclassification. *Abdom. Radiol.* **2021**, *46*, 2699–2711. [CrossRef] [PubMed]
35. Schieda, N.; Davenport, M.S.; Krishna, S.; Edney, E.A.; Pedrosa, I.; Hindman, N.; Baroni, R.H.; Curci, N.E.; Shinagare, A.; Silverman, S.G. Bosniak Classification of Cystic Renal Masses, Version 2019: A Pictorial Guide to Clinical Use. *Radiographics* **2022**, *42*, E33. [CrossRef]
36. Silverman, S.G.; Pedrosa, I.; Ellis, J.H.; Hindman, N.M.; Schieda, N.; Smith, A.D.; Remer, E.M.; Shinagare, A.B.; Curci, N.E.; Raman, S.S.; et al. Bosniak Classification of Cystic Renal Masses, Version 2019: An Update Proposal and Needs Assessment. *Radiology* **2019**, *292*, 475–488. [CrossRef]
37. Sevcenco, S.; Spick, C.; Helbich, T.H.; Heinz, G.; Shariat, S.F.; Klingler, H.C.; Rauchenwald, M.; Baltzer, P.A. Malignancy rates and diagnostic performance of the Bosniak classification for the diagnosis of cystic renal lesions in computed tomography—A systematic review and meta-analysis. *Eur. Radiol.* **2017**, *27*, 2239–2247. [CrossRef]
38. Schoots, I.G.; Zaccai, K.; Hunink, M.G.; Verhagen, P.C.M.S. Bosniak Classification for Complex Renal Cysts Reevaluated: A Systematic Review. *J. Urol.* **2017**, *198*, 12–21. [CrossRef]
39. Israel, G.M.; Bosniak, M.A. Follow-up CT of moderately complex cystic lesions of the kidney (Bosniak category IIF). *AJR Am. J. Roentgenol.* **2003**, *181*, 627–633. [CrossRef]
40. Weibl, P.; Hora, M.; Kollarik, B.; Shariat, S.F.; Klatte, T. Management, pathology and outcomes of Bosniak category IIF and III cystic renal lesions. *World J. Urol.* **2015**, *33*, 295–300. [CrossRef]
41. Weibl, P.; Hora, M.; Kollarik, B.; Kalusova, K.; Pitra, T.; Remzi, M.; Hübner, W.; Balzer, P.; Klatte, T. A practical guide and decision-making protocol forthe management of complex renal cystic masses. *Arab. J. Urol.* **2017**, *15*, 115–122. [CrossRef] [PubMed]
42. Ljungberg, B.; Albiges, L.; Abu-Ghanem, Y.; Bensalah, K.; Dabestani, S.; Montes, S.F.; Gilles, R.H.; Hofmann, F.; Hora, M.; Kuczyk, M.A.; et al. European Association of Urology Guidelines on Renal Cell Carcinoma: The 2019 Update. *Eur. Urol.* **2019**, *75*, 799–810. [CrossRef]

43. Singhai, A.; Babu, S.; Verma, N.; Singh, V. Multilocular cystic renal cell carcinoma: A rare entity. *BMJ Case Rep.* **2013**. [CrossRef]
44. Kuroda, N.; Ohe, C.; Mikami, S.; Inoue, K.; Nagashima, Y.; Cohen, R.J.; Pan, C.-C.; Michal, M.; Hes, O. Multilocular cystic renal cell carcinoma with focus on clinical and pathobiological aspects. *Histol. Histopathol.* **2012**, *27*, 969–974. [PubMed]
45. Montironi, R.; Lopez-Beltran, A.; Cheng, L.; Scarpelli, M. Words of wisdom: Re: Multilocular cystic renal cell carcinoma with focus on clinical and pathobiological aspects. *Eur. Urol.* **2013**, *63*, 400–401. [CrossRef] [PubMed]
46. Williamson, S.R.; Halat, S.; Eble, J.N.; Grignon, D.J.; Lopez-Beltran, A.; Montironi, R.; Tan, P.-H.; Wang, M.; Maclennan, G.T.; Baldridge, L.A.; et al. Multilocular cystic renal cell carcinoma: Similarities and differences in immunoprofile compared with clear cell renal cell carcinoma. *Am. J. Surg. Pathol.* **2012**, *36*, 1425–1433. [CrossRef] [PubMed]
47. von Teichman, A.; Compérat, E.; Behnke, S.; Storz, M.; Moch, H.; Schraml, P. VHL mutations and dysregulation of pVHL- and PTEN-controlled pathways in multilocular cystic renal cell carcinoma. *Mod. Pathol.* **2011**, *24*, 571–578. [CrossRef]
48. Li, G.; Bilal, I.; Gentil-Perret, A.; Feng, G.; Zhao, A.; Peoc'h, M.; Genin, C.; Tostain, J.; Gigante, M. CA9 as a molecular marker for differential diagnosis of cystic renal tumors. *Urol. Oncol.* **2012**, *30*, 463–468. [CrossRef]
49. Gonzalez, M.L.; Alagehbandan, R.; Pivovarcikova, K.; Michalova, K.; Rogala, J.; Martinek, P.; Foix, M.P.; Mundo, E.C.; Comperat, E.; Ulamec, M.; et al. Reactivity of CK7 across the spectrum of renal cell carcinomas with clear cells. *Histopathology* **2019**, *74*, 608–617. [CrossRef]
50. Ostler, D.A.; Prieto, V.G.; Reed, J.A.; Deavers, M.T.; Lazar, A.J.; Ivan, D. Adipophilin expression in sebaceous tumors and other cutaneous lesions with clear cell histology: An immunohistochemical study of 117 cases. *Mod. Pathol.* **2010**, *23*, 567–573. [CrossRef]
51. Kim, S.H.; Park, B.; Joo, J.; Joung, J.Y.; Seo, H.K.; Lee, K.H.; Park, W.S.; Chung, J. Retrospective analysis of 25 immunohistochemical tissue markers for differentiating multilocular cystic renal neoplasm of low malignant potential and multicystic renal cell carcinoma. *Histol. Histopathol.* **2018**, *33*, 589–596.
52. Halat, S.; Eble, J.N.; Grignon, D.J.; Lopez-Beltran, A.; Montironi, R.; Tan, P.H.; Wang, M.; Zhang, S.; MacLennan, G.T.; Cheng, L. Multilocular cystic renal cell carcinoma is a subtype of clear cell renal cell carcinoma. *Mod. Pathol.* **2010**, *23*, 931–936. [CrossRef]
53. Raspollini, M.R.; Castiglione, F.; Martignoni, G.; Cheng, L.; Montironi, R.; Lopez-Beltran, A. Unlike in clear cell renal cell carcinoma, KRAS is not mutated in multilocular cystic clear cell renal cell neoplasm of low potential. *Virchows Arch.* **2015**, *467*, 687–693. [CrossRef] [PubMed]
54. Kim, S.H.; Park, W.S.; Chung, J. *SETD2*, *GIGYF2*, *FGFR3*, *BCR*, *KMT2C*, and *TSC2* as candidate genes for differentiating multilocular cystic renal neoplasm of low malignant potential from clear cell renal cell carcinoma with cystic change. *Investig. Clin. Urol.* **2019**, *60*, 148–155. [CrossRef] [PubMed]
55. Delahunt, B.; Cheville, J.C.; Martignoni, G.; Humphrey, P.A.; Magi-Galluzzi, C.; McKenney, J.; Egevad, L.; Algaba, F.; Moch, H.; Grignon, D.J.; et al. The International Society of Urological Pathology (ISUP) grading system for renal cell carcinoma and other prognostic parameters. *Am. J. Surg. Pathol.* **2013**, *37*, 1490–1504. [CrossRef]
56. Eble, J.N.; Bonsib, S.M. Extensively cystic renal neoplasms: Cystic nephroma, cystic partially differentiated nephroblastoma, multilocular cystic renal cell carcinoma, and cystic hamartoma of renal pelvis. *Semin. Diagn. Pathol.* **1998**, *15*, 2–20. [PubMed]
57. Eble, J.N.; Sauter, G.; Epstein, J.I.; Sesterhenn, I.A. *World Health Organization Classification of Tumours. Pathology and Genetics of Tumours of the Urinary System and Male Genital Organs*; IARC Press: Lyon, France, 2004.
58. Aubert, S.; Zini, L.; Delomez, J.; Biserte, J.; Lemaitre, L.; Leroy, X. Cystic renal carcinomas in adults. Is preoperative recognition of multilocular cystic renal cell carcinoma possible? *J. Urol.* **2005**, *174*, 2115–2119. [CrossRef]
59. Hindman, N.M.; Bosniak, M.A.; Rosenkrantz, A.B.; Lee-Felker, S.; Melamed, J. Multilocular cystic renal cell carcinoma: Comparison of imaging and pathologic findings. *AJR Am. J. Roentgenol.* **2012**, *198*, W20–W26. [CrossRef]
60. Raspollini, M.R.; Montagnani, I.; Montironi, R.; Cheng, L.; Martignoni, G.; Minervini, A.; Serni, S.; Nicita, G.; Carini, M.; Lopez-Beltran, A. A contemporary series of renal masses with emphasis on recently recognized entities and tumors of low malignant potential: A report based on 624 consecutive tumors from a single tertiary center. *Pathol. Res. Pract.* **2017**, *213*, 804–808. [CrossRef]
61. Rübenthaler, J.; Paprottka, K.J.; Marcon, J.; Reiser, M.; Clevert, D.A. MRI and contrast enhanced ultrasound (CEUS) image fusion of renal lesions. *Clin. Hemorheol. Microcirc.* **2016**, *64*, 457–466. [CrossRef]
62. Sanz, E.; Hevia, V.; Gómez, V.; Álvarez, S.; Fabuel, J.J.; Martínez, L.; Rodriguez-Patrón, R.; González-Gordaliza, C.; Burgos, F.-J. Renal Complex Cystic Masses: Usefulness of Contrast-Enhanced Ultrasound (CEUS) in Their Assessment and Its Agreement with Computed Tomography. *Curr. Urol. Rep.* **2016**, *17*, 89. [CrossRef] [PubMed]
63. Katabathina, V.S.; Garg, D.; Prasad, S.R.; Vikram, R. Cystic renal neoplasms and renal neoplasms associated with cystic renal diseases in adults: Cross-sectional imaging findings. *J. Comput. Assist. Tomogr.* **2012**, *36*, 659–668. [CrossRef] [PubMed]

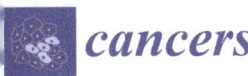

Perspective

Towards Personalized Sampling in Clear Cell Renal Cell Carcinomas

Claudia Manini [1,2], Estíbaliz López-Fernández [3,4] and José I. López [5,*]

1. Department of Pathology, San Giovanni Bosco Hospital, 10154 Turin, Italy; claudia.manini@aslcittaditorino.it
2. Department of Sciences of Public Health and Pediatrics, University of Turin, 10124 Turin, Italy
3. FISABIO Foundation, 46020 Valencia, Spain; estibaliz.lopez@universidadeuropea.es
4. Faculty of Health Sciences, European University of Valencia, 46023 Valencia, Spain
5. Biocruces-Bizkaia Health Research Institute, 48903 Barakaldo, Spain
* Correspondence: joseignacio.lopez@osakidetza.eus or jilpath@gmail.com

Citation: Manini, C.; López-Fernández, E.; López, J.I. Towards Personalized Sampling in Clear Cell Renal Cell Carcinomas. *Cancers* **2022**, *14*, 3381. https://doi.org/10.3390/cancers14143381

Academic Editor: Arndt Hartmann

Received: 27 June 2022
Accepted: 11 July 2022
Published: 12 July 2022

Publisher's Note: MDPI stays neutral with regard to jurisdictional claims in published maps and institutional affiliations.

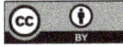

Copyright: © 2022 by the authors. Licensee MDPI, Basel, Switzerland. This article is an open access article distributed under the terms and conditions of the Creative Commons Attribution (CC BY) license (https://creativecommons.org/licenses/by/4.0/).

Simple Summary: Intratumor heterogeneity (ITH) is a constant event in malignant tumors and the cause of most therapeutic failures in modern oncology. Since clear cell renal cell carcinoma (CCRCC) is a paradigm of ITH, an appropriate tumor sampling is mandatory to unveil its histological and genomic complexity. Several strategies have been developed for such a purpose, trading-off cost and benefit. Here, we propose an evolution of the previous multisite tumor sampling (MSTS) strategy based on the last findings in the spatial distribution of metastasizing clones. This new personalized MSTS pays special attention to sample by sectors peripheral zones of the tumor, where ITH is high.

Abstract: Intratumor heterogeneity (ITH) is a constant evolutionary event in all malignant tumors, and clear cell renal cell carcinoma (CCRCC) is a paradigmatic example. ITH is responsible for most therapeutic failures in the era of precision oncology, so its precise detection remains a must in modern medicine. Unfortunately, classic sampling protocols do not resolve the problem as expected and several strategies have been being implemented in recent years to improve such detection. Basically, multisite tumor sampling (MSTS) and the homogenization of the residual tumor tissue are on display. A next step of the MSTS strategy considering the recently discovered patterns of ITH regionalization is presented here, the so-called personalized MSTS (pMSTS). This modification consists of paying more attention to sample the tumor periphery since it is this area with maximum levels of ITH.

Keywords: multisite tumor sampling; intratumor heterogeneity; clear cell renal cell carcinoma

1. Introduction

In these days of highly sophisticated medicine, simple things such as tumor sampling still matter. Pathologists are the specialists responsible for handling and sampling tumor specimens in such a way that crucial information of every tumor can be unveiled. A strategy adaptable to different patterns of tumor evolution, trading-off cost and benefit, is needed to maximize results and to respond to oncologists' expectations [1]. Although tumor sampling is a key point applicable to every tumor type, this narrative focuses specifically on clear cell renal cell carcinoma (CCRCC) because of the previous experience of the authors in this area. In addition, CCRCC is a quite common neoplasm in daily practice and a well-known example of intratumor heterogeneity (ITH). The following paragraphs review the principal arguments supporting the necessity to update tumor sampling strategies and revisit possible alternatives for the progressive implementation of a so-called "precision sampling" [2].

CCRCC ranks in the top 10 list of the most frequent tumors in Western countries and remains a problem of major concern for many health systems. Roughly 79,000 new cases and 14,000 deaths are expected in USA in 2022 [3]. Traditionally chemo- and radio-resistant, only early detection and antiangiogenic and immune checkpoint blockade therapies, alone or in combination, have improved survival of CCRCC patients in the last decade. However, a significant proportion of these patients still die of disease, usually in the context of a metastatic disease.

CCRCC is a paradigmatic example of ITH, which is the cause of most therapeutic failures to date. Genomic analyses have shown that CCRCC is a complex disease in which clonal and sub-clonal diversification is high across the tumor with many genetic alterations involving typically few regions. This fact was unveiled in the seminal paper published by Gerlinger et al. in 2012 [4], in which the authors performed exome sequencing, chromosome aberration analysis, and ploidy profiling in multi-regional samples of four patients with metastatic disease. Since then, a great many studies have brought to light the spatial and temporal dynamics governing the evolution of this tumor type and others.

Although initially considered a purely stochastic process, tumor evolution in CCRCC seems to follow some deterministic pathways. In this sense, a recent analysis of 1206 regions of 101 cases has discovered up to seven evolutionary patterns correlated with patient prognosis [5]. *BAP-1* driven, multiple clonal drivers, and *VHL* wild-type tumors were shown to follow a punctuated evolutionary model with rapid progression and display high levels of chromosomal complexity and low levels of ITH. By contrast, the family of *PBRM1* mutated tumors showed a branched evolution with attenuated progression, with lesser chromosomal complexity and high ITH. An analysis of 575 primary and 335 metastatic regions in 100 CCRCC patients has shown that the metastatic ability of CCRCC is associated with 9p and 14q losses [6]. The same study has also shown that those neoplasms which show a punctuated evolution presented early, multiple metastases while those with a branching pattern develop late, solitary ones.

Punctuated and branching are terms referring to two different patterns of temporal evolution which come from the application of ecological principles to cancer. Under this perspective, a tumor is a huge community of different individuals including neoplastic cells and cells of the tumor microenvironment such as endothelia, tumor-associated fibroblasts, macrophages, tumor-associated lymphocytes, and others. These elements are permanently interacting one each other. At least four models of tumor evolution have been described so far: linear, branching, neutral, and punctuated [7]. Linear, branching, and punctuated are Darwinian-type models whereas neutral is considered non-Darwinian. Linear model refers to a step-wise temporal process in which all cancer cells progressively increase their malignancy. This pattern will generate tumors with very low ITH. In the branching type of evolution, tumor cells coming from the same ancestor temporarily acquire different mutations resulting in different clones which regionalize the tumor in different areas. This pattern will give rise to tumors with high ITH. The punctuated pattern of evolution, also called the "big bang" model, is the result of a genomic aberration generating a dominant clone with high fitness at the very early stages of tumor evolution. As a result, punctuated tumors are typically aggressive and show low levels of ITH. Finally, neutral evolution reflects an evolutionary pattern in which extreme clonal diversity (hyper-branching) develops resulting in tumors with very high ITH.

ITH also impacts tumor microenvironment, including cancer associated fibroblasts, macrophages, and tumor infiltrating lymphocytes. For example, it has been demonstrated that the expression of PD-1, PD-L1, and other immune checkpoint markers may be highly variable across different tumor regions, a feature that can compromise the correct selection of patients for immune checkpoint blockade therapy if the tumor is not appropriately sampled [8]. An incomplete tumor sampling may lead to false negative results, thus ruling out patients for a beneficial therapy. In this sense, Khagi et al. observed non-expected good responses to anti-PD-L1 therapy in up to 17% of cases that apparently did not express PD-L1 in the immunohistochemical study [9] suggesting suboptimal analyses.

2. Classic Sampling Protocols

Classic sampling protocols were designed decades ago when ITH detection was not a key issue for diagnosis and therapy. At that time, the recommendation was to obtain one tumor tissue sample per centimeter of tumor diameter plus samples from the tumor/non-tumor interface and from "suspicious" areas (Figure 1A) [10]. Those sampling protocols are not supported by any scientific observation and surprisingly survive nowadays in the era of precision medicine.

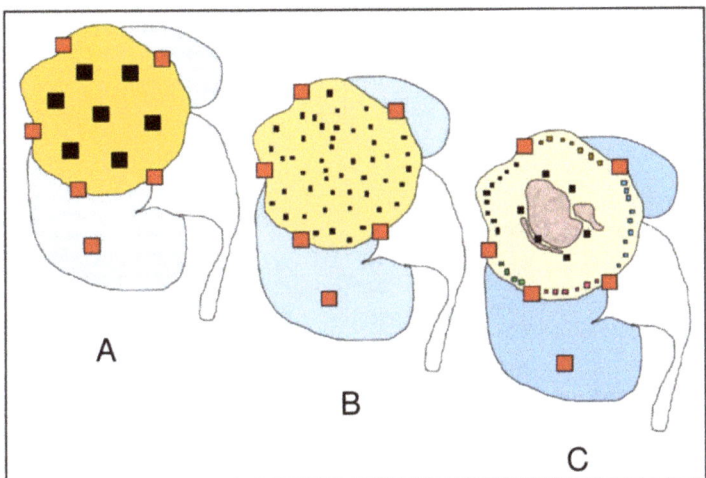

Figure 1. Schematic of tumor sampling evolution in clear cell renal cell carcinoma. The classical sampling protocol (**A**) calls for one block per centimeter of tumor diameter. Multisite tumor sampling (**B**) randomly selects a large number of small tumor samples across the tumor using the same number of blocks as the classic protocol. Advanced multisite tumor sampling (**C**) takes a few samples at the tumor center, where intratumor heterogeneity is low but metastatic genotypes and necrosis (pink areas) are common, and many small samples at the periphery, where intratumor heterogeneity and local invasiveness are high. Here, the small fragments selected are grouped in blocks by sectors, thus enabling the precise location of any key change in any sample to be monitored. Note that tumor/non-tumor, tumor/renal sinus, and tumor/perinephric fat interfaces are similar in the three methods (block shown in red).

Since ITH makes every tumor unique and unrepeatable, and next generation sequencing tools are demonstrating the real dimension of the genetic variability across a single tumor, the main question here should be: how much sampling is needed in every case? Total tumor sampling might be the perfect answer. This strategy may be affordable and advisable in small tumors (<3 cm), but it is not a realistic option in many tumors due to many of them are much larger. Some authors have suggested that sampling three distant regions would suffice to detect with a reliability of 90% of certainty key mutations in CCRCC such as those occurring in *PBRM1*, *SETD2*, *BAP1*, and *KDM5C* genes [11]. However, the number of samples should not be aprioristically fixed since it should vary with the size of the tumor.

3. Multisite Tumor Sampling (MSTS)

Classic sampling protocols seem insufficient in light of subsequent studies, which have suggested the convenience of a more thorough sampling to detect exome-wide driver events [5,6]. For this reason, a new, affordable strategy for trading-off cost and benefit was developed in 2016 [12]. It is called multisite tumor sampling (MSTS) (Figure 1B) and is based on the divide-and-conquer principle [13], a mathematical algorithm successfully used in such widely differing scientific fields as particle physics and medicine. The strategy consists in recursively breaking down a given problem into simpler parts (divide) until they are simple enough to be solved (conquer). Once the simple parts are solved they are all merged to resolve the initial problem. In our example, its application to tumor sampling consists of including six to eight small tissue fragments per block instead of a single large fragment (Figure 2). In this way, MSTS can afford to sample up to 48 tumor regions very distant from each other when sampling a 6 cm-in-diameter tumor, for example. In silico modelling comparing the performances and costs of the classic sampling protocol and MSTS confirms the superiority of the latter in detecting ITH at all temporal stages of tumor evolution [13,14]. A comparison of the performance in detecting histological features of bad prognosis such as high grade and granular eosinophilic cells [15] with both methods in 38 CCRCC showed that MSTS was significantly more informative than routine sampling [16].

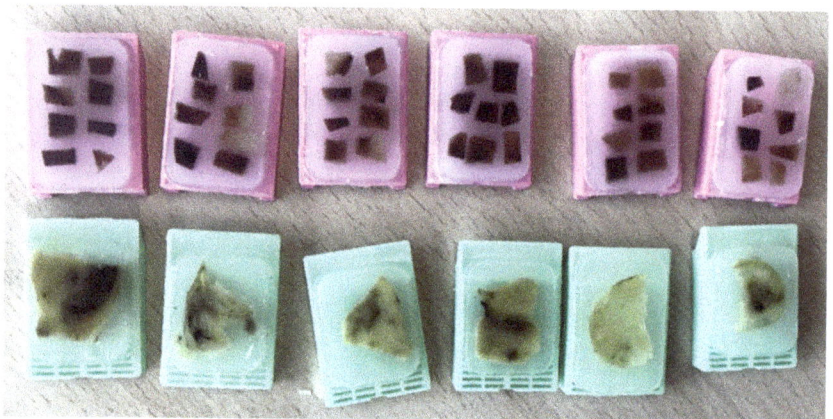

Figure 2. Multisite tumor sampling (pink blocks) consists on including six to eight small tumor tissue fragments in each paraffin block instead of one large tumor fragment proposed by the classic protocol (green blocks). This way, the same number of paraffin blocks sample many more tumor regions.

Aside from CCRCC, the usefulness of MSTS in CCRCC has been confirmed by subsequent histological, immunohistochemical, and molecular studies in ovarian carcinoma, mesothelioma, and head and neck squamous cell carcinoma [17–20]. Lakis et al. [17] have analyzed 294 tumor sections from 70 treatment naïve patients who had undergone cytoreductive surgery of ovarian cancer and have observed not only the high histological variability of tumors across different regions, but also the irregular qualitative and quantitative distribution of tumor-associated lymphocyte, information with obvious prognostic and therapeutic implications. They conclude that ITH in ovarian cancer may limit the usefulness of pre-operative biopsies to make some therapeutic decisions. Meiller et al. [18] underline the usefulness of MSTS in detecting molecular ITH in malignant mesothelioma. MSTS performed in 16 patients from two different hospitals were analyzed both histologically, and by RT-PCR and targeted NGS. Mutational ITH, copy number variations and fusion transcripts, differential gene expression and signal pathway dysregulation, histomolecular heterogeneity, epigenetic ITH, and tumor microenvironment were evaluated. The authors conclude that spatial ITH is high in malignant pleural mesothelioma and stress the convenience of analyzing different topographical areas of the tumor. This policy must be performed to better estimate the patient prognosis and the prediction of response to subsequent treatment. Jie et al. [19] have compared the performance of routine sampling and MSTS in 182 oral and oropharyngeal squamous-cell carcinomas. The authors included in the comparison histological, immunohistochemical, and molecular parameters, and concluded that MSTS was more informative than routine sampling in detecting perineurial permeation, peritumoral vascular/lymphatic growth, necrosis, muscle invasion, PIK3CA mutations (exons 9 and 20), and CDKN2A promoter methylation. Brunelli et al. [20] have recently compared a multi-regional sampling strategy called 3D fusion with routine sampling in 100 CCRCC analyzing the respective performance of both methods in the detection of angiogenic and immune markers. These authors confirm the superiority of 3D fusion sampling and agree that sampling one block/cm of tumor tissue diameter is inadequate to fully characterize ITH in CCRCC. Finally, another in silico study has shown the superiority of an adapted variant of the MSTS method in detecting tumor budding and intramural vasculo-lymphatic invasion in hollow viscera (urinary bladder and digestive) adenocarcinomas [21].

4. Homogenization of the Residual Tumor Tissue

Another attempt to improve genomic ITH detection in solid tumors has recently been made [22]. This method proposes the homogenization of the leftover residual tumor tissue before sequencing, thus guaranteeing the full genomic analysis of the whole tumor. However, this protocol has its limitations because not all surgical specimens generate enough representative leftover tissue after histological sampling. In addition, the topographic localization of the genomic data and its correlation with histology—a point that may be important—is lost after tissue homogenization. As it will be mentioned in the following paragraphs, leftover tissue homogenization will also negatively affect the precise topographic identification of the differences in the tumor microenvironment between tumor center and periphery, which are derived from differences in the hypoxic status, another crucial targetable point.

In a context of high diagnostic pressure, some pathologists may be reluctant to increase the time and cost needed to implement both 3D fusion [20] and the homogenization of the leftover residual tumor [22], a point that may limit their widespread implementation. By contrast, MSTS saves time because it is an *all-in-one* procedure, enabling at the same time the histological analysis with a genomic correlation to take place in the same paraffin block and preserving the formalin-fixed paraffin-embedded material for the future. Also, MSTS is an affordable method in public health systems since it does not increase the cost. If the paraffin block is considered the unit of cost in Pathology Labs, the MSTS's cost is similar to the routine sampling because it employs the same number of blocks. For these reasons, MSTS is superior in terms of trading-off performance obtained and cost.

5. Personalized Multisite Tumor Sampling (pMSTS)

Recent findings on the spatial distribution of CCRCC clones and sub-clones [23,24] also suggest taking a step forward in searching for a more refined tumor sampling strategy. This evolution should look for constraints on cost and time, efficacy in the detection of histological and genomic data, and adaptability to adjust the procedure case by case. It should be noted that tumors are usually sampled without knowing the precise tumor landscape in every case. However, some broad findings in selected cases may supply useful data since predicting the possibility of aggressive forms of CCRCC may help in making sampling decisions. For example, spontaneous tumor necrosis is a common finding in large tumors which can be detected by the naked eye and is always related to high grade. Low ITH at histological and genomic levels are characteristic findings in many aggressive CCRCC [6,25]. In consequence, it can be inferred even in the grossing room that tumors showing areas of necrosis will have high-grade histological features and low levels of ITH.

A study of 756 mapped regions of 101 CCRCC has shown that the copy number alteration burden, percentage of necrosis, and histological grade are higher in the tumor interior, which is also where the metastasizing subclones preferentially develop, probably as a survival response to local environmental hypoxic pressures [23]. Moreover, a model enabling the development of clonal diversity in space and time of these tumors to be understood has been developed based on patterns of tumor growth and necrosis [24]. As a result, high ITH is located at the tumor periphery while the tumor interior remains relatively homogeneous. Since the conditions of hypoxia differ between the tumor center and periphery, tumor microenvironments adapt to the specific local necessities, displaying qualitative and quantitative variations in the innate and adaptive tumor immunities, tumor-associated fibroblasts, and other elements of this tumor compartment [26]. Interestingly, this model or center versus periphery distinction, at least in CCRCC, also has clinical implications since it connects radiological evidence of peripheral tumor budding in the early stages of tumor development with predictable future clonal evolution [24].

A more precise tumor sampling requires investing some extra time in the grossing room paying special attention to the macroscopic characteristics of the tumor, including size and shape, tumor margins, and allowing the detection of other tumor features like tissue consistency and color that usually give additional interesting information. Taking these classic recommendations on mind, together with the latest findings on spatial tumor evolution and regionalization as a whole, an advanced version of the MSTS protocol will provide a more closely adapted approach at the time of sampling CCRCC (Figure 1C). Given that metastasizing clones related to tumor necrosis, high grade, and low ITH are mostly located in the tumor interior, several samples placed in one block would suffice to provide a reliable representation of this tumor area including tumor and non-tumor cells. Also, grey/whitish tumor areas with stiffer consistency indicating sarcomatoid dedifferentiation will be seen by naked-eye and then included within the high-grade tumor blocks. By contrast, the peripheral rim of the tumor is characterized by high levels of ITH [23,24]; for this reason, many small tissue fragments such as those of the MSTS are needed to provide a complete snapshot of the tumor periphery. What is more, these small tissue samples can be included in the blocks distributed by sectors, so the topographic location of any specific molecular alteration associated to prognosis or treatment can be determined with precision in every case.

6. Conclusions

Tumor sampling strategies do impact significantly on the development and success of truly precision oncological therapies. To hit the target and achieve widespread implementation, this strategy must be easily affordable on one hand and trade-off costs and benefits on the other; otherwise, its implementation in many Pathology Labs will be at risk. Two variants of the MSTS adaptable to the macroscopic findings observed in the grossing room and the alternative option of a complete homogenization of the leftover residual tumor tissue are currently available. To note, they appear to be complementary, non-exclusive according to this Perspective.

Author Contributions: C.M., E.L.-F. and J.I.L. have conceived and written this manuscript. All authors have read and agreed to the published version of the manuscript.

Funding: This research received no external funding.

Institutional Review Board Statement: Ethical review and approval were waived for this study due to it was performed as part of the routine analysis necessary to perform the pathological diagnosis.

Informed Consent Statement: Patient consent was waived for this study due to it was performed as part of the routine analysis necessary to perform the pathological diagnosis.

Data Availability Statement: Data sharing is not applicable to this article.

Conflicts of Interest: The authors declare no conflict of interest.

References

1. Soultati, A.; Stares, M.; Swanton, C.; Larkin, J.; Turajlic, S. How should clinicians address intratumour heterogeneity in clear cell renal cell carcinoma? *Curr. Opin. Urol.* **2015**, *25*, 358–366. [CrossRef] [PubMed]
2. Manini, C.; López-Fernández, E.; López, J.I. Precision sampling fuels precision oncology: An evolutionary perspective. *Trends Cancer* **2021**, *7*, 978–981. [CrossRef] [PubMed]
3. Siegel, R.L.; Miller, K.D.; Fusch, H.E.; Jemal, A. Cancer statistics, 2022. *CA A Cancer J. Clin.* **2022**, *72*, 7–33. [CrossRef] [PubMed]
4. Gerlinger, M.; Rowan, A.J.; Horswell, S.; Math, M.; Larkin, J.; Endesfelder, D.; Gronroos, E.; Martinez, P.; Matthews, N.; Stewart, A.; et al. Intratumor heterogeneity and branched evolution revealed by multiregion sequencing. *N. Engl. J. Med.* **2012**, *366*, 883–892. [CrossRef]

5. Turajlic, S.; Xu, H.; Litchfield, K.; Rowan, A.; Horswell, S.; Chambers, T.; O'Brien, T.; Lopez, J.I.; Watkins, T.B.K.; Nicol, D.; et al. Deterministic evolutionary trajectories influence primary tumor growth: TRACERx Renal. *Cell* **2018**, *173*, 595–610. [CrossRef]
6. Turajlic, S.; Xu, H.; Litchfield, K.; Rowan, A.; Chambers, T.; López, J.I.; Nicol, D.; O'Brien, T.; Larkin, J.; Horswell, S.; et al. Tracking cancer evolution reveals constrained routes to metastases: TRACERx Renal. *Cell* **2018**, *173*, 581–594. [CrossRef]
7. Davis, A.; Gao, R.; Navin, N. Tumor evolution: Linear, branching, neutral or punctuated? *Biochim. Biophys. Acta* **2017**, *1867*, 151–161. [CrossRef]
8. Nunes-Xavier, C.E.; Angulo, J.C.; Pulido, R.; López, J.I. A critical insight into the clinical translation of PD-1/PD-L1 blockade therapy in clear cell renal cell carcinoma. *Curr. Urol. Rep.* **2019**, *20*, 1–10. [CrossRef]
9. Khagi, Y.; Kurzrock, R.; Patel, S.P. Next generation predictive biomarkers for immune checkpoint inhibition. *Cancer Metastasis Rev.* **2017**, *36*, 179–190. [CrossRef]
10. Trpkov, K.; Grignon, D.J.; Bonsib, S.M.; Amin, M.B.; Billis, A.; Lopez-Beltran, A.; Samaratunga, H.; Tamboli, P.; Delahunt, B.; Egevad, L.; et al. Handling and staging or renal cell carcinoma: The International Society of Urological Pathology Consensus (ISUP) conference recommendations. *Am. J. Surg. Pathol.* **2013**, *37*, 1505–1517. [CrossRef]
11. Sankin, A.; Hakimi, A.A.; Mikkilineni, N.; Ostrovnaya, I.; Silk, M.T.; Liang, Y.; Mano, R.; Chevinski, M.; Motzer, R.J.; Solomon, S.B.; et al. The impact of genetic heterogeneity on biomarker development in kidney cancer assessed by multiregional sampling. *Cancer Med.* **2014**, *3*, 1485–1492. [CrossRef] [PubMed]
12. López, J.I.; Cortés, J.M. Multisite tumor sampling: A new tumor selection method to enhance intratumor heterogeneity detection. *Hum. Pathol.* **2017**, *64*, 1–6. [CrossRef] [PubMed]
13. López, J.I.; Cortés, J.M. A divide-and-conquer strategy in tumor sampling enhances detection of intratumor heterogeneity in routine pathology: A modeling approach in clear cell renal cell carcinoma. *F1000Reserch* **2016**, *5*, 385. [CrossRef]
14. Erramuzpe, A.; Cortés, J.M.; López, J.I. Multisite tumor sampling enhances the detection of intratumor heterogeneity at all different temporal stages of tumor evolution. *Virchows Arch.* **2018**, *472*, 187–194. [CrossRef]
15. Yoshida, T.; Ohe, C.; Ikeda, J.; Atsumi, N.; Ohsugi, H.; Sugi, M.; Higasa, K.; Saito, R.; Tsuta, K.; Matsuda, T.; et al. Eosinophilic features in clear cell renal cell carcinoma correlate with outcomes of immune checkpoint and angiogenesis blockade. *J. Immun. Ther. Cancer* **2021**, *9*, e002922. [CrossRef]
16. Guarch, R.; Cortés, J.M.; Lawrie, C.H.; López, J.I. Multi-site tumor sampling (MSTS) improves the performance of histological detection of intratumor heterogeneity in clear cell renal cell carcinoma (CCRCC). *F1000Reserch* **2016**, *5*, 2020. [CrossRef]
17. Lakis, S.; Kotoula, V.; Koliou, G.; Efstratiou, I.; Chrisafi, S.; Papanikolaou, A.; Zebekakis, P.; Fountzilas, G. Multisite tumor sampling reveals extensive heterogeneity of tumor and host immune response in ovarian cancer. *Cancer Genom. Proteom.* **2020**, *17*, 529–541. [CrossRef]
18. Meiller, C.; Montagne, F.; Hirsch, T.Z.; Caruso, S.; de Wolf, J.; Bayard, Q.; Assié, J.B.; Meunier, L.; Blum, Y.; Quetel, L.; et al. Multi-site tumor sampling highlights molecular intra-tumor heterogeneity in malignant pleural mesothelioma. *Genome Med.* **2021**, *13*, 1–16. [CrossRef]
19. Jie, W.; Bai, J.; Yan, J.; Chi, Y.; Li, B.B. Multi-site tumour sampling improves the detection of intra-tumour heterogeneity in oral and oropharyngeal squamous cell carcinoma. *Front. Med.* **2021**, *8*, 670305. [CrossRef]
20. Brunelli, M.; Martignoni, G.; Malpeli, G.; Volpe, A.; Cima, L.; Raspollini, M.R.; Barbareschi, M.; Tafuri, A.; Masi, G.; Barzon, L.; et al. Validation of a novel three-dimensional (3D fusion) gross sampling protocol for clear cell renal cell carcinoma to overcome intratumoral heterogeneity: The Meet-Uro 18 study. *J. Pers. Med.* **2022**, *12*, 727. [CrossRef]
21. Cortés, J.M.; de Petris, G.; López, J.I. Detection of intratumor heterogeneity in modern pathology: A multisite tumor sampling perspective. *Front. Med.* **2017**, *4*, 25. [CrossRef] [PubMed]
22. Gallegos, L.L.; Gilchrist, A.; Spain, L.; Stanislaw, S.; Hill, S.M.; Primus, V.; Jones, C.; Agrawal, S.; Tippu, Z.; Barhoumi, A.; et al. A protocol for representative sampling of solid tumors to improve the accuracy of sequencing results. *STAR Protoc.* **2021**, *2*, 100624. [CrossRef] [PubMed]
23. Zhao, Y.; Fu, X.; López, J.I.; Rowan, A.; Au, L.; Fendler, A.; Hazell, S.; Xu, H.; Horswell, S.; Shepherd, S.T.C.; et al. Selection of metastasis competent subclones in the tumour interior. *Nat. Ecol. Evol.* **2021**, *5*, 1033–1045. [CrossRef] [PubMed]
24. Fu, X.; Zhao, Y.; López, J.I.; Rowan, A.; Au, L.; Fendler, A.; Hazell, S.; Xu, H.; Horswell, S.; Shepherd, S.T.C.; et al. Spatial patterns of tumour growth impact clonal diversification in a computational model and the TRACERx Renal study. *Nat. Ecol. Evol.* **2022**, *6*, 88–102. [CrossRef]
25. Manini, C.; López-Fernández, E.; Lawrie, C.H.; Laruelle, A.; Angulo, J.C.; López, J.I. Clear cell renal cell carcinomas with aggressive behavior display low intratumor heterogeneity at the histological level. *Curr. Urol. Rep.* **2022**, *23*, 93–97. [CrossRef]
26. Petrova, V.; Annicchiarico-Petruzzelli, M.; Melino, G.; Amelio, I. The hypoxic tumour microenvironment. *Oncogenesis* **2018**, *7*, 10. [CrossRef]

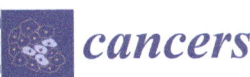

Article

LiKidMiRs: A ddPCR-Based Panel of 4 Circulating miRNAs for Detection of Renal Cell Carcinoma

José Pedro Sequeira [1,2], Vera Constâncio [1,3], Sofia Salta [1,4], João Lobo [1,5,6], Daniela Barros-Silva [1,4], Carina Carvalho-Maia [1], Jéssica Rodrigues [7,8], Isaac Braga [9], Rui Henrique [1,5,6,*,†] and Carmen Jerónimo [1,6,*,†]

1. Cancer Biology and Epigenetics Group, Research Center of IPO Porto (CI-IPOP)/RISE@CI-IPOP (Health Research Network), Portuguese Oncology Institute of Porto (IPO Porto)/Porto Comprehensive Cancer Centre (Porto.CCC), R. Dr. António Bernardino de Almeida, 4200-072 Porto, Portugal; jose.leite.sequeira@ipoporto.min-saude.pt (J.P.S.); vera.salvado.constancio@ipoporto.min-saude.pt (V.C.); sofia.salta@ipoporto.min-saude.pt (S.S.); jpedro.lobo@ipoporto.min-saude.pt (J.L.); daniela.silva@ipoporto.min-saude.pt (D.B.-S.); carina.carvalho.maia@ipoporto.min-saude.pt (C.C.-M.)
2. Master Programme in Oncology, School of Medicine & Biomedical Sciences, University of Porto (ICBAS-UP), Rua Jorge Viterbo Ferreira 228, 4050-513 Porto, Portugal
3. Doctoral Programme in Biomedical Sciences, School of Medicine & Biomedical Sciences, University of Porto (ICBAS-UP), Rua Jorge Viterbo Ferreira 228, 4050-513 Porto, Portugal
4. Doctoral Programme in Molecular Pathology and Genetics, School of Medicine & Biomedical Sciences, University of Porto (ICBAS-UP), Rua Jorge Viterbo Ferreira 228, 4050-513 Porto, Portugal
5. Department of Pathology, Portuguese Oncology Institute of Porto (IPOP), R. Dr. António Bernardino de Almeida, 4200-072 Porto, Portugal
6. Department of Pathology and Molecular Immunology, Institute of Biomedical Sciences Abel Salazar, University of Porto (ICBAS-UP), Rua Jorge Viterbo Ferreira 228, 4050-513 Porto, Portugal
7. Cancer Epidemiology Group, IPO Porto Research Center of IPO Porto (CI-IPOP)/RISE@CI-IPOP (Health Research Network), Portuguese Oncology Institute of Porto (IPO Porto)/Porto Comprehensive Cancer Centre (Porto.CCC), R. Dr. António Bernardino de Almeida, 4200-072 Porto, Portugal; jessica.rocha.rodrigues@ipoporto.min-saude.pt
8. Centre of Mathematics (CMAT), University of Minho, Campus de Gualtar, R. da Universidade, 4710-057 Braga, Portugal
9. Department of Urology & Urology Clinics, Portuguese Oncology Institute of Porto (IPOP), R. Dr. António Bernardino de Almeida, 4200-072 Porto, Portugal; isaac.braga@ipoporto.min-saude.pt
* Correspondence: henrique@ipoporto.min-saude.pt (R.H.); carmenjeronimo@ipoporto.min-saude.pt (C.J.); Tel.: +351-225084000 (C.J.); Fax: +351-225084199 (C.J.)
† These authors contributed equally to this work.

Simple Summary: Early detection of renal cell carcinoma (RCC) significantly increases the likelihood of curative treatment, avoiding the need of adjuvant therapies, associated side effects and comorbidities. Thus, we aimed to discover circulating microRNAs that might aid in early, minimally invasive, RCC detection/diagnosis.

Abstract: Background: Decreased renal cell cancer-related mortality is an important societal goal, embodied by efforts to develop effective biomarkers enabling early detection and increasing the likelihood of curative treatment. Herein, we sought to develop a new biomarker for early and minimally invasive detection of renal cell carcinoma (RCC) based on a microRNA panel assessed by ddPCR. Methods: Plasma samples from patients with RCC ($n = 124$) or oncocytomas ($n = 15$), and 64 healthy donors, were selected. Hsa-miR-21-5p, hsa-miR-126-3p, hsa-miR-155-5p and hsa-miR-200b-3p levels were evaluated using a ddPCR protocol. Results: RCC patients disclosed significantly higher circulating levels of hsa-miR-155-5p compared to healthy donors, whereas the opposite was observed for hsa-miR-21-5p levels. Furthermore, hsa-miR-21-5p and hsa-miR-155-5p panels detected RCC with high sensitivity (82.66%) and accuracy (71.89%). The hsa-miR-126-3p/hsa-miR-200b-3p panel identified the most common RCC subtype (clear cell, ccRCC) with 74.78% sensitivity. Conclusion: Variable combinations of plasma miR levels assessed by ddPCR enable accurate detection of RCC in general, and of ccRCC. These findings, if confirmed in larger studies, provide evidence for a novel ancillary tool which might aid in early detection of RCC.

Keywords: ddPCR; circulating miRNA; renal cell carcinoma; diagnosis; malignancy

1. Introduction

Renal cancer remains one of the leading urologic cancers worldwide, being listed as one of the twenty most common and deadly cancers, especially among men (1.5:1) [1,2].

Renal cell tumors (RCTs) correspond to a set of benign and malignant neoplasms, with extensive diversity at epigenetic, molecular, and clinical levels [3,4]. Among them, about 10% correspond to benign tumors, with oncocytomas constituting the most common benign tumor [1,4]. Concerning malignant RCTs, clear-cell renal cell carcinoma (ccRCC) is the most common subtype (65–75% of all RCCs) [5], followed by papillary renal cell carcinomas (pRCC, ~16%) and chromophobe renal cell carcinomas (chRCC, ~7%)[5]. RCCs derive from nephron epithelial cells [1,6,7] and are characterized by their heterogeneity, both morphological and molecular. Whereas localized RCC is mostly cured by surgery, locally advanced or systemic disease constitute major therapeutic challenges, entailing the need for development not only of biomarkers for early detection, but also novel therapies [8].

In recent years, several studies have been published concerning the use of circulating microRNAs (miRNAs) for early and minimally invasive detection of RCC [1,9]. MiRNAs are small non-coding RNAs involved in cell differentiation, growth, apoptosis, and proliferation, and have been implicated in suppressing gene expression after translation [10,11]. MicroRNA dysregulation has been extensively described in various cancers, including RCC [4,10–13]. Frequently, miRNA levels differ between cancerous and normal tissues, representing an opportunity for biomarker development, both in tissue samples and in liquid biopsies [10,11]. Nonetheless, the biomarker performance of most candidate miRNAs remains suboptimal, and concerns remain as to the most adequate methods for assessment and normalization [14,15]. Indeed, all published studies on the assessment of miRNAs in the liquid biopsies of RCC patients have used qRT-PCR [1,9], a technique which provides relative quantification, thus requiring normalization of the results. Although miR-16 should be the preferential normalizer due to its stability in RCC [15–18], many of the published studies used RNU44, U6, or other similar RNA species instead, which are unstable in liquid biopsies, eventually leading to biased results [14,19–27]. This problem might be solved using a different technology, droplet digital PCR (ddPCR), as it obviates the need for normalization and preamplification. DdPCR is a recent technology that appears to improve miRNA detection, as it is based on sample partitioning before the PCR reaction and on the Poisson distribution, allowing for absolute quantification, in a time-cost effective and reliable manner [28,29]. Furthermore, the time point of data acquisition increases the precision and robustness of the method [28,29].

Thus, in this study, taking advantage of the performance of ddPCR in liquid biopsies, we sought to evaluate, for the first time, the ability of a microRNA panel (hsa-miR-21-5p, hsa-miR-126-3p, hsa-miR-155-5p, and hsa-miR-200b-3p), previously assessed in tissue samples [13,30] to detect RCC using plasma samples.

2. Materials and Methods

2.1. Samples

A total of five plasma samples were included in the technical optimization phase of the study, in which the ddPCR methodology was tested: one oncocytoma, one stage I pRCC, one stage I ccRCC, one stage I chRCC, and one healthy adult blood donor.

After optimizing the ddPCR pipeline, a cohort of 203 plasma samples was assessed, comprising 139 samples collected from RCT patients at the time of diagnosis and 64 healthy blood donors. Regarding RCT patients, 87 corresponded to ccRCC, 22 to chRCC and 15 to pRCC, whereas oncocytoma was diagnosed in the remaining 15. All patients were treated at IPO Porto by the same multidisciplinary team between 2015 and 2021. After peripheral blood collection into EDTA-containing tubes, plasma was separated by centrifugation at

2500 g for 30 min at 4 °C, and subsequently stored at −80 °C in the institutional biobank until further use. All blood samples were processed within 4 h from the time of collection. Relevant clinical and pathological data were analyzed from clinical charts and grouped in an anonymized database specifically constructed for the analysis.

2.2. RNA Extraction and cDNA Synthesis

Total RNA was extracted from 100 µL plasma using a MagMAX mirVana Total RNA Isolation kit (Thermo Fisher, Waltham, MA, USA, A27828), according to the manufacturer's protocol. As a technical control, a non-human synthetic spike-in, ath-miR-159a (0.2 µL per sample of a stock solution at 0.2 nM), was added to the lysis buffer in all samples. The final 50 µL of RNA was collected to a 1.5 mL RNase-free tube. All steps were performed at room temperature, and extracted RNA was stored at −80 °C until further use.

Using TaqMan microRNA reverse transcription kit (Thermo Fisher, 4366596) according to the manufacturer's protocol, five microliters of previously isolated RNA were reversely transcribed in a Veriti thermal cycler (Applied Biosystems™, Waltham, MA, USA) for the miRNAs of interest and the spike-in (ath-miR-159a, hsa-miR-21-5p, hsa-miR-126-3p, hsa-miR-155-5p, hsa-miR-200b-3p).

2.3. Droplet Digital PCR (ddPCR): DigiMir Pipeline

DdPCR reactions were prepared according to the optimizations performed: the volumes of cDNA input [2 µL (ath-miR-159a, hsa-miR-21-5p, hsa-miR-126-3p), 5 µL (hsa-miR-155-5p and hsa-miR-200b-3p)], 11 µL ddPCR Supermix for the probes (Bio-Rad, Hercules, CA, USA, #1863010), and 1 µL TaqMan hsa-miRNA Assay (20×). The volumes of bidistilled water were 8 µL (ath-miR-159a, hsa-miR-21-5p, hsa-miR-126-3p) and 5 µL (hsa-miR-155-5p and hsa-miR-200b-3p); assays: ath-miR-159a—000338, FAM; hsa-miR-21-5p—000397, FAM; hsa-miR-126-3p—002228, VIC; hsa-miR-155-5p—002623, FAM; hsa-miR-200b-3p—002251, FAM. Droplets were generated on the droplet generator QX200 (Bio-Rad, Hercules, CA, USA). The PCR run was set as follows: 95 °C for 10 min, 50 cycles of 94 °C for 30 s, and "Annealing Temperature optimized" for 1 min—ramp rate 2 °C/s—and 98 °C for 10 min. The Annealing Temperature was set at 56 °C for ath-miR-159a and at 55 °C for the other four miRNAs. After PCR reaction, plate was read on the QX200 Droplet Reader (Bio-Rad, Hercules, CA, USA).

The limit of the blank (LOB) and the limit of detection (LOD) were calculated for each target miRNA according to Armsbruster et al. [2]. Additionally, the limit of quantification (LOQ) for the five miRNAs was assessed by performing a 2-fold dilution series of an RCT sample.

2.4. Quality Control Steps

All plasma samples were inspected for hemolysis as previously reported by others [31,32]. Hence, from 238 initial samples, 35 samples that presented absorbance higher than 0.25 at 414 nm were excluded. Appropriate engineering and manual controls were used to prevent contaminations—including a master mix made using a clean hood, clean gloves, PCR reagents and consumables—and reactions were performed in separate dedicated labs. RNA previously extracted from RCC cell lines (HKC8 was obtained from Expasy and Caki-1, 769-P, Caki-2, ACHN, A-498, HEK-293, 786-O were from ATCC), and a pool of them was used as positive control for the four candidate miRNAs. A no-template control (NTC) and no-enzyme control (NEC) were included in all cDNA synthesis and ddPCR stages as negative controls. For ddPCR pipeline optimization, further negative controls ("no-cDNA control" and "no-Supermix control") were included, as recommended [33]. All samples were run in a single reaction for each target.

2.5. Statistical Analysis

Non-parametric tests were performed to compare levels of each miRNA among histologic subtypes and to evaluate associations with clinicopathological features. A Spearman test was used for correlation analyses between two variables. A Mann-Whitney U test was used for comparisons between two groups, whereas a Kruskal-Wallis test was used for multiple groups, followed by a Mann-Whitney U test with Bonferroni's correction for pairwise comparisons. A result was considered statistically significant when the p-value < 0.05.

For each miRNA, samples were categorized as positive or negative based on the cut-off values established using Youden's J index [34,35] (value combining the highest sensitivity and specificity), through Receiver-Operating Characteristic (ROC) curve analysis. Validity estimates (sensitivity, specificity, and accuracy) were determined to assess the detection biomarker performance. To improve the detection performance of the selected miRNAs, panels were constructed considering a positive result whenever at least one target miRNA was plotted as positive in an individual analysis.

A two-tailed p-value calculation and ROC curve analyses (without resampling analysis) were performed using SPSS 27.0 software for Windows (IBM-SPSS Inc., Chicago, IL, USA). All graphics were assembled using GraphPad Prism 8.0 software for Windows (GraphPad Software Inc., LA Jolla, CA, USA). To increase the statistical power through a resampling analysis, multiple ROC curves were constructed to calculate validity estimates for the best miRNA panels, as previously described [36,37]. In brief, samples were randomly divided into training (70%) and validation (30%) sets. Subsequently, the cut-off value was estimated in the training set considering the highest sensitivity and specificity and using this calculated cut-off, validity estimates were calculated in the validation set. The procedure was repeated 1000 times and the mean of the parameters (sensitivity and specificity) were calculated. These calculations were performed using R v3.4.4.

3. Results

3.1. Patients' Cohort Characterization

The relevant clinical-pathological features of optimization and validation cohorts are depicted in Table 1.

According to clinical-demographic factors, a significant, although weak, correlation was found between age and circulating levels of each miRNA—hsa-miR-21-5p, hsa-miR-126-3p and hsa-miR-200b-3p levels ($R^2 = 0.080$ and p-value < 0.001, $R^2 = 0.030$ and p-value = 0.023, $R^2 = 0.020$ and p-value = 0.032, respectively).

3.2. Distribution of Circulating miRNA Levels and Biomarkers Performance for Detection of Malignancy

Initially, target miRNA levels were compared between oncocytoma (a benign tumor) and healthy donor samples, and no significant differences between these groups were found for any of the tested hsa-miRNAs, except for hsa-miR-155-5p (p-value = 0.037).

Due to the clinical relevance of discriminating malignant disease (RCC) from healthy individuals, this comparison was subsequently performed. Interestingly, circulating levels of hsa-miR-21-5p and hsa-miR-155-5p significantly differed between these two groups (p-value < 0.001 and p-value = 0.013, respectively) (Figure 1). Circulating levels of hsa-miR-21-5p disclosed the highest accuracy for identifying malignant tumors, although hsa-miR-155-5p depicted the best specificity (90.63%). Remarkably, a panel comprising hsa-miR-21-5p/hsa-miR-155-5p detected about 83% of the three major RCC subtypes, with 71.89% accuracy (Table 2). Importantly, the same two hsa-miRNAs could discriminate RCTs from healthy individuals (Figures S1 and S2 and Table S1).

Table 1. Clinicopathological data of the technical optimization cohort (5 samples) and LiKidMiRs cohort (composed of 139 Renal Cell Tumors and 64 Healthy donors' samples) used in this study.

Technical Optimization Cohort (*n* = 5 Samples)	
Cases	Description
Sample #1	66 years, Oncocytoma
Sample #2	53 years, pRCC, Stage I
Sample #3	57 years, ccRCC, Stage I
Sample #4	46 years, chRCC, stage I
Sample #5	45 years, healthy blood donor
LiKidMiRs Cohort (*n* = 203 samples)	
Renal cell tumor samples	139
Healthy blood donors	64
Renal cell tumor patients—clinicopathological features	
Age [years (median, interquartile range)]	64 (17.0)
Gender	
Male	96/139 (69.1)
Female	43/139 (30.9)
Size of tumor mass [cm (median, interquartile range)]	4.50 (4.3)
Histology [*n*, (%)]	
ccRCC	87/139 (62.6)
pRCC	15/139 (10.8)
chRCC	22/139 (15.8)
Oncocytoma	15/139 (10.8)
Stage [*n*, (%)]	
I	59/124 (47.6)
II	8/124 (6.5)
III	45/124 (36.3)
IV	12/124 (9.7)
ISUP nuclear grade [*n*, (%)]	
1	7/88 (8.0)
2	47/88 (53.4)
3	24/88 (27.3)
4	10/88 (11.4)
Vital status	
Alive with disease	6/139 (4.3)
Alive without disease	120/139 (86.3)
Death from the disease	13/139 (9.4)
Healthy Blood Donors—clinicopathological features	
Age [years (median, interquartile range)]	46 (4.75)
Gender	
Male	36/64 (56.3)
Female	28/64 (43.8)

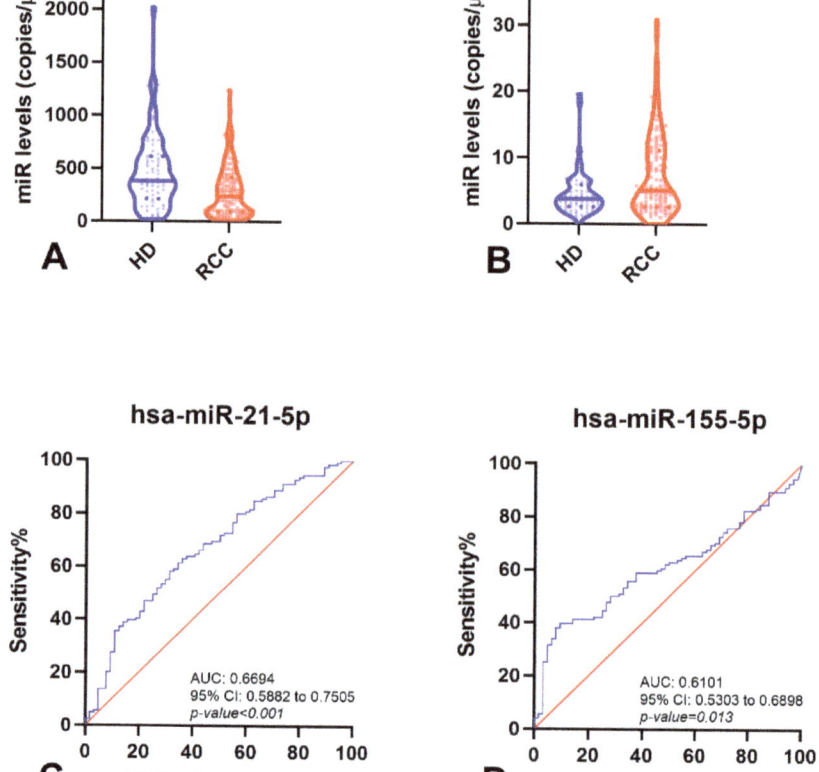

Figure 1. Violin plots with miRNA levels in Healthy Donors (HD) and Renal Cell Carcinoma (RCC) samples of hsa-miR-21-5p (**A**) and hsa-miR-155-5p (**B**), and respective Receiver-Operating Characteristic Curve (without resampling analysis) (**C**,**D**). In violin plots, dashed lines indicate the interquartile range and horizontal line the median of miR levels. In ROC curves, red line indicates the reference line and blue line the identity line for each miRNA. Abbreviations: AUC—Area Under the Curve; CI—Confidence Interval, HD—Healthy Donors, RCC—Renal Cell Carcinoma, *—p-value < 0.05, ***—p-value < 0.0001.

Table 2. Performance of miRNAs as biomarkers for detection of Renal Cell Carcinoma.

miRNAs	SE%	SP%	PPV%	NPV%	Accuracy%
hsa-miR-21-5p	62.90	64.06	77.23	47.13	63.30
hsa-miR-155-5p	39.52	90.63	89.09	43.61	56.91
hsa-miR-21-5p/hsa-miR-155-5p	89.52	54.69	79.29	72.92	77.66
Multiple ROC Curve (hsa-miR-21-5p/hsa-miR-155-5p)	82.66	51.13	77.22	61.76	71.89

Abbreviations: SE—Sensitivity; SP—Specificity; PPV—Positive Predictive Value; NPV—Negative Predictive Value; ROC—Receiver-Operating Characteristic.

When the analysis was restricted to early-stage disease (patients with an organ-confined tumor) and healthy donor samples, hsa-miR-21-5p and hsa-miR-155-5p, but not the other miRNAs, retained statistical difference (*p*-value < 0.01 for both miRNAs) between these two groups (Figure 2A,B). Hence, these two miRNAs were able to detect small RCC (tumors limited to the kidney, without regional lymph node metastasis) with 89.04% sensitivity and high negative predictive value (NPV) (77.68%) (Table 3). Remarkably, the AUC for both miRNAs was higher than 65.00% (Figure 2C,D).

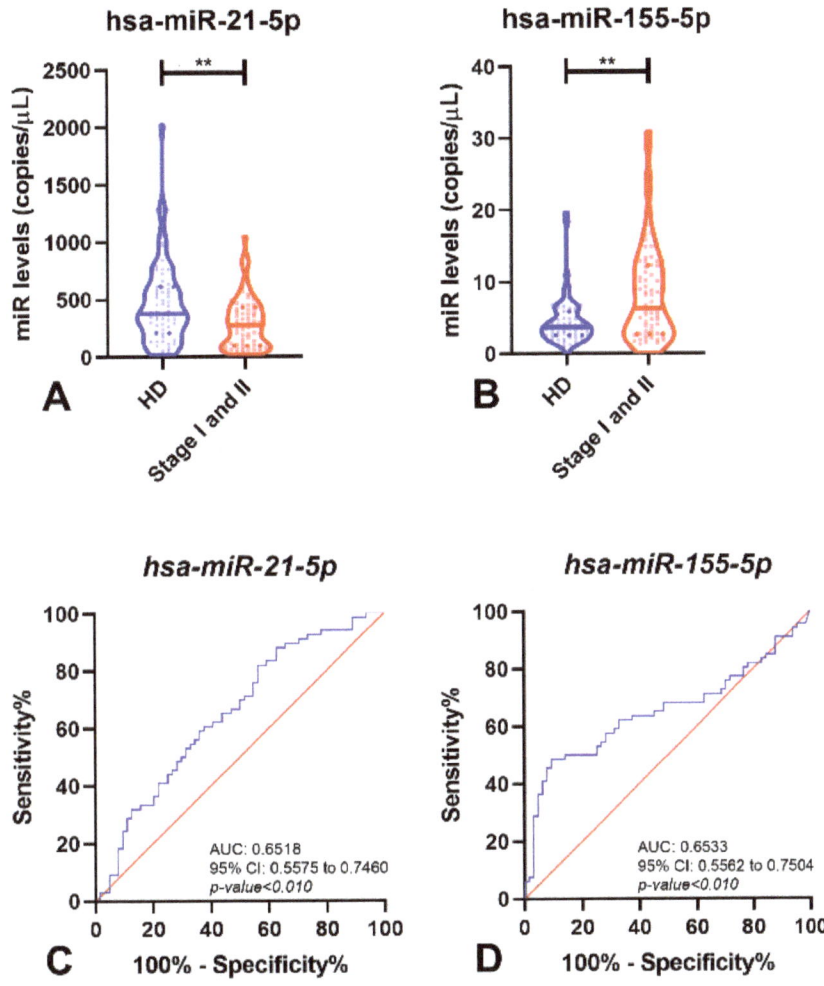

Figure 2. Violin plots of miRNAs levels in Healthy Donor (HD) and early stages of Renal Cell Carcinoma (Stage I and II) samples of hsa-miR-21-5p (**A**) and hsa-miR-155-5p (**B**), and respective Receiver-Operating Characteristic Curve (without resampling analysis) (**C,D**). In violin plots, dashed lines indicate the interquartile range and horizontal line the median of miR levels. In ROC curves, red line indicates the reference line and blue line the identity line for each miRNA. Abbreviations: AUC—Area Under the Curve; CI—Confidence Interval; HD—Healthy Donors, **—*p*-value < 0.001.

Table 3. Performance of miRNAs as biomarkers for identification of early stages Renal Cell Carcinomas.

miRNAs	SE%	SP%	PPV%	NPV%	Accuracy%
hsa-miR-21-5p	81.82	43.75	60.00	70.00	63.08
hsa-miR-155-5p	48.48	90.63	84.21	63.04	69.23
hsa-miR-21-5p/hsa-miR-155-5p	92.42	34.38	59.22	81.48	63.85
Multiple ROC Curve (hsa-miR-21-5p/hsa-miR-155-5p)	89.04	36.23	59.28	77.68	62.88

Abbreviations: SE—Sensitivity; SP—Specificity; PPV—Positive Predictive Value; NPV—Negative Predictive Value; ROC—Receiver-Operating Characteristic.

3.3. MiRNA Levels and Clinicopathological Features

Among RCC subtypes (ccRCC, pRCC and chRCC), significant differences were found for all four miRNAs (hsa-miR-126-3p, hsa-miR-155-5p and hsa-miR-200b-3p, p-value < 0.010; hsa-miR-21-3p, p-value = 0.045, Figure 3).

Furthermore, all four hsa-miRs circulating levels significantly differed between the two major RCC subtypes, ccRCC and pRCC (hsa-miR-126-3p, p-value < 0.001; hsa-miR-155-5p and hsa-miR-200b-3p, p-value < 0.01; hsa-miR-21-5p, p-value = 0.039, Figure 3). Nonetheless, no statistical differences were found between pRCC and chRCC or between ccRCC and chRCC for the tested circulating miRNAs.

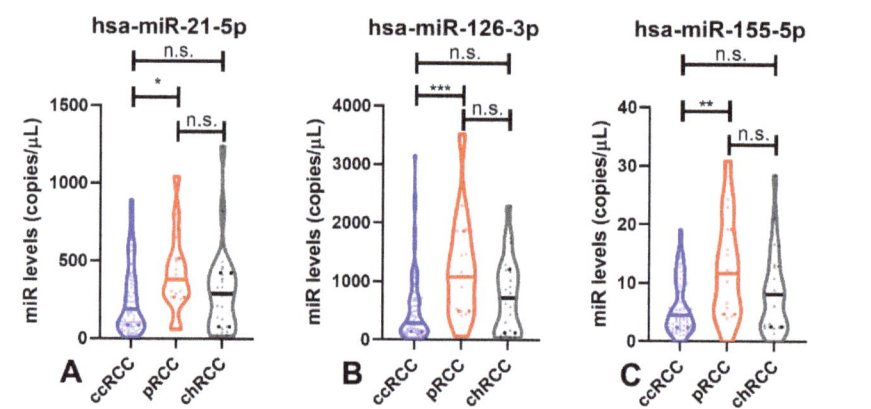

Figure 3. Violin plots of hsa-miR-21-5p (**A**), hsa-miR-126-3p (**B**), hsa-miR-155-5p (**C**) and hsa-miR-200b-3p (**D**) levels in the malignant subtypes (ccRCC, pRCC and chRCC). Dashed lines indicate the interquartile range and horizontal line the median of miR levels. Abbreviations: ccRCC—Clear-Cell Renal Cell Carcinoma; chRCC—Chromophobe Renal Cell Carcinoma; pRCC—Papillary Renal Cell Carcinoma; n.s.—not significant, *—p-value < 0.05, **—p-value < 0.001, ***—p-value < 0.0001.

Due to the poorer outcome and higher incidence of ccRCC, comparisons in circulating hsa-miRNAs were performed between this subtype and the other two RCC subtypes (Figure 4). Interestingly, ccRCC patients displayed significantly lower circulating levels of all hsa-miRs compared to patients diagnosed with the other malignant subtypes (p-value = 0.048 for hsa-miR-21-5p and p-value < 0.01 for hsa-miR-126-3p, hsa-miR-155-5p and hsa-miR-200b-3p—Figure 4).

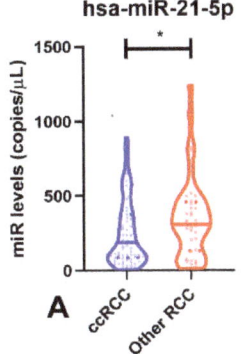 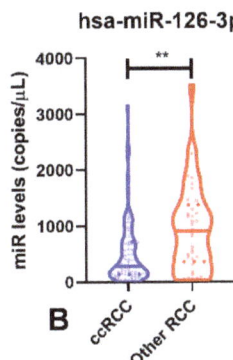 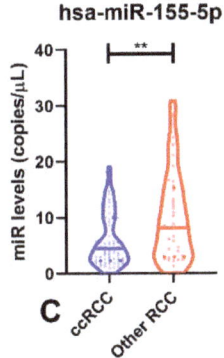 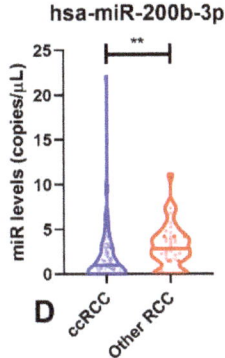

Figure 4. Violin plots of hsa-miR-21-5p (**A**), hsa-miR-126-3p (**B**), hsa-miR-155-5p (**C**) and hsa-miR-200b-3p (**D**) levels in ccRCC and other RCCs (pRCC and chRCC). Dashed lines indicate the interquartile range and horizontal line the median of miR levels. Abbreviations: ccRCC—Clear-Cell Renal Cell Carcinoma; RCC—Renal Cell Carcinomas; n.s.—not significant, *—p-value < 0.05, **—p-value < 0.001.

Moreover, circulating hsa-miR-126-3p and hsa-miR-200b-3p levels discriminated ccRCC from other RCC subtypes with 74.78% sensitivity and 52.95% specificity (Figure 5 and Table 4).

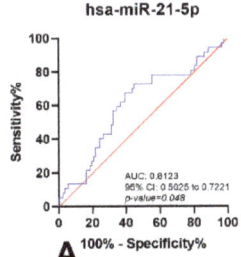 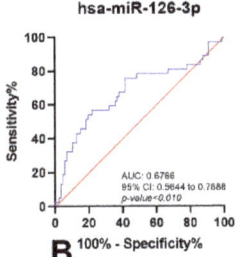 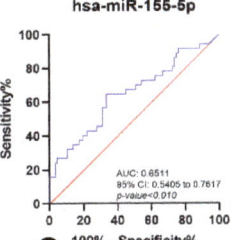 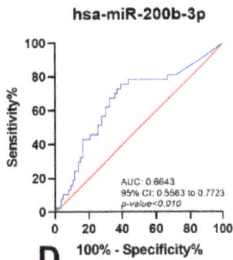

Figure 5. Receiver-Operating Characteristic Curves (without resampling analysis) of hsa-miR-21-5p (**A**), hsa-miR-126-3p (**B**), hsa-miR-155-5p (**C**) and hsa-miR-200b-3p (**D**) in ccRCC and other RCCs (pRCC and chRCC). Red line indicates the reference line and blue line the identity line for each miRNA. Abbreviations: AUC—Area Under the Curve; CI—Confidence Interval.

Table 4. Performance of miRNAs as biomarkers for identification of Clear-Cell Renal Cell Carcinoma.

miRNAs	SE%	SP%	PPV%	NPV%	Accuracy%
hsa-miR-21-5p	60.92	67.57	81.54	42.37	62.90
hsa-miR-126-3p	78.16	56.76	80.95	52.50	71.77
hsa-miR-155-5p	66.67	64.86	81.69	45.28	66.13
hsa-miR-200b-3p	60.92	75.68	85.48	45.16	65.32
hsa-miR-126-3p/hsa-miR-200b-3p	80.46	56.76	81.40	55.26	73.39
Multiple ROC Curve (hsa-miR-126-3p/hsa-miR-200b-3p)	74.78	52.95	79.49	47.46	68.28

Abbreviations: SE—Sensitivity; SP—Specificity; PPV—Positive Predictive Value; NPV—Negative Predictive Value.

4. Discussion

RCC remains a leading cause of cancer-related death worldwide. Alongside prostate and bladder cancers, RCC is one of the most common urological malignancies [38]. Early detection of RCC (ideally at stage I or II) significantly increases the likelihood of a cure through surgical treatment, with a 5-year survival rate of 98%, averting the need for subsequent therapies, which are not curative and often carry significant adverse side effects [15]. Nonetheless, 20–30% of patients display metastatic disease at diagnosis [38,39], and even following curative-intent nephrectomy, the standard of care for localized RCC, metastases develop in up to 20–40% of patients [39]. Notably, the response to medical treatment (mainly targeted therapy or immunotherapy) is rather limited, with a 5-year survival rate lower than 10%. Among RCCs, ccRCC, pRCC, and chRCC represent more than 90% of cases, emphasizing the importance of accurately detecting these tumor subtypes and discriminating them from benign conditions [39,40].

Circulating miRNAs are emergent cancer biomarkers which might be assessed using minimally invasive strategies, eventually constituting promising RCC biomarkers. Nevertheless, only a few studies have addressed this issue, mostly using conventional qPCR techniques [14,15,17–25,41,42]. Owing to the diversity of the results of those studies and the need to overcome the limitations of normalization, we assessed the clinical potential of a circulating miRNA-based panel for RCC detection using ddPCR.

Accurate identification of patients harboring RCC and discrimination from healthy individuals, as well as from carriers of benign renal lesions (including tumors), is pivotal to reliably establishing therapeutic vs. monitoring strategies. Thus, after a first analysis between oncocytomas and healthy donors, we compared healthy donors with RCC patients. Remarkably, two (hsa-miR-21-5p and hsa-miR-155-5p) out of the four candidate miRNAs disclosed statistically significant differences in plasma levels. Although hsa-miR-21-5p has been described to act as oncomiR, we observed lower circulating levels in RCC patients [20,43–45]. This might be due to the distinct miRNAs levels in the different clinical samples. Indeed, higher miRNA levels may be found in tissues compared to body fluid samples [46]. Importantly, increased hsa-miR-21-5p levels were also found in serum samples of RCC patients, further supporting that circulating miRNA levels in serum and plasma may be different [20]. Moreover, differences were also reported for hsa-miR-21-5p levels in serum and plasma among patients with Non-ST-elevation myocardial infarction, a non-cancer-related pathology [47]. Herein, higher hsa-miR-21-5p levels were found in serum when compared with respective control samples, whereas lower levels were observed in plasma samples from the same patients [47]. Of note, plasma has been reported to be the sample of election for translational studies [47–49], as red blood cell lysis during the coagulation process increases discharging of RNA and platelets to the serum, increasing the non-tumor derived circulating miRNAs present in each sample [48]. Importantly, hsa-miR-21-5p is expressed in platelets [47,50] and, thus, an increase of platelets in serum might explain the higher levels found for this miRNA. Furthermore, in breast cancer, lower hsa-miR-30b-5p levels were found in tissue compared with plasma, unveiling the disparities between these two sample sources [51]. Moreover, inadequate normalization and biased results may occur if the normalizer used is not the most suitable. Indeed, U6 is more prone to degradation by serum RNases [1]. Interestingly, in a previous study we found that hsa-miR-21-5p miRNA was significantly downregulated in tissue samples from RCT patients, discriminating RCT patients from healthy donors [13].

Concerning hsa-miR-155-5p, upregulation of this circulating hsa-miR was found in RCC patients, and a panel comprising hsa-miR-155-5p and hsa-miR-21-5p could identify 82.66% of RCC patients with 71.89% accuracy. Interestingly, hsa-miR-155-5p was shown to be upregulated in tissue [13,52] and ccRCC serum samples [18], and is also associated with cancer development [52]. Moreover, an hsa-miR-21-5p/hsa-miR-155-5p panel depicted high sensitivity (89.04%) for identifying organ-confined carcinomas, which might allow for reducing false-negative results and increase the likelihood of curative-intent treatment. To the best of our knowledge, this is the first study that evaluated the biomarker performance of plasma circulating hsa-miRs to detect early-stage RCC. Previously, Wang and colleagues described a 5-miRNA panel (miR-193a-3p, miR-362, miR-572, miR-378, and miR-28-5p) that was able to identify early-stage RCC, albeit in serum samples [22]. Furthermore, our panel achieved a higher NPV than that reported by Wang et al. [22].

We further evaluated whether circulating hsa-miRNAs might also convey relevant information to discriminate ccRCC from the remainder RCC subtypes. Indeed, all four miRNAs were able to differentiate this major RCC subtype from the others. The panel constituted by hsa-miR-126-3p and hsa-miR-200b-3p disclosed the best performance, with 74.78% sensitivity and 52.95% specificity. Since ccRCC is an aggressive RCC subtype, early detection is of major importance, and its accurate identification might improve patient outcomes [20,53]. Although stratification by stage was not performed due to a limited number of cases with advanced stages, for early stages, hsa-miR-126-3p and hsa-miR-200b-3p levels also differed significantly between ccRCC and the remainder RCC subtypes.

Considering that various studies have reported other strategies for RCC identification (including imaging and epigenetic biomarkers), our results seem to offer the best sensitivity for RCC detection [9,54]. Indeed, the methodology we developed uses a lower initial sample volume [15,17,20,22,25,41,42], which is more cost-effective, and the procedure to obtain the sample is better tolerated by patients. Molecular imaging such as ^{18}F-fluorodeoxt-glucose (FDG) positron emission tomography/computed tomography (PET/CT) was reported to detect localized RCC, but it discloses lower sensitivity (only 22%) [54,55]. Despite the superior specificity (85.9%) of ^{124}I-cG250 PET for RCC detection, when compared to our hsa-miR-21-5p/hsa-miR-155-5p panel (51.13%), this monoclonal antibody has a half-life of several days, constituting a significant disadvantage in relation to the protocol reported by us [56]. Moreover, diffusion magnetic resonance imaging was reported to characterize malignant lesions with similar sensitivity (86%) to our panel but with higher specificity (78%) [57]. Nevertheless, it should be noted that despite the better performance, these imaging biomarkers are more costly and less well-tolerated by the patient compared to liquid biopsies [54].

The intense exploration of circulating epigenetic markers such as DNA methylation, miRNAs, and lncRNAs is well illustrated by the more that 60 articles published in this field since 2003 [9]. So far, 10 DNA methylation-based studies (e.g., using *VHL*, *RASSF1A*, *P16*, *P14*, *RARB*, *TIMP3*, *GSTP1*, *APC*) for RCC detection have been published [58–67] and only 33.33% of these had an RCC cohort with more than 50 patients [60,63,64]. Compared with those studies, our results provide higher sensitivity (6–83%). However, DNA methylation-based markers displayed high specificity (53–100%). This was also observed in three lncRNAs studies (e.g., GIHCG, LINC00887) [68–70], in which the diagnostic performance was generally lower than in our study (67.1–87.0%), but the specificity reached values >80% for all biomarkers. Although our biomarker panels disclosed high sensitivity, their specificity is limited. Thus, in an envisaged routine setting, they would ideally be used in first-line screening, requiring complementary use of more specific biomarkers in cases deemed positive. In liquid biopsies, DNA methylation-based markers such as *VHL*, *RASSF1A*, *TIMP3*, *SFRP1*, *SFRP2*, *SFRP4*, *SFRP5*, *PCDH17*, and *TCF21* are highly specific (100%) [58,59,61,62,65–67] and, thus, constitute good candidates as second-line tests, in this setting.

As previously reported, most circulating miRNA studies are based on blood-based liquid biopsies [1]. When compared with our protocol, only a few studies included more than 100 RCC patients, which might, at the least partially, explain the differences in results [9]. Additionally, the discrepant results might also be explained, as described above, by the biased normalization (e.g., spike-in as normalizer miRNA, U6, RNU48) [14,19,20,23,24]. Nevertheless, the sensitivity reported for the most widely studied serum miRNAs (miR-210, miR-1233, and miR-378) was generally lower than our plasma panel [14,17,25]. Indeed, using this less time-consuming and more cost-effective approach, we were able to detect RCC using a minimally invasive technique, with a lower initial quantity of plasma than serum-based studies (although detecting other miRNAs), and obtained similar or even better results, obviating the need for normalization and the associated bias (due to ddPCR absolute quantification) [15,17,20,22,25,41,42]. Hence, our results from multiple ROC curve analysis demonstrate a potential clinical application of this technology to identify RCC, and is the first study to quantify circulating miRNAs in these patients using ddPCR (Figure 6).

These results require validation in more extensive prospective studies. Overall, and notwithstanding our promising results for RCC detection, it should be acknowledged that the lack of long-term follow-up constitutes a significant limitation. Further studies using liquid biopsies should also be considered to further subtype RCC, namely, to distinguish oncocytomas from chRCCs, which will lead to a prioritization of treatments for patients with malignant tumors.

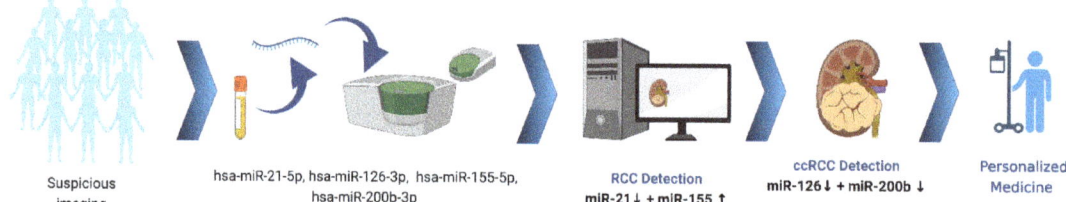

Figure 6. Graphical representation of the potential clinical impact of LiKidMiRs. Created with BioRender.com.

5. Conclusions

Our findings support the research question that a minimally invasive test can be developed to detect RCC, improving patient survival through increased diagnosis at earlier stages. This might help to reduce the morbidity and mortality associated with advanced disease, as well as the lack of curative treatment at those stages. Furthermore, and to the best of our knowledge, this work is the first to report a novel tool to quantify circulating miRNAs in plasma using ddPCR in RCC patients.

Supplementary Materials: The following are available online at https://www.mdpi.com/article/10.3390/cancers14040858/s1, Table S1: Performance of miRNAs as biomarkers for detection of Renal Cell Tumors., Figure S1: Violin plots with all points of miRNAs levels in Healthy Donors (HD) and Renal Cell Tumors (RCT) samples of hsa-miR-21-5p (A), hsa-miR-126-3p (B), hsa-miR-155-5p (C) and hsa-miR-200b-3p (D). Dashed lines indicate the interquartile range and horizontal line the median of miR levels. Abbreviations: HD—Healthy Donors; RCT—Renal Cell Tumors; n.s.—not significant, **—p-value < 0.001, ***—p-value < 0.0001., Figure S2: Receiver Operating Characteristic Curve (without resampling analysis) of hsa-miR-21-5p (A) and hsa-miR-155-5p (B). Red line indicates the reference line and blue line the identity line for each miRNA. Abbreviations: AUC—Area Under the Curve; CI—Confidence Interval.

Author Contributions: J.P.S. performed molecular analyses and wrote the manuscript; J.P.S. and J.L. collected the clinical data; J.P.S., V.C., S.S., D.B.-S. and J.R. analyzed the data; C.C.-M. processed clinical samples; I.B. provided clinical information about the patients; V.C., S.S., D.B.-S., J.L., R.H. and C.J. critically revised the manuscript; R.H. and C.J. supervised the work. All authors have read and agreed to the published version of the manuscript.

Funding: The authors would like to acknowledge the Research Centre of Portuguese Oncology Institute of Porto (CI-IPOP-74-2016). VC received the support of a fellowship from the "la Caixa" Foundation (ID 100010434). The fellowship code is LCF/BQ/DR20/11790013. SS and DB-S are granted with FCT—Fundação para a Ciência e Tecnologia fellowship (SFRH/BD/143717/2019 and SFRH/BD/136007/2018).

Institutional Review Board Statement: This study was approved by the Ethics Committee (CES 518/2010) of the Portuguese Oncology Institute of Porto, Portugal. All procedures performed in tasks involving human participants were in accordance with the ethical standards of the institutional and/or national research committee and with the 1964 Helsinki declaration and its later amendments or comparable ethical standards.

Informed Consent Statement: Written informed consent was obtained from all subjects involved in the study.

Data Availability Statement: All data generated or analyzed during this study are included in this article.

Conflicts of Interest: The authors declare that they have no competing interests.

References

1. Sequeira, J.P.; Constâncio, V.; Lobo, J.; Henrique, R.; Jerónimo, C. Unveiling the World of Circulating and Exosomal microRNAs in Renal Cell Carcinoma. *Cancers* **2021**, *13*, 5252. [CrossRef] [PubMed]
2. Sung, H.; Ferlay, J.; Siegel, R.L.; Laversanne, M.; Soerjomataram, I.; Jemal, A.; Bray, F. Global Cancer Statistics 2020: GLOBOCAN Estimates of Incidence and Mortality Worldwide for 36 Cancers in 185 Countries. *CA Cancer J. Clin.* **2021**, *71*, 209–249. [CrossRef] [PubMed]
3. Maher, E.R. Genomics and epigenomics of renal cell carcinoma. *Semin. Cancer Biol.* **2013**, *23*, 10–17. [CrossRef]
4. Outeiro-Pinho, G.; Barros-Silva, D.; Correia, M.P.; Henrique, R.; Jerónimo, C. Renal Cell Tumors: Uncovering the Biomarker Potential of ncRNAs. *Cancers* **2020**, *12*, 2214. [CrossRef] [PubMed]
5. Shuch, B.; Amin, A.; Armstrong, A.J.; Eble, J.N.; Ficarra, V.; Lopez-Beltran, A.; Martignoni, G.; Rini, B.I.; Kutikov, A. Understanding pathologic variants of renal cell carcinoma: Distilling therapeutic opportunities from biologic complexity. *Eur. Urol.* **2015**, *67*, 85–97. [CrossRef]
6. Arora, R.D.; Limaiem, F. Renal Clear Cell Cancer. In *StatPearls*; StatPearls Publishing: Treasure Island, FL, USA, 2021.
7. Pandey, J.; Syed, W. Renal Cancer. In *StatPearls*; StatPearls Publishing: Treasure Island, FL, USA, 2021.
8. Ricketts, C.J.; De Cubas, A.A.; Fan, H.; Smith, C.C.; Lang, M.; Reznik, E.; Bowlby, R.; Gibb, E.A.; Akbani, R.; Beroukhim, R.; et al. The Cancer Genome Atlas Comprehensive Molecular Characterization of Renal Cell Carcinoma. *Cell Rep.* **2018**, *23*, 313–326. [CrossRef]
9. Kubiliute, R.; Jarmalaite, S. Epigenetic Biomarkers of Renal Cell Carcinoma for Liquid Biopsy Tests. *Int. J. Mol. Sci.* **2021**, *22*, 8846. [CrossRef]
10. Filella, X.; Foj, L. miRNAs as novel biomarkers in the management of prostate cancer. *Clin. Chem. Lab. Med.* **2017**, *55*, 715–736. [CrossRef]
11. Lu, J.; Getz, G.; Miska, E.A.; Alvarez-Saavedra, E.; Lamb, J.; Peck, D.; Sweet-Cordero, A.; Ebert, B.L.; Mak, R.H.; Ferrando, A.A.; et al. MicroRNA expression profiles classify human cancers. *Nature* **2005**, *435*, 834–838. [CrossRef] [PubMed]
12. Guil, S.; Esteller, M. DNA methylomes, histone codes and miRNAs: Tying it all together. *Int. J. Biochem. Cell Biol.* **2009**, *41*, 87–95. [CrossRef] [PubMed]
13. Silva-Santos, R.M.; Costa-Pinheiro, P.; Luis, A.; Antunes, L.; Lobo, F.; Oliveira, J.; Henrique, R.; Jeronimo, C. MicroRNA profile: A promising ancillary tool for accurate renal cell tumour diagnosis. *Br. J. Cancer* **2013**, *109*, 2646–2653. [CrossRef] [PubMed]
14. Wulfken, L.M.; Moritz, R.; Ohlmann, C.; Holdenrieder, S.; Jung, V.; Becker, F.; Herrmann, E.; Walgenbach-Brünagel, G.; von Ruecker, A.; Müller, S.C.; et al. MicroRNAs in Renal Cell Carcinoma: Diagnostic Implications of Serum miR-1233 Levels. *PLoS ONE* **2011**, *6*, e25787. [CrossRef] [PubMed]
15. Iwamoto, H.; Kanda, Y.; Sejima, T.; Osaki, M.; Okada, F.; Takenaka, A. Serum miR-210 as a potential biomarker of early clear cell renal cell carcinoma. *Int. J. Oncol.* **2014**, *44*, 53–58. [CrossRef] [PubMed]
16. Heinemann, F.G.; Tolkach, Y.; Deng, M.; Schmidt, D.; Perner, S.; Kristiansen, G.; Müller, S.C.; Ellinger, J. Serum miR-122-5p and miR-206 expression: Non-invasive prognostic biomarkers for renal cell carcinoma. *Clin. Epigenetics* **2018**, *10*, 11. [CrossRef] [PubMed]
17. Redova, M.; Poprach, A.; Nekvindova, J.; Iliev, R.; Radova, L.; Lakomy, R.; Svoboda, M.; Vyzula, R.; Slaby, O. Circulating miR-378 and miR-451 in serum are potential biomarkers for renal cell carcinoma. *J. Transl. Med.* **2012**, *10*, 55. [CrossRef] [PubMed]
18. Wang, X.; Wang, T.; Chen, C.; Wu, Z.; Bai, P.; Li, S.; Chen, B.; Liu, R.; Zhang, K.; Li, W.; et al. Serum exosomal miR-210 as a potential biomarker for clear cell renal cell carcinoma. *J. Cell Biochem.* **2018**, *120*, 1492–1502. [CrossRef] [PubMed]
19. Mytsyk, Y.; Dosenko, V.; Borys, Y.; Kucher, A.; Gazdikova, K.; Busselberg, D.; Caprnda, M.; Kruzliak, P.; Farooqi, A.A.; Lubov, M. MicroRNA-15a expression measured in urine samples as a potential biomarker of renal cell carcinoma. *Int. Urol. Nephrol.* **2018**, *50*, 851–859. [CrossRef]
20. Tusong, H.; Maolakuerban, N.; Guan, J.; Rexiati, M.; Wang, W.G.; Azhati, B.; Nuerrula, Y.; Wang, Y.J. Functional analysis of serum microRNAs miR-21 and miR-106a in renal cell carcinoma. *Cancer Biomark.* **2017**, *18*, 79–85. [CrossRef]
21. von Brandenstein, M.; Pandarakalam, J.J.; Kroon, L.; Loeser, H.; Herden, J.; Braun, G.; Wendland, K.; Dienes, H.P.; Engelmann, U.; Fries, J.W. MicroRNA 15a, inversely correlated to PKCα, is a potential marker to differentiate between benign and malignant renal tumors in biopsy and urine samples. *Am. J. Pathol.* **2012**, *180*, 1787–1797. [CrossRef]
22. Wang, C.; Hu, J.; Lu, M.; Gu, H.; Zhou, X.; Chen, X.; Zen, K.; Zhang, C.-Y.; Zhang, T.; Ge, J.; et al. A panel of five serum miRNAs as a potential diagnostic tool for early-stage renal cell carcinoma. *Sci. Rep.* **2015**, *5*, 7610. [CrossRef]
23. Yadav, S.; Khandelwal, M.; Seth, A.; Saini, A.K.; Dogra, P.N.; Sharma, A. Serum microRNA Expression Profiling: Potential Diagnostic Implications of a Panel of Serum microRNAs for Clear Cell Renal Cell Cancer. *Urology* **2017**, *104*, 64–69. [CrossRef] [PubMed]
24. Zhai, Q.; Zhou, L.; Zhao, C.; Wan, J.; Yu, Z.; Guo, X.; Qin, J.; Chen, J.; Lu, R. Identification of miR-508-3p and miR-509-3p that are associated with cell invasion and migration and involved in the apoptosis of renal cell carcinoma. *Biochem. Biophys. Res. Commun.* **2012**, *419*, 621–626. [CrossRef] [PubMed]
25. Zhao, A.; Li, G.; Péoc'h, M.; Genin, C.; Gigante, M. Serum miR-210 as a novel biomarker for molecular diagnosis of clear cell renal cell carcinoma. *Exp. Mol. Pathol.* **2013**, *94*, 115–120. [CrossRef] [PubMed]

26. Teixeira, A.L.; Ferreira, M.; Silva, J.; Gomes, M.; Dias, F.; Santos, J.I.; Maurício, J.; Lobo, F.; Medeiros, R. Higher circulating expression levels of miR-221 associated with poor overall survival in renal cell carcinoma patients. *Tumour Biol.* **2014**, *35*, 4057–4066. [CrossRef] [PubMed]
27. Zhang, Q.; Di, W.; Dong, Y.; Lu, G.; Yu, J.; Li, J.; Li, P. High serum miR-183 level is associated with poor responsiveness of renal cancer to natural killer cells. *Tumour Biol.* **2015**, *36*, 9245–9249. [CrossRef]
28. Campomenosi, P.; Gini, E.; Noonan, D.M.; Poli, A.; D'Antona, P.; Rotolo, N.; Dominioni, L.; Imperatori, A. A comparison between quantitative PCR and droplet digital PCR technologies for circulating microRNA quantification in human lung cancer. *BMC Biotechnol.* **2016**, *16*, 60. [CrossRef]
29. Taylor, S.C.; Laperriere, G.; Germain, H. Droplet Digital PCR versus qPCR for gene expression analysis with low abundant targets: From variable nonsense to publication quality data. *Sci. Rep.* **2017**, *7*, 2409. [CrossRef]
30. Di Meo, A.; Saleeb, R.; Wala, S.J.; Khella, H.W.; Ding, Q.; Zhai, H.; Krishan, K.; Krizova, A.; Gabril, M.; Evans, A.; et al. A miRNA-based classification of renal cell carcinoma subtypes by PCR and in situ hybridization. *Oncotarget* **2017**, *9*, 2092–2104. [CrossRef]
31. Androvic, P.; Romanyuk, N.; Urdzikova-Machova, L.; Rohlova, E.; Kubista, M.; Valihrach, L. Two-tailed RT-qPCR panel for quality control of circulating microRNA studies. *Sci. Rep.* **2019**, *9*, 4255. [CrossRef]
32. van Vliet, E.A.; Puhakka, N.; Mills, J.D.; Srivastava, P.K.; Johnson, M.R.; Roncon, P.; Das Gupta, S.; Karttunen, J.; Simonato, M.; Lukasiuk, K.; et al. Standardization procedure for plasma biomarker analysis in rat models of epileptogenesis: Focus on circulating microRNAs. *Epilepsia* **2017**, *58*, 2013–2024. [CrossRef]
33. Stein, E.V.; Duewer, D.L.; Farkas, N.; Romsos, E.L.; Wang, L.; Cole, K.D. Steps to achieve quantitative measurements of microRNA using two step droplet digital PCR. *PLoS ONE* **2017**, *12*, e0188085. [CrossRef]
34. Schisterman, E.F.; Perkins, N.J.; Liu, A.; Bondell, H. Optimal cut-point and its corresponding Youden Index to discriminate individuals using pooled blood samples. *Epidemiology* **2005**, *16*, 73–81. [CrossRef] [PubMed]
35. Youden, W.J. Index for rating diagnostic tests. *Cancer* **1950**, *3*, 32–35. [CrossRef]
36. Baker, S.G.; Kramer, B.S. Identifying genes that contribute most to good classification in microarrays. *BMC Bioinform.* **2006**, *7*, 407. [CrossRef] [PubMed]
37. Nunes, S.P.; Moreira-Barbosa, C.; Salta, S.; Palma de Sousa, S.; Pousa, I.; Oliveira, J.; Soares, M.; Rego, L.; Dias, T.; Rodrigues, J.; et al. Cell-Free DNA Methylation of Selected Genes Allows for Early Detection of the Major Cancers in Women. *Cancers* **2018**, *10*, 357. [CrossRef]
38. Fan, B.; Jin, Y.; Zhang, H.; Zhao, R.; Sun, M.; Sun, M.; Yuan, X.; Wang, W.; Wang, X.; Chen, Z.; et al. MicroRNA-21 contributes to renal cell carcinoma cell invasiveness and angiogenesis via the PDCD4/c-Jun (AP-1) signalling pathway. *Int. J. Oncol.* **2020**, *56*, 178–192. [CrossRef]
39. Carlsson, J.; Christiansen, J.; Davidsson, S.; Giunchi, F.; Fiorentino, M.; Sundqvist, P. The potential role of miR-126, miR-21 and miR-10b as prognostic biomarkers in renal cell carcinoma. *Oncol. Lett* **2019**, *17*, 4566–4574. [CrossRef]
40. Lopez-Beltran, A.; Carrasco, J.C.; Cheng, L.; Scarpelli, M.; Kirkali, Z.; Montironi, R. 2009 update on the classification of renal epithelial tumors in adults. *Int. J. Urol.* **2009**, *16*, 432–443. [CrossRef]
41. Fedorko, M.; Juracek, J.; Stanik, M.; Svoboda, M.; Poprach, A.; Buchler, T.; Pacik, D.; Dolezel, J.; Slaby, O. Detection of let-7 miRNAs in urine supernatant as potential diagnostic approach in non-metastatic clear-cell renal cell carcinoma. *Biochem. Med.* **2017**, *27*, 411–417. [CrossRef] [PubMed]
42. Fedorko, M.; Stanik, M.; Iliev, R.; Redova-Lojova, M.; Machackova, T.; Svoboda, M.; Pacik, D.; Dolezel, J.; Slaby, O. Combination of MiR-378 and MiR-210 Serum Levels Enables Sensitive Detection of Renal Cell Carcinoma. *Int. J. Mol. Sci.* **2015**, *16*, 23382–23389. [CrossRef]
43. Chen, J.; Gu, Y.; Shen, W. MicroRNA-21 functions as an oncogene and promotes cell proliferation and invasion via TIMP3 in renal cancer. *Eur. Rev. Med. Pharmacol. Sci.* **2017**, *21*, 4566–4576. [PubMed]
44. Jung, M.; Mollenkopf, H.J.; Grimm, C.; Wagner, I.; Albrecht, M.; Waller, T.; Pilarsky, C.; Johannsen, M.; Stephan, C.; Lehrach, H.; et al. MicroRNA profiling of clear cell renal cell cancer identifies a robust signature to define renal malignancy. *J. Cell. Mol. Med.* **2009**, *13*, 3918–3928. [CrossRef] [PubMed]
45. Lokeshwar, S.D.; Talukder, A.; Yates, T.J.; Hennig, M.J.P.; Garcia-Roig, M.; Lahorewala, S.S.; Mullani, N.N.; Klaassen, Z.; Kava, B.R.; Manoharan, M.; et al. Molecular Characterization of Renal Cell Carcinoma: A Potential Three-MicroRNA Prognostic Signature. *Cancer Epidemiol. Biomark. Prev.* **2018**, *27*, 464–472. [CrossRef] [PubMed]
46. Nagy, Z.B.; Barták, B.K.; Kalmár, A.; Galamb, O.; Wichmann, B.; Dank, M.; Igaz, P.; Tulassay, Z.; Molnár, B. Comparison of Circulating miRNAs Expression Alterations in Matched Tissue and Plasma Samples During Colorectal Cancer Progression. *Pathol. Oncol. Res.* **2019**, *25*, 97–105. [CrossRef] [PubMed]
47. Mompeón, A.; Ortega-Paz, L.; Vidal-Gómez, X.; Costa, T.J.; Pérez-Cremades, D.; Garcia-Blas, S.; Brugaletta, S.; Sanchis, J.; Sabate, M.; Novella, S.; et al. Disparate miRNA expression in serum and plasma of patients with acute myocardial infarction: A systematic and paired comparative analysis. *Sci. Rep.* **2020**, *10*, 5373. [CrossRef]
48. Wang, K.; Yuan, Y.; Cho, J.-H.; McClarty, S.; Baxter, D.; Galas, D.J. Comparing the MicroRNA spectrum between serum and plasma. *PLoS ONE* **2012**, *7*, e41361. [CrossRef]

49. Dufourd, T.; Robil, N.; Mallet, D.; Carcenac, C.; Boulet, S.; Brishoual, S.; Rabois, E.; Houeto, J.-L.; de la Grange, P.; Carnicella, S. Plasma or serum? A qualitative study on rodents and humans using high-throughput microRNA sequencing for circulating biomarkers. *Biol. Methods Protoc.* **2019**, *4*, bpz006. [CrossRef]
50. Willeit, P.; Zampetaki, A.; Dudek, K.; Kaudewitz, D.; King, A.; Kirkby, N.S.; Crosby-Nwaobi, R.; Prokopi, M.; Drozdov, I.; Langley, S.R.; et al. Circulating MicroRNAs as Novel Biomarkers for Platelet Activation. *Circ. Res.* **2013**, *112*, 595–600. [CrossRef]
51. Adam-Artigues, A.; Garrido-Cano, I.; Simón, S.; Ortega, B.; Moragón, S.; Lameirinhas, A.; Constâncio, V.; Salta, S.; Burgués, O.; Bermejo, B.; et al. Circulating miR-30b-5p levels in plasma as a novel potential biomarker for early detection of breast cancer. *ESMO Open* **2021**, *6*, 100039. [CrossRef]
52. Ji, H.; Tian, D.; Zhang, B.; Zhang, Y.; Yan, D.; Wu, S. Overexpression of miR-155 in clear-cell renal cell carcinoma and its oncogenic effect through targeting FOXO3a. *Exp. Ther. Med.* **2017**, *13*, 2286–2292. [CrossRef]
53. Cheng, T.; Wang, L.; Li, Y.; Huang, C.; Zeng, L.; Yang, J. Differential microRNA expression in renal cell carcinoma. *Oncol. Lett.* **2013**, *6*, 769–776. [CrossRef] [PubMed]
54. Farber, N.J.; Kim, C.J.; Modi, P.K.; Hon, J.D.; Sadimin, E.T.; Singer, E.A. Renal cell carcinoma: The search for a reliable biomarker. *Transl. Cancer Res.* **2017**, *6*, 620–632. [CrossRef] [PubMed]
55. Gofrit, O.N.; Orevi, M. Diagnostic Challenges of Kidney Cancer: A Systematic Review of the Role of Positron Emission Tomography-Computerized Tomography. *J. Urol.* **2016**, *196*, 648–657. [CrossRef] [PubMed]
56. Divgi, C.R.; Uzzo, R.G.; Gatsonis, C.; Bartz, R.; Treutner, S.; Yu, J.Q.; Chen, D.; Carrasquillo, J.A.; Larson, S.; Bevan, P.; et al. Positron emission tomography/computed tomography identification of clear cell renal cell carcinoma: Results from the REDECT trial. *J. Clin. Oncol.* **2013**, *31*, 187–194. [CrossRef]
57. Kang, S.K.; Zhang, A.; Pandharipande, P.V.; Chandarana, H.; Braithwaite, R.S.; Littenberg, B. DWI for Renal Mass Characterization: Systematic Review and Meta-Analysis of Diagnostic Test Performance. *Am. J. Roentgenol.* **2015**, *205*, 317–324. [CrossRef]
58. Battagli, C.; Uzzo, R.G.; Dulaimi, E.; Ibanez de Caceres, I.; Krassenstein, R.; Al-Saleem, T.; Greenberg, R.E.; Cairns, P. Promoter hypermethylation of tumor suppressor genes in urine from kidney cancer patients. *Cancer Res.* **2003**, *63*, 8695–8699.
59. Costa, V.L.; Henrique, R.; Danielsen, S.A.; Eknaes, M.; Patrício, P.; Morais, A.; Oliveira, J.; Lothe, R.A.; Teixeira, M.R.; Lind, G.E.; et al. TCF21 and PCDH17 methylation: An innovative panel of biomarkers for a simultaneous detection of urological cancers. *Epigenetics* **2011**, *6*, 1120–1130. [CrossRef]
60. de Martino, M.; Klatte, T.; Haitel, A.; Marberger, M. Serum cell-free DNA in renal cell carcinoma: A diagnostic and prognostic marker. *Cancer* **2012**, *118*, 82–90. [CrossRef]
61. Hauser, S.; Zahalka, T.; Fechner, G.; Müller, S.C.; Ellinger, J. Serum DNA hypermethylation in patients with kidney cancer: Results of a prospective study. *Anticancer Res.* **2013**, *33*, 4651–4656.
62. Hoque, M.O.; Begum, S.; Topaloglu, O.; Jeronimo, C.; Mambo, E.; Westra, W.H.; Califano, J.A.; Sidransky, D. Quantitative detection of promoter hypermethylation of multiple genes in the tumor, urine, and serum DNA of patients with renal cancer. *Cancer Res.* **2004**, *64*, 5511–5517. [CrossRef]
63. Nuzzo, P.V.; Berchuck, J.E.; Korthauer, K.; Spisak, S.; Nassar, A.H.; Abou Alaiwi, S.; Chakravarthy, A.; Shen, S.Y.; Bakouny, Z.; Boccardo, F.; et al. Detection of renal cell carcinoma using plasma and urine cell-free DNA methylomes. *Nat. Med.* **2020**, *26*, 1041–1043. [CrossRef] [PubMed]
64. Outeiro-Pinho, G.; Barros-Silva, D.; Aznar, E.; Sousa, A.I.; Vieira-Coimbra, M.; Oliveira, J.; Gonçalves, C.S.; Costa, B.M.; Junker, K.; Henrique, R.; et al. MicroRNA-30a-5p(me): A novel diagnostic and prognostic biomarker for clear cell renal cell carcinoma in tissue and urine samples. *J. Exp. Clin. Cancer Res.* **2020**, *39*, 98. [CrossRef] [PubMed]
65. Skrypkina, I.; Tsyba, L.; Onyshchenko, K.; Morderer, D.; Kashparova, O.; Nikolaienko, O.; Panasenko, G.; Vozianov, S.; Romanenko, A.; Rynditch, A. Concentration and Methylation of Cell-Free DNA from Blood Plasma as Diagnostic Markers of Renal Cancer. *Dis. Markers* **2016**, *2016*, 3693096. [CrossRef] [PubMed]
66. Urakami, S.; Shiina, H.; Enokida, H.; Hirata, H.; Kawamoto, K.; Kawakami, T.; Kikuno, N.; Tanaka, Y.; Majid, S.; Nakagawa, M.; et al. Wnt antagonist family genes as biomarkers for diagnosis, staging, and prognosis of renal cell carcinoma using tumor and serum DNA. *Clin. Cancer Res.* **2006**, *12*, 6989–6997. [CrossRef] [PubMed]
67. Xin, J.; Xu, R.; Lin, S.; Xin, M.; Cai, W.; Zhou, J.; Fu, C.; Zhen, G.; Lai, J.; Li, Y.; et al. Clinical potential of TCF21 methylation in the diagnosis of renal cell carcinoma. *Oncol. Lett.* **2016**, *12*, 1265–1270. [CrossRef]
68. He, Z.H.; Qin, X.H.; Zhang, X.L.; Yi, J.W.; Han, J.Y. Long noncoding RNA GIHCG is a potential diagnostic and prognostic biomarker and therapeutic target for renal cell carcinoma. *Eur. Rev. Med. Pharmacol. Sci.* **2018**, *22*, 46–54. [CrossRef]
69. Wu, Y.; Wang, Y.Q.; Weng, W.W.; Zhang, Q.Y.; Yang, X.Q.; Gan, H.L.; Yang, Y.S.; Zhang, P.P.; Sun, M.H.; Xu, M.D.; et al. A serum-circulating long noncoding RNA signature can discriminate between patients with clear cell renal cell carcinoma and healthy controls. *Oncogenesis* **2016**, *5*, e192. [CrossRef]
70. Xie, J.; Zhong, Y.; Chen, R.; Li, G.; Luo, Y.; Yang, J.; Sun, Z.; Liu, Y.; Liu, P.; Wang, N.; et al. Serum long non-coding RNA LINC00887 as a potential biomarker for diagnosis of renal cell carcinoma. *FEBS Open Bio* **2020**, *10*, 1802–1809. [CrossRef]

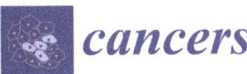

Review

The Next Paradigm Shift in the Management of Clear Cell Renal Cancer: Radiogenomics—Definition, Current Advances, and Future Directions

Nikhil Gopal [1,*], Pouria Yazdian Anari [2], Evrim Turkbey [2], Elizabeth C. Jones [2] and Ashkan A. Malayeri [2]

1. Urologic Oncology Branch, National Cancer Institute, National Institutes of Health, 10 Center Drive, Bethesda, MD 20814, USA
2. Radiology and Imaging Sciences, Clinical Center, National Institutes of Health, 10 Center Drive, Bethesda, MD 20814, USA; pouria.yazdian@nih.gov (P.Y.A.); evrim.turkbey@nih.gov (E.T.); ejones@cc.nih.gov (E.C.J.); ashkan.malayeri@nih.gov (A.A.M.)
* Correspondence: nikhil.gopal@nih.gov

Simple Summary: Radiogenomics is the science of studying imaging–pathology associations on a genomic level. With the potential for improved non-invasive characterization of tumors to predict survival; metastasis; and/or treatment response, it is important for clinicians to have a basic appreciation of this nascent field. The genetic basis for clear cell kidney cancer is more well-defined than many other malignancies, making it an ideal target for radiogenomic analysis. We first define the field of radiogenomics in diagnostic radiology, demonstrating that image biomarkers can be derived either qualitatively or quantitatively, the latter of which often employs machine learning. We then summarize existing literature establishing relationships between image features and single or multiple gene expression patterns in clear cell renal cell carcinoma. Finally, we outline limitations of the scope and methodology of current radiogenomic studies in ccRCC and propose future directions for this field to progress from an experimental setting into the mainstream clinical workflow.

Abstract: With improved molecular characterization of clear cell renal cancer and advances in texture analysis as well as machine learning, diagnostic radiology is primed to enter personalized medicine with radiogenomics: the identification of relationships between tumor image features and underlying genomic expression. By developing surrogate image biomarkers, clinicians can augment their ability to non-invasively characterize a tumor and predict clinically relevant outcomes (i.e., overall survival; metastasis-free survival; or complete/partial response to treatment). It is thus important for clinicians to have a basic understanding of this nascent field, which can be difficult due to the technical complexity of many of the studies. We conducted a review of the existing literature for radiogenomics in clear cell kidney cancer, including original full-text articles until September 2021. We provide a basic description of radiogenomics in diagnostic radiology; summarize existing literature on relationships between image features and gene expression patterns, either computationally or by radiologists; and propose future directions to facilitate integration of this field into the clinical setting.

Keywords: clear cell kidney cancer; radiogenomics; radiomics; machine learning; gene expression

Citation: Gopal, N.; Yazdian Anari, P.; Turkbey, E.; Jones, E.C.; Malayeri, A.A. The Next Paradigm Shift in the Management of Clear Cell Renal Cancer: Radiogenomics—Definition, Current Advances, and Future Directions. *Cancers* 2022, 14, 793. https://doi.org/10.3390/cancers14030793

Academic Editors: Claudia Manini and José I. López

Received: 27 November 2021
Accepted: 28 January 2022
Published: 4 February 2022

Publisher's Note: MDPI stays neutral with regard to jurisdictional claims in published maps and institutional affiliations.

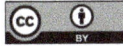

Copyright: © 2022 by the authors. Licensee MDPI, Basel, Switzerland. This article is an open access article distributed under the terms and conditions of the Creative Commons Attribution (CC BY) license (https://creativecommons.org/licenses/by/4.0/).

1. Introduction

Beginning in the late 1980s, our understanding of the pathology of kidney cancer has gradually evolved beyond characterization of histological patterns to identification of specific genetic changes [1,2]. Discovery of pathologically relevant genetic pathways has allowed for discrimination both between and among renal cancer subtypes. The ultimate goal of these endeavors is to create a more personalized approach to predicting disease prognosis and response to treatment. With improved ability to characterize image features, particularly through advances in machine learning, diagnostic radiology is also primed to enter personalized medicine through the field of radiogenomics. Here, we define this nascent field and review available studies in clear cell kidney cancer involving the association of single-gene mutations as well as more complex gene expression patterns with imaging phenotypes.

2. What Is Radiogenomics?

Radiogenomics is the science of identifying the associations between imaging features of a lesion and the underlying genomic signatures. For instance, by developing radiogenomics signatures, one can predict the tumor response to treatment by combining the imaging findings and genomic data. This process can also be used to decode the genetic makeup of a mass seen on imaging that fits the radiogenomic profile developed for that specific mass subtype [3–5]. One of the advantages of this approach is a complete evaluation of the makeup of the mass as opposed to tissue sampling that only evaluates a small portion of the tumor, which may underestimate the dominant molecular pattern given intra-tumoral heterogeneity [6]. Thus, by identifying surrogate imaging biomarkers that represent distinct genotypes with prognostic significance, radiogenomics can improve traditional tumor genetic testing through more comprehensive tumor characterization via wider anatomic coverage. As with current biomarkers, these imaging phenotypes should have prognostic significance; that is, to better define, beyond size and growth rate criteria alone, appropriate candidates for active surveillance and/or systemic treatment regimens in the case of advanced disease.

Imaging characteristics can be obtained either qualitatively (i.e., discrete variables scored by one or more radiologists) or quantitatively. Some of the quantitative variables such as size and degree of contrast uptake/washout can be calculated by the clinicians, while more complex relationships between individual image pixels cannot be ascertained by the naked eye. Conversion of these relationships into mineable quantitative features is the practice of radiomics [5,7,8]. The region of interest (either a single slice or the full volume of the tumor) is marked within an image (segmentation) to be recognized by computer software for image feature extraction. Differential pixel intensities of an image can be captured into either first order features (i.e., frequency distribution of pixel intensities without any spatial information such as skewness or kurtosis) or higher order features (i.e., spatial relationship between different pixel intensities such as gray level discrimination matrix). Given the number of extracted features (at times exceeding 1000) and the assumed nonlinear relationship between features and the dependent variable (i.e., presence or absence of a genetic mutation), machine learning is often employed to establish such relationships. More specifically, the data are split into training and testing sets, with an assigned algorithm developing relationships among relevant features using training data. The ability of the model to accurately classify patients into discrete categories (i.e., mutation or no mutation) is employed on the test data, using the known mutation status as the comparator of efficacy. Typically, prior to model training, the number of extracted features is reduced, either by eliminating redundant features (i.e., those with high intra-class correlation) and inconsistent features (i.e., those not seen if tumor is segmented by a different radiologist), with or without the aid of machine learning. In summary, the steps of a radiomics algorithm are segmentation; feature extraction; feature selection; and, in most cases, machine learning. This workflow is summarized in Figure 1.

Compared to other malignancies, the genetic basis of clear cell kidney cancer is well-established, with a relative paucity of genes implicated in pathogenesis. Thus, kidney cancer is a prime target for initial application of radiogenomics. Below, we review available studies in clear cell renal cell cancer (ccRCC) radiogenomics, focusing on exploratory investigations into relationships between imaging features and mutations in single genes; gene expression patterns; methylation changes in specific genes; and microRNA expression. The goal of each of these investigations is to better predict relevant clinical endpoints, such as overall survival; development of metastasis; and treatment response.

We conducted the review using PubMed, EMBASE, Google Scholar, and Web of Science. We searched by title/abstract in the following databases using the search parameters: "artificial intelligence or radiomics or machine learning or deep learning or radiogenomics" AND "clear cell" AND "kidney or renal". Articles published up to September 2021 were included. Eliminating redundant articles, 354 articles were identified from our search parameters. Titles from articles were screened out if they did not involve a correlation of imaging features to gene expression patterns. Through this manner, we identified 20 full text, original study articles that were incorporated into this review. See Figure 2 for a summary of the workflow for inclusion of studies for this review. Table 1 summarizes these studies with their relevant findings.

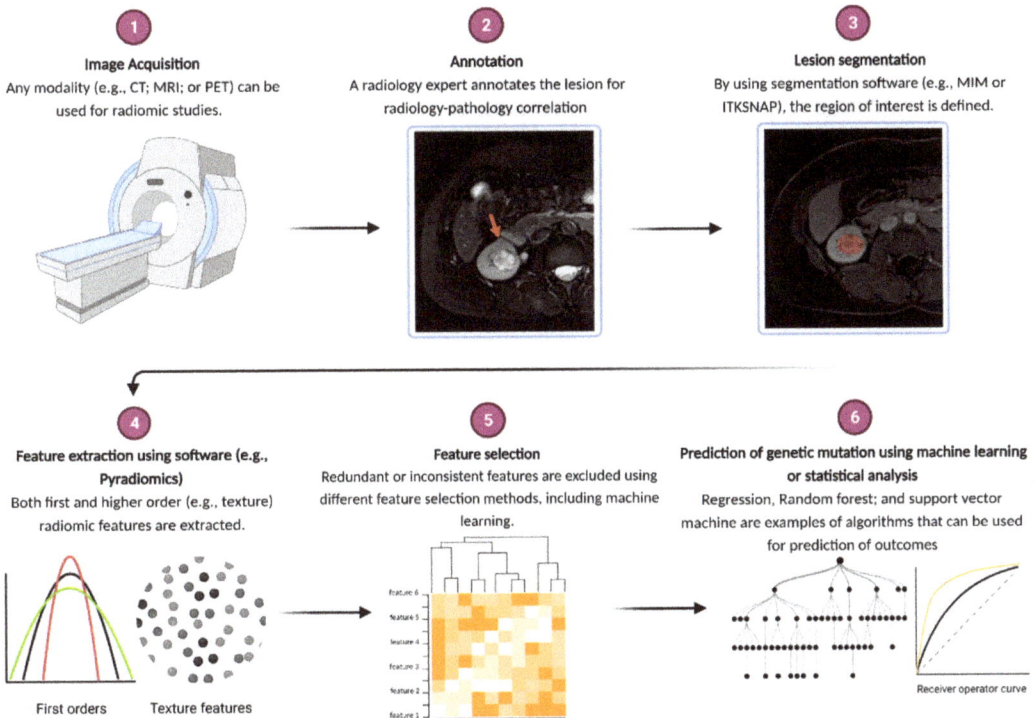

Figure 1. Outline of workflow for radiomic studies. Annotation is particularly important for multifocal masses to ensure matching of radiologically identified lesion with appropriate pathological specimen. Classification of machine learning algorithms is typically binary and thus analyzed using receiver operated curve (ROC), with area under the curve (AUC) used as benchmark for machine performance. Image created using BioRender.com (accessed on 26 November 2021).

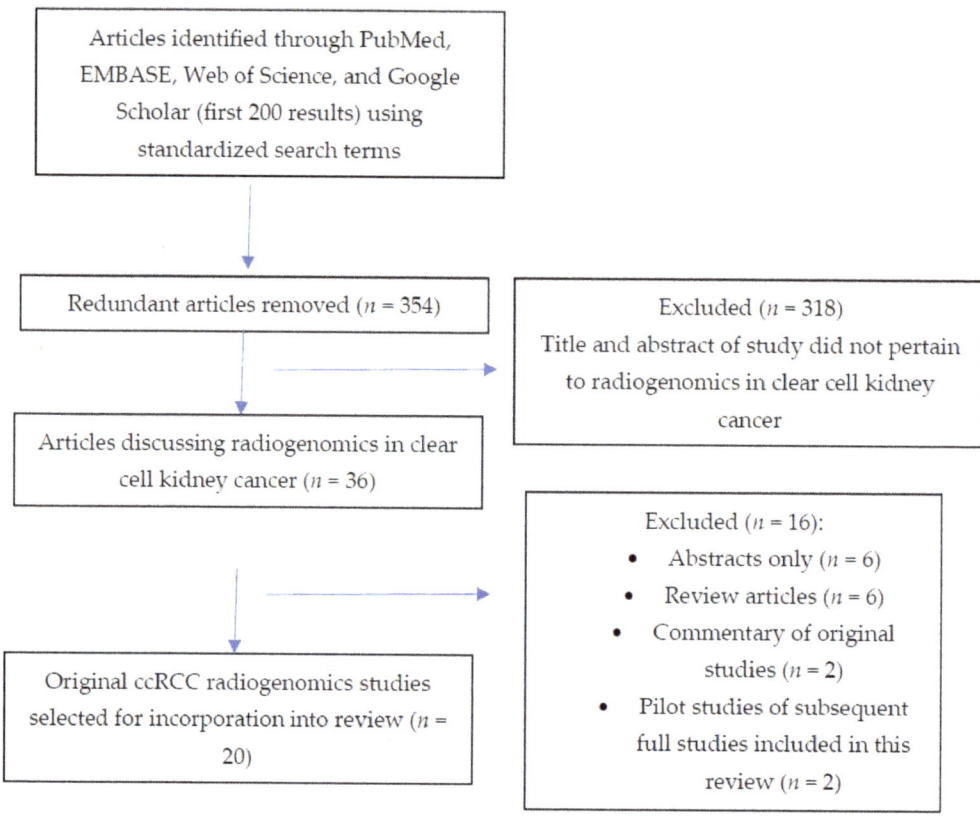

Figure 2. Flowchart demonstrating the search strategy and selection criteria for the articles included in this review.

Table 1. Summary of 20 reviewed articles on radiogenomics in clear cell renal cell carcinoma. Nature of feature extraction is indicated by "Radiologist" if features are scored by one or more radiologists. Elsewise, software derived features are indicated by "Computational". Number of selected features indicated in parenthesis. TAT (total adipose tissue), VAT (visceral adipose tissue), AUC (area under the curve), OR (odds ratio), HR (hazard ratio), CSS (cancer specific survival), OS (overall survival), PFS (progression free survival).

Author	Title	Year of Publication	Patient #	Feature Extraction (Number)	±Machine Learning	Image Phase Used	Genes Studied	Outcome
Karlo et al. [9]	Radiogenomics of Clear Cell Renal Cell Carcinoma: Associations between CT Imaging Features and Mutations	2014	233	Radiologist (10)	—	CT	BAP1 VHL KD5MC	BAP1 and KD5MC: renal vein invasion (OR 3.50 and 3.89) VHL: ill-defined margin (OR 0.49), nodular enhancement (OR 2.33), intratumoral vasculature (OR 0.51)
Shinagare et al. [10]	Radiogenomics of clear cell renal cell carcinoma: Preliminary findings of the cancer genome atlas–renal cell carcinoma (TCGA–RCC) imaging research group	2015	103	Radiologist (6)	—	Contrast-enhanced CT	BAP1 MUC-4	BAP1: Ill-defined margin and calcification MUC4: Exophytic growth
Greco et al. [11]	Relationship between visceral adipose tissue and genetic mutations (VHL and KDM5C) in clear cell renal cell carcinoma	2021	97	Computational (3)	—	CT	KDM5C vs. VHL	KDM5C higher TAT and VAT area than VHL
Feng et al. [12]	Identifying BAP1 Mutations in Clear-Cell Renal Cell Carcinoma by CT Radiomics: Preliminary Findings	2020	54	Computational (58)	+ (Random Forest)	CT	BAP1	AUC 0.77
Kocak et al. [13]	Machine learning-based unenhanced CT texture analysis for predicting BAP1 mutation status of clear cell renal cell carcinomas	2020	65	Computational (6)	+ (Random Forest)	CT	BAP1	AUC 0.897

Table 1. *Cont.*

Author	Title	Year of Publication	Patient #	Feature Extraction (Number)	±Machine Learning	Image Phase Used	Genes Studied	Outcome
Ghosh et al. [14]	Imaging-genomic pipeline for identifying gene mutations using three-dimensional intra-tumor heterogeneity features	2015	78	Computational (1636)	+ (Random Forest)	CT nephrographic phase	BAP1	AUC 0.71
Kocak et al. [15]	Radiogenomics in Clear Cell Renal Cell Carcinoma: Machine Learning-Based High-Dimensional Quantitative CT Texture Analysis in Predicting PBRM1 Mutation Status	2019	45	Computational (10)	+ (Random Forest)	CT	PBRM1	AUC 0.987
Chen et al. [16]	Reliable gene mutation prediction in clear cell renal cell carcinoma through multi-classifier multi-objective radiogenomics model	2018	57	Computational (43)	+ (6 classifier composite)	CT	VHL PBRM1 BAP1	AUC 0.88 0.86 0.93 Mutation status prediction
Marigliano et al. [17]	Radiogenomics in clear cell renal cell carcinoma: correlations between advanced CT imaging (texture analysis) and microRNAs expression	2019	20	Computational (6)	−	CT	miR-21-5p	$R^2 = 0.25$ between entropy and change in miR-21-5p expression between tumor and surrounding parenchyma
Cen et al. [18]	Renal cell carcinoma: predicting RUNX3 methylation level and its consequences on survival with CT features	2019	106	Radiologist (9)	−	CT	RUNX3 methylation	High methylation: left side (OR 2.70), ill-defined margin (OR 2.69), intratumoral vascularity (OR 3.29)—AUC of 0.73

Table 1. Cont.

Author	Title	Year of Publication	Patient #	Feature Extraction (Number)	±Machine Learning	Image Phase Used	Genes Studied	Outcome
Yu et al. [19]	Renal Cell Carcinoma: Predicting DNA Methylation Subtyping and Its Consequences on Overall Survival With Computed Tomography Imaging Characteristics	2020	212	Radiologist (12)	—	CT	Tumor methylation (M1-M3 subtype)	M1: >7 cm (OR 2.45), necrosis (OR 4.76) M2: necrosis (OR 0.047), enhancement (OR 0.083) M3: Long axis > median (OR 0.30), necrosis (OR 3.26)
Jamshidi et al. [20]	The radiogenomic risk score: construction of a prognostic quantitative, noninvasive image-based molecular assay for renal cell carcinoma	2015	70	Radiologist (4)	—	Contrast CT	SPC gene signature	RRS correlation with SPC (R = 0.45), HR 3.32 for CSS after surgery
Jamshidi et al. [4]	The radiogenomic risk score stratifies outcomes in a renal cell cancer phase 2 clinical trial	2016	41	Radiologist (4)	—	Contrast CT	SPC gene signature	PFS: 6 mo (high RRS) vs. >25 mo (low RRS)—After bevacizumab tx OS: 25 mo (high RRS) vs. >37 months (low RRS)
Bowen et al. [21]	Radiogenomics of clear cell renal cell carcinoma: associations between mRNA-based subtyping and CT imaging features	2019	177	Computational (8)	—	CT	mRNA subtyping (m1-m4)	M1: OR 2.1—well-defined margin M3: OR 0.42 (well-defined margin), OR 2.12 (renal vein involvement)
Yin et al. [22]	Integrative radiomics expression predicts molecular subtypes of primary clear cell renal cell carcinoma	2018	8	Computational (4)	+ (Fisher's linear discriminant analysis)	PET and MRI	Molecular subtype of ccRCC (ccA vs. ccB)	Accuracy of classification—86.96%

Table 1. *Cont.*

Author	Title	Year of Publication	Patient #	Feature Extraction (Number)	±Machine Learning	Image Phase Used	Genes Studied	Outcome
Lee et al. [23]	Integrative radiogenomics approach for risk assessment of post-operative metastasis in pathological T1 renal cell carcinoma: a pilot retrospective cohort study	2020	58	Computational (4)	+ (Random Forest)	Contrast CT	Multiple gene-mediated pathways	AUC 0.955—Metastasis
Zhao et al. [24]	Validation of CT radiomics for prediction of distant metastasis after surgical resection in patients with clear cell renal cell carcinoma: exploring the underlying signaling pathways	2021	547	Computational (9)	+ (Logistic regression)	CT	19 gene pathway signatures	AUC 0.84—Metastasis
Lin et al. [25]	Radiomic profiling of clear cell renal cell carcinoma reveals subtypes with distinct prognoses and molecular pathways	2021	160	Computational (122)	+ (Consensus clustering)	Unenhanced CT	VHL, MUC16, FBN2, and FLG Cell cycle related pathways	C1: Lower OS and PFS than C2 and C3 C1: Lower VHL expression C3: Higher FBN2 expression
Huang et al. [26]	Exploration of an integrated prognostic model of radiogenomics features with underlying gene expression patterns in clear cell renal cell carcinoma	2021	205	Computational (4)	+ (LASSO/SVM for feature selection, random forest for classification)	Contrast CT	Gene modules	AUC 0.837, 0.806 and 0.751—1-, 3-, and 5-year OS (combined radiogenomic model)

Table 1. *Cont.*

Author	Title	Year of Publication	Patient #	Feature Extraction (Number)	±Machine Learning	Image Phase Used	Genes Studied	Outcome
Zeng et al. [27]	Integrative radiogenomics analysis for predicting molecular features and survival in clear cell renal cell carcinoma	2021	207	Computational (4)	+ (Random Forest)	Contrast CT	VHL, BAP1, PBRM1, SETD2, molecular subtypes (m1–m4)	AUC 0.846—5-year OS (Combined radiogenomic model)

The # refers to number (as in number of patients).

3. Associations between Image Features and Mutations in Single Genes Commonly Implicated in ccRCC

While mutations in Von-Hippel Lindau (VHL) gene have long been implicated in the pathogenesis of ccRCC [1,2], the Cancer Genome Atlas (TCGA) helped identify additional causative genes, including those in the chromosome 3p region adjacent to VHL, such as polybromo-1 (PBRM1); BRCA associated protein 1 (BAP1); and SET domain containing 2 (SETD2) [28]. Indeed, while 90% of sporadic clear cell kidney cancers are associated with 3p chromosomal deletions, a minority of these tumors have wild type VHL expression, indicating the independent role of other genes within this region in tumorigenesis. Additional relevant genes for ccRCC identified by TCGA include lysine specific demethylase 5C (KDM5C) and mucin 4 (MUC-4) [29,30]. Although the presence of a VHL mutation itself has not been shown to have any predictive or prognostic value, important clinical differences emerge with respect to the mutational status of other genes. For instance, PBRM1 mutational status may determine response to immune checkpoint therapy [31,32]; BAP1 mutations are associated with more aggressive tumors [28,33]; tumors with SETD2 and KDM5C mutations are linked to unfavorable prognosis in the localized setting [34–36]; and tumors with MUC4 mutation have a favorable prognosis [37].

Karlo and others [9] sought to assess whether mutations in VHL; KDM5C; SETD2; and/or BAP1 were associated with any image features from computed tomography (CT). A total of 233 patients from two cohorts (i.e., MSKCC and the Cancer Imaging Archive (TCIA)) with available CT and genomic analysis had their corresponding tumors scored on eight qualitative (e.g., presence of necrosis) and two quantitative (e.g., tumor size) features via consensus from three radiologists. Significant image-genotype correlations were seen with VHL, KDM5C, and BAP1 mutations. Tumors with VHL mutations were associated with a well-defined tumor margin; nodular enhancement; and presence of intratumoral vascularity. KDM5C and BAP1 mutations were more predominant in tumors with renal vein invasion. Finally, KDM5C mutant tumors tended to be hypo-enhancing relative to the renal cortex in the CT nephrographic phase.

Shinagare et al. [10] performed a similar type of hypothesis-generating study; here, 103 patients exclusively from the Cancer Imaging Archive (TCIA) had six imaging features on either contrast-enhanced CT (79% of cohort) or MRI assessed by three radiologists. For each feature, the median or most common score (depending on whether the variable was qualitative or quantitative) was used to determine an association with tumor genotype. Despite the overlap in image features and patients with Karlo et al. [9], different results were obtained. With respect to VHL; KDM5C; and BAP1 mutational status, there was a significant association only with BAP1. Namely, tumors with BAP1 mutations were more likely to have ill-defined margins and calcifications. Additionally, MUC-4 mutation was associated with an exophytic tumor growth pattern.

Despite the inconsistency in results between these two studies, plausible biological explanations can be ascertained for these surrogate imaging biomarkers. For instance, BAP1 mutations confer aggressive traits to renal tumors, which may increase the likelihood of renal vein invasion as well as promote de-differentiation and increased proliferation, both of which can account for a poorly visualized tumor margin. The unregulated HIF expression with VHL mutation, resulting in upregulation of angiogenesis factors, can explain the prominence of intratumoral vascularity seen in these tumors.

Greco et al. [11] sought to characterize differences, if any, between patients with VHL and KDM5C mutant tumors in terms of abdominal fat content. With 52 VHL and 10 KDM5C mutant tumors derived from the TCIA cohort, patients with KDM5C mutations had higher total and visceral abdominal fat content than those with VHL tumor mutations. The authors also included a cohort of patients with no renal tumors ($n = 35$) and noted that ccRCC overall is associated with higher total and visceral fat content. There is evidence that fat deposits in obese individuals may promote oncogenesis and tumor progression through a chronic inflammatory state created through adipokines [38,39], which may explain the study results, given the negative prognostic biomarker of localized KDM5C mutant tumors.

Apart from qualitative and quantitative scoring derived from radiologists, associations between image features and single gene alterations have also been studied using radiomics and machine learning. For instance, Feng et al. [12] used a random forest classifier to assign tumors from 54 TCIA patients (45 BAP1 wildtype and 9 BAP1 mutants) to either presence or absence of BAP1 mutation based on 58 quantitatively derived radiomics features, with an AUC of 0.77. Image features from this study were derived from the nephrogenic CT phase, with the most predictive being a higher order feature (gray level run length matrix—number of consecutive voxels of a similar gray level intensity within a given direction [8]. Kock et al. [13] also used a random forest classifier to predict BAP1 tumor mutational status but used an unenhanced CT for easier availability and improved homogeneity between image studies, the latter of which is relevant in the multi-institutional collaboration of TCIA. Utilizing CTs of 65 patients (13 BAP1 mutant tumors and 52 BAP1 wildtype tumors), the random forest classifier was trained on 6 selected features, achieving an AUC of 0.897. Although Ghosh et al. had previously shown features extracted from nephrographic phase as opposed to unenhanced phase to be most predictive of BAP1 mutation [14], it should be noted that different extracted features from Feng et al. [12] were used to train this model; indeed, the dominant feature class was first-order. Nevertheless, half of the selected features [13] were higher order, indicating that region of interest (ROI) analysis without taking into account the spatial relationship of encapsulated voxels (i.e., utilizing only first order features) was insufficient for optimal prediction of BAP1 mutation status.

In addition, to study results potentially being affected by the image phase used and features selected, the type of machine learning algorithm can have an impact on the predictive performance of the model classifier. For instance, Kocak et al. [15] assessed the differential performance of two algorithms (random forest classifier and artificial neural network) in predicting the presence or absence of a PBRM1 mutation. In studying 45 patients (29 PBRM1 tumor wild-type and 16 PBRM1 mutants) from the TCIA using the corticomedullary phase of CT, the random forest classifier outperformed the artificial neural network in predicting tumor genotype, with AUC of 0.987 and 0.925, respectively. In this study, a machine learning algorithm was used to select the extracted radiomic features as well as train the model using the selected features. In other words, while 828 initial features were extracted from the CT, the final features used to train the model classifier differed depending on the algorithm (i.e., 10 features selected by artificial neural network and 4 features by random forest classifier). Indeed, only three selected features were shared by both algorithms, accounting for discrepancy in results beyond the intrinsic properties of the algorithms themselves. Regardless, two out of the top three features most predictive of PBRM1 mutation status were a higher order for both types of model classifiers. Across both types of algorithms, tumors with the PBRM1 mutation had greater pixel heterogeneity of gray level intensity.

Rather than comparing different machine learning algorithms, Chen et al. [16] used six different types of classifiers to generate the composite probability of different tumor genetic mutations. Here, 43 selected features from corticomedullary phase CT scan (a total of 57 patients from TCIA) were used to train and test each model classifier (support vector machine; logistic regression; discriminant analysis; decision tree; K-nearest neighbor; and naïve Bayesian). The predictive capability of the multi-classifier algorithm was superior to any single classifier, with AUC for predicting VHL; PBRM1; and BAP1 mutations being 0.88; 0.86; and 0.93, respectively. The selected features common to all six classifiers that discriminated VHL mutational status were both first order (mean and kurtosis). Tumors with VHL mutation had lower mean voxel intensity and had less variation in pixel intensity values (i.e., less tailedness or kurtosis). On the other hand, a relatively equivalent proportion of first and higher order features were selected across all six classifiers for distinguishing PBRM1 mutation class. Finally, more higher order features were common to all six classifiers for BAP1 classification, with BAP1 mutant tumors having greater heterogeneity in terms of voxel intensity.

4. Beyond Mutations in Common Pathogenic Single Genes in Clear Cell Kidney Cancer: Establishing Image Biomarkers for Epigenetic, Regulatory, and Multiple Gene Expression Signatures

Despite single gene mutations being implicated in renal cancer pathogenesis, kidney cancer development is reliant not just on any one aberrant gene product, but also on changes in regulatory molecules for both the gene product and its downstream effectors. While our understanding of these modulators of gene expression is in its infancy, preliminary investigations into relationships between imaging features and these molecules have been conducted.

For instance, Marigliano et al. [17] sought to determine whether there was any association between intensity-based pixel features (e.g., mean pixel attenuation) of ccRCCs seen on contrast CT and the amount of mi-21-5p, a micro-RNA whose expression was previously shown to be correlated with poor cancer specific survival following RCC resection [40]. Unlike previous studies, image features were extracted from both the tumor and the surrounding normal renal parenchyma. In 20 patients, the authors found a significant positive correlation between change in miR-21-5p expression from tumor to adjacent normal parenchyma and degree of image entropy (i.e., variation in pixel intensity within the tumor) [17].

Another regulatory factor implicated in several carcinomas is RUNX3 (runt related transcription factor 3), which belongs to a family of transcription factors that modulate major developmental pathways [41,42]. Methylation of this tumor suppressor RUNX3 has been negatively associated with overall survival in other carcinomas [43,44]. Cen et al. [18] scored 106 ccRCCs from the TCIA cohort on 9 qualitative CT imaging features and found, on multivariate regression, that ill-defined tumor margin, left sided tumors, and presence of intratumoral vascularity significantly predicted elevated RUNX3 methylation levels (AUC of 0.725). Furthermore, patients with higher methylation levels had lower median overall survival. The laterality bias is difficult to explain, with additional validation needed, but intratumoral vascularity and ill-defined margin are both imaging markers associated with aggressive tumors, which is in line with the negative prognosis associated with RUNX3 methylation.

Other tumor suppressor genes that can be susceptible to methylation-induced silencing in RCC have been identified, such as Dickkopf1 (DKK1); WNT pathway regulatory genes; and secreted frizzed related protein (SFRP1) [45,46]. Through the TCGA, three DNA methylation subgroups in ccRCC (M1-M3) with prognostic implications were identified, with the M1 subtype found to have the worst overall survival [28]. In assessing tumors from 212 patients (180 ccRCC cases) from the TCIA cohort on 12 different qualitative CT imaging features, Yu et al. [19] noted that, on multivariate analysis, a long axis >7 cm and presence of necrosis was associated with the unfavorable M1 subtype, with an AUC of 0.68. While M2 subtype was mostly characterized by absence of necrosis, the presence of necrosis was a significant independent predictor of the M3 subtype on multivariate logistic regression, limiting the utility of that imaging parameter.

As illustrated above, characterizing tumors by a panel of molecular markers, as opposed to a single entity, may more accurately capture the full extent of their biological behavior. In this manner, Zhao et al. [47] described 259 genes that predicted survival after ccRCC surgery independent of grade; stage; and performance status, creating the so-called SPC (supervised principal components) gene signature. Jamshidi et al. [20] used available CT and genetic data from 70 patients from a single institution to develop a radiogenomic risk score (RRS) using the top 4 qualitative CT imaging features that were best associated with expression of genes within the SPC signature. This score was independently validated in 77 patients from the same institution at a later time point. In a separate phase II trial assessing the role of neoadjuvant bevacizumab prior to cytoreductive nephrectomy, RRS using pre-treatment CT features was able to predict radiological progression free survival after anti-angiogenic administration [4].

The Cancer Genome Atlas also helped identify four unique mRNA-based subgroups in clear cell renal cell cancer: m1–m4 [48]. For instance, M1 contains gene sets involved with chromatin remodeling and a higher proportion of PBRM1 mutations. On the other hand, higher deletions of PTEN are seen in the m3 subtype. Bowen et al. scored tumors from 177 patients from TCIA on 8 CT imaging features and noted that a well-defined tumor margin was a significant positive predictor of m1 subtype vs. others, whereas the opposite was true of the m3 subtype [21]. As seen in other qualitative studies, the margin status of the m1 subtype is in line with its prognostically favorable outcome with respect to overall survival.

Further genetic expression analysis of ccRCC tumors have revealed two distinct molecular subtypes that are captured by a 34-signature gene model (ClearCode34): ccA and ccB. CCA is characterized by upregulation of genes involved in angiogenesis, while ccB tumors have higher cellular differentiation activity (i.e., epithelial to mesenchymal signaling). CCB tumors are more aggressive, based on higher Furhman grade; increased nodal metastasis; and worsened cancer specific as well as overall survival [49,50]. Unfortunately, the utility of this biomarker is hindered due to high intra-tumoral heterogeneity [51], limiting radiogenomic studies derived from biopsy samples. Yin et al. [22] circumvented this problem by performing radiomic and genetic expression analysis on different areas of the tumor from the same patient. A total of 168 features were extracted from 23 tumor ROIs on a PET/MRI from 8 patients; using sparse partial least analysis (SPLA), 4 radiomic features (2 first order and 2 higher order) were selected and found to correctly classify the ccRCC molecular subtype 86.96% of the time.

Thus far, radiomic signatures have been linked to molecular factors with established prognostic associations; for instance, BAP1 mutation with aggressive tumor phenotype or ccB with worsened cancer specific survival. However, radiomic analysis can be used for gene discovery, with associated prognostic and therapeutic implications. That is, machine learning algorithms can group image features into those that are found to differ based on clinical outcomes such as metastasis free or overall survival. The genotype of tumors within each imaging group can then be interrogated to determine the underlying biology of different image classes, with identification of distinct genetic pathways helping to usher, for instance, development of new drugs.

Lee et al. [23] used three different machine learning algorithms (i.e., random forest classifier; logistic regression; and support vector machine) and a training set of 58 patients with a contrast CT prior to partial or radical nephrectomy to determine differential contributions of 4 selected image features (only 1 of which was higher order) towards prediction of postsurgical metastasis. This model was independently validated on 28 patients from the TCIA with an AUC of 0.89–0.95. Genetic expression analysis was performed on tumors, with specific image features correlating with genes involved with translation regulation; ECM interaction; focal adhesion; PI3K-AKT pathway; signaling by notch receptor 1 (NOTCH1); Wnt signaling pathway; and regulation of actin cytoskeleton. Differences in fibroblast growth factor expression and amount of T cells were found to correlate with image features, which have therapeutic implications (i.e., preferential FGFR inhibitor or immunotherapy for metastatic disease).

In a similar study, Zhao et al. [24] used nine radiomic features selected by machine learning (eight of which were higher order) to predict development of postoperative metastasis with AUC of 0.86. With genetic expression analysis and correlation with 9 image features, 19 gene signatures (ECM interaction; focal adhesion; and PI3K-AKT pathway were similar sets of genes from the previous study) were constructed that independently accurately predicted metastasis (AUC of 0.84). Additionally, Lin et al. [25] developed three distinct radiomic feature classes that, independent of tumor grade and patient age, differed based on overall survival from unenhanced CT scans of 160 patients. Genetic analysis revealed that classes differed based on underlying genetic mutations. For instance, class 1 with the lowest overall survival had reduced VHL mutation expression relative to the other two classes. Class 3 had higher FBN2 expression, which has been previously associated with improved overall survival [52,53]. Finally, Huang et al. [26] unearthed a gene expression module (comprised of 256 genes) that was associated with four selected radiomic features (75% higher-order) derived from 205 ccRCC patients from the TCIA. These genes mediate tumor angiogenesis, cell adhesion, and extracellular structure organization. The top four correlated genes within this module (RPS6KA2, CYYR1, KDR, and GIMAP6) were selected for incorporation into a machine learning algorithm. A decision classifier integrating both radiomic and genomic factors was a better predictor of 1-, 3-, and 5-year overall survival than a classifier using only radiomic features (5-year survival AUC 0.75 and 0.69, respectively).

5. Limitations and Future Directions

While radiogenomics has the potential to revolutionize a clinician's diagnostic capabilities, several existing limitations in this field will need to be addressed to allow these advances to proceed beyond the experimental setting. First, many of the institutional-based studies fail to have an external validation set from an outside institution, limiting the generalizability of their findings. In a recent review, only 7% of studies utilizing radiomic analysis of renal masses had this type of validation [54].

Despite not having an independent validation set, studies attempt to nonetheless seek generalizability by relying on cohorts from TCIA, which are comprised of images from multiple institutions. However, as institutions differ in image processing protocols, a different problem emerges, particularly for radiomic analysis, with the type and quantity of features extracted dependent on the specific way an image is acquired and processed (e.g., number of slices used for segmentation) [5,54].

A significant time burden in the radiomics workflow is manual segmentation, especially if more than one slice is considered. Manual segmentation is also subject to inter-observer variability [55,56]; although, some studies have tried to address this issue through multi-reader segmentation. As software to achieve reliable automated segmentation improves and becomes more available, large imaging sets can not only managed efficiently, but segmentation of tumor for radiomic analysis can be performed prospectively as part of the diagnostic radiologist's clinical workflow [5].

Apart from image acquisition differences, other aspects of heterogeneity within radiomic studies can be seen, accounting for discrepancies in results. For instance, studies investigating the same question (i.e., whether radiomic features can predict the presence of BAP1 mutations) use different phases of CT (i.e., nephrographic vs. excretory vs. unenhanced). Radiomic studies have been inconsistent in the CT phase most predictive of outcomes. As was illustrated above, features derived from CT nephrographic phase was most predictive of BAP-1 mutation status [14]; however, Nguyen et al. found that features from the corticomedullary phase was most predictive of renal mass characterization (e.g., RCC vs. benign) [57]. Just as is performed by the practicing radiologist, the optimal strategy may be to incorporate features from all CT phases into radiomic analysis.

Studies also differ in the extent of feature extraction, with some not obtaining higher order features from image filtration. Additionally, there is variability in the manner through which feature selection is performed, with some but not others employing machine learning to eliminate redundant and/or inconsistent features. Another important, yet underutilized, consideration for feature selection is that predictive model performance may be improved if features related to slice thickness and tumor size are also eliminated [58]. The former is an important consideration with studies relying on multi-institutional databases such as TCIA. With regard to the latter, as radiomics is meant to augment current diagnostic capability, development of radiomic signatures should only involve features that are not easily calculable in the clinical setting.

Thus, for radiomic studies to be reliably compared against each other, standardization of image processing (including acquisition and segmentation); feature extraction; and feature selection needs to be established. Perhaps an international consensus conference can be conducted for this purpose, with stakeholders from different fields outlining guidelines (i.e., radiologists; computer scientists; technicians; physicists; and treating clinicians). Standardization will also ensure that multi-disciplinary collaboration can be robustly performed from high quality and well curated images. Large sample sizes are necessary to improve generalizability of machine learning classifiers. With low sample size (i.e., <1:10 ratio of features: number of patients/tumors in a particular group [5]), overfitting of data can occur, preventing the model from performing well on other types of data, both within and outside a given institution. Additionally, in order to further promote replication of results in other institutions, source code of decision classifiers should be made public, which is not routine practice at present [59].

Currently, the vast majority of current radiomic and radiogenomic studies focus on CT. This approach is sensible at present, given that this imaging modality is the predominant means of evaluating renal masses worldwide. However, with its lack of radiation, MRI has grown in popularity, particularly as more serial imaging is incorporated into kidney tumor evaluation (i.e., active surveillance or treatment response in metastatic disease). The main advantage of MRI is the additional information that can be obtained from a variety of imaging sequences, such as T2 or DWI, which may improve image prediction models by providing additional radiomic features. Only one study reviewed here utilized MRI for computational image feature extraction; it is hoped that additional studies utilizing MRI for radiogenomic analysis will be conducted as experience and/or availability of this imaging modality grows.

In terms of scope of study, radiogenomic analysis thus far has largely focused on molecular features of the tumor itself. However, the tumor exists within a microenvironment that modulates its growth and development. For instance, Zhong et al. [60] identified two subtypes of ccRCC from analysis of the TCGA that differed based on checkpoint inhibitor and lymphocyte expression. These differences in immune-related tumor microenvironment have prognostic relevance; for instance, the subtype with elevated checkpoint inhibitor expression was predicted to have reduced response to immunotherapy. Some preliminary radiogenomic work characterizing the tumor ecosystem has been employed, such as Greco et al. [11] characterizing visceral fat content with ccRCC mutation as well as Marigliano et al. [17] and Lee et al. [23] also incorporating the surrounding normal parenchyma in feature extraction. It is hoped that as the field of radiogenomics evolves along with our understanding of the biology of the tumor microenvironment, additional radiomic analysis of the parenchyma and perinephric fat surrounding a tumor can be performed to establish more comprehensive surrogate imaging biomarkers.

While a clear advantage of establishing imaging biomarkers of underlying genetic activity is that images provide wider anatomical coverage than can be procured by a biopsy sample, many radiogenomic studies still correlate image features of an entire tumor with genetic information from a biopsy specimen. Furthermore, most of the time, the exact location of the biopsy is not known, preventing radiomic analysis of the corresponding area of a tumor to achieve a more optimal association study given genetic intra-tumor heterogeneity [61]. For this reason, the study by Yin et al. [22] was unique in that radiomic analysis was performed at different areas of a single tumor, with each area having distinct genetic testing and thus a known gene expression pattern. Future studies should also perform radiogenomic analysis within tumors as opposed to simply between different tumors. In the era of digital pathology utilizing quantitative image analysis and machine learning, models characterizing spatial heterogeneity of genetic mutations and surrounding microenvironment (i.e., T lymphocyte expression) within a tumor have been developed [62]. Provided that these models can be validated across institutions, they can be integrated into radiomic studies to provide more robust imaging–pathology associations.

Although the majority of presented studies here utilize tumors of different stages in image analysis, the genetic information is generally derived from the primary kidney tumor. That being said, the assumption of genetic homogeneity between the primary tumor and metastatic deposits may not necessarily hold. In a recent study using ClearCode34 to classify primary and metastatic tumor sites into different molecular subtypes (i.e., clear cell type A and B), there was a 43% discordance in subtype between the primary tumor and metastatic deposits within the same patient [63]. On the other hand, for a given patient, the molecular subtypes were similar among different metastatic sites. Thus, future radiogenomic studies incorporating patients with metastatic disease should have tumor sampling from metastatic sites to obtain a more reliable genotype within which to develop image biomarkers for prognostically relevant outcomes such as treatment response. It is clear that feature extraction from radiomic analysis provides more information about a tumor than can be ascertained by any radiologist (i.e., higher order features). However, with greater complexity comes greater abstraction of data from traditional biological or clinical understanding. Seeking to understand higher order features in clinical terms is challenging. However, "de-mystifying" these features can be accomplished through studying associations between qualitative and quantitative image variables. For instance, ill-defined tumor margin is associated with unfavorable genotypes, such as BAP1 mutation; methylation of RUNX3; and SPC gene signature. Determining which radiomic higher order features relate to these qualitative variables will allow for better integration of the literature and to improve clinical relevance of these features.

Given that tumor genetic testing does not often encompass the entire tumor (i.e., biopsy), radiomic analysis may provide additional prognostic information beyond the procured molecular signature [64]. Thus, rather than determining radiomic–genomic correlations alone, studies should incorporate both radiomic and genomic factors into prognostic models. Additional integration of existing clinical predictors and other -omic analysis into these models will also help improve prediction of clinically relevant outcomes. For instance, Zeng et al. [27] demonstrated that a combined radiomic, genomic, transcriptomic, and proteomic model had higher AUC than any single model alone in predicting overall survival of patients with ccRCC. Additionally, Yin et al. [22] showed that a model combining radiomic and clinical features (tumor size; stage; and grade) outperformed a radiomics only model in predicting ccRCC molecular subtype (91.3% vs. 86.96% accuracy). Finally, Huang et al. [26] developed an integrative nomogram of ccRCC survival incorporating tumor stage, gender, and a risk score incorporating both prognostic radiomic and genetic factors.

6. Conclusions

Radiogenomics represents the next paradigm shift in diagnostic medicine, and just as with the Human Genome Project, kidney cancer is one of the lead malignancies with which to apply advances from this field. Initial work in radiogenomics of clear cell kidney cancer has been promising, with relationships seen between imaging features and single and multiple gene expression patterns. Not only can image phenotypes be linked to prognostically relevant molecular signatures, but they can also be used to facilitate identification of associated gene expression pathways (i.e., biological basis of image differences) and can augment existing clinico-pathologic nomograms. Establishing non-invasive surrogate imaging biomarkers will no doubt increase the non-invasive diagnostic armamentarium of the clinician, with both prognostic and therapeutic implications, and has been greatly facilitated with radiomics and machine learning, which can elucidate the complex patterns within an image in an objective, quantifiable manner, unlike qualitative scoring by radiologists.

Future directions include feature extraction of the surrounding tumor environment; utilization of modalities other than CT; incorporating spatial tumor genetic heterogeneity in radiomic analysis; and integration of multi-omic (i.e., transcriptomic) and clinical information to create more powerful decision tools. Most importantly, consensus guidelines on radiomic and machine learning analysis need to be employed to facilitate comparison among studies and collaboration among institutions to allow advances in radiogenomics to be implemented in the clinical setting.

Author Contributions: Literature review: P.Y.A. and N.G.; Writing manuscript—N.G.; Figure and table—P.Y.A. and N.G.; Editing—P.Y.A., A.A.M., E.C.J. and E.T. All authors have read and agreed to the published version of the manuscript.

Funding: The APC was funded by the Intramural Research programs of The Center for Cancer Research, National Cancer Institute, and the National Institutes of Health Clinical Center, Bethesda, Maryland, USA.

Conflicts of Interest: The authors declare no conflict of interest.

References

1. Schmidt, L.S.; Linehan, W.M. Genetic predisposition to kidney cancer. *Semin. Oncol.* **2016**, *43*, 566–574. [CrossRef] [PubMed]
2. Latif, F.; Tory, K.; Gnarra, J.; Yao, M.; Duh, F.M.; Orcutt, M.L.; Stackhouse, T.; Kuzmin, I.; Modi, W.; Geil, L.; et al. Identification of the von Hippel-Lindau disease tumor suppressor gene. *Science* **1993**, *260*, 1317–1320. [CrossRef] [PubMed]
3. Alessandrino, F.; Shinagare, A.B.; Bossé, D.; Choueiri, T.K.; Krajewski, K.M. Radiogenomics in renal cell carcinoma. *Abdom. Radiol.* **2019**, *44*, 1990–1998. [CrossRef] [PubMed]
4. Jamshidi, N.; Jonasch, E.; Zapala, M.; Korn, R.L.; Brooks, J.D.; Ljungberg, B.; Kuo, M.D. The radiogenomic risk score stratifies outcomes in a renal cell cancer phase 2 clinical trial. *Eur. Radiol.* **2016**, *26*, 2798–2807. [CrossRef] [PubMed]
5. Gillies, R.J.; Kinahan, P.E.; Hricak, H. Radiomics: Images are more than pictures, they are data. *Radiology* **2016**, *278*, 563–577. [CrossRef] [PubMed]
6. Katabathina, V.S.; Marji, H.; Khanna, L.; Ramani, N.; Yedururi, S.; Dasyam, A.; Menias, C.O.; Prasad, S.R. Decoding genes: Current update on radiogenomics of select abdominal malignancies. *RadioGraphics* **2020**, *40*, 1600–1626. [CrossRef]
7. Lubner, M.G.; Smith, A.D.; Sandrasegaran, K.; Sahani, D.V.; Pickhard, P.J. CT texture analysis: Definitions, applications, biologic correlates, and challenges. *Radiographics* **2017**, *37*, 1483–1503. [CrossRef]
8. Davnall, F.; Yip, C.S.; Ljungqvist, G.; Selmi, M.; Ng, F.; Sanghera, B.; Ganeshan, B.; Miles, K.A.; Cook, G.J.; Goh, V. Assessment of tumor heterogeneity: An emerging imaging tool for clinical practice? *Insights Into. Imaging* **2012**, *3*, 573–589. [CrossRef]
9. Karlo, C.A.; Di Paolo, P.L.; Chaim, J.; Hakimi, A.A.; Ostrovnaya, I.; Russo, P.; Hricak, H.; Motzer, R.; Hsieh, J.J.; Akin, O. Radiogenomics of clear cell renal cell carcinoma: Associations between CT imaging features and mutations. *Radiology* **2014**, *270*, 464–471. [CrossRef]
10. Shinagare, A.B.; Vikram, R.; Jaffe, C.; Akin, O.; Kirby, J.; Huang, E.; Freymann, J.; Sainani, N.I.; Sadow, C.A.; Bathala, T.K.; et al. Radiogenomics of clear cell renal cell carcinoma: Preliminary findings of the cancer genome atlas–renal cell carcinoma (TCGA-RCC) imaging research group. *Abdom. Imaging* **2015**, *40*, 1684–1692. [CrossRef]
11. Greco, F.; Mallio, C.A. Relationship between visceral adipose tissue and genetic mutations (VHL and KDM5C) in clear cell renal cell carcinoma. *La Radiol. Med.* **2021**, *126*, 645–651. [CrossRef] [PubMed]
12. Feng, Z.; Zhang, L.; Qi, Z.; Shen, Q.; Hu, Z.; Chen, F. Identifying BAP1 mutations in clear-cell renal cell carcinoma by CT radiomics: Preliminary findings. *Front. Oncol.* **2020**, *10*, 279. [CrossRef] [PubMed]
13. Kocak, B.; Durmaz, E.S.; Kaya, O.K.; Kilickesmez, O. Machine learning-based unenhanced CT texture analysis for predicting BAP1 mutation status of clear cell renal cell carcinomas. *Acta Radiol.* **2020**, *61*, 856–864. [CrossRef] [PubMed]
14. Ghosh, P.; Tamboli, P.; Vikram, R.; Rao, A. Imaging-genomic pipeline for identifying gene mutations using three-dimensional intra-tumor heterogeneity features. *J. Med. Imaging* **2015**, *2*, 041009. [CrossRef]
15. Kocak, B.; Durmaz, E.S.; Ates, E.; Ulusan, M.B. Radiogenomics in clear cell renal cell carcinoma: Machine learning–based high-dimensional quantitative CT texture analysis in predicting PBRM1 mutation status. *Am. J. Roentgenol.* **2019**, *212*, W55–W63. [CrossRef]
16. Chen, X.; Zhou, Z.; Hannan, R.; Thomas, K.; Pedrosa, I.; Kapur, P.; Brugarolas, J.; Mou, X.; Wang, J. Reliable gene mutation prediction in clear cell renal cell carcinoma through multi-classifier multi-objective radiogenomics model. *Phys. Med. Biol.* **2018**, *63*, 215008. [CrossRef]
17. Marigliano, C.; Badia, S.; Bellini, D.; Rengo, M.; Caruso, D.; Tito, C.; Miglietta, S.; Palleschi, G.; Pastore, A.L.; Carbone, A.; et al. Radiogenomics in clear cell renal cell carcinoma: Correlations between advanced CT imaging (texture analysis) and microRNAs expression. *Technol. Cancer Res. Treat.* **2019**, *18*, 1533033819878458. [CrossRef]
18. Cen, D.; Xu, L.; Zhang, S.; Chen, Z.; Huang, Y.; Li, Z.; Liang, B. Renal cell carcinoma: Predicting RUNX3 methylation level and its consequences on survival with CT features. *Eur. Radiol.* **2019**, *29*, 5415–5422. [CrossRef]
19. Yu, T.; Lin, C.; Li, X.; Quan, X. Renal Cell Carcinoma: Predicting DNA Methylation Subtyping and Its Consequences on Overall Survival With Computed Tomography Imaging Characteristics. *J. Comput. Assist. Tomogr.* **2020**, *44*, 737–743. [CrossRef]
20. Jamshidi, N.; Jonasch, E.; Zapala, M.; Korn, R.L.; Aganovic, L.; Zhao, H.; Tumkur Sitaram, R.; Tibshirani, R.J.; Banerjee, S.; Brooks, J.D.; et al. The radiogenomic risk score: Construction of a prognostic quantitative, noninvasive image-based molecular assay for renal cell carcinoma. *Radiology* **2015**, *277*, 114–123. [CrossRef]
21. Bowen, L.; Xiaojing, L. Radiogenomics of clear cell renal cell carcinoma: Associations between mRNA-based subtyping and CT imaging features. *Acad. Radiol.* **2019**, *26*, e32–e37. [CrossRef] [PubMed]
22. Yin, Q.; Hung, S.-C.; Rathmell, W.K.; Shen, L.; Wang, L.; Lin, W.; Fielding, J.R.; Khandani, A.H.; Woods, M.E.; Milowsky, M.I.; et al. Integrative radiomics expression predicts molecular subtypes of primary clear cell renal cell carcinoma. *Clin. Radiol.* **2018**, *73*, 782–791. [CrossRef] [PubMed]

23. Lee, H.W.; Cho, H.-H.; Joung, J.-G.; Jeon, H.G.; Jeong, B.C.; Jeon, S.S.; Lee, H.M.; Nam, D.H.; Park, W.Y.; Kim, C.K. Integrative radiogenomics approach for risk assessment of post-operative metastasis in pathological T1 renal cell carcinoma: A pilot retrospective cohort study. *Cancers* **2020**, *12*, 866. [CrossRef] [PubMed]
24. Zhao, Y.; Liu, G.; Sun, Q.; Zhai, G.; Wu, G.; Li, Z.-C. Validation of CT radiomics for prediction of distant metastasis after surgical resection in patients with clear cell renal cell carcinoma: Exploring the underlying signaling pathways. *Eur. Radiol.* **2021**, *31*, 5032–5040. [CrossRef] [PubMed]
25. Lin, P.; Lin, Y.-Q.; Gao, R.-Z.; Wen, R.; Qin, H.; He, Y.; Yang, H. Radiomic profiling of clear cell renal cell carcinoma reveals subtypes with distinct prognoses and molecular pathways. *Transl. Oncol.* **2021**, *14*, 101078. [CrossRef] [PubMed]
26. Huang, Y.; Zeng, H.; Chen, L.; Luo, Y.; Ma, X.; Zhao, Y. Exploration of an Integrative Prognostic Model of Radiogenomics Features With Underlying Gene Expression Patterns in Clear Cell Renal Cell Carcinoma. *Front. Oncol.* **2021**, *11*, 330. [CrossRef] [PubMed]
27. Zeng, H.; Chen, L.; Wang, M.; Luo, Y.; Huang, Y.; Ma, X. Integrative radiogenomics analysis for predicting molecular features and survival in clear cell renal cell carcinoma. *Aging* **2021**, *13*, 9960. [CrossRef]
28. Ricketts, C.J.; De Cubas, A.A.; Fan, H.; Smith, C.C.; Lang, M.; Reznik, E.; Bowlby, R.; Gibb, E.A.; Akbani, R.; Beroukhim, R.; et al. The cancer genome atlas comprehensive molecular characterization of renal cell carcinoma. *Cell Rep.* **2018**, *23*, 313–326. [CrossRef]
29. Sato, Y.; Yoshizato, T.; Shiraishi, Y.; Maekawa, S.; Okuno, Y.; Kamura, T.; Shimamura, T.; Sato-Otsubo, A.; Nagae, G.; Suzuki, H.; et al. Integrated molecular analysis of clear-cell renal cell carcinoma. *Nat. Genet.* **2013**, *45*, 860–867. [CrossRef]
30. Brugarolas, J. Molecular genetics of clear-cell renal cell carcinoma. *J. Clin. Oncol.* **2014**, *32*, 1968. [CrossRef]
31. Joseph, R.W.; Kapur, P.; Serie, D.J.; Parasramka, M.; Ho, T.H.; Cheville, J.C.; Frenkel, E.; Parker, A.S.; Brugarolas, J. Clear cell renal cell carcinoma subtypes identified by BAP1 and PBRM1 expression. *J. Urol.* **2016**, *195*, 180–187. [CrossRef] [PubMed]
32. Hsieh, J.J.; Chen, D.; Wang, P.I.; Marker, M.; Redzematovic, A.; Chen, Y.-B.; Selcuklu, S.D.; Weinhold, N.; Bouvier, N.; Huberman, K.H.; et al. Genomic biomarkers of a randomized trial comparing first-line everolimus and sunitinib in patients with metastatic renal cell carcinoma. *Eur. Urol.* **2017**, *71*, 405–414. [CrossRef] [PubMed]
33. Ge, Y.-Z.; Xu, L.-W.; Zhou, C.-C.; Lu, T.-Z.; Yao, W.-T.; Wu, R.; Zhao, Y.C.; Xu, X.; Hu, Z.K.; Wang, M.A.; et al. BAP1 mutation-specific microRNA signature predicts clinical outcomes in clear cell renal cell carcinoma patients with wild-type BAP1. *J. Cancer* **2017**, *8*, 2643. [CrossRef] [PubMed]
34. Liu, W.; Fu, Q.; An, H.; Chang, Y.; Zhang, W.; Zhu, Y.; Xu, L.; Xu, J. Decreased expression of SETD2 predicts unfavorable prognosis in patients with nonmetastatic clear-cell renal cell carcinoma. *Medicine* **2015**, *94*, e2004. [CrossRef]
35. Manley, B.J.; Reznik, E.; Ghanaat, M.; Kashan, M.; Becerra, M.F.; Casuscelli, J.; Tennenbaum, D.; Redzematovic, A.; Carlo, M.I.; Sato, Y.; et al. Characterizing recurrent and lethal small renal masses in clear cell renal cell carcinoma using recurrent somatic mutations. *Urol. Oncol. Semin. Orig. Investig.* **2019**, *37*, 12–17. [CrossRef]
36. Hakimi, A.; Ostrovnaya, I.; Reva, B.; Schultz, N.; Chen, Y.; Gonen, M.; Liu, H.; Takeda, S.; Voss, M.H.; Tickoo, S.K.; et al. ccRCC Cancer Genome Atlas (KIRC TCGA) Research Network investigators Adverse outcomes in clear cell renal cell carcinoma with mutations of 3p21 epigenetic regulators BAP1 and SETD2: A report by MSKCC and the KIRC TCGA research network. *Clin. Cancer Res.* **2013**, *19*, 3259–3267. [CrossRef]
37. Fu, H.; Liu, Y.; Xu, L.; Chang, Y.; Zhou, L.; Zhang, W.; Yang, Y.; Xu, J. Low expression of mucin-4 predicts poor prognosis in patients with clear-cell renal cell carcinoma. *Medicine* **2016**, *95*, e3225. [CrossRef]
38. Gati, A.; Kouidhi, S.; Marrakchi, R.; El Gaaied, A.; Kourda, N.; Derouiche, A.; Chebil, M.; Caignard, A.; Perier, A. Obesity and renal cancer: Role of adipokines in the tumor-immune system conflict. *Oncoimmunology* **2014**, *3*, e27810. [CrossRef]
39. Rajandram, R.; Perumal, K.; Yap, N.Y. Prognostic biomarkers in renal cell carcinoma: Is there a relationship with obesity? *Transl. Androl. Urol.* **2019**, *8*, S138. [CrossRef]
40. Tang, K.; Xu, H. Prognostic value of meta-signature miRNAs in renal cell carcinoma: An integrated miRNA expression profiling analysis. *Sci. Rep.* **2015**, *5*, 1–12. [CrossRef]
41. Chen, F.; Liu, X.; Cheng, Q.; Zhu, S.; Bai, J.; Zheng, J. RUNX3 regulates renal cell carcinoma metastasis via targeting miR-6780a-5p/E-cadherin/EMT signaling axis. *Oncotarget* **2017**, *8*, 101042. [CrossRef] [PubMed]
42. Chen, F.; Bai, J.; Li, W.; Mei, P.; Liu, H.; Li, L.; Pan, Z.; Wu, Y.; Zheng, J. RUNX3 suppresses migration, invasion and angiogenesis of human renal cell carcinoma. *PLoS ONE* **2013**, *8*, e56241. [CrossRef]
43. Yan, C.; Kim, Y.W.; Ha, Y.S.; Kim, I.Y.; Kim, Y.J.; Yun, S.J.; Moon, S.K.; Bae, S.C.; Kim, W.J. RUNX3 methylation as a predictor for disease progression in patients with non-muscle-invasive bladder cancer. *J. Surg. Oncol.* **2012**, *105*, 425–430. [CrossRef] [PubMed]
44. Richiardi, L.; Fiano, V.; Vizzini, L.; De Marco, L.; Delsedime, L.; Akre, O.; Tos, A.G.; Merletti, F. Promoter methylation in APC, RUNX3, and GSTP1 and mortality in prostate cancer patients. *J. Clin. Oncol.* **2009**, *27*, 3161–3168. [CrossRef] [PubMed]
45. Ueno, K.; Hirata, H.; Majid, S.; Chen, Y.; Zaman, M.S.; Tabatabai, Z.L.; Hinoda, Y.; Dahiya, R. Wnt antagonist DICKKOPF-3 (Dkk-3) induces apoptosis in human renal cell carcinoma. *Mol. Carcinog.* **2011**, *50*, 449–457. [CrossRef] [PubMed]
46. Urakami, S.; Shiina, H.; Enokida, H.; Hirata, H.; Kawamoto, K.; Kawakami, T.; Kikuno, N.; Tanaka, Y.; Majid, S.; Nakagawa, M.; et al. Wnt antagonist family genes as biomarkers for diagnosis, staging, and prognosis of renal cell carcinoma using tumor and serum DNA. *Clin. Cancer Res.* **2006**, *12*, 6989–6997. [CrossRef]
47. Zhao, H.; Ljungberg, B.; Grankvist, K.; Rasmuson, T.; Tibshirani, R.; Brooks, J.D. Gene expression profiling predicts survival in conventional renal cell carcinoma. *PLoS Med.* **2006**, *3*, e13. [CrossRef]
48. Network CGAR. Comprehensive molecular characterization of clear cell renal cell carcinoma. *Nature* **2013**, *499*, 43. [CrossRef]

49. De Velasco, G.; Culhane, A.C.; Fay, A.P.; Hakimi, A.A.; Voss, M.H.; Tannir, N.M.; Tamboli, P.; Appleman, L.J.; Bellmunt, J.; Kimryn Rathmell, W.; et al. Molecular subtypes improve prognostic value of international metastatic renal cell carcinoma database consortium prognostic model. *Oncologist* **2017**, *22*, 286. [CrossRef]
50. Brannon, A.R.; Reddy, A.; Seiler, M.; Arreola, A.; Moore, D.T.; Pruthi, R.S.; Wallen, E.M.; Nielsen, M.E.; Liu, H.; Nathanson, K.L.; et al. Molecular stratification of clear cell renal cell carcinoma by consensus clustering reveals distinct subtypes and survival patterns. *Genes Cancer* **2010**, *1*, 152–163. [CrossRef]
51. Gulati, S.; Martinez, P.; Joshi, T.; Birkbak, N.J.; Santos, C.R.; Rowan, A.J.; Pickering, L.; Gore, M.; Larkin, J.; Szallasi, Z.; et al. Systematic evaluation of the prognostic impact and intratumour heterogeneity of clear cell renal cell carcinoma biomarkers. *Eur. Urol.* **2014**, *66*, 936–948. [CrossRef] [PubMed]
52. Ricketts, C.J.; Hill, V.K.; Linehan, W.M. Tumor-specific hypermethylation of epigenetic biomarkers, including SFRP1, predicts for poorer survival in patients from the TCGA Kidney Renal Clear Cell Carcinoma (KIRC) project. *PLoS ONE* **2014**, *9*, e85621. [CrossRef] [PubMed]
53. Morris, M.R.; Ricketts, C.; Gentle, D.; McRonald, F.; Carli, N.; Khalili, H.; Brown, M.; Kishida, T.; Yao, M.; Banks, R.E.; et al. Genome-wide methylation analysis identifies epigenetically inactivated candidate tumour suppressor genes in renal cell carcinoma. *Oncogene* **2011**, *30*, 1390–1401. [CrossRef] [PubMed]
54. Kocak, B.; Durmaz, E.S.; Erdim, C.; Ates, E.; Kaya, O.K.; Kilickesmez, O. Radiomics of renal masses: Systematic review of reproducibility and validation strategies. *Am. J. Roentgenol.* **2020**, *214*, 129–136. [CrossRef]
55. Velazquez, E.R.; Aerts, H.J.; Gu, Y.; Goldgof, D.B.; De Ruysscher, D.; Dekker, A.; Korn, R.; Gillies, R.J.; Lambin, P. A semiautomatic CT-based ensemble segmentation of lung tumors: Comparison with oncologists' delineations and with the surgical specimen. *Radiother. Oncol.* **2012**, *105*, 167–173. [CrossRef]
56. van Dam, I.E.; de Koste, J.R.v.S.; Hanna, G.G.; Muirhead, R.; Slotman, B.J.; Senan, S. Improving target delineation on 4-dimensional CT scans in stage I NSCLC using a deformable registration tool. *Radiother. Oncol.* **2010**, *96*, 67–72. [CrossRef]
57. Nguyen, K.; Schieda, N.; James, N.; McInnes, M.D.; Wu, M.; Thornhill, R.E. Effect of phase of enhancement on texture analysis in renal masses evaluated with non-contrast-enhanced, corticomedullary, and nephrographic phase–enhanced CT images. *Eur. Radiol.* **2021**, *31*, 1676–1686. [CrossRef]
58. Lu, L.; Ahmed, F.S.; Akin, O.; Luk, L.; Guo, X.; Yang, H.; Yoon, J.; Hakimi, A.A.; Schwartz, L.H.; Zhao, B. Uncontrolled Confounders May Lead to False or Overvalued Radiomics Signature: A Proof of Concept Using Survival Analysis in a Multicenter Cohort of Kidney Cancer. *Front. Oncol.* **2021**, *11*, 1397. [CrossRef]
59. Kocak, B.; Kaya, O.K.; Erdim, C.; Kus, E.A.; Kilickesmez, O. Artificial intelligence in renal mass characterization: A systematic review of methodologic items related to modeling, performance evaluation, clinical utility, and transparency. *Am. J. Roentgenol.* **2020**, *215*, 1113–1122. [CrossRef]
60. Zhong, W.; Li, Y.; Yuan, Y.; Zhong, H.; Huang, C.; Huang, J.; Lin, Y.; Huang, J. Characterization of Molecular Heterogeneity Associated With Tumor Microenvironment in Clear Cell Renal Cell Carcinoma to Aid Immunotherapy. *Front. Cell Dev. Biol.* **2021**, *9*, 736540. [CrossRef]
61. Gullo, R.L.; Daimiel, I.; Morris, E.A.; Pinker, K. Combining molecular and imaging metrics in cancer: Radiogenomics. *Insights Into. Imaging* **2020**, *11*, 1–17. [CrossRef]
62. Baxi, V.; Edwards, R.; Montalto, M.; Saha, S. Digital pathology and artificial intelligence in translational medicine and clinical practice. *Mod. Pathol.* **2022**, *35*, 23–32. [CrossRef] [PubMed]
63. Serie, D.J.; Joseph, R.W.; Cheville, J.C.; Ho, T.H.; Parasramka, M.; Hilton, T.; Thompson, R.H.; Leibovich, B.C.; Parker, A.S.; Eckel-Passow, J.E. Clear cell type A and B molecular subtypes in metastatic clear cell renal cell carcinoma: Tumor heterogeneity and aggressiveness. *Eur. Urol.* **2017**, *71*, 979–985. [CrossRef] [PubMed]
64. Mazurowski, M.A. Radiogenomics: What it is and why it is important. *J. Am. Coll. Radiol.* **2015**, *12*, 862–866. [CrossRef] [PubMed]

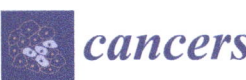

Review

First-Line Treatment of Metastatic Clear Cell Renal Cell Carcinoma: What Are the Most Appropriate Combination Therapies?

Yann-Alexandre Vano [1,*], Sylvain Ladoire [2], Réza Elaidi [3], Slimane Dermeche [4], Jean-Christophe Eymard [5], Sabrina Falkowski [6], Marine Gross-Goupil [7], Gabriel Malouf [8], Bérangère Narciso [9], Christophe Sajous [10], Sophie Tartas [10], Eric Voog [11] and Alain Ravaud [12]

1. Georges Pompidou European Hospital, 75015 Paris, France
2. Georges François Leclerc Centre, 21000 Dijon, France; sladoire@cgfl.fr
3. Association for the Research of Innovative Therapeutics in Cancerology (ARTIC), 75015 Paris, France; relaidi@gmail.com
4. Paoli Calmettes Institute, 13009 Marseille, France; DERMECHES@ipc.unicancer.fr
5. Jean Godinot Institute, 51100 Reims, France; jc.eymard@reims.unicancer.fr
6. Limoges Polyclinic, 87000 Limoges, France; s.falkowski@polyclinique-limoges.fr
7. Saint André Hospital, Bordeaux University Hospital, 33000 Bordeaux, France; marine.gross-goupil@chu-bordeaux.fr
8. Institute of Cancerology of Strasbourg (ICANS), 67200 Strasbourg, France; maloufg@igbmc.fr
9. Tours University Hospital, 37000 Tours, France; berengere.narciso@univ-tours.fr
10. Lyon Civil Hospices Institute of Cancerology, Pierre Bénite, 69002 Lyon, France; christophe.sajous@chu-lyon.fr (C.S.); sophie.tartas@chu-lyon.fr (S.T.)
11. Victor Hugo Clinic, Inter-Regional Institute of Cancerology, 72000 Le Mans, France; e.voog@ilcgroupe.fr
12. Bordeaux University Hospital, 33000 Bordeaux, France; alain.ravaud@chu-bordeaux.fr
* Correspondence: yann.vano@aphp.fr

Simple Summary: First-line treatment options for metastatic clear cell renal cell carcinoma have significantly increased. The current recommended therapeutic strategy is based on a combination, but monotherapy remains an alternative. However, the choice of the type of combination, i.e., dual immunotherapy or immunotherapy combined with an antiangiogenic drug, has not been clearly standardized. A strategy based on the International Metastatic Database Consortium (IMDC) classification is currently recommended with pembrolizumab + axitinib, cabozantinib + nivolumab, and lenvatinib + pembrolizumab (for all patients) or nivolumab + ipilimumab (for patients with intermediate or poor risk), which are the first-line treatment standards of care. This review summarizes all recent data from the main combinations evaluated in first-line treatment and discusses the choice of drugs according to the patient's profile and the benefit/risk balances of each combination.

Abstract: The development of antiangiogenic treatments, followed by immune checkpoint inhibitors (ICI), has significantly changed the management of metastatic clear cell renal cell cancer. Several phase III trials show the superiority of combination therapy, dual immunotherapy (ICI-ICI) or ICI plus tyrosine kinase inhibitors (TKI) of the vascular endothelium growth factor (VEGF) over sunitinib monotherapy. The question is therefore what is the best combination for a given patient? A strategy based on the International Metastatic Database Consortium (IMDC) classification is currently recommended with pembrolizumab + axitinib, cabozantinib + nivolumab, and lenvatinib + pembrolizumab (for all patients) or nivolumab + ipilimumab (for patients with intermediate or poor risk), which are the first-line treatment standards of care. However, several issues remain unresolved and require further investigation, such as the PD-L1 status, the relevance of possible options based on the patient's profile, and consideration of second-line and subsequent treatments.

Keywords: metastatic clear cell renal cell carcinoma; first-line treatment; immunotherapy; tyrosine kinase inhibitors; combinations

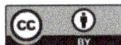

1. Introduction

Clear cell renal cell carcinoma (ccRCC) used to be associated with a very poor prognosis when diagnosed at an advanced stage. The last 15 years have provided dramatic improvements in this field, thanks to the development of vascular endothelial growth factor (VEGF) tyrosine kinase inhibitors (TKI) followed by immune checkpoint inhibitors (ICIs) [1,2]. ICIs are monoclonal antibodies directed against immune checkpoints and enable the reversal of tumor-induced immunosuppression. Currently, the anti-checkpoint agents used in oncology target inhibitory receptors present on the surface of lymphocytes such as programmed cell death 1 (PD-1) and cytotoxic T lymphocyte–associated protein 4 (CTLA-4) or their ligands (PD-L1, programmed cell death ligand 1) [3,4]. Combining therapies to further improve survival and response rates has been tested in large phase III randomized trials, in particular CheckMate-214 (nivolumab (PD-1) + ipilimumab (CTLA-4) vs. sunitinib (TKI)), JAVELIN Renal 101 (axitinib (TKI) + avelumab (PD-L1), vs. sunitinib), KEYNOTE-426 (axitinib + pembrolizumab (PD-1) vs. sunitinib), CheckMate 9ER (nivolumab + ipilimumab vs. sunitinib) and CLEAR (lenvatinib (TKI) + pembrolizumab) [5–12]. These trials were positive, showing the superiority of the combination, i.e., dual immunotherapy (ICI-ICI) or ICI plus TKI (ICI-TKI) over sunitinib monotherapy. A recent meta-analysis including these trials confirms that immune-based combinations are more effective than sunitinib monotherapy with a three-fold increase in the complete response rate [4]. According to the recently updated European guidelines, lenvatinib + pembrolizumab joins other VEGFR+PD-1 inhibitor-targeted combinations (axitinib + pembrolizumab or cabozantinib + nivolumab) to be recommended for first-line treatment of advanced ccRCC irrespective of International Metastatic RCC Database Consortium (IMDC) risk groups. Ipilimumab + nivolumab also continues to be recommended for first-line treatment of IMDC intermediate- and poor-risk (I/P) patients [13,14]. One of the most critical emerging questions now is how to select the best option for a given patient? A recent article suggested treatment algorithms for first-line treatment in metastatic ccRCC (mccRCC) with a wide spectrum of treatment recommendations based on multiple decision criteria demonstrated. Significant inter-expert variations were observed [15]. Herein, we review recent data and discuss how, for a given patient, the best strategy should be chosen. Our approach integrates data available in routine clinical practice, such as effectiveness data, IMDC groups, PD-L1 status, tolerability of treatments and perspectives of treatment sequence.

2. Overview of Studies in First-Line Metastasis

Today, the European Society for Medical Oncology (ESMO) recommends dual immunotherapy (ICI-ICI) or a combination of immunotherapy and antiangiogenics (ICI-TKI) for patients with mccRCC. Dual immunotherapy is recommended only for patients with an intermediate or poor risk tumor, which constitutes approximately 80% of patients with advanced ccRCC (Figure 1) [13,14].

This combination improves survival outcome in these patients with mccRCC. The CheckMate-214 study comparing nivolumab + ipilimumab (NIVO + IPI) to sunitinib (SUN) showed results in favor of the combination, which was confirmed by updated results over four years [5,6]. Overall survival (OS) (hazard ratio (HR); 95% confidence interval (CI)) remained superior with NIVO + IPI compared with SUN in the intention-to-treat (ITT) population (0.69; 0.59 to 0.81) and particularly in patients with I/P disease (0.65; 0.54 to 0.78). Four-year progression-free survival (PFS) rates were 31.0% vs. 17.3% (ITT) and 32.7% vs. 12.3% (I/P) in the NIVO + IPI group vs. SUN. The objective response rate (ORR) remained higher with NIVO + IPI vs. SUN in the ITT population (39.1% vs. 32.4%) and in the I/P risk group (41.9% vs. 26.8%). Similarly, the complete response rate (CR) was 10.7% vs. 2.6% in the ITT population and 10.4% vs. 1.4% in the I/P risk population for the NIVO + IPI groups vs. SUN, respectively.

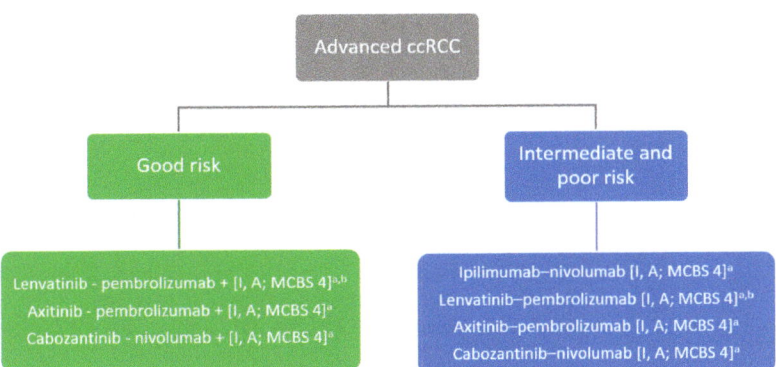

Figure 1. ESMO Clinical Practice Guideline update: Systemic first-line treatment of clear cell renal cell carcinoma (ccRCC) [14]. ccRCC, clear cell renal cell cancer; EMA, European Medicines Agency; ESMO-MCBS, European Society for Medical Oncology-Magnitude of Clinical Benefit Scale; FDA, Food and Drug Administration; IMDC, International Metastatic RCC Database Consortium; MCBS, ESMO-Magnitude of Clinical Scale; VEGFR, vascular endothelial growth factor receptor. a ESMO-MCBS v1.1 score for new therapy/indication approved by the EMA or FDA. The score has been calculated by the ESMO-MCBS Working Group and validated by the ESMO Guidelines Committee; b FDA approved; not currently EMA approved.

The first major trial for the ICI plus VEGFR TKI with axitinib combination was KEYNOTE-426. The first results at 14 months and then at 30 months were clearly in favor of the pembrolizumab + axitinib (PEMBRO + AXI) combination [9,10]. The 42.8-month update confirmed the superiority over all endpoints in the ITT population: median OS of 45.7 vs. 40.1 months (HR 0.73 [95% CI: 0.60, 0.88], $p < 0.001$), median PFS of 15.7 vs. 11.1 months (HR 0.68 [0.58–0.80], $p < 0.0001$) and ORR 60% (10% CR) vs. 40% (3.5% CR) ($p < 0.0001$), respectively [16]. These results confirmed the status of PEMBRO + AXI as a first-line treatment standard for all patients according to the latest European recommendations [13,14]. Another immunotherapy combination trial—the JAVELIN Renal 101 trial—reported, with 13 months of follow-up, superior PFS of avelumab + axitinib (AVE + AXI) vs. SUN, whether in patients with PD-L1 positive (PD-L1$^+$) tumors (HR 0.61; $p < 0.0001$; 13.8 vs. 7.2 months) or in the overall population (HR 0.69; $p < 0.0001$; 13.8 vs. 8.4 months). This combination did not appear in the recommendations due to a lack of OS benefit [7,8]. A third interim analysis over more than two years confirmed these data, with a non-statistically significant OS benefit and a PFS of 13.9 vs. 8.5 months (HR 0.67; $p < 0.0001$) [17]. More recently, the CheckMate 9ER study evaluated the cabozantinib and nivolumab (CABO + NIVO) combination and showed an OS benefit compared with SUN monotherapy (HR 0.6; 95% CI: 0.4–0.49; $p = 0.001$) and PFS (16.6 vs. 8.3 months; HR 0.51; 95% CI: 0.41–0.64; $p < 0.0001$) with an ORR of 55.7%, including 8% of CR [11]. With an 18-month follow-up, this trial was largely positive for survival and response rates. Only 6% of patients were progressive from the outset, and this combination was therefore also promising. The last combination of interest was lenvatinib + pembrolizumab (LENVA + PEMBRO) compared with SUN monotherapy in the phase III CLEAR study in 1069 treatment-naïve patients with mccRCC [12]. With a median follow-up of 27 months, this study was clearly positive for its primary endpoint with a median PFS of 23.9 months (20.8–27.7) in the LENVA + PEMBRO arm versus 9.2 months (6.0–11.0) in the SUN arm (HR 0.39; 0.32–0.49; $p < 0.001$). PFS was improved regardless of the IMDC subgroup or sarcomatoid contingent. Lenvatinib + everolimus also met the primary endpoint, with median PFS of 14.7 months versus 9.2 months for SUN, representing a 35% improvement in favor of this combination. The LENVA + PEMBRO combination significantly improved OS compared to SUN (HR 0.66; 0.49–0.69; $p = 0.005$) with a particularly marked benefit in IMDC poor risk group

(HR 0.30). The ORR in the LENVA + PEMBRO arm was 71%, including 16% of CR. Only 5.4% of patients experienced immediate progression following the introduction of LENVA + PEMBRO. It should be noted that in this study a high proportion of patients had a good prognosis, with a spontaneously more favorable history. Nevertheless, this combination provided the longest PFS or OS durations ever reported in a pivotal phase III trial (Table 1).

3. Pending Questions and Impact on Clinical Practice

3.1. Comparisons of Combinations

Given the number of effective first-line treatment options and the absence of direct comparison studies, the major question is which combination to prescribe to which patients? A recent meta-analysis indirectly compared the three combinations NIVO + IPI, PEMBRO + AXI, and AVE + AXI in terms of PFS, OS, and ORR, with a trend in favor of the PEMBRO + AXI combination [18]. However, this meta-analysis did not include the last two combinations and was based solely on published, non-individual data. The IMDC consortium compared the NIVO + IPI or ICI (anti-PD-(L)1)-TKI combinations in 723 patients including 546 with I/P risk [19]. This retrospective analysis of a large number of patients required very careful interpretation as the quality of the data collected varied. The ORR was 37% vs. 59% in the NIVO + IPI and ICI-TKI arms, respectively, which was quite similar to the phase III data. In contrast, CR rates were similar in both arms, but lower than those in trials at only 4%. OS was not significantly different between the two types of treatment received: 40.2 vs. 39.7 months for NIVO + IPI vs. ICI-TKI (HR adjusted 0.92, $p = 0.71$), respectively. Based on the OS parameter alone, this analysis showed that there was no combination more effective than another in this poorly selected population. But it seemed that the benefit in OS was maintained over time for NIVO + IPI (constant HR), while the HR increased for the PEMBRO + AXI association. Finally, the meta-analysis of Quhal et al.—incorporating six studies (CheckMate-214, Keynote-426, IMmotion-151, JAVELIN Renal 101, Checkmate-9ER, and CLEAR), i.e., 5121 patients—suggested that ICI-TKI combinations provided superior PFS, ORR, and OS vs. ICI-ICI combinations, independent of the IMDC group [20]. Based on treatment classification analysis, NIVO + CABO was most likely to provide maximum OS (p-score 0.7573). These comparisons remain indirect and limited by the variability of patient characteristics in the trials evaluated (prognostic risk categories and PD-L1 expression) and differences in subsequent treatments received that may influence OS outcomes.

Table 1. Phase III trials of the immune checkpoint-based regimens evaluated in treatment-naïve mccRCC.

Parameter	CheckMate-214 [5,6]	JAVELIN Renal-101 [7,8]	KEYNOTE-426 [9,16]	CheckMate-9ER [11]	CLEAR [12]
Number of patients	1096	886	861	651	1069
Treatment arms	Nivolumab + ipilimumab (n = 550) vs. sunitinib (n = 546)	Avelumab + axitinib (n = 442) vs. sunitinib (n = 444)	Pembrolizumab + axitinib (n = 432) vs. sunitinib (n = 429)	Nivolumab + cabozantinib (n = 323) vs. sunitinib (n = 328)	Lenvatinib + pembrolizumab (n = 355) vs. lenvatinib + everolimus (n = 357) vs. sunitinib (n = 357)
Primary outcome	ORR, PFS and OS in I/P risk patients	PFS and OS in PD-L1+ patients	PFS and OS	PFS	PFS
Median follow-up, mo	55	13	42.8	18.1	27
Median OS, mo	ITT group: NR vs. 38.4 HR 0.69; 95% CI 0.59, 0.81 I/P-risk: 48.1 vs. 26.6 HR 0.65; 95% CI 0.54, 0.78	PD-L1+: NE vs. 28.6 HR 0.83; 95% CI 0.60, 1.15; p = 0.1301 ITT group: NE vs. NE HR 0.80; 95% CI, 0.62, 1.03 p = 0.0392	45.7 vs. 40 HR 0.73; 95% CI 0.60, 0.88; p < 0.001	NR vs. NR HR 0.60; 95% CI 0.40, 0.89; p = 0.0010	NR vs. NR vs. NR HR vs. Sun = 0.66; 95% CI 0.49, 0.69; p = 0.005
Median PFS, mo	ITT group: 12.2 vs. 12.3 HR 0.89; 95% CI 0.76, 1.05 I/P-risk: 11.2 vs. 8.3 HR 0.74; 95% CI 0.62, 0.88	PD-L1+: 13.8 vs. 7.0 HR 0.62; 95% CI 0.49, 0.78; p < 0.0001 ITT group: 13.3 vs. 8.0 HR 0.69; 95% CI, 0.57, 0.83; p < 0.0001	15.7 vs. 11.1 HR 0.68; 95% CI 0.58, 0.80; p < 0.0001	16.6 vs. 8.3 HR 0.51; 95% CI 0.41, 0.64; p < 0.0001	23.9 vs. 14.7 vs. 9.2 HR vs. Sun: 0.39; 95% CI 0.32, 0.49; p < 0.001
ORR, %	ITT group: 39.1 vs. 32.4 I/P risk: 41.9 vs. 26.8	PD-L1+: 55.9 vs. 27.2 ITT group: 52.5 vs. 27.3	60.4 vs. 39.6	55.7 vs. 27.1	71.0 vs. 53.5 vs. 36.1
Complete response, %	ITT group: 10.7 vs. 2.6 I/P risk: 10.4 vs. 1.4	PD-L1+: 5.6 vs. 2.4 Overall pop: 3.8 vs. 2.0	10.0 vs. 3.5	8.0 vs. 4.6	16.1 vs. 9.8 vs. 4.2
Partial response, %	ITT group: 28.4 vs. 29.9 I/P risk: 31.5 vs. 25.4	PD-L1+: 50.4 vs. 24.8 Overall pop: 48.6 vs. 25.2	50.5 vs. 36.1	47.7 vs. 22.6	54.9 vs. 43.7 vs. 31.9
Stable disease, %	ITT group: 36.0 vs. 42.1 I/P risk: 30.8 vs. 44.3	PD-L1+: 27.0 vs. 41.4 Overall pop: 28.3 vs. 43.7	22.9 vs. 35.4	32.2 vs. 42.1	19.2 vs. 33.6 vs. 38.1
Progressive disease, %	ITT group: 17.6 vs. 14.1 I/P risk: 19.3 vs. 16.8	PD-L1+: 11.5 vs. 22.4 Overall pop: 12.4 vs. 19.4	11.3 vs. 17.0	5.6 vs. 13.7	5.4 vs. 7.3 vs. 14.0
Toxicities Events, %	All grades: 94.0 vs. 97.4 G3/4: 47.9 vs. 64.1	All grades: 99.5 vs. 99.3 G3/4: 71.2 vs. 71.5	All grades: 96.3 vs. 97.6 G3/5: 67.8 vs. 63.8	All grades: 100 vs. 99 G3/4: 75 vs. 71	All grades: 96.9 vs. 97.7 vs. 92.1 G3/4: 71.6 vs. 73.0 vs. 58.8

CI, confidence interval; HR, hazard ratio; I/P, intermediate/poor risk; ITT, intention-to-treat population; mccRCC, metastatic clear cell renal cell carcinoma; NE, not estimable; NR, not reached; ORR, objective response rate; OS, overall survival; PFS, progression-free survival.

3.2. IMDC Groups

The patient's prognostic profile based on the IMDC risk score is a criterion that must be considered. The magnitude of the PFS benefit of the CABO + NIVO combination seemed particularly marked in patients with poor risk: HR 0.37 vs. 0.62 and 0.54 for patients with a good and intermediate risk, respectively. Similarly, OS benefits were greater in patients with poor risk, with a 63% reduction in the risk of death (HR 0.37 vs. 0.84 and 0.70 for a good and intermediate risk, respectively) [11]. The LENVA + PEMBRO combination presented similar results with a particularly significant OS benefit in the IMDC poor risk group (HR 0.30) and important response rates: 71% ORR and 16% CR. Given the significant percentage of CR, it may be an objective in its own right, but it remains to be seen whether it is influenced by the rather favorable population included in the trial or whether it is confirmed in real life or in other trials [12]. Moreover, the percentages of progression from the outset of both combinations were very low, at around 4–5% compared to 18% with NIVO + IPI [6,11,12]. Thus, in a patient at risk of rapid progression or presenting a threatening disease (e.g. threatening epiduritis with a high risk for spinal cord compression or bronchial compression) with a limited life expectancy, obtaining a rapid and important response could tip the decision towards an ICI-TKI combination (CABO + NIVO or LENVA + PEMBRO). Based on available data, it is still difficult to speculate whether the addition of CABO offers the combination a gain in efficacy on predominant or major bone lesions. Finally, an FDA analysis pooled individual data from 3447 patients from four randomized phase III trials of ICI-ICI ($n = 1$) or ICI-TKI ($n = 3$) combinations. Improvement in OS with combinations vs. SUN was found in I/P risk patients (HR 0.696; 95% CI: 0.62, 0.78) but not in patients with a good prognosis (HR 0.953; 95% CI: 0.72, 1.27) [21]. However, it should be noted that the monitoring, still too short in the trials, has not, for the time being, shown a benefit in OS or even PFS for the ICI-TKI combinations in these patients with a good prognosis, with only a benefit in ORR being found so far. In addition, IMDC favorable patients will be prone to receive first-line treatment for a long period of time, leading to an increased risk of experiencing cumulative TKI toxicities. Thus, in these patients, TKI is frequently interrupted which would be harmful, since it has been shown that their tumors are pro-angiogenic and highly sensitive to angiogenesis inhibitors [22]. As for ICI-ICI, PFS, and TR were lower than for TKI monotherapy, but the CR rates were higher and OS was comparable. According to the post-hoc analysis of the CheckMate 214 study performed according to the number of IMDC risk factors, a benefit of treatment with NIVO + IPI on SUN was found for all patients at intermediate risk, including those with one or two risk factors (ORR (40–44% vs. 16–38%), OS (HR 0.50–0.72), and PFS (HR 0.44–0.86)) [23]. All of these data favored combinations, including in patients with a good prognosis. Overall, it seemed relevant to have the second-line strategy in perspective when choosing the first-line treatment. Thus, in a patient without significant tumor volume and risk of rapid worsening, the criteria for the choice of treatment should include tolerance, continuation of treatment, and possible second-line treatment, leading the strategy towards ICI-ICI vs. ICI-TKI. Nevertheless, as part of a prolonged follow-up, the impact on the response rate—and possibly on OS—also leads us to consider an ICI-TKI combination.

3.3. Potential Impact of PD-L1 Status

PD-L1 status is a recognized prognostic factor, but its predictive response value to ICI remains to be demonstrated [24,25]. The meta-analysis of Mori et al. [26] investigated the predictive value of PD-L1 expression in patients with mccRCC treated with first-line ICI combinations. Based on key clinical outcomes, including response rate and PFS, the authors found that PD-L1$^+$ patients benefited more from ICI combinations than from SUN, with a PFS of 22 months vs. 6 months (HR 0.65, 95% CI: 0.57, 0.74, $p < 0.001$). In PD-L1$^+$ patients, NIVO + IPI resulted in a more significant improvement in efficacy criteria compared with ICI-TKI for all IMDC risk groups. Examined study by study, in the I/P subgroup of the CheckMate-214 study [5], OS was significantly better in the NIVO + IPI arm compared to SUN regardless of PD-L1 status, although the magnitude of OS benefit was greater in the PD-L1$^-$ subgroup (HR 0.73 vs. 0.45 for PD-L1$^+$). For ICI-TKI, the data were heterogeneous [7–11]. In KEYNOTE-426, the superiority of PEMBRO + AXI over SUN was maintained regardless of PD-L1 status (HR 0.54 for PD-L1$^+$ vs. HR 0.59 for PD-L1$^-$). Conversely, the CHECKMATE-9ER trial showed an impact of PD-L1 status, with a lower HR for OS in the PD-L1$^-$ population (0.51 vs. 0.80 for PD-L1$^+$). Similarly, in the CLEAR study, the OS benefit was particularly pronounced for PD-L1$^-$ status (HR 0.50 vs. HR 0.76 for PD-L1$^+$) [12]. However, these comparisons are questionable since the methods used to assess PD-L1 status differed according to the CheckMate-214/CheckMate-9ER, JAVELIN Renal 101 and KEYNOTE-426 studies: 28-8 clone (Dako), PD-L1 $\geq$ 1% in tumor cells, SP263 clone (Ventana), PD-L1 $\geq$ 1% in immune cells and 22C3 clone (Dako), Combined Positive Score (CPS) > 1% tumor cells plus immune cells, respectively [5–11]. This can probably partly explain why the proportion of the PD-L1$^+$ population varied so widely from study to study. In addition, a biomarker analysis was performed using data from the CheckMate-214 study [27], in which the PD-L1 status was defined on tumor cells, but also according to the CPS combining tumor cells and immune cells. The recovered PD-L1$^+$ level was 25% for tumor cells and 60% by CPS. The results of this analysis showed that when the proportion of positive patients increased, the OS benefit vs. SUN remained, but was of lower magnitude. Overall, the results diverged and harmonization of techniques in the future would allow a better comparison between the populations studied. To date, PD-L1 status does not seem to be a formal decision criterion in the choice of treatment, but it can be considered during the ICI-ICI vs. ICI-TKI decision. If PD-L1 status is assessed, it seems preferable to do so on tumor cells only since the most discriminant outcomes according to PD-L1 status has been shown in the CheckMate-214 study with ICI-ICI [27].

3.4. Tolerance Profile/Quality of Life

Tolerance and quality of life (QoL) are also important criteria for choosing the therapeutic strategy, especially as the potential lifespan increases. The type of adverse events (AEs) differs depending on the treatment or combination considered: there are more AEs with the ICI-TKI combination compared to ICI-ICI over the long term; however, when they occur in ICI-ICI, they may be more acute and unpredictable. Based on a meta-analysis that included four trials (CheckMate-214, Keynote-426, IMmotion-151 and JAVELIN Renal 101), ICI-based combinations were associated with a higher risk of all-grade pruritus (HR 3.11) and all-grade rash (HR 1.44) compared to patients treated with SUN. However, the combinations presented less grade 3/4 fatigue (HR 0.49) and nausea (HR 0.60) vs. SUN [28]. Another more recent meta-analysis incorporated the Checkmate-9ER and CLEAR studies [20]. Compared to the SUN, LENVA + PEMBRO was associated with the highest probability of treatment-related AEs of grade $\geq$3 (OR 1.84, 95% CI: 1.28, 2.64) and discontinuations (OR 3.55, 95% CI: 2.46, 5.12) [12]. NIVO + IPI was associated with the lowest rates of grade $\geq$3 AEs, but with a higher probability of endocrine-related AEs [20]. A higher probability of high-grade diarrhea was associated with PEMBRO + AXI and AVE + AXI. The duration of AEs was also different: in the CheckMate-214 study, ICI-ICI-related toxicity occurred mainly during the first four months of the study and subsequently stabilized while in the SUN arm, the rate of AEs remained more stable throughout the study, particularly for vascular, digestive, and hematological toxicities [5,6]. It should be noted that the benefit/risk balance of immunotherapy should be discussed in the first-line treatment for certain patient profiles, particularly those with inflammatory colitis, especially if they are active [29,30]. In patients over 75 years of age, OS was comparable but AEs were more frequent than in younger patients; however, this did not contraindicate the use of immunotherapy in these patients [6,31]. Given the small number of elderly patients enrolled in the trials, data from other or real-life trials remain necessary.

In terms of QoL, patient-reported outcomes (PROs) were assessed as an exploratory criterion in the CheckMate-214 trial and showed that combined treatment resulted in fewer symptoms and a better QoL than with SUN [32]. In the Checkmate-9ER study,

QoL was sustained over time with NIVO + CABO, while constant deterioration was observed with SUN. Combination therapy improved symptoms up to week 91 unlike SUN [11]. In an analysis of a secondary endpoint of HRQoL (Health-Related QoL) scores in the CLEAR trial, LENVA + PEMBRO demonstrated a similar time to first deterioration (TTD) in 14 out of 18 HRQoL and disease-related symptom scores, and a delay in TTD for physical functioning, dyspnea, appetite loss, and EQ-5D visual analog scale compared to SUN [33]. Overall, QoL improved when treated with ICI-ICI, but not with ICI-TKI due to continuous administration of antiangiogenics. It should be noted that in practice, induction of treatment with ICI-ICI requires close monitoring due to the specific nature of the AEs and access to a network of specialists and dedicated multidisciplinary consultative meetings (such as ImmunoTox).

3.5. Treatment Sequence: Second-Line and Subsequent Therapies

The therapeutic strategy is crucial for patients with a good prognosis: they have a life expectancy of several years and therefore a higher probability of receiving many lines unlike I/P patients. For the time being, there is no gain in OS, so it is too early to know whether a sequential approach with an antiangiogenic in the first-line treatment, based on the often-predominant angiogenic profile, and then immunotherapy in the second-line treatment, would really be inferior to a combination strategy from the outset. In patients with a good prognosis and a small-volume tumor for which a CR is achievable, the notion of the second-line treatment and the strategy of subsequent lines are important to consider. Based on data from the favorable prognostic patient group in the CheckMate-214 study [6], more than 50% of patients survived at 48 months (with an HR for OS of 0.69 in the NIVO + IPI arm vs. 0.65 in the SUN arm). However, there are numerous treatment options after a first-line treatment of SUN or post-NIVO + IPI, but fewer after CABO + NIVO or PEMBRO + LENVA. Indeed, after treatment with CABO, which has a strong anti-VEGFR2 effect, no solid data suggest the efficacy of SUN or AXI. It should be noted that HIF (Hypoxia Inducible Factor) inhibitors are being evaluated after these first-line strategies [34].

In patients with I/P risk who have received a first-line therapy with ICI-ICI combination, the question that arises is which TKI to choose for second-line therapy? A retrospective trial in 33 patients in the CheckMate 214 trial who received second-line TKI after ICI-ICI reported a median PFS of 8 months for first-generation TKI (sunitinib/pazopanib) and 7 months for second-generation TKI (axitinib/cabozantinib) (p = 0.66) [35]. This retrospective trial did not validate the feasibility of a second-line treatment by TKI after ICI-ICI or the choice of the first- or second-generation TKI molecule. Dudani et al. [36], using IMDC data, compared the efficacy of second-line treatment after ICI-ICI NIVO + IPI or after ICI-TKI. A total of 113 patients received ICI-TKI and 75 ICI-ICI in the first-line treatment, and 34 patients (30%) in the ICI-TKI group and 30 patients (40%) in the ICI-ICI group received a second-line treatment, mainly VEGF TKI (axitinib, cabozantinib, lenvatinib + everolimus, pazopanib and sunitinib). The second line response rate was 15% in the ICI-TKI group vs. 45% post-ICI-ICI (p = 0.04); however, the time to treatment failure (TTF) was not statistically different (3.7 vs. 5.4 months; p = 0.4). Updating of data in 142 patients, 103 of whom had received the second-line treatment, confirmed these results with a response rate that remained higher after ICI-ICI (37% vs. 12%, p < 0.01), but with no difference in OS or TTF [37]. Finally, a phase II study evaluating PEMBRO + LENVA after ICI, presented by Lee et al at ASCO 2020, reported an ORR of 47% in the 38 patients who received NIVO + IPI in first line [38]. The choice of TKI must therefore consider the patient's profile and the fact that a proportion of patients will not reach a third-line treatment. However, the optimal sequence remains to be validated in the trials.

Another question is: Is the introduction of an anti-CTLA-4 in salvage therapy after a lack of response to an anti-PD-1 monotherapy (NIVO or PEMBRO) in the first-line treatment of interest? To date, the only data on the use of NIVO + IPI after prior anti-PD-(L)1 failure are based on four non-randomized phase II trials that were presented at the ESMO 2019

(TITAN-RCC) and ASCO 2020 (FRACTION-RCC, OMNIVORE, and HCRN GU16-260) congresses [39–42]. The pooled analysis of the four studies ($n = 237$ patients) confirmed a low response rate of 10.0% associated with 27.0% of grade ≥ 3 AEs [43]. Finally, a small retrospective study of 45 patients reported results of the combination of NIVO + IPI in second-line treatment post-anti-PD-1 alone or in combination and/or post-TKI: after a median follow-up of 12 months, the ORR was 20% and the median PFS was 4 months (0.8–19 months) [44]. Overall, the combination of NIVO (anti-PD-1) + IPI (anti-CTLA-4) in patients who have already received anti-PD-(L)1 treatment, but no anti-CTLA-4, did not seem an option to retain and supported administering anti-CTLA-4 only in the setting of first-line treatment.

4. Outlook

Beyond sequential therapeutic strategy trials, researching biomarkers predictive of response to ICI is also essential. Among the biomarkers studied is the PD-L1 status, but also the molecular profiling of the tumor. Thus, the BIONIKK study assessed personalized treatments with ICI alone or ICI-ICI or TKI according to tumor molecular characteristics in mccRCC [45]. Using an expression signature of 35 genes, patients were divided into four molecular groups (1 to 4). Patients in groups 1 and 4 were randomized to receive NIVO alone or NIVO + IPI (four administrations) followed by NIVO alone. Patients in groups 2 and 3 were randomized to receive either NIVO + IPI followed by NIVO alone or a TKI (sunitinib or pazopanib) according to the investigator. The study questioned the interest of establishing a routine tumor molecular profile to optimize the choice of treatment between immunotherapy monotherapy, or an ICI-ICI or ICI-TKI combination. First results presented at the 2019 ESMO meeting were encouraging [46].

Finally, other developments in the therapeutic arsenal are expected in the coming years with, on one hand, potential intensification with first-line triplet CABO + NIVO + IPI and, on the other, the introduction of anti-PD-1 in the adjuvant setting [47] which may increase survival but will also impact subsequent lines. Furthermore, the time to progression (within 6–12 months or more than 12 months after the end of anti-PD-1) will likely influence the choice.

5. Conclusions

To conclude, currently the PEMBRO + AXI, CABO + NIVO (for all patients), and NIVO + IPI (for patients with I/P risk) combinations constitute the first-line management standard for mccRCC. However, multiplication of first-line treatment options continues and now no less than five combinations have robust data, with unfortunately no direct comparison study of the different combinations available. The choice of strategy must therefore be based on efficacy criteria, but also on the patient's risk profile and tolerance to each treatment (Table 2), while keeping the options of the subsequent lines in perspective. Given the complexity of choice, therapeutic sequence data with second-line combinations will become essential to guide the therapeutic strategy. Even if these combinations were approved regardless of the tumor PD-L1 status, the use of predictive biomarkers of response to ICI could, in the future, help determine the best personalized treatment strategy for each patient.

Table 2. Parameters guiding the choice of strategy between ICI/ICI and ICI/TKI combinations.

Parameter		ICI-ICI	ICI-TKI
Prolonged follow-up		✓	✓
Efficacy: overall	CR, OS	✓	✓
	ORR, PFS	✓	✓
Efficacy: subgroups	IMDC favorable	✗	✓
	IMDC intermediate/poor	✓	✓
	PD-L1+	✓	✓
	PD-L1-	✓	✓
Tolerability	Overall	✓	✗
	Cardiovascular	✓	✗
	Immune-mediated	✗	✓
Quality of life		✓	✓
Subsequent line options		✓	✗

Green check mark: in favor; Orange check mark: lacks information or does not allow to conclude; Red cross: rather in disfavor; CR, complete response rate; ICI, immune checkpoint inhibitors; IMDC, International Metastatic RCC Database Consortium; ORR, objective response rate; OS, overall survival; PD-L1, Programmed cell death ligand 1; PFS, progression free-survival; TKI, tyrosine kinase inhibitors.

Author Contributions: Y.-A.V., S.L. and A.R. contributed to the development of the outline, drafted, revised, and edited the manuscript. R.E., S.D., J.-C.E., S.F., M.G.-G., G.M., B.N., C.S., S.T. and E.V. reviewed the manuscript. All authors have read and agreed to the published version of the manuscript.

Funding: Medical writing support was provided by Celine Rouger of Medical Education Corpus Agency and was funded by Pfizer.

Conflicts of Interest: Yann-Alexandre Vano has received honoraria for advisory board from Bristol-Myers Squibb, Pfizer, Novartis, Ipsen, Merck, MSD, Janssen, Sanofi, Astellas Pharma, and Roche, and travel expenses/accommodations from Bristol-Myers Squibb, Pfizer, MSD, and Roche. Sylvain Ladoire has received research funding from Novartis, honoraria for consultancy from Lilly, Pfizer, Novartis, Bristol-Myers Squibb, Astellas Pharma, Roche, Ipsen, Janssen Oncology, and Sanofi, and travel expenses/accommodations from Pfizer, Novartis, AstraZeneca, Sanofi, Astellas Pharma, Janssen Oncology, Ipsen, Bristol-Myers Squibb. Reza Elaidi has received honoraria for advisory board from Pfizer. Slimane Dermeche has received honoraria for advisory board from Pfizer. Jean-Christophe Eymard has received honoraria for consultancy from Bristol-Myers Squibb, Pfizer, Ipsen, Novartis, Janssen, Astellas and Sanofi, and travel expenses/accommodations from Bristol-Myers Squibb and Pfizer. Sabrina Falkowski has received honoraria for advisory board from Bristol-Myers Squibb, Pfizer, Sanofi, MSD, Janssen, AstraZeneca and Astellas, and travel expenses/accommodations from Pfizer, Sanofi, MSD, and Janssen. Marine Gross-Goupil has received honoraria for advisory board/consultancy from Bristol-Myers Squibb, MSD, Pfizer, Merck, Ipsen, and Novartis, and as a speaker from Roche and AstraZeneca, and travel expenses/accommodations from Bristol-Myers Squibb, Pfizer, and Ipsen. Gabriel Malouf has received honoraria for consultancy from Pfizer, Bristol-Myers Squibb, Astellas Pharma, and Ipsen. Berangere Narciso has received honoraria for advisory board from Janssen, Ipsen, Bristol-Myers Squibb and MSD. Christophe Sajous has received honoraria for advisory board from Pfizer, for consultancy from AstraZeneca, and as a speaker from Lilly. Sophie Tartas has received honoraria for advisory board from Pfizer. Eric Voog has received honoraria for advisory board from Pfizer. Alain Ravaud has received honoraria for advisory board/consultancy from Bristol-Myers Squibb, Pfizer, Novartis, Ipsen, Merck, MSD, AstraZeneca and Roche, and travel expenses/accommodations from Pfizer, Novartis, Bristol-Myers Squibb, Astra Zeneca, Ipsen, and MSD.

References

1. Lalani, A.-K.A.; McGregor, B.A.; Albiges, L.; Choueiri, T.K.; Motzer, R.; Powles, T.; Wood, C.; Bex, A. Systemic Treatment of Metastatic Clear Cell Renal Cell Carcinoma in 2018: Current Paradigms, Use of Immunotherapy, and Future Directions. *Eur. Urol.* **2019**, *75*, 100–110. [CrossRef] [PubMed]
2. Salgia, N.J.; Dara, Y.; Bergerot, P.; Salgia, M.; Pal, S.K. The Changing Landscape of Management of Metastatic Renal Cell Carcinoma: Current Treatment Options and Future Directions. *Curr. Treat. Options Oncol.* **2019**, *20*, 41. [CrossRef]
3. Pardoll, D.M. The blockade of immune checkpoints in cancer immunotherapy. *Nat. Rev. Cancer* **2012**, *12*, 252–264. [CrossRef]
4. Massari, F.; Rizzo, A.; Mollica, V.; Rosellini, M.; Marchetti, A.; Ardizzoni, A.; Santoni, M. Immune-based combinations for the treatment of metastatic renal cell carcinoma: A meta-analysis of randomised clinical trials. *Eur. J. Cancer* **2021**, *154*, 120–127. [CrossRef]
5. Motzer, R.J.; Tannir, N.M.; McDermott, D.F.; Arén Frontera, O.; Melichar, B.; Choueiri, T.K.; Plimack, E.R.; Barthélémy, P.; Porta, C.; George, S.; et al. Nivolumab plus Ipilimumab versus Sunitinib in Advanced Renal-Cell Carcinoma. *N. Engl. J. Med.* **2018**, *378*, 1277–1290. [CrossRef]
6. Albiges, L.; Tannir, N.M.; Burotto, M.; McDermott, D.; Plimack, E.R.; Barthélémy, P.; Porta, C.; Powles, T.; Donskov, F.; George, S.; et al. Nivolumab plus ipilimumab versus sunitinib for first-line treatment of advanced renal cell carcinoma: Extended 4-year follow-up of the phase III CheckMate 214 trial. *ESMO Open* **2020**, *5*, e001079. [CrossRef] [PubMed]
7. Motzer, R.J.; Penkov, K.; Haanen, J.; Rini, B.; Albiges, L.; Campbell, M.T.; Venugopal, B.; Kollmannsberger, C.; Negrier, S.; Uemura, M.; et al. Avelumab plus Axitinib versus Sunitinib for Advanced Renal-Cell Carcinoma. *N. Engl. J. Med.* **2019**, *380*, 1103–1115. [CrossRef] [PubMed]
8. Choueiri, T.; Motzer, R.; Rini, B.; Haanen, J.; Campbell, M.; Venugopal, B.; Kollmannsberger, C.; Gravis-Mescam, G.; Uemura, M.; Lee, J.; et al. Updated efficacy results from the JAVELIN Renal 101 trial: First-line avelumab plus axitinib versus sunitinib in patients with advanced renal cell carcinoma. *Ann. Oncol.* **2020**, *31*, 1030–1039. [CrossRef]
9. Rini, B.I.; Plimack, E.R.; Stus, V.; Gafanov, R.; Hawkins, R.; Nosov, D.; Pouliot, F.; Alekseev, B.; Soulières, D.; Melichar, B.; et al. Pembrolizumab plus Axitinib versus Sunitinib for Advanced Renal-Cell Carcinoma. *N. Engl. J. Med.* **2019**, *380*, 1116–1127. [CrossRef] [PubMed]
10. Powles, T.; Plimack, E.R.; Soulières, D.; Waddell, T.; Stus, V.; Gafanov, R.; Nosov, D.; Pouliot, F.; Melichar, B.; Vynnychenko, I.; et al. Pembrolizumab plus axitinib versus sunitinib monotherapy as first-line treatment of advanced renal cell carcinoma (KEYNOTE-426): Extended follow-up from a randomised, open-label, phase 3 trial. *Lancet Oncol.* **2020**, *21*, 1563–1573. [CrossRef]
11. Choueiri, T.K.; Powles, T.; Burotto, M.; Escudier, B.; Bourlon, M.T.; Zurawski, B.; Oyervides-Juárez, V.M.; Hsieh, J.J.; Basso, U.; Shah, A.Y.; et al. Nivolumab plus Cabozantinib versus Sunitinib for Advanced Renal-Cell Carcinoma. *N. Engl. J. Med.* **2021**, *384*, 829–841. [CrossRef] [PubMed]
12. Motzer, R.J.; Porta, C.; Eto, M.; Powles, T.; Grünwald, V.; Hutson, T.E.; Alekseev, B.; Rha, S.Y.; Kopyltsov, E.; Méndez-Vidal, M.J.; et al. Phase 3 trial of lenvatinib (LEN) plus pembrolizumab (PEMBRO) or everolimus (EVE) versus sunitinib (SUN) monotherapy as a first-line treatment for patients (pts) with advanced renal cell carcinoma (RCC) (CLEAR study). *JCO* **2021**, *39*, 269. [CrossRef]
13. Escudier, B.; Porta, C.; Schmidinger, M.; Rioux-Leclercq, N.; Bex, A.; Khoo, V.; Grünwald, V.; Gillessen, S.; Horwich, A.; ESMO Guidelines Committee. Renal Cell Carcinoma: ESMO Clinical Practice Guidelines for Diagnosis, Treatment and Follow-Up. *Ann. Oncol.* **2019**, *30*, 706–720. [CrossRef] [PubMed]
14. Powles, T.; Albiges, L.; Bex, A.; Grünwald, V.; Porta, C.; Procopio, G.; Schmidinger, M.; Suárez, C.; de Velasco, G.; ESMO Guidelines Committee. ESMO Clinical Practice Guideline Update on the Use of Immunotherapy in Early Stage and Advanced Renal Cell Carcinoma. *Ann. Oncol.* **2021**. [CrossRef] [PubMed]
15. Aeppli, S.; Schmaus, M.; Eisen, T.; Escudier, B.; Grünwald, V.; Larkin, J.; McDermott, D.; Oldenburg, J.; Porta, C.; Rini, B.I.; et al. First-line treatment of metastatic clear cell renal cell carcinoma: A decision-making analysis among experts. *ESMO Open* **2021**, *6*, 100030. [CrossRef]
16. Rini, B.I.; Plimack, E.R.; Stus, V.; Waddell, T.; Gafanov, R.; Pouliot, F.; Nosov, D.; Melichar, B.; Soulieres, D.; Borchiellini, D.; et al. Pembrolizumab (Pembro) plus Axitinib (Axi) versus Sunitinib as First-Line Therapy for Advanced Clear Cell Renal Cell Carcinoma (CcRCC): Results from 42-Month Follow-up of KEYNOTE. *JCO* **2021**, *39*, 4500. [CrossRef]
17. Haanen, J.B.A.G.; Larkin, J.; Choueiri, T.K.; Albiges, L.; Rini, B.I.; Atkins, M.B.; Schmidinger, M.; Penkov, K.; Thomaidou, D.; Wang, J.; et al. Efficacy of Avelumab + Axitinib (A + Ax) versus Sunitinib (S) by IMDC Risk Group in Advanced Renal Cell Carcinoma (ARCC): Extended Follow-up Results from JAVELIN Renal. *JCO* **2021**, *39*, 4574. [CrossRef]
18. ElAidi, R.; Phan, L.; Borchiellini, D.; Barthelemy, P.; Ravaud, A.; Oudard, S.; Vano, Y. Comparative Efficacy of First-Line Immune-Based Combination Therapies in Metastatic Renal Cell Carcinoma: A Systematic Review and Network Meta-Analysis. *Cancers* **2020**, *12*, 1673. [CrossRef]
19. Gan, C.L.; Dudani, S.; Wells, J.C.; Schmidt, A.L.; Bakouny, Z.; Szabados, B.; Parnis, F.; Wong, S.; Lee, J.-L.; de Velasco, G.; et al. Outcomes of first-line (1L) immuno-oncology (IO) combination therapies in metastatic renal cell carcinoma (mRCC): Results from the International mRCC Database Consortium (IMDC). *JCO* **2021**, *39*, 276. [CrossRef]
20. Quhal, F.; Mori, K.; Remzi, M.; Fajkovic, H.; Shariat, S.F.; Schmidinger, M. Adverse events of systemic immune-based combination therapies in the first-line treatment of patients with metastatic renal cell carcinoma: Systematic review and network meta-analysis. *Curr. Opin. Urol.* **2021**, *31*, 332–339. [CrossRef]

21. Lee, D.; Gittleman, H.; Weinstock, C.; Suzman, D.L.; Bloomquist, E.; Agrawal, S.; Brave, M.H.; Brewer, J.R.; Singh, H.; Tang, S.; et al. An FDA-pooled analysis of frontline combination treatment benefits by risk groups in metastatic renal cell carcinoma (mRCC). *J. Clin. Oncol.* **2021**, *39*, 4559. [CrossRef]
22. Verbiest, A.; Renders, I.; Caruso, G.; Couchy, G.; Job, S.; Laenen, A.; Verkarre, V.; Rioux-Leclercq, N.; Schöffski, P.; Vano, Y.A.; et al. Clear-cell Renal Cell Carcinoma: Molecular Characterization of IMDC Risk Groups and Sarcomatoid Tumors. *Clin. Genitourin. Cancer* **2019**, *17*, e981–e994. [CrossRef]
23. Escudier, B.; Motzer, R.J.; Tannir, N.M.; Porta, C.; Tomita, Y.; Maurer, M.A.; McHenry, M.B.; Rini, B.I. Efficacy of Nivolumab plus Ipilimumab According to Number of IMDC Risk Factors in CheckMate. *Eur. Urol.* **2020**, *77*, 449–453. [CrossRef]
24. Flaifel, A.; Xie, W.; Braun, D.A.; Ficial, M.; Bakouny, Z.; Nassar, A.H.; Jennings, R.B.; Escudier, B.; George, D.J.; Motzer, R.J.; et al. PD-L1 Expression and Clinical Outcomes to Cabozantinib, Everolimus, and Sunitinib in Patients with Metastatic Renal Cell Carcinoma: Analysis of the Randomized Clinical Trials METEOR and CABOSUN. *Clin. Cancer Res.* **2019**, *25*, 6080–6088. [CrossRef] [PubMed]
25. Iacovelli, R.; Nolè, F.; Verri, E.; Renne, G.; Paglino, C.; Santoni, M.; Cossu Rocca, M.; Giglione, P.; Aurilio, G.; Cullurà, D.; et al. Prognostic Role of PD-L1 Expression in Renal Cell Carcinoma. A Systematic Review and Meta-Analysis. *Target. Oncol.* **2016**, *11*, 143–148. [CrossRef] [PubMed]
26. Mori, K.; Abufaraj, M.; Mostafaei, H.; Quhal, F.; Fajkovic, H.; Remzi, M.; Karakiewicz, P.I.; Egawa, S.; Schmidinger, M.; Shariat, S.F.; et al. The Predictive Value of Programmed Death Ligand 1 in Patients with Metastatic Renal Cell Carcinoma Treated with Immune-checkpoint Inhibitors: A Systematic Review and Meta-analysis. *Eur. Urol.* **2021**, *79*, 783–792. [CrossRef]
27. Motzer, R.J.; Choueiri, T.K.; McDermott, D.F.; Powles, T.; Yao, J.; Ammar, R.; Papillon-Cavanagh, S.; Saggi, S.S.; McHenry, B.M.; Ross-Macdonald, P.; et al. Biomarker analyses from the phase III CheckMate 214 trial of nivolumab plus ipilimumab (N+I) or sunitinib (S) in advanced renal cell carcinoma (aRCC). *JCO* **2020**, *38*, 5009. [CrossRef]
28. Massari, F.; Mollica, V.; Rizzo, A.; Cosmai, L.; Rizzo, M.; Porta, C. Safety evaluation of immune-based combinations in patients with advanced renal cell carcinoma: A systematic review and meta-analysis. *Expert Opin. Drug Saf.* **2020**, *19*, 1329–1338. [CrossRef]
29. Abu-Sbeih, H.; Faleck, D.M.; Ricciuti, B.; Mendelsohn, R.B.; Naqash, A.R.; Cohen, J.V.; Sellers, M.C.; Balaji, A.; Ben-Betzalel, G.; Hajir, I.; et al. Immune Checkpoint Inhibitor Therapy in Patients With Preexisting Inflammatory Bowel Disease. *J. Clin. Oncol.* **2020**, *38*, 576–583. [CrossRef]
30. Haanen, J.; Ernstoff, M.; Wang, Y.; Menzies, A.; Puzanov, I.; Grivas, P.; Larkin, J.; Peters, S.; Thompson, J.; Obeid, M. Autoimmune diseases and immune-checkpoint inhibitors for cancer therapy: Review of the literature and personalized risk-based prevention strategy. *Ann. Oncol.* **2020**, *31*, 724–744. [CrossRef]
31. Araujo, D.V.; Wells, J.C.; Hansen, A.R.; Dizman, N.; Pal, S.K.; Beuselinck, B.; Donskov, F.; Gan, C.L.; Yan, F.; Tran, B.; et al. Efficacy of immune-checkpoint inhibitors (ICI) in the treatment of older adults with metastatic renal cell carcinoma (mRCC) – an International mRCC Database Consortium (IMDC) analysis. *J. Geriatr. Oncol.* **2021**, *12*, 820–826. [CrossRef]
32. Cella, D.; Grünwald, V.; Escudier, B.; Hammers, H.J.; George, S.; Nathan, P.; Grimm, M.-O.; Rini, B.I.; Doan, J.; Ivanescu, C.; et al. Patient-reported outcomes of patients with advanced renal cell carcinoma treated with nivolumab plus ipilimumab versus sunitinib (CheckMate 214): A randomised, phase 3 trial. *Lancet Oncol.* **2019**, *20*, 297–310. [CrossRef]
33. Motzer, R.J.; Porta, C.; Alekseev, B.; Rha, S.Y.; Choueiri, T.K.; Mendez-Vidal, M.J.; Hong, S.-H.; Kapoor, A.; Goh, J.C.; Eto, M.; et al. Health-related quality-of-life (HRQoL) analysis from the phase 3 CLEAR trial of lenvatinib (LEN) plus pembrolizumab (PEMBRO) or everolimus (EVE) versus sunitinib (SUN) for patients (pts) with advanced renal cell carcinoma (aRCC). *JCO* **2021**, *39*, 4502. [CrossRef]
34. Choueiri, T.K.; Bauer, T.M.; Papadopoulos, K.P.; Plimack, E.R.; Merchan, J.R.; McDermott, D.F.; Michaelson, M.D.; Appleman, L.J.; Thamake, S.; Perini, R.F.; et al. Inhibition of hypoxia-inducible factor-2α in renal cell carcinoma with belzutifan: A phase 1 trial and biomarker analysis. *Nat. Med.* **2021**, *27*, 802–805. [CrossRef]
35. Auvray, M.; Auclin, E.; Barthelemy, P.; Bono, P.; Kellokumpu-Lehtinen, P.; Gross-Goupil, M.; De Velasco, G.; Powles, T.; Mouillet, G.; Vano, Y.A.; et al. Second-line targeted therapies after nivolumab-ipilimumab failure in metastatic renal cell carcinoma. *Eur. J. Cancer* **2019**, *108*, 33–40. [CrossRef] [PubMed]
36. Dudani, S.; Graham, J.; Wells, J.C.; Bakouny, Z.; Pal, S.K.; Dizman, N.; Donskov, F.; Porta, C.; de Velasco, G.; Hansen, A.; et al. First-line Immuno-Oncology Combination Therapies in Metastatic Renal-cell Carcinoma: Results from the International Metastatic Renal-cell Carcinoma Database Consortium. *Eur. Urol.* **2019**, *76*, 861–867. [CrossRef] [PubMed]
37. Stukalin, I.; Dudani, S.; Wells, C.; Gan, C.L.; Pal, S.K.; Dizman, N.; Powles, T.; Donskov, F.; Wood, L.; Bakouny, Z.; et al. Second-line VEGF TKI after IO combination therapy: Results from the International Metastatic Renal Cell Carcinoma Database Consortium (IMDC). *JCO* **2020**, *38*, 684. [CrossRef]
38. Lee, C.-H.; Shah, A.Y.; Hsieh, J.J.; Rao, A.; Pinto, A.; Bilen, M.A.; Cohn, A.L.; Di Simone, C.; Shaffer, D.R.; Sarrio, R.G.; et al. Phase II trial of lenvatinib (LEN) plus pembrolizumab (PEMBRO) for disease progression after PD-1/PD-L1 immune checkpoint inhibitor (ICI) in metastatic clear cell renal cell carcinoma (mccRCC). *JCO* **2020**, *38*, 5008. [CrossRef]
39. Grimm, M.-O.; Schmidinger, M.; Martinez, I.D.; Schinzari, G.; Esteban, E.; Schmitz, M.; Schumacher, U.; Baretton, G.; Barthelemy, P.; Melichar, B.; et al. Tailored immunotherapy approach with nivolumab in advanced renal cell carcinoma (TITAN-RCC). *Ann. Oncol.* **2019**, *30*, v892. [CrossRef]

40. Atkins, M.B.; Jegede, O.; Haas, N.B.; McDermott, D.F.; Bilen, M.A.; Drake, C.G.; Sosman, J.A.; Alter, R.S.; Plimack, E.R.; Rini, B.I.; et al. Phase II study of nivolumab and salvage nivolumab + ipilimumab in treatment-naïve patients (pts) with advanced renal cell carcinoma (RCC) (HCRN GU16-260). *J. Clin. Oncol.* **2020**, *38*, 5006. [CrossRef]
41. McKay, R.R.; McGregor, B.A.; Xie, W.; Braun, D.A.; Wei, X.; Kyriakopoulos, C.E.; Zakharia, Y.; Maughan, B.L.; Rose, T.L.; Stadler, W.M.; et al. Optimized Management of Nivolumab and Ipilimumab in Advanced Renal Cell Carcinoma: A Response-Based Phase II Study (OMNIVORE). *J. Clin. Oncol.* **2020**, *38*, 4240–4248. [CrossRef] [PubMed]
42. Choueiri, T.K.; Kluger, H.M.; George, S.; Tykodi, S.S.; Kuzel, T.M.; Perets, R.; Nair, S.; Procopio, G.; Carducci, M.A.; Castonguay, V.; et al. FRACTION-RCC: Innovative, high-throughput assessment of nivolumab + ipilimumab for treatment-refractory advanced renal cell carcinoma (aRCC). *JCO* **2020**, *38*, 5007. [CrossRef]
43. Carril-Ajuria, L.; Lora, D.; Carretero-González, A.; Martín-Soberón, M.; Rioja-Viera, P.; Castellano, D.; De Velasco, G. Systemic Analysis and Review of Nivolumab-ipilimumab Combination as a Rescue Strategy for Renal Cell Carcinoma After Treatment With Anti-PD-1/PD-L1 Therapy. *Clin. Genitourin. Cancer* **2021**, *19*, 95–102. [CrossRef] [PubMed]
44. Gul, A.; Stewart, T.F.; Mantia, C.M.; Shah, N.J.; Gatof, E.S.; Long, Y.; Allman, K.D.; Ornstein, M.C.; Hammers, H.J.; McDermott, D.F.; et al. Salvage Ipilimumab and Nivolumab in Patients With Metastatic Renal Cell Carcinoma After Prior Immune Checkpoint Inhibitors. *J. Clin. Oncol.* **2020**, *38*, 3088–3094. [CrossRef] [PubMed]
45. Epaillard, N.; Simonaggio, A.; Elaidi, R.; Azzouz, F.; Braychenko, E.; Thibault, C.; Sun, C.-M.; Moreira, M.; Oudard, S.; Vano, Y.-A. BIONIKK: A phase 2 biomarker driven trial with nivolumab and ipilimumab or VEGFR tyrosine kinase inhibitor (TKI) in naïve metastatic kidney cancer. *Bull. Cancer* **2020**, *107*, eS22–eS27. [CrossRef]
46. Vano, Y.; ElAidi, R.; Bennamoun, M.; Chevreau, C.; Borchiellini, D.; Pannier, D.; Maillet, D.; Gross-Goupil, M.; Tournigand, C.; Laguerre, B.; et al. LBA25 Results from the phase II biomarker driven trial with nivolumab (N) and ipilimumab or VEGFR tyrosine kinase inhibitor (TKI) in naïve metastatic kidney cancer (m-ccRCC) patients (pts): The BIONIKK trial. *Ann. Oncol.* **2020**, *31*, S1157. [CrossRef]
47. Choueiri, T.K.; Tomczak, P.; Park, S.H.; Venugopal, B.; Ferguson, T.; Chang, Y.-H.; Hajek, J.; Symeonides, S.N.; Lee, J.L.; Sarwar, N.; et al. Adjuvant Pembrolizumab after Nephrectomy in Renal-Cell Carcinoma. *N. Engl. J. Med.* **2021**, *385*, 683–694. [CrossRef]

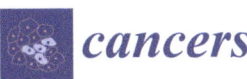

Article

Soluble PD-L1 Is an Independent Prognostic Factor in Clear Cell Renal Cell Carcinoma

Gorka Larrinaga [1,2,3,*], Jon Danel Solano-Iturri [3,4,5], Peio Errarte [2,3], Miguel Unda [6], Ana Loizaga-Iriarte [6], Amparo Pérez-Fernández [6], Enrique Echevarría [2], Aintzane Asumendi [7], Claudia Manini [8], Javier C. Angulo [9,10] and José I. López [3,11]

1. Department of Nursing, Faculty of Medicine and Nursing, University of the Basque Country (UPV/EHU), 48940 Leioa, Spain
2. Department of Physiology, Faculty of Medicine and Nursing, University of the Basque Country (UPV/EHU), 48940 Leioa, Spain; peio@onenameds.com (P.E.); enrique.etxebarria@ehu.eus (E.E.)
3. BioCruces-Bizkaia Health Research Institute, 48903 Barakaldo, Spain; jondanel.solanoiturri@osakidetza.eus (J.D.S.-I.); joseignacio.lopez@osakidetza.eus (J.I.L.)
4. Department of Pathology, Donostia University Hospital, 20014 San Sebastian-Donostia, Spain
5. Department of Medical-Surgical Specialities, Faculty of Medicine and Nursing, University of the Basque Country (UPV/EHU), 48940 Leioa, Spain
6. Department of Urology, Basurto University Hospital, University of the Basque Country (UPV/EHU), 48013 Bilbao, Spain; jesusmiguel.undaurzaiz@osakidetza.eus (M.U.); ana.loizagairiarte@osakidetza.eus (A.L.-I.); amparo.perezfernandez@osakidetza.eus (A.P.-F.)
7. Department of Cellular Biology and Histology, Faculty of Medicine and Nursing, University of the Basque Country (UPV/EHU), 48940 Leioa, Spain; aintzane.asumendi@ehu.eus
8. Department of Pathology, San Giovanni Bosco Hospital, 10154 Turin, Italy; claudia.manini@aslcittaditorino.it
9. Clinical Department, Faculty of Medical Sciences, European University of Madrid, 28670 Villaviciosa de Odón, Spain; javier.angulo@universidadeuropea.es
10. Department of Urology, University Hospital of Getafe, 28907 Getafe, Spain
11. Department of Pathology, Cruces University Hospital, 48903 Barakaldo, Spain
* Correspondence: gorka.larrinaga@ehu.eus

Citation: Larrinaga, G.; Solano-Iturri, J.D.; Errarte, P.; Unda, M.; Loizaga-Iriarte, A.; Pérez-Fernández, A.; Echevarría, E.; Asumendi, A.; Manini, C.; Angulo, J.C.; et al. Soluble PD-L1 Is an Independent Prognostic Factor in Clear Cell Renal Cell Carcinoma. *Cancers* **2021**, *13*, 667. https://doi.org/10.3390/cancers13040667

Academic Editor: Jörg Ellinger
Received: 27 November 2020
Accepted: 4 February 2021
Published: 7 February 2021

Publisher's Note: MDPI stays neutral with regard to jurisdictional claims in published maps and institutional affiliations.

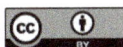

Copyright: © 2021 by the authors. Licensee MDPI, Basel, Switzerland. This article is an open access article distributed under the terms and conditions of the Creative Commons Attribution (CC BY) license (https://creativecommons.org/licenses/by/4.0/).

Simple Summary: Renal cell carcinoma (RCC) is a heterogeneous and complex disease with almost no response to chemotherapy. Immune checkpoint inhibitors have achieved great clinical success but no interesting circulating markers of clinical use have developed so far in clear cell renal cell carcinoma (CCRCC). We investigate the diagnostic and prognostic role of plasma PD-1 (sPD-1) and PD-L1 (sPD-L1) proteins for the first time together with the immunohistochemical expression counterpart of these proteins within the tumor front and tumor center in the same sample of patients with renal cancer undergoing surgery. We also investigate these plasma and tissue markers in the population of metastatic patients according to International mRCC Database Consortium (IMDC) prognostic groups and the response to systemic therapy. The independent role of sPD-L1 as a predictor of prognosis and treatment response is demonstrated.

Abstract: (1). *Background*: Immunohistochemical (IHC) evaluation of programmed death-1 (PD-1) and its ligand (PD-L1) is being used to evaluate advanced malignancies with potential response to immune checkpoint inhibitors. We evaluated both plasma and tissue expression of PD-1 and PD-L1 in the same cohort of patients, including non-metastatic and metastatic clear cell renal cell carcinoma (CCRCC). Concomitant plasma and tissue expression of PD-1 and PD-L1 was evaluated with emphasis on diagnostic and prognostic implications. (2) *Methods*: we analyzed PD-1 and PD-L1 IHC expression in tumor tissues and soluble forms (sPD-1 and sPD-L1) in plasma from 89 patients with CCRCC, of which 23 were metastatic and 16 received systemic therapy. The primary endpoint was evaluation of overall survival using Kaplan-Meier analysis and the Cox regression model. Plasma samples from healthy volunteers were also evaluated. (3) *Results*: Interestingly, sPD-1 and sPD-L1 levels were lower in cancer patients than in controls. sPD-1 and sPD-L1 levels and their counterpart tissue expression both at the tumor center and infiltrating front were not associated. Higher expression of both PD-1 and PD-L1 were associated with tumor grade, necrosis and tumor size. PD-1 was associated to tumor stage (pT) and PD-L1 to metastases. sPD-1 and sPD-L1 were not associated with clinico-pathological parameters, although both were higher in patients with synchronous metastases compared to metachronous ones and sPD-L1 was also higher for metastatic patients compared to non-metastatic patients. sPD-1 was also associated with the International Metastatic Renal Cell Cancer Database Consortium (IMDC) prognostic groups in metastatic CCRCC and also to the Morphology, Attenuation, Size and Structure (MASS) response criteria in metastatic patients treated with systemic therapy, mainly tyrosine-kinase inhibitors. Regarding prognosis, PD-L1 immunostaining at the tumor center with and without the tumor front was associated with worse survival, and so was sPD-L1 at a cut-off >793 ng/mL. Combination of positivity at both the tissue and plasma level increased the level of significance to predict prognosis. (4) *Conclusions*: Our findings corroborate the role of PD-L1 IHC to evaluate prognosis in CCRCC and present novel data on the usefulness of plasma sPD-L1 as a promising biomarker of survival in this neoplasia.

Keywords: clear cell renal cell carcinoma; prognosis; plasma; PD-1; PD-L1

1. Introduction

Clear cell renal cell carcinoma (CCRCC) is a very prevalent disease and a clinical problem of major concern in Western countries due to its biological aggressiveness and its well-known resistance to chemotherapy and radiotherapy regimes [1–3]. Traditionally, radical surgery coupled with early diagnosis has been the only strategy with a direct impact on patient survival [4]. CCRCC is a model of hypoxia-related disease. *VHL* gene malfunction is detected in the overwhelming majority of the cases, resulting in a pseudo-hypoxic status that promotes angiogenesis [5]. The implementation of antiangiogenic therapies with tyrosine kinase inhibitors has improved the prognosis of many of these patients [6,7]. However, its efficacy is limited due to the development of resistant-to-therapy cell clones [8].

Immune checkpoint blockade of PD-1 and its ligand PD-L1 have been implemented in advanced lung, renal (CCRCC) and bladder carcinomas, as well as in melanoma, with promising results in several trials [9,10]. In CCRCC the immunohistochemical evaluation is selectively performed in the intratumor lymphoid inflammatory infiltrates. However, the patient selection for such a form of therapy is difficult, since this evaluation is subjected to interobserver variability [11]. In fact, up to 17% of patients with negative immuno-histochemistry results do respond to this therapy [12]. Other important limitations for the development of immune checkpoints inhibitors targeting the PD-1 pathway are that responses rates are low and biomarkers are needed for the prediction of treatment responses [13,14].

To overcome the aforementioned difficulties, composite biomarkers have been investigated including tumor mutational burden, profiling of tumor infiltrating lymphocytes, molecular subtypes and the characterization of ligand PD-L2. Distinct tumor microenvironment immune types have been described, mainly based on the level of CD8A and PD-1 expression, with the intention to standardize a more comprehensive score to be used as a prognostic marker [15]. Combination with other composite biomarkers is currently under investigation [16]. Another interesting strategy to maximize the clinical benefit and predict treatment toxicity is the characterization of gastrointestinal microbiome [17]. Surprisingly, not much attention has been given to the evaluation of soluble PD-1 (sPD-1) and PD-L1 (sPD-L1) in plasma as potential biomarkers in patients with CCRCC, a heterogeneous neoplasm in serious need of identification of molecular markers that clinicians could use to facilitate an earlier diagnosis, to monitor the disease and to predict prognosis and clinical response to different therapies.

We evaluate plasma and tissue expression of PD-1 and PD-L1 in the same cohort of patients and analyze the relationship between them, also taking into account the non-metastatic and metastatic samples. Within metastatic CCRCC, plasma and tissue expression of PD-1 and PD-L1 were analyzed according to the IMDC risk classification and also according to the Morphology, Attenuation, Size and Structure (MASS) response criteria in patients receiving systemic therapy for metastatic disease. Also, we provide a very interesting simultaneous evaluation of sPD-1 and sPD-L1 and its concomitant expression in the tumor center and infiltrating front, with emphasis on the prognostic implication of these categories. The potential use of sPD-L1 as a tumor marker itself is also discussed, and its relation to other clinical and pathological variables that predict prognosis in CCRCC and treatment response in metastatic CCRCC, according to MASS criteria, is investigated.

2. Results

2.1. PD-L1 and PD-1 Tissue Expression and Plasma Levels Are Not Correlated with the Gender and Age of CCRCC Patients

To assess whether the expression in tumors and plasma levels of these biomarkers varies according to the gender or age of the patients, the non-parametric Rho Spearman test was performed. There was not any statistically significant correlation in any case (Table S1). Therefore, it can concluded that the sample has no gender or age bias.

2.2. The Expression of PD-L1 and PD-1 at the Tumour Centre and at the Infiltrating Front Is Correlated

We analyzed the expression of PD-L1 and PD-1 in lymphocytes at both the tumor center and front (Figure 1). The expression correlated positively in all cases (Table S2). Thus, the higher the percentage of PD-L1 or PD-1 positives at the tumor center, the higher the percentage was at the tumor front. Moreover, PD-L1 correlated positively with the expression of PD-1.

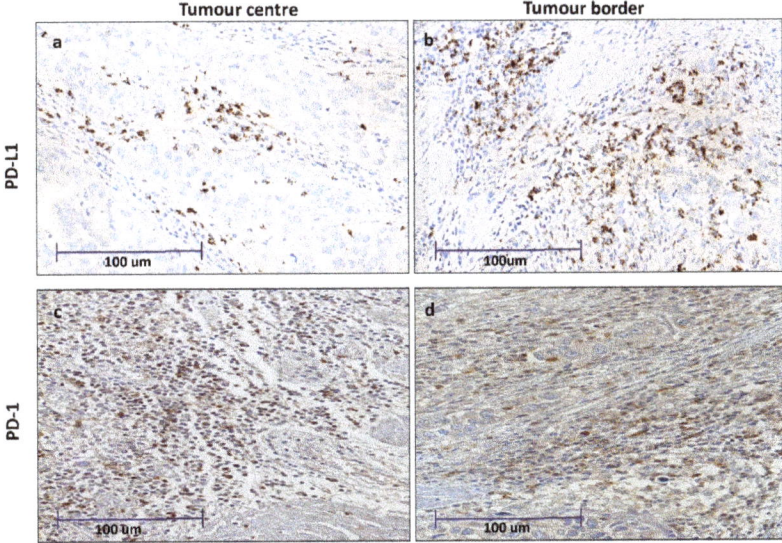

Figure 1. Immunohistochemical expression of PD-1 (sPD-1) and PD-L1 (sPD-L1) staining in inflammatory cells in clear cell renal cell carcinoma (CCRCC) samples, both in the tumor center (**a,c**) and infiltrating front (**b,d**).

Although there was a significant positive correlation between the expression of both biomarkers at the tumor center and edge, this does not mean that there was a concomitant expression in all cases. Therefore, we also evaluated the simultaneous positive staining of PD-L1 and PD-1 at both areas of tumors and stratified the rest of data, taking this characteristic into account. Thus, simultaneous positivity of PD-L1 at tumor center and front was found to be correlated with simultaneous expression of PD-1 at both areas (Table S2).

2.3. Plasma PD-L1 Levels Are Lower in CCRCC Patients than in Control Subjects

Plasma levels of sPD-L1 and sPD-1 from CCRCC patients were compared to plasma from 46 controls (Table 1). sPD-L1 levels were significantly lower in patients than in healthy subjects. Plasma sPD-1 levels showed high variability both in patients and in controls. These levels were higher in patients than in controls; however, the result was not statistically significant.

Table 1. sPD-L1 and sPD-1 levels in plasma samples from clear cell renal cell carcinoma (CCRCC) patients and healthy controls. Values are means ± standard errors. Significant p value in bold.

sPD-L1 (ng/mL)			sPD-1 (ng/mL)		
CCRCC	Controls	Mann-U ($p=$)	CCRCC	Controls	Mann-U ($p=$)
902.8 ± 139.7	989.1 ± 155.9	**0.048**	1304.7 ± 306.3	941.3 ± 300.3	0.33

We also aimed to analyze the association between plasma levels of these two biomarkers according to their expression at the tumor center, at the infiltration front and, simultaneously, at both areas (Table 2). We observed higher plasma PD-L1 levels in patients whose tumors were PD-L1 positive at the tumor center, border and at both areas. However, this trend was not statistically significant. We did not find any significant association between sPD-1 levels and PD-1 expression in CCRCC tissues.

Table 2. Plasma sPD-L1 and sPD-1 levels in CCRCC patients in terms of PD-L1 and PD-1 expression in CCRCC tissues.

	PD-L1 Expression at Tumour Centre			PD-L1 Expression at Infiltrating Front		
	Negative	Positive	Mann-U, $p=$	Negative	Positive	Mann-U, $p=$
Plasma sPD-L1 (ng/mL)	849.1 ± 148.3	1182.1 ± 412.7	0.13	905.9 ± 184.5	1035.7 ± 353.1	0.99
	PD-1 at Tumour Centre			PD-1 at Infiltrating Front		
	Negative	Positive	Mann-U, $p=$	Negative	Positive	Mann-U, $p=$
Plasma sPD-1 (ng/mL)	1151.6 ± 344.4	1545.5 ± 576.5	0.61	1480.8 ± 446.6	983 ± 424.5	0.88
	PD-L1 Expression in Both Areas			PD-1 Expression in Both Areas		
	Negative	Positive	Mann-U, $p=$	Negative	Positive	Mann-U, $p=$
Plasma sPD-L1 (ng/mL)	845.1 ± 137.3	1439.5 ± 684.5	0.44	-	-	-
Plasma sPD-1 (ng/mL)	-	-	-	1383.2 ± 367.4	1103 ± 562.6	0.94

2.4. Tissue Expression of PD-L1 and PD-1 as Well as Plasma sPD-L1 and sPD-1 Are Associated with CCRCC Aggressiveness

We stratified results by clinical parameters tightly related to tumor aggressiveness such as the Fuhrman histological grade, tumor necrosis, size, local invasion (pT), presence/absence of affected lymph nodes (N) and time of presentation of distant metastasis (M). Data are shown in Figures 2 and 3. Data in metastatic patients was also evaluated according to IMDC categories predictive of prognosis and also in metastatic patients receiving systemic therapies, mainly tyrosine kinase inhibitors (TKIs) in sequential use (Table S3), results were evaluated according to the tumor response to treatment following the MASS criteria.

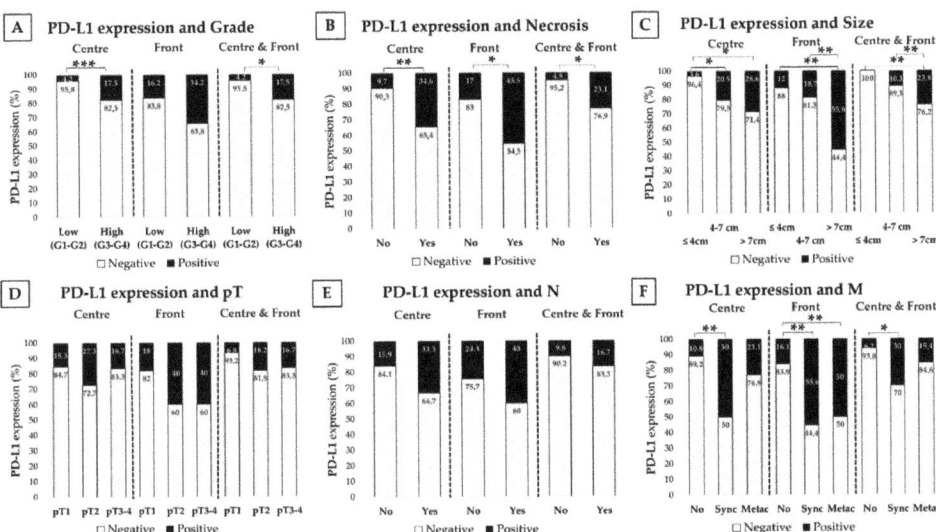

Figure 2. Immunohistochemical PD-L1 staining in terms of the CCRCC aggressiveness. PD-L1 immunostaining at the tumor center, infiltrating front and simultaneously at both areas depending on histological grade (**A**), tumor necrosis (**B**), diameter (**C**), local invasion or pT (**D**), lymph node metastasis or N (**E**), and distant metastasis or M (**F**). PD-L1 staining intensity was scored as negative or positive. Chi-Square test * $p < 0.05$; ** $p < 0.01$, *** $p < 0.001$.

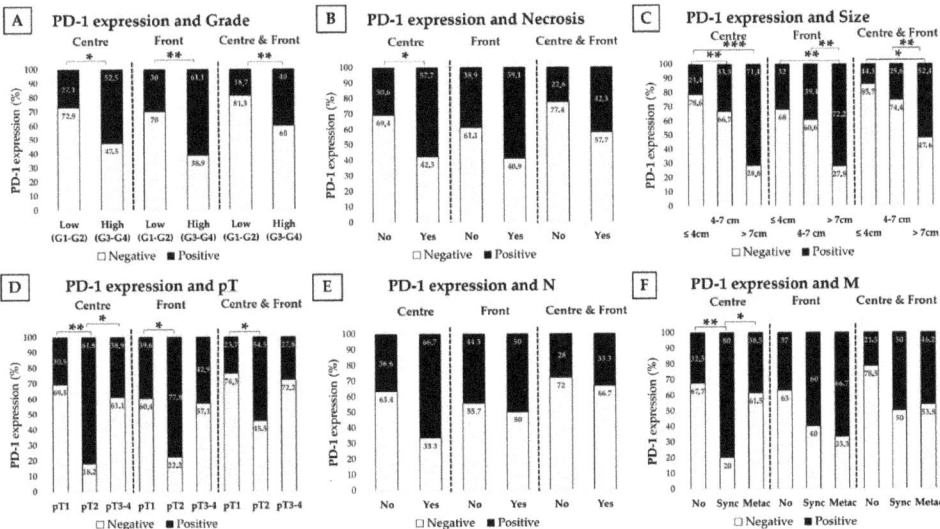

Figure 3. Immunohistochemical PD-1 staining according to CCRCC aggressiveness. PD-1 immunostaining at the tumor center, infiltrating simultaneously at both areas depending on the histological grade (**A**), tumor necrosis (**B**), diameter (**C**), local invasion or pT (**D**), lymph node metastasis or N (**E**) and distant metastasis or M (**F**). PD-1 staining intensity was scored as negative or positive. Chi-Square test * $p < 0.05$; ** $p < 0.01$, *** $p < 0.001$.

2.4.1. PD-L1 and PD-1 Expression Is Higher in High-Grade Tumors

Tumors were stratified as having a low Fuhrman grade (G1–G2) and a high-grade (3–4). High-grade CCRCCs showed higher PD-L1 and PD-1 expression than low-grade tumors, both at the center and at the infiltrating front. Simultaneous positive expression at both areas was also higher in high grade CCRCCs (Figure 2A or Figure 3A).

Plasma sPD-L1 and sPD-1 showed opposite pattern, with higher levels in patients with low grade tumors; however, these results were not statistically significant (Table 3).

Table 3. Plasma sPD-L1 and sPD-1 levels in terms of pathological parameters of CCRCC aggressiveness. The Mann-Whitney test was used for comparisons between two groups and Kruskal-Wallis for more than two groups. Values are represented as means ± standard errors. [a] sPD-L1 synchronous vs. No, Mann-U $p = 0.038$; [b] sPD-L1 synchronous vs. Metachronous, Mann-U $p = 0.008$; [c] sPD-1 synchronous vs. Metachronous, Mann-U $p = 0.037$. Statistically significant values are highlighted in bold.

CCRCC Patients	n=	sPD-L1 (ng/mL)	p=	sPD-1 (ng/mL)	p=
Fuhrman Grade					
Low-Grade (G1-G2)	49	982 ± 215	0.53	1795 ± 474	0.23
High-Grade (G3-G4)	40	806 ± 168		678 ± 348	
Necrosis					
No	63	754 ± 248	0.55	1472 ± 371	0.15
Yes	26	964 ± 169		876 ± 537	
Size					
≤4 cm	28	1143 ± 353		1880 ± 644	
>4 to 7 cm	39	685 ± 104	0.37	1021 ± 394	0.95
>7 cm	22	982 ± 289		1024 ± 587	
Local Invasion (pT)					
pT1	59	896 ± 179		1467 ± 402	
pT2	12	1049 ± 512	0.41	1414 ± 1089	0.95
pT3–pT4	18	826 ± 157		760 ± 364	
Lymph node invasion (N)					
No	83	885 ± 148	0.08	1322 ± 328	0.14
Yes	6	1148 ± 305		1089 ± 524	
Distant metastasis (M)					
No	66	977 ± 184		1583 ± 395	
Synchronous	10	1014 ± 191	**0.034** [a,b]	824 ± 369	0.14 [c]
Metachronous	13	438 ± 76		130 ± 68	

2.4.2. PD-L1 and PD-1 Are Highly Expressed in CCRCC Tumors with Necrosis

These series had 26 necrotic tumors. PD-L1 expression at the center and border was higher in these tumors. Simultaneous expression of PD-L1 at both areas was more frequent in necrotic CCRCCs (Figure 2B). PD-1 expression showed a similar staining pattern, but data only reached statistical significance at the tumor center (Figure 3B). Plasma sPD-L1 and sPD-1 levels did not show any significant difference depending on the necrosis status of CCRCCs (Table 3).

2.4.3. PD-L1 and PD-1 Positive Staining Is More Frequent in Larger CCRCCs

We classified tumors in three groups: tumors with 4 cm or smaller, 4 to 7 cm and larger than 7 cm. We observed that the larger the tumor was, the higher the positive staining of both biomarkers (Figure 2C or Figure 3C). However, these results in tumor tissues were not reflected in plasma, since sPD-L1 and sPD-1 did not vary significantly (Table 3).

2.4.4. PD-1 Expression Is Associated to Local Invasion (pT)

The limited number of pT4 cases led us to stratify the local invasion in three groups: pT1 (organ-confined tumors smaller than 7 cm), pT2 (organ-confined tumors larger than 7 cm) and pT3-pT4 (non-organ-confined tumors). Percentages of PD-1 positive staining were significantly higher in pT2 tumors than in pT1 (Figure 3D). PD-L1 staining was also higher in pT2 tumors; however, data did not reach statistical significance (Figure 2D). Plasma analyses did not provide any significant results (Table 3).

2.4.5. PD-L1 and PD-1 Tissue Expression and Plasma sPD-L1 and sPD-1 Are Higher in Patients with Synchronous Distant Metastasis

Data were also stratified by lymph node (N) and distant metastasis (M). Plasma sPD-L1 levels were higher in patients with lymph node invasion; however, the number of patients with this characteristic was limited ($n = 6$) and the result did not reach statistical significance (Table 3). PD-L1 and PD-1 expression in tissue and sPD-1 in plasma did not show any relevant difference (Figure 2E or Figure 3E).

With respect to distant metastases, we first compared primary tumors with (M1) or without (M0) metastases at the moment of the first diagnosis of CCRCC. PD-L1 expression at the tumor center (Chi-square test, $p = 0.004$), front ($p = 0.029$) and simultaneously at both areas ($p = 0.03$) was higher in primary tumors with onset as metastatic lesions than in not metastasized ones. PD-1 in the center of tumors also predicted metastasis ($p = 0.005$) (data not shown in figures or tables).

We also classified distant metastases as early synchronous (metastases that debuted within 6 months of the first primary cancer) and late metachronous (relapse of the disease with distant metastases more than 6 months later), and compared them with tumors that did not metastasize during follow-up. Thus, primary CCRCCs with synchronous metastases showed higher percentages of positive staining of PD-L1 (tumor center, front and simultaneous) and PD-1 (center) than in tumors that did not metastasize (Figure 2F or Figure 3F). PD-L1 in tumor front was also higher in metachronous ones than in tumors without metastases.

Plasma analyses showed that sPD-L1 levels were higher in patients that manifested with metastasis at the onset of the disease (M0: 857 ± 157 ng/mL vs. M1: 1014 ± 191, Mann-U test, $p = 0.017$). Furthermore, levels were also higher in patients with synchronous metastases than in patients without (Table 3). Both sPD-L1 and sPD-1 levels were also higher in patients with early metastases than with metachronous ones (Table 3).

2.5. PD-L1 and PD-1 Expression and Plasma Levels in Terms of the Overall Survival (OS) of CCRCC Patients

PD-L1 positive immunostaining at the tumor center and simultaneously at both the center and front was associated with a worse 5-year OS of CCRCC patients (Figure 4A,B). The expression of PD-L1 at the infiltrating front showed a similar result but it did not reach statistical significance (Log-rank test, $p = 0.068$). PD-1 expression at the center (Log-rank test, $p = 0.29$), front ($p = 0.24$) and concomitantly at both areas ($p = 0.23$) was not associated to OS.

A Classification and Regression Tree (CRT) was employed to obtain cut-off values of plasma sPD-L1 and sPD-1 for OS analyses (Figure S1). A plasma sPD-L1 value of 793 ng/mL determined two nodes with significant differences in the percentage of dead patients: 14.1% of deaths in the group of patients had plasma levels below this cut-off and 48.8% of deaths in the group had sPD-L1 levels above this cut-off ($p = 0.047$) (Figure S1A). Thus, Kaplan-Meier curves demonstrated that CCRCC patients with sPD-L1 levels above 793 ng/mL had worse 5-year OS than patients with lower levels (Figure 4C).

With regard to sPD-1, the CRT selected a cut-off value of 27ng/mL ($p = 0.017$) (Figure S1B). Kaplan-Meier curves showed a trend towards worse survival in CCRCC patients with plasma sPD-1 levels below this cut-off; however, the difference did not reach statistical significance (Log-rank test, $p = 0.073$).

Tumors and plasmas were obtained from the same patients. Therefore, taking into account the significant results with PD-L1 and its soluble isoform predicting patients' 5-year OS, we also performed Kaplan-Meier curves by combining data of tissue expression and plasma levels. Thus, two groups were created: (1) PD-L1 positive cases at the center of tumors, at the infiltrating front or simultaneously at both areas, together with sPD-L1 levels above 793 ng/mL; and (2) the rest of the possible combinations (PD-L1-/sPD-

L1 ≤793 ng/mL; PD-L1-/sPD-L1 >793 ng/mL; PD-L1+/sPD-L1 ≤793 ng/mL). CCRCC patients with tumor PD-L1 positivity and plasma levels above 793 ng/mL had significantly worse 5-year OS than patients with the rest of combinations (Figure 4D–F).

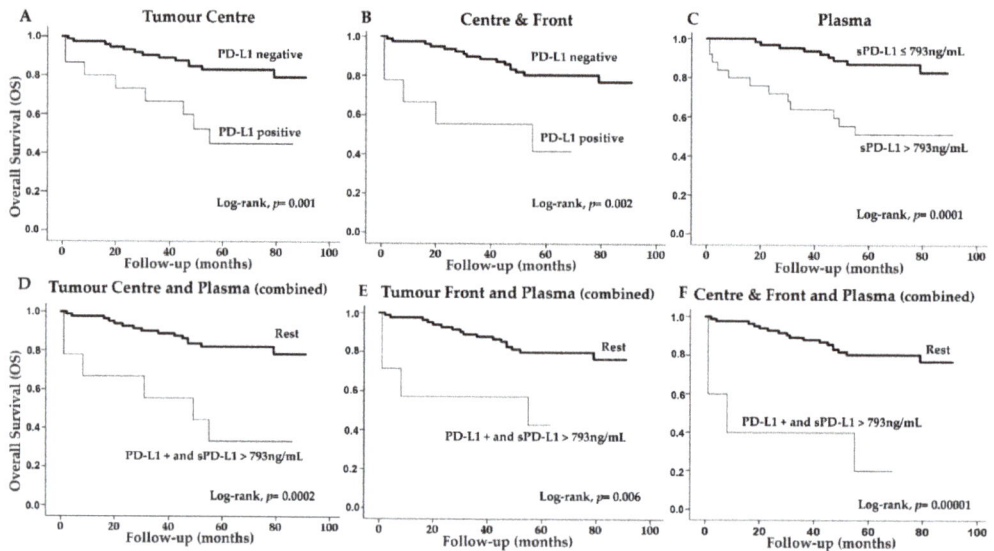

Figure 4. Immunohistochemical PD-L1 expression and plasma sFAP levels according to CCRCC patients' 5-year overall survival (OS). Kaplan-Meier curves and univariate Log-rank test showed that PD-L1 expression at tumor center (**A**) and concomitant expression at center and border (**B**) is associated to worse OS. (**C**) CCRCC patients with sPD-L1 above 793 ng/mL had worse OS. The expression of PD-L1 at tumor center (**D**), front (**E**) or at both areas (**F**) together with plasma sPD-L1 levels above 793 ng/mL are associated with worse OS.

Multivariate Cox regression analyses were performed to determine whether PD-L1 expression in tumor center, concomitantly at both center and front, sPD-L1 plasma levels (cut-off 793 ng/mL) or the combination of both isoforms are independent prognostic factors for 5-year OS. The logistic model resulting from a backward Wald stepwise elimination of variables revealed that the expression of PD-L1 at the tumor center, concomitant expression at both areas and plasma sPD-L1 were independent prognostic factors for 5-year OS (Table 4). Moreover, combinations of PD-L1 positivity in tumor tissues and plasma sPD-L1 were also explanatory independent variables for patients' OS. Complete multiple Cox regression is shown as supplementary material (Table S4).

2.6. PD-L1 and PD-1 Tissue Expression and Plasma Levels in Patients with Metastatic CCRCC According to IMDC Model and Response to Therapy

Twenty-three patients with metastatic CCRCC were stratified according to the IMDC model for classification of patients at different risks of death. PD-L1 and PD-1 tissue expression and plasma levels of sPD-L1 and sPD-1 were also stratified according to IMDC categories. With the limited number of patients in this subseries, the percentage of patients with positive PD-L1 and PD-1 tissular expression did not associate with IMDC groups; however, if the favorable and intermediate groups are pooled together, then PD-L1 expression in tumor center was higher in patients with poor prognosis and approached statistical significance ($p = 0.056$) (Table 5). Also, median sPD-L1 levels almost correlated with IMDC groups ($p = 0.062$) and did so again when favorable and intermediate median sPD-L1 levels discriminated against prognostic groups ($p = 0.021$) (Table 5).

Table 4. Cox Regression model for 5-year overall survival (OS) prediction in CCRCC patients, final step of the Wald Method. Selected pathologic variables for analyses were: Fuhrman grade or G (low vs. high grade), tumor necrosis (no/yes), local invasion pT (pT1 vs. pT2 vs. pT3-pT4), lymph node metastasis N (no/yes) and distant metastases M (no vs. synchronous vs. metachronous). Exponentiation of the B coefficient (ExpB) with confidence interval (CI) is also included. Statistically significant values are highlighted in bold. PD-L1c: combination of tissue and soluble isoforms of PD-L1.

5-Year OS	Variables	Tumour Centre				Centre-Front				Plasma		
		p	ExpB	CI		p	ExpB	CI		p	ExpB	CI
	pT	**0.04**	1.9	1	3.5	0.09	1.65	0.92	9	**0.004**	2.24	1.3	3.86
	N	**0.02**	4.09	1.2	13.9	**0.001**	6.68	2.1	21.4	-		
	M	**0.01**	2	1.19	3.38	**0.005**	2.07	1.24	3.46	8×10^{-6}	2.83	1.68	4.75
	PD-L1	0.06	2.74	0.96	7.78	**0.026**	3.34	1.15	9.66	1×10^{-5}	8.67	3.26	23.1

5-Year OS	Variables	Tumour Centre and Plasma				Front and Plasma				Centre-Front and Plasma		
		p	ExpB	CI		p	ExpB	CI		p	ExpB	CI
	pT	**0.002**	4.66	1.77	12.22	**0.01**	1.83	1.34	9.12	**0.017**	3.3	1.24	8.66
	N	**0.02**	4.29	1.21	15.17	**0.002**	3.28	1.96	21.7	**0.005**	5.85	1.69	20.2
	M	**0.001**	2.33	1.4	3.89	**0.0001**	5.13	1.6	4.5	**0.0001**	2.63	1.57	4.4
	PD-L1c	**0.03**	3.5	1.09	11.28	**0.009**	2.56	1.53	19.7	**0.003**	7.98	2.05	31

Table 5. PD-L1 and PD-1 expression and sPD-L1 and sPD-1 levels in the subgroup of metastatic CCRCC classified according to the International Metastatic Renal Cell Cancer Database Consortium (IMDC) score (* Favorable and Intermediate pooled together). Chi-x^2, Mann-Whitney and Kruskal Wallis tests were used. Statistically significant values are highlighted in bold.

		Tumor Centre			Tumor Front			Plasma
		PD-L1 n (%)			PD-L1 n (%)			
	Variables	Negative	Positive	Total	Negative	Positive	Total	sPD-L1 (ng/mL)
IMDC score	Favorable	7 (77.8)	2 (22.2)	9	3 (42.9)	4 (52.1)	7	488 ± 112.9
	Intermediate	6 (75)	2 (25)	8	5 (71.4)	2 (28.6)	7	705.4 ± 259.4
	Poor	2 (33.3)	4 (66.7)	6	1 (20)	4 (80)	5	967 ± 135.4
	Total	15	8	23	9	10	19	688.6 ± 109.5
		$p = 0.161 / p = 0.056$ *			$p = 0.203$			$p = 0.062 / p = \mathbf{0.021}$ *

		Tumor Center			Tumor Front			Plasma
		PD-1 n (%)			PD-1 n (%)			
	Variables	Negative	Positive	Total	Negative	Positive	Total	sPD-1 (ng/mL)
IMDC score	Favorable	5 (55.6)	4 (44.4)	9	3 (33.3)	6 (66.7)	9	154.3 ± 93
	Intermediate	3 (37.5)	5 (62.5)	8	2 (28.6)	5 (71.4)	7	618.1 ± 294.8
	Poor	2 (33.3)	4 (66.7)	6	3 (50)	3 (50)	6	650 ± 532.3
	Total	15	8	23	8	14	22	442.1 ± 182.8
		$p = 0.637$			$p = 0.704$			$p = 0.341$

Sixteen patients received systemic therapy for metastatic CCRCC and response to therapy was evaluated according to the MASS criteria. PD-L1 and PD-1 expression and sPD-L1 and sPD-1 levels were investigated according to the three categories of favorable, indeterminate and unfavorable responses (Table 6).

The percentage of patients with positive PD-L1 and PD-1 tissular expression did not associate with MASS response groups to systemic therapy; however, if the indeterminate and unfavorable response groups are pooled together, then PD-L1 expression in the tumor front was more often negative and the association approached statistical significance ($p = 0.079$) (Table 6). However, median sPD-L1 levels correlated with the different IMDC groups ($p = 0.014$) and did so again when favorable and intermediate are gathered ($p = 0.021$). The discrimination level was even enhanced if indeterminate and unfavorable responses were pooled together and compared to patients with a favorable response ($p = 0.005$). These data suggest that sPD-L1 could be a marker of treatment response in patients with metastatic CCRCC receiving systemic therapy (Table 6).

Table 6. PD-L1 and PD-1 expression and sPD-L1 and sPD-1 levels in patients with treated metastatic CCRCC according to Morphology, Attenuation, Size and Structure (MASS) classification of response to therapy (* Favorable and Indeterminate responses pooled together; ** Indeterminate and Unfavorable responses pooled together). Chi-x^2, Mann-Whitney and Kruskal Wallis tests were used. Statistically significant values are highlighted in bold.

		Tumour Centre			Tumour Front			Plasma
		PD-L1 n (%)			PD-L1 n (%)			
	Variables	Negative	Positive	Total	Negative	Positive	Total	sPD-L1 (ng/mL)
MASS Response	Favorable	6 (60)	4 (40)	10	2 (28.6)	5 (71.4)	7	387.5 ± 89.1
	Indeterminate	2 (66.7)	1 (33.3)	3	2 (66.7)	1 (33.3)	3	811.4 ± 78.1
	Unfavorable	2 (66.7)	1 (33.3)	3	2 (100)	0 (0)	2	1621 ± 442.9
	Total	10	6	16	6	6	12	698.3 ± 151.2
		$p = 0.965$			$p = 0.164 / p = 0.079$ **			$p = 0.014$ / $p = 0.021$ */ $p = 0.005$ **
		Tumour Centre			Tumour Front			Plasma
		PD-1 n (%)			PD-1 n (%)			
	Variables	Negative	Positive	Total	Negative	Positive	Total	sPD-1 (ng/mL)
MASS Response	Favorable	5 (50)	5 (50)	10	3 (33.3)	6 (66.7)	9	268.9 ± 129.9
	Indeterminate	2 (66.7)	1 (33.3)	3	1 (33.3)	2 (66.7)	3	433.1 ± 265.7
	Unfavorable	1 (33.3)	3 (66.7)	3	3 (100)	0 (0)	3	1743.6 ± 935.1
	Total	8	8	16	7	8	15	647.1 ± 267
		$p = 0.717$			$p = 0.117$			$p = 0.33$

3. Discussion

The T-cell coinhibitory receptor programmed death (PD-1) protein and one of its ligands, PD-L1, play an important role in the evasion of the immune system by tumor cells. Both PD-1 and PD-L1 suppress T cell function and immune tolerance [18]. Recent clinical commercialization of PD-1 pathway inhibitors (nivolumab, pembrolizumab, atezolizumab, durvalumab, avelumab) has raised interest in PD-1 and PD-L1 expression as potential markers of response to immune checkpoint therapy in several malignancies, including CCRCC [19]. Identification and validation of biomarkers will be crucial to optimize first-line selection of treatment and also treatment sequences.

In this sense, it has been demonstrated that PD-1 and PD-L1 expression is associated with adverse clinico-pathological features in CCRCC, such as a large tumor size, high nuclear grade, tumor necrosis and presence of sarcomatoid differentiation [20]. What is more, PD-1 expression has been suggested as one of the most interesting biomarkers denoting poor outcomes in patients with metastatic CCRCC receiving molecular targeted therapies, while conflicting results have been shown for PD-L1 in the same population [20,21]. Both PD-1 and PD-L1 are expressed in intra-tumor inflammatory lymphocytes [22]. PD-1 and PD-L1 expression associates with CD4+, CD8+ and FOXP3+ tumor infiltrating lymphocytes related to poor survival in CCRCC [20,23,24]. However, the identification of patients that are likely to obtain a benefit from PD-1/PD-L1 inhibition therapy remains a challenge [25].

Metastatic CCRCC with a long-term response to sunitinib has been characterized as a distinct phenotype independently associated with low PD-L1 expression [26]. However, the inherent heterogeneity of CCRCC includes a very variable expression of positive and negative regions of PD-L1 expression within each tumor [27]. Also, differential expression of PD-1 and PD-L1 has been confirmed between primary and metastatic sites within the same case [28–30]. This conflicting scenario can be worsened as the different expression across primary and metastatic tumor for PD-L1 could be associated with metastatic tumor timing. In fact, larger differences between their primary and metastatic tumor pairs have been detected in synchronous metastatic patients in comparison to the metachronous metastatic ones, and this could be explained by the fact that distant metachronous metastasis may have evolved independently of the primary tumor [31].

PD-L1 expression has been used as surrogate marker of response to immune checkpoint inhibitors and, indirectly, as marker of prognosis as well. In fact, despite all the limitations mentioned to evaluate responses to therapy based on PD-1/PD-L1 expression, a tendency towards a higher PD-L1 expression has been confirmed in responders but without a good correlation [32]. For this reason, PD-L1 assessment is not required so far to initiate immune checkpoint inhibition therapy in patients with CCRCC. On the other hand, strong evidence is accumulating to consider PD-L1 expression as a likely strong prognosticator in patients with CCRCC not only in metastatic cases receiving anti-PD-1 antibodies, but also receiving sunitinib or pazopanib [33]. In the series that we present here, PDL-1 expression in CCRCC and sPD-L1 levels were predictors of overall survival, and the combination of both tissue expression and plasma levels was an independent predictor of prognosis. It should be stressed that most of the patients in this series were only treated surgically and therefore, we cannot directly infer that PD-L1 (either tissular or plasmatic) is an independent prognostic marker in patients with metastatic CCRCC treated with systemic therapies. Also, as the tissue and plasma samples analyzed in this series belong to the TKI era (checkpoint immune inhibitors were only used in a small number of patients after progression on TKI). Even though the number of patients with metastatic CCRCC in this series is small, we can confirm that PD-L1 expression in tumor center is higher in metastatic patients within the IMDC poor prognosis group ($p = 0.056$) and also that sPD-L1 levels better discriminate poor prognosis for this population of ($p = 0.021$).

Circulating sPD-L1 can be determined by ELISA in normal human serum and in supernatants of different cells including CD4+, CD8+, CD19+, CD14+ and CD56+ T cells, and may play an important role in immunoregulation [34]. sPD-L1 have been described in several malignancies including renal cell cancer, pancreatic cancer, rectal cancer, B-cell lymphoma, multiple myeloma and melanoma [35–39]. It has been hypothesized that sPD-L1 may act as a paracrine negative immune regulator within the tumor [40]. However, the sources of sPD-L1 in patients with cancer is unclear, as it may derive from protumor inflammatory responses, antitumor immune-responses and also intrinsic splicing variants in tumor cells. It is also unclear whether sPD-L1 is associated with clinical characteristics such as patient age, sex or treatment response. In our series sPD-L1 is higher in controls than in patients with CCRCC and the level of sPD-L1 in cancer patients is associated with metastatic disease, but not with conventional prognosticators of CCRCC. Interestingly, higher levels of sPD-L1 in CCRCC are an independent predictor of prognosis. Other authors have investigated the role of several immune checkpoint-related proteins as predictors of tumor recurrence and survival in CCRCC and sustain sTIM3 and sBTLA, but did not predict worse survival for sPD-L1 [41].

According to our experience, both PD-1 and PD-L1 immunohistochemical expression are associated with well-recognized histopathologic parameters of tumor aggressiveness and PD-L1 is also an independent marker of prognosis in our series, both on the tumor center and invasive fronts. Notably, this is a population of patients with CCRCC including all stages and not necessarily treated with antiangiogenic therapy or immune checkpoint inhibition therapy. What is more, we have simultaneously evaluated PD-1 and PD-L1 both in the tumor and serum of the same cohort of patients and have confirmed that sPD-L1 is definitely an independent prognostic factor that is non-associated with the tumor size, Fuhrman grade or histopathological staging. Multivariate analysis revealed that sPD-L1 > 793 ng/mL is associated with worse survival (HR 8.67), together with pT category (HR 2.24) or presence of metastasis (HR 2.83). We also confirmed a major variation in sPD-L1 levels according to the time of the metastatic event, with a much higher expression in synchronous metastases than in metachronous ones. No less interesting is the fact that a positive PD-L1 expression in the tumor center and the invading tumor front— as well as as PD-L1 level > 793 ng/mL—leads to a worse overall survival rate in CCRCC patients. However, what is even more interesting in our experience is that sPDL-1 levels appear to represent a good surrogate of a response criteria to systemic therapy administered in metastatic CCRCC. In this context, there are many limitations to consider when deciding to treat CCRCC patients with immune checkpoint inhibitors based on the immunohistochemical detection of PD-1/PD-L1 positivity alone [11,27], while the search of markers to anticipate the response to immunotherapy continues [42–44]. A new trial (UMIN000027873) has been recently launched to evaluate the therapeutic effect of nivolumamb as a second-line therapy for advanced CCRCC based on the concentrations of serum sPD-L1. The hypothesis of this study is that patients with high blood levels of sPD-L1 will experience a greater therapeutic effect during nivolumab treatment [45].

The limitations of our study include its retrospective nature, despite the fact that the cases were prospectively followed after tumor and serum samples were obtained. Patients were treated using state-of-the art procedures, and size of the sample was also relatively small, especially when different subsets of patients were specifically analyzed. Also, our finding that sPD-1 levels in controls are higher than in CCRCC patients could be explained by a confounding effect of disparity levels in CCRCC patients due to the fact that the sample includes patients with all stages of disease. It also could have been due to inappropriateness of the control sample as a result of unknown factors. Regardless, we did not test the hypothesis that sPD-L1 can be a tumor marker for the diagnosis of CCRCC, but we did show evidence supporting the idea that it can be a good marker to evaluate prognosis for CCRCC patients when they are taken as a whole, and also in the subset of metastatic patients being treated with the IMDC model. Also, we support its use as a marker of prognosis in metastatic patients treated with systemic therapies, mainly TKIs.

Future studies should try to evaluate the role of sPD-L1 and other soluble immune checkpoint-related proteins to elucidate their role as intrinsic tumor markers with utility in prognostic evaluation involving CCRCC as a malignancy without markers of clinical value, despite the great therapeutic success that has been achieved in the last decade.

4. Materials and Methods

The present study including all of its experiments comply with current Spanish and European Union legal regulations. The Basque Biobank for Research-OEHUN (www.biobancovasco.org) was employed the source of samples and data from patients that could be used for research purposes. Each patient signed a specific document which had been approved by the Ethical and Scientific Committees of the Basque Country Public Health System (Osakidetza) (PI + CES-BIOEF 2018-04).

4.1. Patients

Plasma samples and tumor tissues were obtained from 89 CCRCC patients that were surgically treated at Basurto University Hospital from 2012 to 2016. The plasma samples were preoperatively collected for the study. Patients with non-metastatic CCRCC were treated surgically and patients with metastatic disease received nephrectomy and systemic therapy according to their ICDM classification, age and clinical condition.

Sixty patients were males (mean age: 60.83 years; range: 36–82) and 29 were females (mean age: 62.69; range: 32–80). Pathological characteristics are summarized in Table 3. Plasma from 46 healthy volunteers with no clinical history of neoplastic diseases was used as control samples (male/female 28/18, age 55.8/61.8 years).

Samples from the center ($n = 88$) and the infiltration front ($n = 75$) of tumors from these patients were distinguished in the histopathological department and included in tissue microarrays (TMAs) for further immunohistochemical analyses. American Joint Committee on Cancer (AJCC) [19] and Furhman's [20] methods were applied to assign the relevant stage and grade, respectively.

During the follow-up (mean: 59.9 months, range: 1–91 months), 21 patients were found to no longer be alive and 68 were still alive. All patients were prospectively followed until death or the last-follow-up. The cause and date of death was taken as specified in clinical records and overall survival (OS) was investigated.

4.2. IMDC Model and MASS Response Criteria for Patients with Metastatic CCRCC

The International mRCC Database Consortium (IMDC) represents the largest collection of real-world data on patients with advanced kidney cancer treated with targeted therapies. The IMDC prognostic model has been used to stratify patients in contemporary clinical trials and to provide risk-directed treatment selection in everyday clinical practice. This model classifies metastatic patients into three categories at different risk of death: favorable, intermediate and poor risk [46]. We used the IMDC to evaluate the group of patients with metastatic CCRCC in this series ($n = 23$).

In order to evaluate the response assessment to systemic therapy in metastatic CCRCC receiving treatments other than nephrectomy ($n = 16$), the Morphology, Attenuation, Size and Structure (MASS) criteria was used to distinguish between the three categories of patients. Patients with a favorable response to therapy are those with no new lesions displayed on imaging modalities and any of the following outcomes: i. A decrease in the tumor size of $\geq 20\%$; ii. One or more predominantly solid enhancing lesions showed marked central necrosis or marked decreased attenuation (≥ 40 Hounsfield units). Patients with an unfavorable response are those with either: i. An increase in the tumor size of $\geq 20\%$ in the absence of marked central necrosis or marked decreased attenuation; ii. New metastases, marked central fill-in or new enhancement of a previously homogeneously hypoattenuating non-enhancing mass. Patients with an indeterminate response are those who do not fit the criteria for favorable or unfavorable responses [47].

4.3. Immunohistochemistry

PD-L1 and PD-1 was analyzed in formalin-fixed and paraffin-embedded material using specific antibodies (PD-1 (Ventana, clone NAT105, ready-to-use) and PD-L1 (Ventana, clone SP-142, ready-to-use)). Immunostaining was performed using an automated immunostainer (Benchmark Ultra, Ventana, Roche, AZ, USA) following the protocols recommended by the manufacturer.

We documented the presence (+) or absence (−) of PD-L1 and PD-1 immunolabels in inflammatory cells [27] using a Nikon Eclipse 80i microscope (Nikon, Tokyo, Japan). All specimens were independently evaluated by two observers; in the event of discrepancies, samples were re-evaluated to arrive at a final conclusion.

4.4. ELISA Assays

Levels of soluble PD-L1 and PD-1 were evaluated using the human B7-H1 and PD-1 DuoSet ELISA kits (R&D Systems, DY156 and DY1086, respectively) according to the manufacturer's protocols [37]. Briefly, 96 well plates were coated with capture antibodies diluted in PBS and incubated overnight at 4 °C. After washing, plates were blocked in order to avoid unspecific binding. Standards (100 µL) together with optimized plasma sample dilutions (1/8 for sPD-L1 and 1/4 for sPD-1) and controls were added to the wells and incubated for 2 h at room temperature (RT). After washing the plate, 100 µL/well of biotinylated detection antibody was added and incubated for 1 h at RT. Subsequently, Streptavidin-HRP A solution was added and the mixture was incubated for 20 min. Finally, following multiple washes, the wells were incubated with 100 µL/well of Substrate Solution and were stopped after 20 min with 2N H2SO4. The readout was made by reading the absorbance at 450 nm with a FluoStar Optima plate reader (BMG Labtech). The amount of protein of interest in the sample was estimated using a standard curve after applying the dilution factor.

4.5. Statistical Analysis

The statistical analysis was performed by using SPSS® 24.0 software. In order to assess whether data obtained from the tissue and plasma samples followed a normal distribution, we applied a Kolmogorov-Smirnov test. Based on this information, data were further analyzed using parametric or non-parametric tests.

The Spearman Rho test was used to test the correlation between tumor tissue PD-L1 and PD-1 expression, sPD-L1 and sPD-1 levels and patient age and gender. Comparison of plasma levels of sPD-L1 and sPD-1 between two groups or more (respectively) was carried out using the Mann-Whitney (Mann-U) and Kruskal-Wallis tests. To analyze categorical tissue expression of PD-L1 and PD-1 (negative/positive) and to test the association of differences with pathological variables, we used the Chi-square (χ^2) test.

Overall survival (OS) analyses were performed following the establishing of groups by cut-off points, following different methods: (I) for tissue analyses, cut-off points were based on the categorical expression of PD-L1 and PD-1 (negative (<1% staining) vs. positive ($\geq$1% staining)); (II) a classification and regression tree (CRT) method was employed for the analysis of plasma sPD-L1 and sPD-1; (III) in order to evaluate the OS of CCRCC patients, Kaplan-Meier curves and log-rank tests were utilized; (IV) to evaluate the independent effects of PD-L1 and PD-1 expression and plasma levels of soluble isoforms and pathological variables on OS, we employed multivariate analyses (the Cox regression model with the backward Wald stepwise method).

5. Conclusions

There is a major need to identify new molecular markers in CCRCC which are useful from the clinical perspective. We corroborated the value of PD-L1 immunostaining in lymphocytic infiltrate both in the tumor center and in the border of neoplastic tissue to predict worse overall survival in patients with CCRCC undergoing surgery which were not necessarily treated with immune-checkpoint inhibitors. We also advocate for the clinical utility of sPD-L1 level > 793ng/mL as an independent and novel predictor of prognosis in clinical practice for the same patients. In addition, we determined that the sPD-L1 level increased for IMDC prognostic groups in the population of patients with metastatic CCRCC, and was also associated with the clinical response of patients with metastatic CCRCC receiving systemic therapy.

These findings could be of primary importance because they indicate that the determination of sPD-L1 can be widely performed in clinical practice. Our results should be validated in prospective studies and possibly incorporated into predictive nomograms that have clinical transcendence in patients with CCRCC.

Supplementary Materials: The following materials are available online at https://www.mdpi.com/2072-6694/13/4/667/s1, Figure S1: Classification and Regression Tree (CRT) for both sPD-L1 and sP-D1, and CCRCC patients' 5-year overall survival (OS), Table S1: Correlation between age and sex, and PD-L1 and PD-1 CCRCC expression and plasma levels (Spearman Rho test). PD-L1 and PD-1 expression in the centre of the tumour (c), infiltration front (f) and in both areas (cf), and plasma levels of sPD-L1 and sPD-1 were not correlated with sex and age of CCRCC patients, Table S2: Correlation between PD-L1 and PD-1 expression at the tumor center and at the infiltration front (Spearman Rho test), Table S3: Systemic therapies received by 16 patients with metastatic CCRCC, Table S4: Cox Regression model for 5-year overall survival (OS) prediction in CCRCC patients (complete table with the first step and the final step of Wald method).

Author Contributions: Conceptualization, G.L., J.C.A. and J.I.L.; Data curation, E.E., A.A., A.L.-I. and J.D.S.-I.; Formal analysis, J.D.S.-I., P.E., C.M. and J.I.L.; Funding acquisition, G.L., A.A., J.C.A. and J.I.L.; Investigation, J.D.S.-I., P.E., M.U., A.L.-I., A.P.-F., C.M. and J.I.L.; Methodology, J.D.S.-I., P.E. and C.M.; Project administration, G.L., A.A., J.C.A. and J.I.L.; Supervision, G.L., J.C.A. and J.I.L.; Writing—original draft, G.L., J.C.A. and J.I.L.; Writing—review & editing, G.L., J.D.S.-I., P.E., A.A., E.E., M.U., A.L.-I., A.P.-F., C.M., J.C.A. and J.I.L. All authors have read and agreed to the published version of the manuscript.

Funding: The work was funded by the Basque Government (ELKARTEK KK2018-00090 and KK-2020/00069).

Institutional Review Board Statement: The present study including all its experiments comply with current Spanish and European Union legal regulations. The Basque Biobank for Research-OEHUN (www.biobancovasco.org) was the source of samples and the data from patients employed could possibly be used for research purposes. The study was approved by the Ethical and Scientific Committees of the Basque Country Public Health System (Osakidetza) (PI+CES-BIOEF 2018-04).

Informed Consent Statement: Informed consent was obtained from all subjects involved in the study.

Data Availability Statement: Full data will be available from the Corresponding Author upon reasonable request.

Acknowledgments: The authors want to thank Arantza Pérez Dobaran (UPV/EHU) for her technical support.

Conflicts of Interest: The authors declare no conflict of interest. The funders had no role in the design of the study; in the collection, analyses, or interpretation of data; in the writing of the manuscript, or in the decision to publish the results.

References

1. Bray, F.; Ferlay, J.; Soerjomataram, I.; Siegel, R.L.; Torre, L.A.; Jemal, A. Global cancer statistics 2018: GLOBOCAN estimates of incidence and mortality worldwide for 36 cancers in 185 countries. *CA Cancer J. Clin.* **2018**, *68*, 394–424. [CrossRef]
2. Siegel, R.L.; Miller, K.D.; Jemal, A. Cancer statistics, 2020. *CA Cancer J Clin.* **2020**, *70*, 7–30. [CrossRef] [PubMed]
3. MacLennan, G.T.; Cheng, L. Neoplasms of the kidney. In *Urologic Surgical Pathology*, 3rd ed.; Bostwick, D.G., Cheng, L., Eds.; Saunders: Saunders Park, PA, USA, 2014; pp. 76–156.
4. Tomita, Y. Early renal cell cancer. *Int. J. Clin. Oncol.* **2006**, *11*, 22–27. [CrossRef] [PubMed]
5. Mitchell, T.J.; Turajlic, S.; Rowan, A.; Nicol, D.; Farmery, J.H.; O'Brien, T.; Martincorena, I.; Tarpey, P.; Angelopoulos, N.; Yates, L.R.; et al. Timing the Landmark Events in the Evolution of Clear Cell Renal Cell Cancer: TRACERx Renal. *Cell* **2018**, *173*, 611–623.e17. [CrossRef] [PubMed]
6. Angulo, J.C.; Lawrie, C.H.; López, J.I. Sequential treatment of metastatic renal cancer in a complex evolving landscape. *Ann. Transl. Med.* **2019**, *7*, S272. [CrossRef]
7. Santoni, M.; Heng, D.Y.C.; Bracarda, S.; Procopio, G.; Milella, M.; Porta, C.; Matrana, M.; Cartenì, G.; Crabb, S.J.; de Giorgi, U.; et al. Real-World Data on Cabozantinib in Previously Treated Patients with Metastatic Renal Cell Carcinoma: Focus on Sequences and Prognostic Factors. *Cancers* **2019**, *12*, 84. [CrossRef]
8. Mollica, V.; di Nunno, V.; Gatto, L.; Santoni, M.; Scarpelli, M.; Cimadamore, A.; Montironi, R.; Cheng, L.; Battelli, N.; Montironi, R.; et al. Resistance to Systemic Agents in Renal Cell Carcinoma Predict and Overcome Genomic Strategies Adopted by Tumor. *Cancers* **2019**, *11*, 830. [CrossRef] [PubMed]
9. Atkins, M.B.; Tannir, N.M. Current and emerging therapies for first-line treatment of metastatic clear cell renal cell carcinoma. *Cancer Treat. Rev.* **2018**, *70*, 127–137. [CrossRef]
10. Angulo, J.C.; Shapiro, O. The Changing Therapeutic Landscape of Metastatic Renal Cancer. *Cancers* **2019**, *11*, 1227. [CrossRef] [PubMed]
11. Nunes-Xavier, C.E.; Angulo, J.C.; Pulido, R.; Lopez, J.I. A Critical Insight into the Clinical Translation of PD-1/PD-L1 Blockade Therapy in Clear Cell Renal Cell Carcinoma. *Curr. Urol. Rep.* **2019**, *20*, 1. [CrossRef] [PubMed]
12. Khagi, Y.; Kurzrock, R.; Patel, S.P. Next generation predictive biomarkers for immune checkpoint inhibition. *Cancer Metastasis Rev.* **2017**, *36*, 179–190.
13. Zhu, J.; Armstrong, A.J.; Friedlander, T.W.; Kim, W.; Pal, S.K.; George, D.J.; Zhang, T. Biomarkers of immunotherapy in urothelial and renal cell carcinoma: PD-L1, tumor mutational burden, and beyond. *J. Immunother. Cancer* **2018**, *6*, 4. [CrossRef] [PubMed]
14. Lecis, D.; Sangaletti, S.; Colombo, M.P.; Chiodoni, C. Immune Checkpoint Ligand Reverse Signaling: Looking Back to Go Forward in Cancer Therapy. *Cancers* **2019**, *11*, 624. [CrossRef]
15. Ock, C.Y.; Keam, B.; Kim, S.; Lee, J.S.; Kim, M.; Kim, T.M. Pan-cancer immunogenomic perspective on the Tumour microenvironment based on PD-L1 and CD8 T-Cell infiltration. *Clin. Cancer Res.* **2016**, *22*, 2261–2270. [CrossRef]
16. Miao, D.; Margolis, C.A.; Gao, W.; Voss, M.H.; Li, W.; Martini, D.J.; Norton, C.; Bossé, D.; Wankowicz, S.M.; Cullen, D.; et al. Genomic correlates of response to immune checkpoint therapies in clear cell renal cell carcinoma. *Science* **2018**, *359*, 801–806. [CrossRef]
17. Dubin, K.; Callahan, M.K.; Ren, B.; Khanin, R.; Viale, A.; Ling, L.; No, D.; Gobourne, A.; Littmann, E.; Huttenhower, B.R.C.; et al. Intestinal microbiome analyses identify melanoma patients at risk for checkpoint-blockade-induced colitis. *Nat. Commun.* **2016**, *7*, 10391. [CrossRef] [PubMed]

18. Topalian, S.L.; Hodi, F.S.; Brahmer, J.R.; Gettinger, S.N.; Smith, D.C.; McDermott, D.F. Five-year survival and correlates among patients with advanced melanoma, renal cell carcinoma, or non-small cell lung cancer treated with nivolumab. *JAMA Oncol.* **2019**, *5*, 1411–1420. [CrossRef] [PubMed]
19. Wu, X.; Gu, Z.; Chen, Y.; Chen, B.; Chen, W.; Weng, L.; Liu, X. Application of PD-1 Blockade in Cancer Immunotherapy. *Comput. Struct. Biotechnol. J.* **2019**, *17*, 661–674. [CrossRef] [PubMed]
20. Ueda, K.; Suekane, S.; Kurose, H.; Chikui, K.; Nakiri, M.; Nishihara, K.; Matsuo, M.; Kawahara, A.; Yano, H.; Igawa, T. Prognostic value of PD-1 and PD-L1 expression in patients with metastatic clear cell renal cell carcinoma. *Urol. Oncol. Semin. Orig. Investig.* **2018**, *36*, 499.e9–499.e16. [CrossRef] [PubMed]
21. Hara, T.; Miyake, H.; Fujisawa, M. Expression pattern of immune checkpoint-associated molecules in radical nephrectomy specimens as a prognosticator in patients with metastatic renal cell carcinoma treated with tyrosine kinase inhibitors. *Urol. Oncol.* **2017**, *35*, 363–369. [CrossRef]
22. Taube, J.M.; Klein, A.; Brahmer, J.R.; Xu, H.; Pan, X.; Kim, J.H. Association of PD-1, PD-1 ligands, and other features of the tumour immune microenvironment with response to anti-PD-1 therapy. *Clin. Cancer Res.* **2014**, *20*, 5064–5074. [CrossRef] [PubMed]
23. Nakano, O.; Sato, M.; Naito, Y.; Suzuki, K.; Orikasa, S.; Aizawa, M. Proliferative activity of intratumoural CD8(+) T-lymphocytes as a prognostic factor in human renal cell carcinoma: Clinicopathologic demonstration of antitumour immunity. *Cancer Res.* **2001**, *61*, 5132–5136.
24. Liotta, F.; Gacci, M.; Frosali, F.; Querci, V.; Vittori, G.; Lapini, A.; Santarlasci, V.; Serni, S.; Cosmi, L.; Maggi, L.; et al. Frequency of regulatory T cells in peripheral blood and in tumour-infiltrating lymphocytes correlates with poor prognosis in renal cell carcinoma. *BJU Int.* **2010**, *107*, 1500–1506. [CrossRef] [PubMed]
25. Hayashi, H.; Nakagawa, K. Combination therapy with PD-1 or PD-L1 inhibitors for cancer. *Int. J. Clin. Oncol.* **2020**, *25*, 818–830. [CrossRef]
26. Kammerer-Jacquet, S.-F.; Deleuze, A.; Saout, J.; Mathieu, R.; Laguerre, B.; Verhoest, G.; Dugay, F.; Belaud-Rotureau, M.-A.; Bensalah, K.; Rioux-Leclercq, N. Targeting the PD-1/PD-L1 Pathway in Renal Cell Carcinoma. *Int. J. Mol. Sci.* **2019**, *20*, 1692. [CrossRef]
27. Lopez, J.I.; Pulido, R.; Cortes, J.M.; Angulo, J.; Lawrie, C.H. Potential impact of PD-L1 (SP-142) immunohistochemical heterogeneity in clear cell renal cell carcinoma immunotherapy. *Pathol. Res. Pract.* **2018**, *214*, 1110–1114. [CrossRef]
28. Jilaveanu, L.B.; Shuch, B.; Zito, C.R.; Parisi, F.; Barr, M.; Kluger, Y.; Chen, L.; Kluger, H.M. PD-L1 Expression in Clear Cell Renal Cell Carcinoma: An Analysis of Nephrectomy and Sites of Metastases. *J. Cancer* **2014**, *5*, 166–172. [CrossRef]
29. Basu, A.; Yearley, J.H.; Annamalai, L.; Pryzbycin, C.; Rini, B. Association of PD-L1, PD-L2, and Immune Response Markers in Matched Renal Clear Cell Carcinoma Primary and Metastatic Tissue Specimens. *Am. J. Clin. Pathol.* **2018**, *151*, 217–225. [CrossRef]
30. Zhang, X.; Yin, X.; Zhang, H.; Sun, G.; Yang, Y.; Chen, J.; Zhu, X.; Zhao, P.; Zhao, J.; Liu, J.; et al. Differential expressions of PD-1, PD-L1 and PD-L2 between primary and metastatic sites in renal cell carcinoma. *BMC Cancer* **2019**, *19*, 1–10. [CrossRef] [PubMed]
31. Eckel-Passow, J.E.; Ho, T.H.; Serie, D.J.; Cheville, J.C.; Houston-Thompson, R.; Costello, B.A. Concordance of PD-1 and PD-L1 (B7-H1) in paired primary and metastatic clear cell renal cell carcinoma. *Cancer Med.* **2020**, *9*, 1152–1160. [CrossRef]
32. Stenzel, P.J.; Schindeldecker, M.; Tagscherer, K.E.; Foersch, S.; Herpel, E.; Hohenfellner, M. Prognostic and predictive value of tumour-infiltrating leukocytes and of immune checkpoint molecules PD1 and PDL1 in clear cell renal cell carcinoma. *Transl. Oncol.* **2020**, *13*, 336–345. [CrossRef] [PubMed]
33. Choueiri, T.K.; Figueroa, D.J.; Fay, A.P.; Signoretti, S.; Liu, Y.; Gagnon, R. Correlation of PD-L1 tumour expression and treatment outcomes in patients with renal cell carcinoma receiving sunitinib or pazopanib: Results from COMPARZ, a randomized controlled trial. *Clin. Cancer Res.* **2015**, *21*, 1071–1077. [CrossRef]
34. Chen, Y.; Wang, Q.; Shi, B.; Xu, P.; Hu, Z.; Bai, L.; Zhang, X. Development of a sandwich ELISA for evaluating soluble PD-L1 (CD274) in human sera of different ages as well as supernatants of PD-L1+ cell lines. *Cytokine* **2011**, *56*, 231–238. [CrossRef]
35. Rossille, D.; Gressier, M.; Damotte, D.; Maucort-Boulch, D.; Pangault, C.; Semana, G. High level of soluble programmed cell death ligand 1 in blood impacts overall survival in aggressive diffuse large B-Cell lymphoma: Results from a French multicentre clinical trial. *Leukemia* **2014**, *28*, 2367–2375. [CrossRef]
36. Zhou, J.; Mahoney, K.M.; Giobbie-Hurder, A.; Zhao, F.; Lee, S.; Liao, X.; Rodig, S.; Li, J.; Wu, X.; Butterfield, L.H.; et al. Soluble PD-L1 as a Biomarker in Malignant Melanoma Treated with Checkpoint Blockade. *Cancer Immunol. Res.* **2017**, *5*, 480–492. [CrossRef] [PubMed]
37. Kruger, S.; Legenstein, M.-L.; Rösgen, V.; Haas, M.; Modest, D.P.; Westphalen, C.B.; Ormanns, S.; Kirchner, T.; Heinemann, V.; Holdenrieder, S.; et al. Serum levels of soluble programmed death protein 1 (sPD-1) and soluble programmed death ligand 1 (sPD-L1) in advanced pancreatic cancer. *eCollection* **2017**, *6*, e1310358. [CrossRef] [PubMed]
38. Tominaga, T.; Akiyoshi, T.; Yamamoto, N.; Taguchi, S.; Mori, S.; Nagasaki, T.; Fukunaga, Y.; Ueno, M. Clinical significance of soluble programmed cell death-1 and soluble programmed cell death-ligand 1 in patients with locally advanced rectal cancer treated with neoadjuvant chemoradiotherapy. *PLoS ONE* **2019**, *14*, e0212978. [CrossRef] [PubMed]
39. Bian, B.; Fanale, D.; Dusetti, N.; Roque, J.; Pastor, S.; Chretien, A.-S.; Incorvaia, L.; Russo, A.; Olive, D.; Iovanna, J.L. Prognostic significance of circulating PD-1, PD-L1, pan-BTN3As, BTN3A1 and BTLA in patients with pancreatic adenocarcinoma. *OncoImmunology* **2019**, *8*, e1561120. [CrossRef] [PubMed]

40. Mahoney, K.M.; Shukla, S.A.; Patsoukis, N.; Chaudhri, A.; Browne, E.P.; Arazi, A.; Eisenhaure, T.M.; Pendergraft, W.F.; Hua, P.; Pham, H.C.; et al. A secreted PD-L1 splice variant that covalently dimerizes and mediates immunosuppression. *Cancer Immunol. Immunother.* **2019**, *68*, 421–432. [CrossRef] [PubMed]
41. Wang, Q.; Zhang, J.; Tu, H.; Liang, D.; Chang, D.W.; Ye, Y.; Wu, X. Soluble immune checkpoint-related proteins as predictors of tumor recurrence, survival, and T cell phenotypes in clear cell renal cell carcinoma patients. *J. Immunother. Cancer* **2019**, *7*, 334. [CrossRef] [PubMed]
42. Raimondi, A.; Sepe, P.; Zattarin, E.; Mennitto, A.; Stellato, M.; Claps, M.; Guadalupi, V.; Verzoni, E.; de Braud, F.; Procopio, G. Predictive Biomarkers of Response to Immunotherapy in Metastatic Renal Cell Cancer. *Front. Oncol.* **2020**, *10*, 1644. [CrossRef] [PubMed]
43. Paver, E.C.; Cooper, W.A.; Colebatch, A.J.; Ferguson, P.M.; Hill, S.K.; Lum, T.; Shin, J.-S.; O'Toole, S.; Anderson, L.; Scolyer, R.A.; et al. Programmed death ligand-1 (PD-L1) as a predictive marker for immunotherapy in solid tumours: A guide to immunohistochemistry implementation and interpretation. *Pathology* **2021**, *53*, 141–156. [CrossRef] [PubMed]
44. Simonaggio, A.; Epaillard, N.; Pobel, C.; Moreira, M.; Oudard, S.; Vano, Y.-A. Tumor Microenvironment Features as Predictive Biomarkers of Response to Immune Checkpoint Inhibitors (ICI) in Metastatic Clear Cell Renal Cell Carcinoma (mccRCC). *Cancers* **2021**, *13*, 231. [CrossRef]
45. Bando, Y.; Hinata, N.; Omori, T.; Fujisawa, M. A prospective, open-label, interventional study protocol to evaluate treatment efficacy of nivolumab based on serum-soluble PD-L1 concentration for patients with metastatic and unresectable renal cell carcinoma. *BMJ Open* **2019**, *9*, e030522. [CrossRef] [PubMed]
46. Heng, D.Y.C.; Xie, W.; Regan, M.M.; Harshman, L.C.; A Bjarnason, G.; Vaishampayan, U.N.; MacKenzie, M.; Wood, L.; Donskov, F.; Tan, M.-H.; et al. External validation and comparison with other models of the International Metastatic Renal-Cell Carcinoma Database Consortium prognostic model: A population-based study. *Lancet Oncol.* **2013**, *14*, 141–148. [CrossRef]
47. Smith, A.D.; Shah, S.N.; Rini, B.I.; Lieber, M.L.; Remer, E.M. Morphology, Attenuation, Size, and Structure (MASS) Criteria: Assessing Response and Predicting Clinical Outcome in Metastatic Renal Cell Carcinoma on Antiangiogenic Targeted Therapy. *Am. J. Roentgenol.* **2010**, *194*, 1470–1478. [CrossRef]

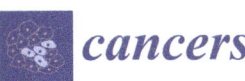

Review

Molecular Mechanisms of Resistance to Immunotherapy and Antiangiogenic Treatments in Clear Cell Renal Cell Carcinoma

Pablo Álvarez Ballesteros [1], Jesús Chamorro [1], María San Román-Gil [1], Javier Pozas [1], Victoria Gómez Dos Santos [2], Álvaro Ruiz Granados [1], Enrique Grande [3], Teresa Alonso-Gordoa [4,*] and Javier Molina-Cerrillo [4,*]

1. Medical Oncology Department, Ramón y Cajal University Hospital, 28034 Madrid, Spain; palvarezb@salud.madrid.org (P.Á.B.); jchamorro@salud.madrid.org (J.C.); mariavictoria.san@salud.madrid.org (M.S.R.-G.); Javier.pozas@salud.madrid.org (J.P.); agranados@salud.madrid.org (Á.R.G.)
2. Urology Department, Ramón y Cajal University Hospital, Alcala University, 28034 Madrid, Spain; vgomezd@salud.madrid.org
3. MD Anderson Cancer Center, 28033 Madrid, Spain; egrande@oncomadrid.com
4. Medical Oncology Department, Ramón y Cajal University Hospital, Medical School, Alcala University, 28034 Madrid, Spain
* Correspondence: talonso@oncologiahrc.com (T.A.-G.); jmolinac@salud.madrid.org (J.M.-C.)

Simple Summary: Renal cell carcinoma is particularly characterized by its high vascularization and dense immune cells infiltration. The angiogenesis blockade in combination with immune checkpoint inhibitors have supposed milestones in the treatment landscape of this tumor. This article gathers the available data on the mechanisms of resistance to current treatments, as well as new strategies under development to overcome these resistances.

Abstract: Clear cell renal cell carcinoma (ccRCC) is the most common histological subtype arising from renal cell carcinomas. This tumor is characterized by a predominant angiogenic and immunogenic microenvironment that interplay with stromal, immune cells, and tumoral cells. Despite the obscure prognosis traditionally related to this entity, strategies including angiogenesis inhibition with tyrosine kinase inhibitors (TKIs), as well as the enhancement of the immune system with the inhibition of immune checkpoint proteins, such as PD-1/PDL-1 and CTLA-4, have revolutionized the treatment landscape. This approach has achieved a substantial improvement in life expectancy and quality of life from patients with advanced ccRCC. Unfortunately, not all patients benefit from this success as most patients will finally progress to these therapies and, even worse, approximately 5 to 30% of patients will primarily progress. In the last few years, preclinical and clinical research have been conducted to decode the biological basis underlying the resistance mechanisms regarding angiogenic and immune-based therapy. In this review, we summarize the insights of these molecular alterations to understand the resistance pathways related to the treatment with TKI and immune checkpoint inhibitors (ICIs). Moreover, we include additional information on novel approaches that are currently under research to overcome these resistance alterations in preclinical studies and early phase clinical trials.

Keywords: renal cell cancer; treatment resistance; immunotherapy; angiogenesis; tumor microenvironment

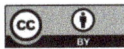

1. Introduction

Renal cell carcinoma (RCC) represents around 3% of all cancers in adults showing an incidence of more than 400,000 cases and being responsible for approximately 175,000 deaths worldwide in 2020 [1–3]. Approximately 25% of patients present with metastatic disease at initial diagnosis and between 20–40% relapse after nephrectomy for localized disease [4]. Overall, mortality rates for RCC increased until the early 1990s, with rates generally stabilizing or declining thereafter (actually 2.2 renal cancer related deaths per 100.000 population) [5].

Clear cell renal cell carcinoma (ccRCC) is the most common histologic subtype that arises in approximately 75% of RCC [6].

From a molecular point of view, genetic alterations are common in RCC and various genes are involved in its development and progression. Inactivation of the *VHL* gene function by deletion of chromosome 3p, mutation, and/or promoter methylation is a predominant feature of ccRCC [7,8] and leads to abnormal accumulation of hypoxia-inducible factors (HIF-1α and HIF-2α) and activation of the angiogenesis program with increased levels of VEGF [9,10]. However, *VHL* loss itself is insufficient for tumorigenesis, and additional genomic aberrations, such as mutations in 3p-associated genes *PBRM1*, *SETD2*, and *BAP1*; loss of *CDKN2A* and *CDKN2B* genes via focal or arm-level deletion of the 9p21 locus; and alterations in *KDM5C*, *TP53*, *MTOR*, or *PTEN* have been implicated in disease progression and degree of aggressiveness [7].

Over the last 15 years, treatment for metastatic RCC (mRCC) has focused on targeting the VEGF signaling pathway with tyrosine kinase receptor inhibitors (TKI), such as sunitinib, pazopanib, cabozantinib, axitinib or lenvatinib, or monoclonal antibodies that block VEGF, such as bevacizumab. Although VEGF pathway blockade is effective in many patients, it is associated with the development of acquired resistance mechanisms [11,12].

Furthermore, ccRCC is also distinguished as a highly inflamed tumor, with high levels of tumor infiltrating lymphocytes, and a predominant expression of immune checkpoints, such as PD-L1 and CTLA-4 [13,14]. Under this rationale of hypervascularity linked with an immunologically hot tumor microenvironment, inhibitors of the VEGF pathway and the PD-(L)1 axis as monotherapy or in combination, have contribute a noteworthy improvement in terms of survival and quality of life in patients with advanced RCC [6]. Unfortunately, there is an important group of patients who do not respond or lose achieved responses.

In this review we aim to summarize key molecular alterations in RCC to understand the resistance to TKI and immunotherapy treatments, as well as the basis for the development of new drugs that potentially overcome these resistances.

2. Molecular Pathways Associated with Resistance to Treatment with Tyrosine-Kinase Inhibitors

2.1. Hypoxia as a Resistance Inductor

Heterogeneity is a pivotal characteristic of RCC, as different genomic and transcriptomic profiles can be observed between primary renal and metastatic lesions [15]. Furthermore, this intratumoral heterogeneity comprises a fundamental feature that hinder efficacy of TKIs. Hypoxia also participates in that inner heterogeneity since RCC tissues show different blood flow conditions.

Anti-VEGF therapies interfere in tumor angiogenesis inducing hypoxic cell death. In consequence, hypoxia enhances epithelial–mesenchymal transition (EMT), causes microenvironmental cells like tumor associated endothelial cells (TECs) and tumor associated macrophages and fibroblasts (TAMs/TAFs) to thrive, increases the expression of proteins involved in lysosomal sequestration of TKIs, interferes with drug penetration, activates many VEGF- and PDGF-independent proangiogenic cascades and alternative pathways that lead to HIF pathway stimulation, and induces alternative modes of vascularization. Moreover, cell glycolysis promoted by hypoxia increases lactic acid levels which is an obstacle for immune cells functions [16]. In this sense, belzutifan, a HIF-2α inhibitor, is currently under development with promising results in disease control rate and duration of response as monotherapy or in combination with other TKI in patients with previously treated mccRCC (NCT03634540, NCT04195750, and NCT 03634540). Indeed, this drug has been approved by the FDA this year, for adult patients with von Hippel–Lindau (VHL) disease who require systemic therapy. Its role in combination with other ICI and in the first line setting is also under research (NCT04736706). However, other novel drugs targeting metabolism, such as telaglenastat, have not shown an additional benefit when analyzed in clinical trails, such as the CANTATA and ENTRATA trials (Figure 1).

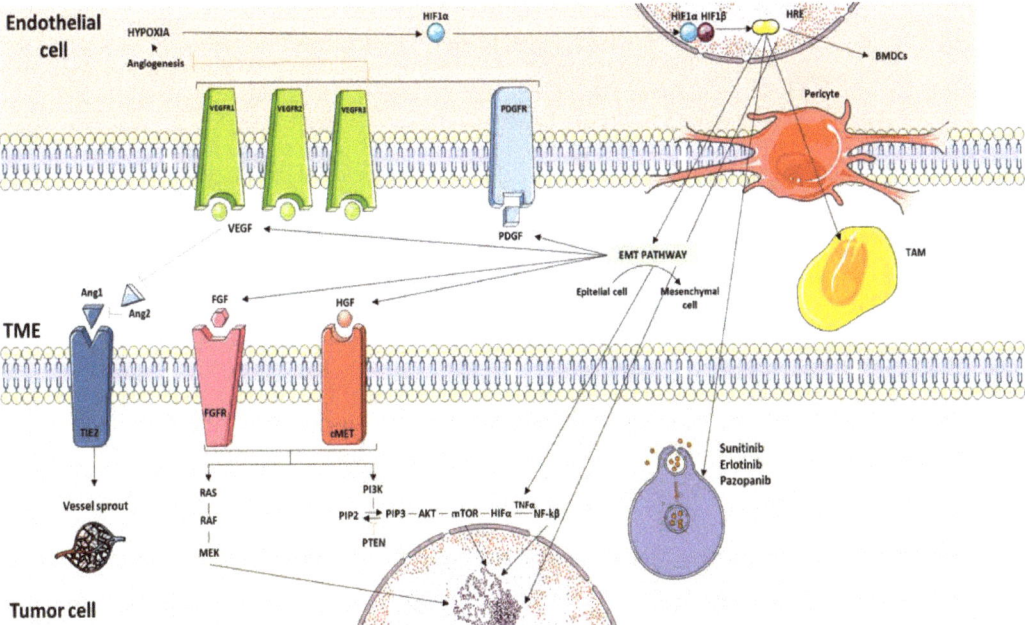

Figure 1. In this figure we illustrate the most preponderant mechanisms of resistance to TKIs: hypoxia-induced activation of alternative proangiogenic pathways, TME factors, EMT, and TKI-induced autophagy.

2.2. Angiogenic Switch

There is robust evidence that describes several non-angiogenic mechanisms which enable tumors to keep growing when angiogenesis is blocked. The first one is known as vessel co-option and lies in the ability of tumor cells to harness normal tissues vessels to maintain oxygen availability [17,18]. It is hypothesized that the initiation of the neoplasm is driven by this angiogenesis-independent strategy, forming the center of the neoplasm. Therefore, co-opted vessels trigger self-apoptosis in order to induce tumor necrosis. Meanwhile, the neoplasm is able to counteract this host defense mechanism by developing neoangiogenesis in the periphery. This process also allows the tumor to initiate metastatic invasion [17].

Vasculogenic mimicry is another less common alternative mode of vascularization that consists in forming channels to provide oxygen to tumor cells. These channels are formed by the tumor cells itself, which can simulate endothelial cells by increasing matrix metalloproteinases in order to modulate tumor microenvironment. This process was mainly described in aggressive melanomas [19].

Another noteworthy way of vascularization is intussusceptive angiogenesis, where no endothelial proliferation is needed and therefore is difficult to counteract with anti-angiogenic drugs. This mechanism is complex and poorly understood since it happens within preexisting vessels. It starts with the interaction of the vessels of opposite walls, forming an interendothelial junction at their edge in the "kissing contact" process. Mesenchymal stem cells, pericytes, and myofibroblasts come into play, taking up the gap formed by the new vessels, creating a new extracellular matrix, and forming the interstitial pillar. Hence, two new transvascular pillars are formed without endothelial proliferation. This mode of vascularization is a rapid and efficient procedure to expand existing vasculature [20,21].

2.3. Epithelial–Mesenchymal Transition (EMT)

Epithelial–mesenchymal transition is a well-studied process where the tumor is skilled to change the phenotype of polarized epithelial cells to a mesenchymal one through different molecular and biochemical changes. These empowered cells unhitch from the primary site and invade peritumoral tissues as well as systemic circulation in order to spread across distant places. In addition to these migratory functions, EMT also awards higher resistance to apoptosis and increases extracellular matrix [22].

Sunitinib has different ways to enhance EMT. One of the main pathways that unleash and orchestrate EMT is HIF1-α, accompanied by other molecular pathways such as HGF, EGF or PDGF. HIF-α increases the expression of ZEB1 and ZEB2 which facilitates loss of adhesion of epithelial cells by repressing E-cadherin. [23,24]. Snail and Slug are proteins that participate as well in E-cadherin repression. Sunitinib can favor invasiveness and progression of renal cell carcinoma by stimulating Snail expression and subsequent E-cadherin inhibition. The Akt/GSK3/β–catenin pathway also promotes EMT when activated by cytokines like IL-6, IL-8, and TNF-α [25].

EMT also participates in sarcomatoid differentiation in RCC patients by N-cadherin, Snail and Sparc stimulation and dissociation of β- catetin from cell membrane [26].

2.4. Activating Bypass Pathways

2.4.1. VEGF

Sustained treatment with antiangiogenic therapeutics would conduct enhancement of alternative cell signaling pathways that avoids TKIs' effect. Between the VEGF receptors, VEGFR2 has been the main target for primary TKIs designed, leaving free activity to other VEGFR proteins like VEGFR 1 and VEGFR 3. Furthermore, there are some non-VEGF alternative pathways that allow the tumor to uphold its growth [27].

2.4.2. PTEN

Phosphate and tensin homolog (*PTEN*) are tumor suppressors that have a down regulating function over PI3K/Akt/mTOR pathway. Even though *PTEN* mutations are rarely described in RCC [28], studies have demonstrated that patients with resistance to sunitinib show low expression of *PTEN*, thus constitutively Akt/mTOR expression.

2.4.3. FGF

FGFR pro-angiogenic function is led by upregulation of MAPK/ERK, PI3K/Akt and STAT pathways as well as IP3 and DAG and PKC signaling. Upregulation of FGF2 has been directly related to resistance to sunitinib and constitutes one of the major growth factors able to drive sunitinib resistance. Sunitinib is able to suppress phosphorylation of MEK1/2 and ERK 1/2 conducted by VEGF. However, when FGF2 is overexpressed, strong phosphorylation of MEK $\frac{1}{2}$ and ERK1/2 occurs despite sunitinib administration [29].

2.4.4. Axl and c-MET

Both Axl and c-MET are implicated in antiangiogenic resistance of VEGF targeted therapies and are also related to poor prognosis and decreased overall survival [30–32]. Zhou et al. studied the relation between sunitinib resistance and Axl and MET pathways. They demonstrated that in the first phases of treatment, it is able to suppress MET function, but when sunitinib is administered chronically, MET activity is enhanced. Moreover, this activity is maintained once sunitinib is withdrawn. They also proved that treatment with sunitinib increased Axl protein levels. Both Axl and MET are able to promote angiogenesis through activation of ERK and PI3K/AKT signaling and increment of VEGF secretion. Furthermore, sunitinib stimulates Axl and MET dependent EMT and favors cell migration and invasion [30].

2.4.5. TNF-α

Tumor necrosis factor (TNF- α) pathway is involved in multiple physiologic functions like immune response or hematopoiesis, but also plays a key role in tumor pathogenesis. For instance, it is implicated in EMT, activating the nuclear factor κB (NF-κB) pathway through the binding of TNF receptor 1 (TNFR1) and GSK3β activation [33,34].

The involvement of TNF- α in acquired resistances of certain treatments had already been hinted at in breast and lung cancer [35,36], but its implication in RCC remained scarcely explored. In 2020, Hwang et al. discovered that tumor tissues that have acquired TKI resistance express high expression of *TNFR1SF1A* gene. They also related high-*TNFR1* expression in intrinsic-resistance tumors as well as sarcomatoid dedifferentiation [37]. Nevertheless, to which extension TNF-α is involved in TKI resistance in RCC remains to be elucidated and further studies are needed.

2.4.6. Angiopoietin/Tie Pathway

Ang/Tie is a key signaling cascade which constitutes a significant alternative antiangiogenic pathway able to regulate endothelial maturation and vascularization. Angiopoietin 2 (Ang2) has a dual function depending on VEGF presence. When VEGF is inhibited, it binds to Tie2 and inhibits Ang1/Tie2 pathway, consequently promoting vascular degradation and cell death. Wang et al. demonstrated that at the beginning of treatment with sunitinib, the levels of Ang 2 decreased progressively, as long as the tumor was sensitive to sunitinib. Inversely, they showed that patients with sunitinib resistance expressed elevated Ang 2 levels. This fact was correlated with tumor progression, acting Ang2 as an angiogenic escape mechanism [38,39].

2.4.7. Enhancer of Zeste Homologue 2 (EZH2)

The enhancer of zeste homologue 2 (EZH2) is a histone methyltransferase that participates in the methylation of lysine 27 on histone 3 producing gene repression [40].

EZH2 is one of the major epigenetic mechanisms of resistance to TKI in RCC. It enhances EMT, impeding the expression of E-cadherin and therefore favoring invasiveness and migration [40]. Adelaiye et al. exposed in their studies that EZH2 overexpression leads to methylation of promoter regions of anti-angiogenic factors and subsequently favors tumor vascularization and therefore sunitinib resistance. Furthermore, EZH2 can induce adaptive kinase reprogramming through epigenetic changes, allowing tumor cells to find alternative pathways such as FAK, SCR, MET, FGFR2, EGFR, IGF-1R, and ERBB2 [41]. Nevertheless, this resistance mechanism can be counteracted by dose escalation [42].

2.5. Lysosomal Sequestration of TKIs

Lysosomal sequestration is the process by which sunitinib is accumulated within the lysosome structure. Most TKIs can traverse lysosomal membrane easily because they are weak bases. Once the molecule is internalized, it finds an acid environment achieved by proton pumping vacuolar ATPases. This environment protonates the molecule and sequestrates it inside the lysosome. Therefore, it is unable to exert its function [43].

Certain TKIs, such as erlotinib and pazopanib, can also be exposed to lysosomal sequestration [44]. Sorafenib comprises a different kind of molecule with differential characteristics that does not permit free travel across lysosomal membranes. Because of this fact, other lysosomal sequestration mechanisms have been proposed for Sorafenib. It was demonstrated that drug pumps like ABC transporter P-glycoprotein can mediate not only sunitinib sequestration but sorafenib too. In the frame of this thinking, P-gp inhibitors like verapamil or elacridar have been studied in preclinical models of CCR showing enhancement of antitumor activity of sunitinib [45–47].

Moreover, lysosome sequestration is a multidrug resistance (MDR) mechanism that can lead to a feedback process where the exposure to tyrosine kinase inhibitors reinforces lysosome biogenesis. The increased lysosomal gene expression and lysosomal enzyme activity lead to augmented drug sequestration and MDR. Lysosomal biogenesis seems to be driven by the nuclear transcription of transcription factor EF (TFEB) [48]. This process is ultimately commanded by mTORC1 [49]

2.6. Noncoding RNAs (ncRNA) and Single Nucleotide Polymorphisms

Circulating noncoding RNAs have raised interest in many oncologic fields. They have been studied as potential biomarkers in early stages of RCC as well as prognostic and predictive treatment response biomarkers [50–52].

Micro RNA (miRNA), a particular class of ncRNA, have been studied as molecules able to carry out TKIs resistance, concretely miRNA-15b, which overexpression has been described as a mechanism of resistance to sunitinib [53]. Other miRNA like miRNA-575, miRNA-642b-3p and miRNA-4430 were detected in cultures of RCC cells resistant to sunitinib [54]. Regulation of miR-141 and miR-429 also contributes to EMT and its development [55].

Le Qu et al. described a sunitinib resistance mechanism based on intercellular transfer by exosomes of long noncoding RNA (lncRNA) called lncARSR. Long-noncoding RNA are a class of ncRNA with a minimum length of 200 bases involved in gene transcription by multiple regulation functions such as recruitment of chromatin-modifying complexes and post-transcriptional modulation [56,57].

Le Qu's analysis confirmed high levels of lncARSR in sunitinib-resistant RCC tumor cells as well as endothelial cells. LncASRS seemed to be upregulated by the activation of the AKT pathway and ultimately the inhibition of FOXO1 and FOXO3a. LncASRS is packed into exosomes via heterogeneous nuclear ribo-nuclear protein A2B1 (hnRNP A2B1) and afterwards transferred to surrounding cells disseminating sunitinib resistance. The authors hypothesized and confirmed that lncASRS functioned like competing endogenous RNA (ceRNA) for miR-34 and miR-449, whose targets are Axl and c-MET. This competitive binding increased the expression of Axl and c-MET, hence the stimulation of STAT3, AKT, and ERC pathways and subsequent sunitinib resistance.

Single nucleotide polymorphisms (SNPs) are the most common genetic variation and are defined as a single base pair variation that reaches at least 1% of the population. SNPs related to sunitinib pharmacokinetics (ABCB1, NR1/2, and NR 1/3) and pharmacodynamics (VEGFR3 and FGFR3) had already been described by Beuselinck et al. as determinants of sunitinib outcome in RCC patients [58]. Their effect in CYP3A4 is essential in the metabolism of sunitinib. SNPs in NR1I2 and NR1I3 suppressed CYP3A4 function and were associated with shorter PFS. Inversely, SNPs in CYP3A4 were associated with increased PFS as a result of increased metabolism of sunitinib [58,59].

2.7. Tumor Microenvironment Factors Related to Resistance to TKIs

Tumor microenvironment (TME) is constituted by several components such as the tumor cells itself, extracellular matrix (ECM), fibroblasts, vascular endothelial cells, immune cells, and several other stromal cells. Tumor microenvironment is an essential participant of tumor progression and maintenance of its pathogenesis [60].

Robust evidence has been constructed in recent years supporting the importance of tumor microenvironment in development of resistance to TKIs.

2.7.1. Tumor Endothelial Cells (TECs)

Tumor endothelial cells are an important element of TME and participate actively in tumor development. They blossom in hypoxic conditions and can also drive resistance to targeted therapeutics. A study reflected that sunitinib was able to increase VEGF and vascular cell adhesion molecule-1 (sVCAM) as well as levels of circulating endothelial cell-related proteins like Ang-2. The increase of these proteins and TECs were described in patients with acquired resistance to sunitinib [61]. Notch ligand Delta-like 4 (Dll4) has been also related to TECs and the expression of this pathway exerts downstream inhibition of VEGF [62,63].

2.7.2. Bone Marrow-Derived Proangiogenic Inflammatory Cell Recruitment

Hypoxic conditions lead to recruitment of different bone marrow-derived cells (BMDCs) and it is known that this environment is enhanced by antiangiogenic agents. BMDC can participate in the formation of a premetastatic niche environment by crafting new vessels that supply oxygen tumor requirements.

Myeloid-derived suppressor cells (MDSC) is a class of BMDCs worth highlighting. This major component of TME is able to induce resistance to TKIs by enhancing VEGF-independent angiogenesis. This is carried out by GM-CSF availability in tumor tissue and is a STAT5 dependent mechanism, since it was objectified that START 5ab (null/null) MDSC were not able to induce sunitinib resistance [64,65].

2.7.3. Pericyte Coverage

By their attachment around blood vessels and expression of proangiogenic factors like VEGF, pericytes promote proliferation and maintenance of tumorigenesis. When they are pathologically activated, abnormal micro-vessel networks embedding the tumor cells are formed. It is known that increase of pericyte coverage favors antiangiogenic resistance enhancing survival of endothelial cells and making them less sensitive to VEGF inhibition [66].

2.7.4. Tumor-Associated Fibroblasts (TAFs)

There is strong evidence that tumor-associated fibroblasts (TAFs) are able to interact with multiple signaling pathways in RCC cells and promote angiogenesis, tumor invasion, and TKI resistance through paracrine mechanisms. For instance, it can enhance HIF-1α accumulation in RCC through CXCR4 upregulation favoring resistance to treatments. CXCR4 is a molecular proangiogenic pathway expressed by many components of TME such as TAFs. This process is induced by *VHL* malfunction, which is inherent to RCC pathogenesis [67,68]. TAFs can promote resistance to anti-angiogenic molecules promoting activation alternative pathways such as MAPK/ERK and Akt [69].

They also interact with interstitial fluid pressure inside the tumor and are capable of nullifying the travel of drugs through tumor cells. They also mediate induction of aggressive phenotypes of RCC as a result of increased recruitment of macrophages and remodeling of TME [70,71].

Crawford et al. showed that TAFs stimulate expression of PDGF-C and consequently generate angiogenesis and treatment resistance [72].

2.7.5. Tumor-Associated Macrophages

Tumor-associated macrophages (TAMs) have been lately attributed an important role in tumor induction and progression. Nevertheless, they can have a twofold function being able to enhance tumor growth as well as produce anti-tumor signals [73]. It is known that hypoxia prompts tumor-associated macrophages to favor tumor progression through secretion of different molecules like MMP-9, CSC chemokines, IL-6, TNF-α, and VEGF which not only promotes angiogenesis but also participate in TME regulation. All this angiogenic storm can aid the tumor to find alternative pathways and lessen the effect of anti-angiogenic therapies [74].

3. Molecular Pathways Associated with Resistance to Treatment with Immune Checkpoint Inhibitors

Many factors have been described as relevant in the resistance to immunotherapy in different tumors, leading to two main forms of resistance (primary resistance and secondary). Primary resistance makes reference to intrinsic resistance (probably related to the tumor) and secondary to acquired resistance (probably related to microenvironment changes) in patients with initial response to treatments. For simplicity, these factors have been classified into "intrinsic tumor mechanisms" and "microenvironment related" (Figure 2).

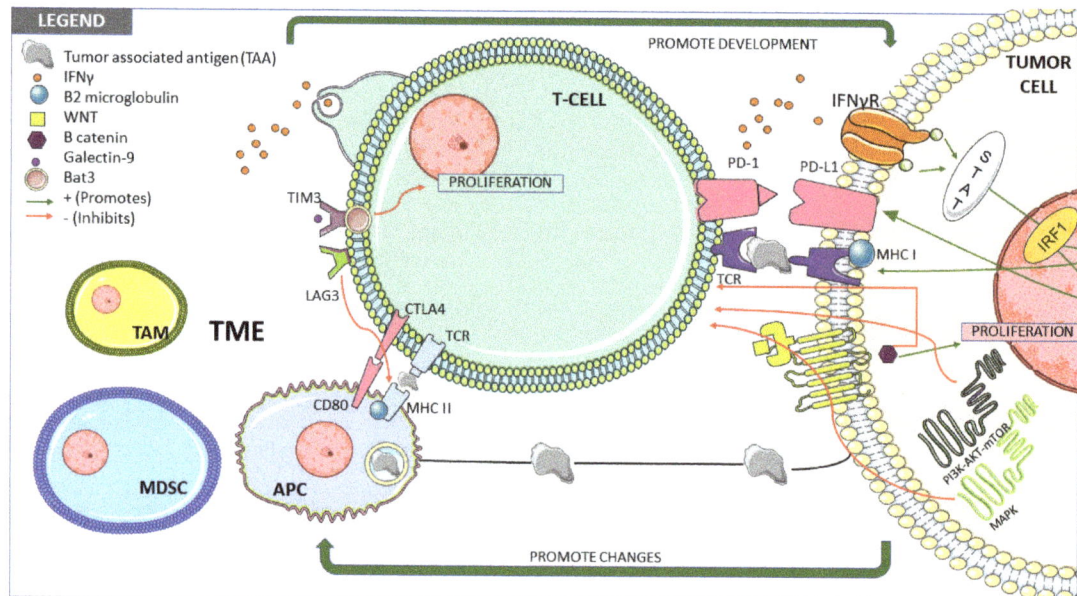

Figure 2. Among the key mechanisms described we can mainly distinguish tumor-intrinsic factors and factors associated to tumor microenvironment (TME). In the first subgroup it is important to outline the alterations of antitumor immune response pathways (e.g., aberrant expression of tumor antigens), variations in the antigen presentation pathways (e.g., β2-microglobulin mutations leading to loss of MHC) or defective signaling pathways (e.g., IFNγ-STAT-IRF1 signaling pathway); What is more, these intrinsic factors promote the formation of an immunosuppressive microenvironment through the mutations of functional genes such as Wnt/β-catenin, MAPK, or PI3K-AKT-mTOR pathways and the modifications of the metabolism of TME (e.g., hypoxic conditions); The second subgroup (factors associated to TME) includes the presence of immunosuppressive cells (e.g., MDSCs or TAM) as well as the activation of coinhibitory receptors (e.g., TIM-3, LAG-3).

3.1. Tumor Cells-Intrinsic Factors

3.1.1. Interferon Gamma Signaling Pathway

The intrinsic interferon gamma (INFγ) pathway plays a key role in the T-cell response against a tumor antigen. The activation of the INFγ membrane receptor results in the downstream interaction with the Janus Kinase (JAK) signal transducer, the activator of transcription (STAT) and the interferon regulatory factor 1 (IRF1), leading to PD-L1 expression. Genetic disorders in the INFγ signaling pathway have been revealed as resistance-associated to treatment with ICI [75]. Moreover, INFγ enhances MHC-I antigen presentation. In MHC-deficient tumor cells, treatment with INFγ is necessary to express the antigen processing machinery and has been able to induce tumor-specific T-cell responses [76]. INFγ pathway also promote the recruitment of immune cells and has direct effects over the tumoral cells, leading to anti-proliferative and proapoptotic signals [77]. Recently, loss-of-function truncating mutations in genes *JAK1* and *JAK2* have been associated with lack of response to INFγ, as well as PD-1 inhibitors' inefficacy [78].

3.1.2. Wnt/β-catenin Pathway

The Wnt/β-catenin pathway is associated with different biological processes, such as stem cell development, embryogenesis, cell differentiation, and immune regulation. In most cancers, Wnt/β-catenin is overexpressed. In several tumoral models not including renal cell carcinoma, this overactivation is correlated to absence of T cell gene expression signatures and T-cell exclusion, leading to "immune-desert" tumors, conditioning resistance to immune checkpoint inhibitors. [79–82]. Wnt/β-catenin is also involved in the regulation of IDO1 and the PPARgamma receptor, both inducing immunosuppressive effects [83]. A role in tumor stemness and dedifferentiation is also well-described [84].

3.1.3. Mitogen-Activated Protein Kinases (MAPK) Pathway

The MAPK pathway is associated with VEGF, IL-6, IL-8, and IL-10 production and has been related with the inhibition of T cell functions and immune cells recruitment. Furthermore, MAPK pathway mediates in the negative regulation of MHC expression and antigen presentation, as well as a reduced responsiveness to the anti-proliferative effects of IFNγ and TNFα [75,85].

3.1.4. PI3K/AKT/m-TOR Pathway

PI3K/AKT pathway has been identified as one of the most altered pathways in ccRCC, following the molecular characterization performed by The Cancer Genome Atlas Program. The loss of expression of PTEN has been pointed out as another relevant alteration [86]. These alterations have been associated with expression of immunosuppressive cytokines and inhibition of the autophagosome, resulting in a decreased T-cell infiltration at tumor sites, poor T-cell recruitment, and failure of T-cell-mediated cell death. PTEN loss has also been correlated with worst outcomes with anti PD-1 inhibitor therapy [87].

3.1.5. Cell Cycle Checkpoint Pathway

Cyclin dependent kinase 4 and 6 (CDK4/6) and their co-factors D-type cyclins are principal drivers of the cell cycle from G1 to S phase and have been associated with tumoral progression. Several studies have emphasized the impact of CDK 4/6 inhibition enhancing the immune response. Thus, the CDK4/6 inhibitor abemaciclib in combination with immune checkpoint blockade had a substantially greater capacity to induce pronounced responses in mouse breast cancer models than either agent alone [88,89]. A substantial IL-2 expression and increased T-cell tumor infiltration was observed in these models and have been connected to the beneficial effect of CDK4 inhibition on antitumoral immunity [90].

3.1.6. Loss of MHC

The loss of MHC I and II molecules favors the tumoral immune escape by incapacitating the T-cells to recognize the tumoral antigens. Many genetic and epigenetic alterations that involves the antigen processing and presenting machinery have been potentially associated with this event. Truncating mutations in the gene encoding B2-microglobulin has shown a loss of expression of MHC I in the cell surface, resulting in an absence of response to ICI in melanoma patients [88,91]. In addition, loss of heterozygosity at the B2-microglobulin locus was associated with lower overall survival in melanoma patients receiving immune checkpoint inhibitors [92].

3.2. Tumor Microenvironment Related Factors and their Role in Resistance to Immune Response

3.2.1. T Cells

RCC is one of the most T cell-enriched tumors. The high densities of CD8+ tumor-infiltrating lymphocytes (TILs) is associated with a poorer prognosis, compared to other tumor types [93,94]. Amongst the many hypotheses that underlie this contra-intuitive prognosis on the impact of CD8 in ccRCC, it has been demonstrated that co-expression of PD-1 and LAG-3 induced by a lack of antigen presentation by dysfunctional dendritic cells results in CD8 TILs exhaustion in ccRCC [95].

However, recently the controversial role of tumor infiltrating T cells has started to be clarified. In the phase III trial JAVELIN RENAL 101 (comparing the combination of anti PD-L1 antibody avelumab + TKI axitinib vs sunitinib in monotherapy), an association between large CD8 infiltration and poor PFS in patients treated with sunitinib was observed. However, these outcomes were not reflected in patients treated with the combination, suggesting that CD8 infiltration has prognostic value in TKI-treated ccRCC but loses it when the patient is treated with ICI [96].

In 2017, Giraldo et al. [97] proposed a classification of primary ccRCCs depending on their dominant immune profile. They studied 40 tumors, dividing them in three different profiles: 1. The immune regulated, represented by polyclonal cytotoxic CD8+ PD-1+ Tim-3+ Lag 3+ TILs and CD4+ ICOS+ cells with a Treg phenotype, characterized by highly infiltrated tumors with notable proportion of dysfunctional dendritic cells expressing PD-L1. 2. The immune activated, distinguished by oligoclonal/ CD8+ PD-1+ Tim-3+ TILs, that represented 22% of the patients. 3. The immune silent, enriched in TILs revealing a RIL-like (renal infiltrating lymphocytes) phenotype, constituting the majority of tumors of the cohort (56% of the patients analyze).

The immune regulated and immune activated tumors have been connected with distinctive phenotypic signatures, which confer aggressive histologic properties and high risk of relapse or progression. These findings support the hypothesis that these selected patients could benefit from adjuvant treatment with ICIs [97].

Subsequently, molecular biomarkers evaluated in the IMmotion 150 phase II trial (comparing first line treatment in mccRCC with the combination of atezolizumab + bevacizumab versus standard therapy with sunitinib) showed distinct biological subgroups based on levels of angiogenesis, immune infiltration, and myeloid inflammation. In addition, the subgroup with high expression of the Angio gene signature ($Angio^{High}$) was characterized by higher vascular density and was associated with improved response within the sunitinib arm. The $Angio^{Low}$ subgroup showed better response to atezolizumab + bevacizumab versus sunitinib. Moreover, high expression of the T-effector (T_{eff}) gene signature was positively associated with expression of PD-L1 and CD8 T-cell infiltration. The T_{eff}^{High} subgroup had an improved ORR and PFS with atezolizumab + bevacizumab compared with T_{eff}^{Low} subgroup. High Teff gene signature was also related to improve PFS with atezolizumab + bevacizumab versus sunitinib, and showed no difference with atezolizumab in monotherapy, which can highlight the role of Teff gene signature in response and resistance to immunotherapy. Complementary, differential expression of genes associated with myeloid inflammation within the T_{eff}^{High} and T_{eff}^{Low} subgroups was observed. Atezolizumab monotherapy had worse activity in the $T_{eff}^{High}Myeloid^{High}$ tumors compared with the $T_{eff}^{High}Myeloid^{Low}$ group [98].

Motzer et al. characterized seven molecular subtypes of ccRCC using a large RNA-seq dataset from the IMmotion 151 phase III trial [99]. They identified and refined transcriptionally defined subgroups using non-negative matrix factorization, an unsupervised clustering algorithm. Patient tumors in clusters 1 (Angiogenic/Stromal) and 2 (Angiogenic) were characterized as highly angiogenic, with enrichment of VEGF pathway-related genes. These tumors showed the longest PFS in both treatment arms, suggesting better outcomes regardless of treatment. However, no differences between the combination treatment with atezolizumab + bevacizumab versus sunitinib were observed, which suggests that these groups essentially benefit from treatment with antiangiogenics. Clusters 4 (T-effector/Proliferative), 5 (Proliferative), and 6 (Stromal/Proliferative) were characterized by enrichment of cell cycle transcriptional programs, and lower expression of angiogenesis-related genes. Atezolizumab + bevacizumab treatment showed improved ORR and PFS over sunitinib in tumors from clusters 4 and 5, confirming the contribution of pre-existing intratumoral adaptive immune presence described in these patients. However, cluster 6 was associated with a poor outcome.

At last, cluster 3 (Complement/Ω-oxidation cluster) presents lower expression of both angiogenesis and immune genes and has been associated with poor prognosis. Cluster 7 (snoRNA) is characterized by expression of snoRNA (small nucleolar RNA, a group of RNA molecules of variable length, that guide modifications processes of other RNAs, mainly ribosomal RNA maturation), especially C/D box snoRNAs which have been implicated in alterations of epigenetic and translation programs. This last cluster improved PFS with atezolizumab + bevacizumab, but the biological basis of this effect remains to be elucidated.

Additionally, IDO-1 upregulation was described as a key driver of T cell nutrient deprivation. IDO-1 overexpression in tumor endothelial cells is associated with better response and PFS in patients treated with nivolumab and has been proposed as a new biomarker [100].

3.2.2. Innate Immune System

Macrophages can undergo M1 (classical) or M2 (alternative) activation in result of the inflammatory triggering signal. The M1 type are characterized by producing high levels of inflammatory cytokines, such as IL-12, IL-23, and IL-6. M2 macrophages can be subdivided into different subsets called M2a, M2b, M2c, and M2d [101,102]. Th2 cytokines IL-4 and IL-13 stimulate the macrophages to develop M2a phenotype; M2b are induced by activation of Toll-like receptors; and IL-10 polarizes the M2c subtype. M2d subtype is also known as tumor-associated, due to the ability of tumor cells to switch the potential phenotype of macrophages into this subtype. Tumor associated macrophages express multiple receptors or ligands of immune inhibitory pathways, such as PD-L1, PD-L2, and B7-1 [101]. In RCC, poor survival outcomes have been identified in tumors with high expression of anti-inflammatory macrophage phenotype (M2) [103]. Moreover, extensive tumor-associated macrophage (M2d) infiltration into the RCC microenvironment leads the recruitment of Tregs to the tumor site by secreting CCL20 or CCL22 and has been linked with enhancement of angiogenesis, tumor proliferation, and metastatic cellular migration and invasion.

3.2.3. B Cells and Tertiary Lymphoid Structures

B cells and tertiary lymphoid structures (TLS) have recently arisen as an important feature in cancer biology. B cells have been analyzed within the tumor and the microenvironment, showing a strong memory response against tumor associated antigens [104]. Bregs are a specific population of B cells with a regulatory role that have been marked as inmunosupressive cells, due to their capacity to secrete inhibitory molecules, like IL-10 and TGFβ, which regulate T-reg differentiation [105]. In ccRCC, higher expression of B cell related genes, measured by microarrays profiling of baseline tumor samples, have been associated with better response to ICIs [106]. In sarcoma, a cluster of patients (known as "immune and TLS high") which predominantly express the B lineage signature, has demonstrated a significant improvement in life expectancy with anti PD-1 treatment [107].

Tertiary lymphoid structures are ectopic lymph-like structures whose structure varies from an aggregation on B and T cells to more complex structures. Generally, these TLS are constituted by a T cell zone with mature dendritic cells covering a follicular zone rich in proliferating and differentiating B cells. These structures play an important (and still largely unknown) role against tumor immunity and are associated with better prognosis in patients with several cancers, including ccRCC. Typically, these structures can develop a niche which supports the appearance of transformed cells and activated T regs, favoring the immune response [93,108].

3.2.4. Proinflammatory Cytokines

The RCC microenvironment is associated with pro-inflammatory conditions. Among the factors associated with this fact, the release of pro-inflammatory molecules and cytokines induced by tissue damage emerges as the most important one. Upper concentrations of molecules, such as adenosine triphosphate, IL-6, IL-8, macrophage inflammatory protein 1-alpha, tumor necrosis factor alpha (TNFα), or IFNγ promote the angiogenesis, genomic instability, cellular proliferation, and the epithelial–mesenchymal transition, as well as increase the recruitment of immune cells, leading to a pro-tumorigenic microenvironment.

Furthermore, it is important to notice that this recruitment promotes immunosuppression leading by the increased expression of PD-1 on T cells which is induced by IFNγ also [109]. This sustained expression of PD-1 is responsible for T cell exhaustion via the SHP2 recruitment. Transcriptional factors such as STAT-3 and IRF1, induced by pro-inflammatory conditions, also modulate the expression of PDL1 and PDL2, favoring this exhaustion process. Additionally, IL-1, IL-6, IL-11, IL-17, and TNF alpha promote Treg expansion and increase T cell exhaustion [110,111].

3.2.5. Hypoxia

RCC is characterized as being one of the most vascularized tumors. However, this vascularization is composed of fragile, disorganized vessels, causing an erratic nutrient and oxygen intake, which leads to hypoxia and a lower pH, facilitating tumor progression [112]. Furthermore, hypoxia induces the activation of different genes, which are involved in differentiation of tumor associated macrophages, Treg recruitment and infiltration of myeloid-derived suppressor cells. These immune structural changes favor the inhibition of T cells [113,114]. Furthermore, HIF-1a and HIF-2a induce increased expression of PD-L1 in tumor cells [115,116]. An immune escape pathway is developed by increased levels of HIF-1 and HIF-2, which enables the generation of VEGF, which in turn increase the expression of the immune checkpoints CTLA-4, TIM-3, and LAG-3 on T cells, and PD-L1 on dendritic cells [114,117]. Finally, hypoxic tissues are enriched in adenosine, which suppress the effect of T cells, contributing to immune escape [118].

3.2.6. Protein Polybromo-1(PBRM-1) Expression

PBRM-1 is a specific subunit of the PBAF form of the SWI/SNF chromatin remodeling complex. Loss-of-function mutations in this complex are recurrent in many cancers, including ccRCC, which appears in around 40% of patients [119,120]. In ccRCC, low expression of PBRM1 and high tumor grade imply a worse prognosis. In vitro studies performing the inactivation of PBRM1 using CRISPR-Cas9, have shown a larger production of chemokines in response to IFNγ, which recruits effector T cells and promotes sensibilization of treatment-resistant mouse melanoma cells to immunotherapy [119]. Other studies involving whole exome sequencing have remarked that the loss-of-function mutation in the *PBRM1* gene has been linked with improved PFS and OS in patients receiving antiPD-1 treatment [121–123]. However, recent studies have demonstrated that ccRCC with low expression of PBRM-1 are related with lower CD4-CD8 tumor infiltration, lower expression levels of CXCL10, CCL12, ICAM-1, and other cell migration-related molecules, and in the end, with poorer outcomes with anti-PD1 treatment compared with PBRM-1 high tumors [124]. These new findings reveal the potential of PBRM-1 as a therapeutic target.

3.2.7. Immune Escape Related to Other Immune Checkpoints

T-cell immunoglobulin and mucin domain 3 (TIM-3) is a type I trans-membrane protein that was originally discovered in an effort to identify novel cell surface molecules that would mark IFN-γ-producing Th1 and Tc1 cells. Tim-3 plays a key role in inhibiting Th1 responses and the expression of cytokines such as TNF and INF-γ, leading to the suppression of tumoral immune response [125]. On T-cell activation, TIM-3 is recruited to the immunological synapse with B-associated transcript 3 (Bat3) bound to the cytoplasmic tail of TIM-3. When TIM-3 is engaged by a ligand, in most cases galectin-9, the conserved tyrosine residues in the cytoplasmic tail become phosphorylated, leading to the release of Bat3 and activates the downregulation of TCR signaling and suppression of T-cell proliferation and survival [126]. In ccRCC, TIM-3 and PD-1 co-expression on CD8 T cells is associated with worse outcomes including higher TNM stage, larger tumor size and lower PFS [127].

Lymphocyte activation gene-3 (LAG-3, also known as CD223) is a cell surface molecule that belongs to the immunoglobulin superfamily and is located near CD4. Like CD4, LAG-3 binds to major histocompatibility complex-II (MHC-II) on antigen presenting cells (APCs), but with a much stronger affinity [128], which prohibits the binding of the same MHC molecule to TCR and CD4, thus directly hampering TCR signaling in immune response [129]. LAG-3 is expressed in the membrane of multiple immune cells, including CD4 T cells, CD8 T cells, and T-reg cells. Several studies have delineated that LAG-3 is over-expressed on tumor-infiltrating CD8 T cells in various tumor types, including renal cell carcinomas [130]. LAG-3 overexpression leads to CD8 T cells exhaustion and resistance to anti PD-1 inhibitors [131]. This interaction occurs without binding to MHC-II, which have given rise to the discovery of additional tumor-related ligands, such as galectin-3 and liver sinusoidal endothelial cell lectin (LSECtin). These ligands seem to play an important role in the TME, although it remains unclear [132]. LAG-3 expression tends to be associated with a lower OS in RCC [120,133].

T cell immunoglobulin and ITIM domain (TIGIT) is a membrane protein with an extracellular IgV ligand-binding domain and an intracellular immune-receptor domain. TIGIT is primarily expressed on T cells and NK cells and binds to the poliovirus receptor PVR (CD155) and Nectin-2 (CD112) as a competitor to DNAM-1. DNAM-1 enhances cytotoxicity of T lymphocytes and NK cells, and TIGIT blocks its function acting like an immune suppressor. TIGIT has been found to be expressed on subsets of exhausted intratumoral CD8+ T cells [134,135].

4. Discussion

Resistance to systemic therapies in RCC, either intrinsic due to presence of resistance genes or acquired after initial tumor regression can directly impact the clinical course and additional treatment approach of these patients. This review highlights the new insights into key biological pathways underlying treatment resistance.

At the beginning of this century, treatment with TKIs that block the VEGFR has revolutionized the RCC treatment landscape, resulting in a significant increase in terms of life expectancy and quality of life for these patients. However, the benefit shown by these initial treatments was limited.

Looking at initial resistance to VEGFR2 inhibition by enhanced activity from other VEGFR receptors, multiple VEGFR inhibitors have been designed trying to overcome this obstacle. Moreover, the inhibition of the PI3K/Akt/mTOR pathway has become an option to overcome PTEN downregulation. Thus, preclinical studies combining sunitinib with PI3K/mTOR inhibitors, mTOR inhibitors or pan-AKT inhibitors, can restore sunitinib effect and induce apoptosis in those PTEN-negative cells [136,137]. However, in the clinical setting these combinations were related with increased toxicity requiring dose attenuation, and efficacy was less than expected in comparison with single-agent sunitinib at full doses [138].

In the FGF overexpression setting, lenvatinib, an oral inhibitor of FGFR, VEGF 1-3, PDGFR α, RET, and KIT, is able to overcome the FGF resistance mechanism and has demonstrated activity in the first line setting in combination with pembrolizumab and in subsequent treatment lines in combination with everolimus of patients with advanced RCC [139]. Inhibiting the FGF pathway with brivanib (a first-class dual inhibitor of VEGR2-3/FGFR1-2-3) in mice with pancreatic neuroendocrine tumors has resulted in promising activity after failure to anti-VEGF treatment [140].

Other TKIs have been developed in the last few years. Cabozantinib has been designed as a multi-tyrosine kinase inhibitor against VEGFR, KIT, RET, Tie2, cMET, and Axl inhibitor among others. Molecular testing from tumor samples by Zhou et al. demonstrated that cabozantinib could suppress Axl and MET activation including AKT and ERK downstream cascades induced by chronic sunitinib treatment [30]. Therefore, cabozantinib has been included in the therapeutic algorithm of patients with advanced RCC [141]. Crizotinib, a MET inhibitor, has been also studied in combination with axitinib, showing decrement in vascularity density along with suppressed tumor growth [142]. The role of crizotinib has been focused on the subtype papillary RCC due to its MET inhibition, but clinical results have not shown greater antitumor activity over other TKI VEGFR driven [143].

New pathways are being explored in order to reverse the resistance to TKIs. Ang/Tie pathway has indeed become an interesting target for new drug development, as MEDI 3671 (a monoclonal antibody against Ang2), trebananib (fusion protein which hampers the binding of Ang1/2 to Tie 1/2) or CovX bodies have demonstrated the ability to inhibit tumor growth and decrease vascular density [144–147].

Alternatively, the regulation of epigenetic alterations has also been spotted as a target. Tazemetostat is an EZH2 inhibitor studied in multiple solid tumors with promising results [148,149].

Lysosomal sequestration is a reversible resistance mechanism. A study conducted in sunitinib resistant RCC cells revealed that lysosomal function was suppressed when sunitinib was withdrawn from the cell cultures and drug sensitivity was retrieved [150]. Furthermore, alkalinizing lysosomes with an H+-ATPase inhibitor like bafilomycin has been also studied for reversing sunitinib resistance since pH gradient plays a key role in its sequestration. Notwithstanding, the excessive toxicity of this molecule constitutes a hindrance for its use in vivo. Following this rationale, chloroquine is being studied in preclinical assays showing interesting results in pancreatic neuroendocrine tumors (P-NET) combined with sunitinib [151].

Looking at the future, ncRNA expression and SNPs seem to be new paths to explore in further years. Long noncoding RNA lncASRS targeting with locked nucleic acids has provided evidence that could overcome the resistance and restore sunitinib response. However, further studies are needed to elucidate the role of lncASRS as potential therapeutic target as well as a clinical biomarker [57].

TME modulation has gained strength as a strategy to overcome resistance to TKIs. Pericytes have been conceived as interesting new targets to design novel drugs [66]. Pericyte coverage is regulated by PDGFs family molecules and inhibiting PDGFRβ in combination with antiangiogenic drugs can reduce pericyte coverage and inhibit tumor growth in mouse model P-NETs [152]. However, decrement of pericyte can likewise increase risk of metastatic dissemination and these strategies should always live in an intricate equilibrium where tumoral progression can be favored. Moreover, TME regulation focusing on the tumor endothelial cells with new molecules targeting the Ang-2 pathway and Dll4 inhibitors have demonstrated anti-tumor activity in sunitinib and sorafenib resistant RCCs [62,63,153].

In recent years, strategies enhancing the immune system with the inhibition of immune checkpoint proteins PD-1/PDL-1 and CTLA-4 have revolutionized the RRC therapeutic landscape [128,140,154–157]. Nevertheless, there is still an important number of patients who never benefit from these treatments or lose this benefit in a short period of time. Taking this in consideration, big efforts have been taken in order to shed some light on the resistance mechanisms which lead to tumor insensitivity to ICIs and disease progression.

Novel immune checkpoints (such as TIM-3 and LAG-3) have been analyzed as potential targets, due to their responsibility in lymphocyte exhaustion and tumor immune evasion. Thus, TIM-3 has been targeted alone or in combination with anti-PD-1/PD-L1, with four ongoing phase I trials assessing antiTIM-3 antibodies in metastatic solid tumors (NCT02608268, NCT02817633, NCT03099109, and NCT03066648) [158].

Furthermore, several clinical trials targeting LAG-3 (alone or in combination with anti PD-1) in metastatic solid tumors including mccRCC patients are ongoing [159]. Relatlimab, an anti-LAG3 antibody with promising results in metastatic melanoma, is under investigation in combination with nivolumab (NCT02996110). Eftilagimod-α (IMP321), a soluble LAG-3 immunoglobulin fusion protein agonist has been evaluated in a phase I clinical trial, showing a promising activity inducing memory CD8+ T cells, as well as an acceptable toxicity [160]. XmAb22841, a bispecific antibody targeting CTLA-4 and LAG-3 is being evaluated in monotherapy or combination with pembrolizumab in select patients with advanced solid tumors, including mccRCC (NCT03849469).

Other immune checkpoints are under research. In phase Ia/Ib and randomized phase II clinical trials, tiragolumab (an anti-TIGIT antibody) had a tolerable safety profile with promising efficacy (most notably in patients with non-small-cell lung cancer), and clinical trials designed to assess the safety and efficacy of TIGIT inhibitors in patients with RCC are currently ongoing. An early-phase trial exploring a V-domain immunoglobulin suppressor of T cell activation (VISTA) inhibitor in patients with advanced-stage solid tumors is also ongoing [161].

Additionally, IDO-1 targeting has been one of the most promising approaches in the last years. The phase I/II ECHO-202/KEYNOTE 037 where the combination of the oral IDO-1 inhibitor epacadostat and PD-1 inhibitor pembrolizumab was tested, result in an objective response in 25 of 62 patients (40%), including eight complete responses and 13 patients with stable disease. In the mccRCC set, two patients presented responses out of 11 [162]. However, the ECHO-301/KEYNOTE-252 phase III study (epacadostat + pembrolizumab vs placebo in patients with unresectable or metastatic melanoma) failed to improve PFS or OS [163]. These results have led to the withdrawal in the development of IDO-1 inhibitors for the moment.

IFNγ pathway activation has been pointed out for its important role in sustaining the immune response. STING and RIG-1 are basic mediators in the detection of cytosolic DNA. The STING pathway activates nuclear factor-kappa B (NF-κB) and interferon regulatory factor 3 (IRF-3) through the activity of IκB, enhancing the IFNγ pathway and increasing the production of proinflammatory cytokines [164]. RIG-1 contributes to the stimulation of the immune system, favoring the production and activation of NK and CD8+ T cells [165]. Two phase I trials evaluating a STING agonist and a RIG-1 agonist as monotherapy or in combination with ICI respectively, in patients with metastatic solid tumors including mccRCC are ongoing (NCT03010176 and NCT03739138).

IL-2 is another promising target in the horizon of renal cancer treatment. Decades ago, high-dose IL2 was commonly used to treat mccRCC, achieving complete and durable responses in a subset of patients. However, the life-threatening toxicity associated with high-dose IL2 restricted this therapy to a limited number of young patients without underlying comorbidities. Bempegaldesleukin is a pegylated IL2 which preferentially binds to the beta-gamma subunit of the IL2 receptor. This interaction has shown a promotion of IL2 effects on T-effector cells, enhancing the expansion of effector elements, as well as depletes intratumoral T-reg cells. In phase I studies, bempegaldesleukin has been well tolerated with low grade 1-2 manageable adverse events, such as hypotension and edema. Despite clinical efficacy in randomized trials has still not been proven, data from tumor and blood analysis support the combinatorial use of bempegaldesleukin with ICI [166,167]. Other studies evaluating the utility of modified versions of IL2 and combinations with ICIs are also ongoing (NCT03861793, NCT03875079, NCT02989714, and NCT02964078).

Macrophage reprogramming is another promising approach nowadays, as diverse therapeutic strategies have been suggested to suppress tumor-associated macrophage recruitment, switching them back to the antitumor M1 phenotype [121]. Nevertheless, several studies have reported that high M2 macrophage tumor infiltration is associated with a more durable response to anti-PD-1 therapy [116,168]. This association was not found in patients treated with TKIs. Colony stimulating factor 1 receptor (CSF1R) expression has a key role allowing the switching of M1 macrophages into M2 tumor-associated macrophages [169]. Combinations of CSF1R inhibitors and ICI are under investigation in phase I trials (NCT02718911, NCT02526017).

Personalized neoantigen-based vaccines are a new compelling immunotherapy approach. Neoantigens are products of diverse tumoral mutations that can trigger tumor-specific T cell responses since they are exclusively expressed by cancer cells, thus avoiding vaccine "off target" effects. They can also propel immunological memory that boosts long term responses and delay disease recurrence. Despite being associated with a moderate tumor mutational burden, RCCs have an important proportion of frameshift indels and T cell infiltration, and are likely to have several candidate neoantigens for vaccine development. Phase I clinical trials with neoantigen-based vaccines in combination with ICIs or IL2 enhancers are currently being explored in RCC (NCT02950766, NCT03289962, NCT03548467, and NCT03633110) [170].

Finally, precision immunotherapy targeting surface antigens with chimeric antigen receptor (CAR) T cells and MHC antigens with tumor infiltrating lymphocytes (TILs) are under early development in RCC (NCT02830724, NCT03393936, and NCT03638206) [161].

Probably, combination strategies between novel immunotherapies and approaches in combination with "older" treatments such as TKIs could reverse the resistance mechanism in RCC. However, it is necessary to point out, that these investigational combinations with positive results in vitro/in vivo have to demonstrate efficacy and safety in further clinical trials. Moreover, we need to develop predictive biomarkers to current therapies in order to guide clinical decisions.

Predictive biomarkers of response to this target and immune-based therapies have been largely studied and have become one of the major challenges in ccRCC treatment. Currently, only the IMDC risk model (based on clinical features and initially designed as a prognostic model) has been validated as a robust tool for treatment selection not only for immunotherapy but also for TKI treatment [171–179]. Despite the PD-L1 expression and tumor mutational burden (TMB) have been broadly studied in many other tumors as a ICIs predictive biomarker, their applicability in ccRCC have not been demonstrated, mainly due to their unclear cutoff for positivity, intratumoral heterogeneity and inconsistency between primary tumor and metastasis [172]. Other promising predictive biomarkers have not bridged the investigational and clinical stages yet. Among these, neutrophil/lymphocyte ratio (NLR) [173,174], PBMR and molecular gene signatures [175,177] are worth highlighting.

5. Conclusions

New therapeutic options for RCC have expanded rapidly over the past decade, with the combination of TKIs and ICIs being the new cornerstone. Understanding the underlying resistance mechanisms to these treatments is a driving force for survival improvement in metastatic RCC.

Counteracting alternative modes of vascularization, EMT, lysosomal sequestration, and alternative molecular pathways can overcome TKIs resistance and restore sensitivity to these molecules. Tumor microenvironment modulation constitutes another fundamental approach, since it participates in both resistance to TKI and ICI. Finally, novel immune checkpoints like LAG-3 and TIM-3, as well as a renewed approach in cytokine therapy with IL-2 are promising targets in development.

Further investigation is warranted to improve our knowledge of RCC biological behavior and to develop successful treatment approaches.

Author Contributions: Conceptualization: J.M.-C., T.A.-G., P.Á.B. and J.C.; Methodology, J.M.-C. and T.A.-G., Validation, J.M.-C., T.A.-G. and E.G.; Formal analysis and investigation, P.Á.B., J.C., Á.R.G., V.G.D.S., M.S.R.-G. and J.P.; Resources, T.A.-G.; Data curation, J.M.-C.; Writing: P.Á.B., J.C., M.S.R.-G. and J.P.; Supervision, T.A.-G., E.G. and J.M.-C.; Project administration: P.Á.B., J.C., M.S.R.-G., J.P., V.G.D.S., Á.R.G., E.G., T.A.-G and J.M.-C. All authors have read and agreed to the published version of the manuscript.

Funding: This research received no external funding.

Conflicts of Interest: EG has received honoraria for speaker engagements, advisory roles or funding of continuous medical education from Adacap, AMGEN, Angelini, Astellas, Astra Zeneca, Bayer, Blueprint, Bristol Myers Squibb, Caris Life Sciences, Celgene, Clovis-Oncology, Eisai, Eusa Pharma, Genetracer, Guardant Health, HRA-Pharma, IPSEN, ITM-Radiopharma, Janssen, Lexicon, Lilly, Merck KGaA, MSD, Nanostring Technologies, Natera, Novartis, ONCODNA (Biosequence), Palex, Pharmamar, Pierre Fabre, Pfizer, Roche, Sanofi-Genzyme, Servier, Taiho, and Thermo Fisher Scientific. EG has received research grants from Pfizer, Astra Zeneca, Astellas, and Lexicon Pharmaceuticals. JMC declares consultant, advisory or speaker roles for IPSEN, Roche, Pfizer, Sanofi, Janssen, and BMS. JMC has received research grants from Pfizer, IPSEN and Roche. TAG declares consultant, advisory or speaker roles for Ipsen, Pfizer, Roche, Bayer, Sanofi-Genzyme, Adacap, Janssen, Eisai, Bristol-Myers Squibb. TAG has received research grants from Pfizer, IPSEN and Roche. The other authors declare no conflicts of interest or state.

References

1. Sung, H.; Ferlay, J.; Siegel, R.L.; Laversanne, M.; Soerjomataram, I.; Jemal, A.; Bray, F. Global Cancer Statistics 2020: GLOBOCAN Estimates of Incidence and Mortality Worldwide for 36 Cancers in 185 Countries. *CA Cancer J. Clin.* **2021**, *71*, 209–249. [CrossRef]
2. Ferlay, J.; Colombet, M.; Soerjomataram, I.; Dyba, T.; Randi, G.; Bettio, M.; Gavin, A.; Visser, O.; Bray, F. Cancer incidence and mortality patterns in Europe: Estimates for 40 countries and 25 major cancers in 2018. *Eur. J. Cancer* **2018**, *103*, 356. [CrossRef] [PubMed]
3. Capitanio, U.; Bemsalah, K.; Bex, A.; Boorjian, S.A.; Bray, F.; Coleman, J.; Gore, J.L.; Sun, M.; Wood, C.; Russo, P. Epidemiology of Renal Cell Carcinoma. *Eur. Urol.* **2019**, *75*, 74. [CrossRef] [PubMed]
4. Dabestani, S.; Thorstenson, A.; Lindblad, P.; Harmenberg, U.; Ljungberg, B.; Lundstam, S. Renal cell carcinoma recurrences and metastases in primary non-metastatic patients: A population-based study. *World J. Urol.* **2016**, *34*, 1081–1086. [CrossRef] [PubMed]
5. Levi, F.; Ferlay, J.; Galeone, C.; Lucchini, F.; Negri, E.; Boyle, P.; La Vecchia, C. The changing pattern of kidney cancer incidence and mortality in Europe. *BJU Int.* **2008**, *101*, 949. [CrossRef]
6. Choueiri, T.K.; Motzer, R.J. Systemic therapy for metastatic renal cell carcinoma. *N. Engl. J. Med.* **2017**, *376*, 354–366. [CrossRef]
7. Cancer Genome Atlas Research, N. Comprehensive molecular characterization of clear cell renal cell carcinoma. *Nature* **2013**, *499*, 43–49. [CrossRef] [PubMed]
8. Gnarra, J.R.; Tory, K.; Weng, Y.; Schmidt, L.; Wei, M.H.; Li, H.; Latif, F.; Liu, S.; Chen, F.; Duh, F.M.; et al. Mutations of the VHL tumour suppressor gene in renal carcinoma. *Nat. Genet.* **1994**, *7*, 85–90. [CrossRef] [PubMed]
9. Kaelin, W.G., Jr. The von Hippel-Lindau tumour suppressor protein and clear cell renal cell carcinoma. *Clin. Cancer Res.* **2007**, *13*, 680s–684s. [CrossRef]
10. Semenza, G.L. HIF-1 mediates metabolic responses to intratumoral hypoxia and oncogenic mutations. *J. Clin. Invest.* **2013**, *123*, 3664–3671. [CrossRef]
11. Motzer, R.J.; Nosov, D.; Eisen, T.; Bondarenko, I.; Lesovoy, V.; Lipatov, O.; Tomczak, P.; Lyulko, O.; Alyasova, A.; Harza, M.; et al. Tivozanib versus sorafenib as initial targeted therapy for patients with metastatic renal cell carcinoma: Results from a phase III trial. *J. Clin. Oncol.* **2013**, *31*, 3791–3799. [CrossRef] [PubMed]
12. Clark, J.I.; Wong, M.K.K.; Kaufman, H.L.; Daniels, G.; Morse, M.A.; McDermott, D.F.; Agarwala, S.S.; Lewis, L.D.; Stewart, J.H. Vaishampayan, U.; et al. Impact of sequencing targeted therapies with high-dose interleukin-2 immunotherapy: An analysis of outcome and survival of patients with metastatic renal cell carcinoma from an on-going observational Il-2 clinical trial: PROCLAIMSM. *Clin. Genitourin. Cancer* **2017**, *15*, 31–41.e4. [CrossRef] [PubMed]
13. Rooney, M.S.; Shukla, S.A.; Wu, C.J.; Getz, G.; Hacohen, N. Molecular and genetic properties of tumors associated with local immune cytolytic activity. *Cell* **2015**, *160*, 48–61. [CrossRef] [PubMed]
14. Senbabaoglu, Y.; Gejman, R.S.; Winer, A.G.; Liu, M.; van Allen, E.M.; de Velasco, G.; Miao, D.; Ostrovnaya, I.; Drill, E.; Luna, A.; et al. Tumor immune microenvironment characterization in clear cell renal cell carcinoma identifies prognostic and immunotherapeutically relevant messenger RNA signatures. *Genome Biol.* **2016**, *17*, 231. [CrossRef]
15. Dietz, S.; Sultmann, H.; Du, Y.; Reisinger, E.; Riediger, A.L.; Volckmar, A.L.; Stenzinger, A.; Schlesner, M.; Jäger, D.; Hohenfellner, M.; et al. Patient-specific molecular alterations are associated with metastatic clear cell renal cell cancer progressing under tyrosine kinase inhibitor therapy. *Oncotarget* **2017**, *8*, 74049–74057. [CrossRef]
16. Ahmed, N.; Escalona, R.; Leung, D.; Chan, E.; Kannourakis, G. Tumour microenvironment and metabolic plasticity in cancer and cancer stem cells: Perspectives on metabolic and immune regulatory signatures in chemoresistant ovarian cancer stem cells. *Semin. Cancer Biol.* **2018**, *53*, 265–281. [CrossRef]
17. Donnem, T.; Reynolds, A.R.; Kuczynski, E.A.; Gatter, K.; Vermeulen, P.B.; Kerbel, R.S.; Harris, A.L.; Pezzella, F. Non-angiogenic tumours and their influence on cancer biology. *Nat. Rev. Cancer* **2018**, *18*, 323–336. [CrossRef]
18. Pezzella, F.; Ribatti, D. Vascular co-option and vasculogenic mimicry mediate resistance to antiangiogenic strategies. *Cancer Rep.* **2020**, e1318. [CrossRef] [PubMed]
19. Seftor, R.E.; Seftor, E.A.; Koshikawa, N.; Meltzer, P.S.; Gardner, L.M.; Bilban, M.; Stetler-Stevenson, W.G.; Quaranta, V.; Hendrix, M.J. Cooperative interactions of laminin 5 gamma2 chain, matrix metalloproteinase-2, and membrane type-1-matrix/metalloproteinase are required for mimicry of embryonic vasculogenesis by aggressive melanoma. *Cancer Res.* **2001**, *61*, 6322–6327.
20. Saravanan, S.; Vimalraj, S.; Pavani, K.; Nikarika, R.; Sumantran, V.N. Intussusceptive angiogenesis as a key therapeutic target for cancer therapy. *Life Sci.* **2020**, *252*, 117670. [CrossRef]
21. Mentzer, S.J.; Mentzer, M.A. Konerding Intussuceptive angiogenesis: Expansion and remodeling of microvascular networks. *Angiogenesis* **2014**, *17*, 499–509. [CrossRef] [PubMed]
22. He, H.; Magi-Galluzzi, C. Epithelial-to-mesenchymal transition in renal neoplasms. *Adv. Anat. Pathol.* **2014**, *21*, 174–180. [CrossRef] [PubMed]
23. Krishnamachary, B.; Zagzag, D.; Nagasawa, H.; Rainey, K.; Okuyama, H.; Baek, J.H.; Semenza, G.L. Hypoxia-inducible Factor-1-dependent repression of E-cadherin in von Hippel-Lindau tumor suppressor–null renal cell carcinoma mediated by TCF3, ZFHX1A, and ZFHX1B. *Cancer Res.* **2006**, *66*, 2725–2731. [CrossRef]
24. Kalluri, R.; Neilson, E.G. Epithelial-mesenchymal transition and its implications for fibrosis. *J. Clin. Investig.* **2003**, *112*, 1776–1784. [CrossRef] [PubMed]

25. Chen, Q.; Yang, D.; Zong, H.; Zhu, L.; Wang, L.; Wang, X.; Zhu, X.; Song, X.; Wang, J. Growth-induced stress enhances epithelial-mesenchymal transition induced by IL-6 in clear cell renal cell carcinoma via the Akt/GSK-3β/β-catenin signaling pathway. *Oncogenesis* **2017**, *6*, e375. [CrossRef]
26. Boström, A.K.; Möller, C.; Nilsson, E.; Elfving, P.; Axelson, H.; Johansson, M.E. Sarcomatoid conversion of clear cell renal cell carcinoma in relation to epithelial-to-mesenchymal transition. *Hum. Pathol.* **2012**, *43*, 708–719. [CrossRef] [PubMed]
27. Tammela, T.; Zarkada, G.; Wallgard, E.; Murtomäki, A.; Suchting, S.; Wirzenius, M.; Waltari, M.; Hellström, M.; Schomber, T.; Peltonen, R.; et al. Blocking vegfr-3 suppresses angiogenic sprouting and vascular network formation. *Nature* **2008**, *454*, 656–660. [CrossRef]
28. van der Mijn, J.C.; Mier, J.W.; Broxterman, H.J.; Verheul, H.M. Predictive biomarkers in renal cell cancer: Insights in drug resistance mechanisms. *Drug Resist. Updates* **2014**, *17*, 77–88. [CrossRef]
29. Welti, J.C.; Gourlaouen, M.; Powles, T.; Kudahetti, S.C.; Wilson, P.; Berney, D.M.; Reynolds, A.R. Fibroblast growth factor 2 regulates endothelial cell sensitivity to sunitinib. *Oncogene* **2011**, *30*, 1183–1193. [CrossRef]
30. Zhou, L.; Liu, X.D.; Sun, M.; Falcón, B.; Hashizume, H.; Yao, L.C.; Aftab, D.T.; McDonald, D.M. Targeting MET and AXL overcomes resistance to sunitinib therapy in renal cell carcinoma. *Oncogene* **2016**, *35*, 2687–2697. [CrossRef]
31. Gustafsson, A.; Martuszewska, D.; Johansson, M.; Ekman, C.; Hafizi, S.; Ljungberg, B.; Dahlbäck, B. Differential expression of Axl and Gas6 in renal cell carcinoma reflecting tumor advancement and survival. *Clin. Cancer Res. Off. J. Am. Assoc. Cancer Res.* **2009**, *15*, 4742–4749. [CrossRef] [PubMed]
32. Gibney, G.T.; Aziz, S.A.; Camp, R.L.; Conrad, P.; Schwartz, B.E.; Chen, C.R.; Kelly, W.K.; Kluger, H.M. c-Met is a prognostic marker and potential therapeutic target in clear cell renal cell carcinoma. *Ann. Oncol. Off. J. Eur. Soc. Med. Oncol./ESMO.* **2013**, *24*, 343–349. [CrossRef] [PubMed]
33. Balkwill, F. Tumour necrosis factor and cancer. *Nat. Rev. Cancer.* **2009**, *9*, 361–371. [CrossRef]
34. Ho, M.Y.; Tang, S.J.; Chuang, M.J.; Cha, T.L.; Li, J.Y.; Sun, G.H.; Sun, K.H. TNF-α induces epithelial-mesenchymal transition of renal cell carcinoma cells via a GSK3β-dependent mechanism. *Mol. Cancer Res.* **2012**, *10*, 1109–1119. [CrossRef] [PubMed]
35. Gong, K.; Guo, G.; Gerber, D.E.; Gao, B.; Peyton, M.; Huang, C.; Minna, J.D.; Hatanpaa, K.J.; Kernstine, K.; Cai, L. TNF-driven adaptive response mediates resistance to EGFR inhibition in lung cancer. *J. Clin. Invest.* **2018**, *128*, 2500–2518. [CrossRef]
36. Zhang, Z.; Lin, G.; Yan, Y.; Li, X.; Hu, Y.; Wang, J.; Yin, B.; Wu, Y.; Li, Z.; Yang, X.P. Transmembrane TNF-alpha promotes chemoresistance in breast cancer cells. *Oncogene* **2018**, *37*, 3456–3470. [CrossRef]
37. Hwang, H.S.; Park, Y.Y.; Shin, S.J.; Go, H.; Park, J.M.; Yoon, S.Y.; Lee, J.L.; Cho, Y.M. Involvement of the TNF-α Pathway in TKI Resistance and Suggestion of TNFR1 as a Predictive Biomarker for TKI Responsiveness in Clear Cell Renal Cell Carcinoma. *J. Korean Med. Sci.* **2020**, *35*, e31. [CrossRef]
38. Rigamonti, N.; Kadioglu, E.; Keklikoglou, I.; Rmili, C.W.; Leow, C.C.; de Palma, M. Role of angiopoietin-2 in adaptive tumor resistance to VEGF signaling blockade. *Cell Rep.* **2014**, *8*, 696–706. [CrossRef]
39. Wang, X.; Bullock, A.J.; Zhang, L.; Wei, L.; Yu, D.; Mahagaokar, K.; Alsop, D.C.; Mier, J.W.; Atkins, M.B.; Coxon, A.; et al. The role of angiopoietins as potential therapeutic targets in renal cell carcinoma. *Transl. Oncol.* **2014**, *7*, 188–195. [CrossRef]
40. Liu, L.; Xu, Z.; Zhong, L.; Wang, H.; Jiang, S.; Long, Q.; Xu, J.; Guo, J. Enhancer of zeste homolog 2 (EZH2) promotes tumour cell migration and invasion via epigenetic repression of E-cadherin in renal cell carcinoma. *BJU Int.* **2016**, *117*, 351–362. [CrossRef]
41. Adelaiye-Ogala, R.; Budka, J.; Damayanti, N.P.; Arrington, J.; Ferris, M.; Hsu, C.C.; Chintala, S.; Orillion, A.; Miles, K.M.; Shen, L.; et al. EZH2 Modifies Sunitinib Resistance in Renal Cell Carcinoma by Kinome Reprogramming. *Cancer Res.* **2017**, *77*, 6651–6666. [CrossRef]
42. Adelaiye, R.; Ciamporcero, E.; Miles, K.M.; Sotomayor, P.; Bard, J.; Tsompana, M.; Conroy, D.; Shen, L.; Ramakrishnan, S.; Ku, S.Y.; et al. Sunitinib dose escalation overcomes transient resistance in clear cell renal cell carcinoma and is associated with epigenetic modifications. *Mol. Cancer* **2015**, *14*, 513–522. [CrossRef] [PubMed]
43. Gotink, K.J.; Broxterman, H.J.; Labots, M.; de Haas, R.R.; Dekker, H.; Honeywell, R.J.; Rudek, M.A.; Beerepoot, L.V.; Musters, R.J.; Jansen, G.; et al. Lysosomal sequestration of sunitinib: A novel mechanism of drug resistance. *Clin. Cancer Res.* **2011**, *17*, 7337–7346. [CrossRef] [PubMed]
44. Gotink, K.J.; Rovithi, M.; de Haas, R.R.; Honeywell, R.J.; Dekker, H.; Poel, D.; Azijli, K.; Peters, G.J.; Broxterman, H.J.; Verheul, H.M.W. Cross-resistance to clinically used tyrosine kinase inhibitors sunitinib, sorafenib and pazopanib. *Cell Oncol.* **2015**, *38*, 119–129. [CrossRef] [PubMed]
45. Azijli, K.; Gotink, K.J.; Verheul, H.M.W. The Potential Role of Lysosomal Sequestration in Sunitinib Resistance of Renal Cell Cancer. *J. Kidney Cancer VHL.* **2015**, *2*, 195–203. [CrossRef]
46. Giuliano, S.; Cormerais, Y.; Dufies, M.; Grépin, R.; Colosetti, P.; Belaid, A.; Parola, J.; Martin, A.; Lacas-Gervais, S.; Mazure, N.M.; et al. Resistance to sunitinib in renal clear cell carcinoma results from sequestration in lysosomes and inhibition of the autophagic flux. *Autophagy* **2015**, *11*, 1891–1904. [CrossRef]
47. Sato, H.; Siddig, S.; Uzu, M.; Suzuki, S.; Nomura, Y.; Kashiba, T.; Gushimiyagi, K.; Sekine, Y.; Uehara, T.; Arano, Y.; et al. Elacridar enhances the cytotoxic effects of sunitinib and prevents multidrug resistance in renal carcinoma cells. *Eur. J. Pharm.* **2015**, *746*, 258–266. [CrossRef]
48. Zhitomirsky, B.; Assaraf, Y.G. Lysosomal sequestration of hydrophobic weak base chemotherapeutics triggers lysosomal biogenesis and lysosome-dependent cancer multidrug resistance. *Oncotarget* **2015**, *6*, 1143–1156. [CrossRef]

49. Settembre, C.; Zoncu, R.; Medina, D.L.; Vetrini, F.; Erdin, S.; Erdin, S.; Huynh, T.; Ferron, M.; Karsenty, G.; Vellard, M.C.; et al. A lysosome-to-nucleus signalling mechanism senses and regulates the lysosome via mTOR and TFEB. *EMBO J.* **2012**, *31*, 1095–1108. [CrossRef]
50. Zhao, A.; Li, G.; Péoc'h, M.; Genin, C.; Gigante, M. Serum miR-210 as a novel biomarker for molecular diagnosis of clear cell renal cell carcinoma. *Exp. Mol. Pathol.* **2013**, *94*, 115–120. [CrossRef]
51. Dias, F.; Teixeira, A.L.; Ferreira, M.; Adem, B.; Bastos, N.; Vieira, J.; Fernandes, M.; Sequeira, M.I.; Maurício, J.; Lobo, F.; et al. Plasmatic miR-210, miR-221 and miR1233 profile: Potential liquid biopsies candidates for renal cell carcinoma. *Oncotarget* **2017**, *8*, 103315–103326. [CrossRef] [PubMed]
52. Wang, C.; Wu, C.; Yang, Q.; Ding, M.; Zhong, J.; Zhang, C.; Ge, J.; Wang, J.; Zhang, C. miR-28-5p acts as a tumor suppressor in renal cell carcinoma for multiple antitumor effects by targeting RAP1B. *Oncotarget* **2016**, *7*, 73888–73902. [CrossRef] [PubMed]
53. Lu, L.; Li, Y.; Wen, H.; Feng, C. Overexpression of miR-15b promotes resistance to Sunitinib in renal cell carcinoma. *J. Cancer* **2019**, *10*, 3389–3396. [CrossRef]
54. Yamaguchi, N.; Osaki, M.; Onuma, K.; Yumioka, T.; Iwamoto, H.; Sejima, T.; Kugoh, H.; Takenaka, A.; Okada, F. Identification of MicroRNAs involved in resistance to Sunitinib in renal cell carcinoma cells. *Anticancer Res.* **2017**, *37*, 2985–2992.
55. Yoshino, H.; Enokida, H.; Itesako, T.; Tatarano, S.; Kinoshita, T.; Fuse, M.; Kojima, S.; Nakagawa, M.; Seki, N. Epithelial–mesenchymal transition-related microRNA-200s regulate molecular targets and pathways in renal cell carcinoma. *J. Hum. Genet.* **2013**, *58*, 508–516. [CrossRef]
56. Kourembanas, S. Exosomes: Vehicles of intercellular signaling, biomarkers, and vectors of cell therapy. *Annu. Rev. Physiol.* **2015**, *77*, 13–27. [CrossRef]
57. Qu, L.; Ding, J.; Chen, C.; Wu, Z.J.; Liu, B.; Gao, Y. Exosome-Transmitted lncARSR Promotes Sunitinib Resistance in Renal Cancer by Acting as a Competing Endogenous RNA. *Cancer Cell* **2016**, *29*, 653–668. [CrossRef] [PubMed]
58. Beuselinck, B.; Karadimou, A.; Lambrechts, D.; Claes, B.; Wolter, P.; Couchy, G.; Berkers, J.; Paridaens, R.; Schöffski, P.; Méjean, A.; et al. Single-nucleotide polymorphisms associated with outcome in metastatic renal cell carcinoma treated with sunitinib. *Br. J. Cancer* **2013**, *108*, 887–900. [CrossRef]
59. Diekstra, M.H.; Swen, J.J.; Boven, E.; Castellano, D.; Gelderblom, H.; Mathijssen, R.H.J.; Rodríguez-Antona, C.; García-Donas, J.; Rini, B.I.; Guchelaar, H.-J. Cyp3a5 and abcb1 polymorphisms as predictors for sunitinib outcome in metastatic renal cell carcinoma. *Eur. Urol.* **2015**, *68*, 621–629. [CrossRef]
60. Makhov, P.; Joshi, S.; Ghatalia, P.; Kutikov, A.; Uzzo, R.G.; Kolenko, V.M. Resistance to Systemic Therapies in Clear Cell Renal Cell Carcinoma: Mechanisms and Management Strategies. *Mol. Cancer Ther.* **2018**, *17*, 1355–1364. [CrossRef]
61. van der Veldt, A.A.; Vroling, L.; de Haas, R.R.; Koolwijk, P.; van den Eertwegh, A.J.; Haanen, J.B.A.G.; van Hinsbergh, V.W.M.; Broxterman, H.J.; Boven, E. Sunitinib-induced changes in circulating endothelial cell-related proteins in patients with metastatic renal cell cancer. *Int. J. Cancer* **2012**, *131*, E484–E493. [CrossRef]
62. Miles, K.M.; Seshadri, M.; Ciamporcero, E.; Adelaiye, R.; Gillard, B.; Sotomayor, P.; Attwood, K.; Shen, L.; Conroy, D.; Kuhnert, F.; et al. Dll4 blockade potentiates the anti-tumor effects of VEGF inhibition in renal cell carcinoma patient-derived xenografts. *PLoS ONE* **2014**, *9*, e112371.
63. Xiao, W.; Gao, Z.; Duan, Y.; Yuan, W.; Ke, Y. Notch signaling plays a crucial role in cancer stem-like cells maintaining stemness and mediating chemotaxis in renal cell carcinoma. *J. Exp. Clin. Cancer Res.* **2017**, *36*, 41. [CrossRef]
64. Shojaei, F.; Wu, X.; Qu, X.; Kowanetz, M.; Yu, L.; Tan, M.; Meng, Y.G.; Ferrara, N. G-CSF-initiated myeloid cell mobilization and angiogenesis mediate tumor refractoriness to anti-VEGF therapy in mouse models. *Proc. Natl. Acad. Sci. USA* **2009**, *106*, 6742–6747. [CrossRef]
65. Ko, J.S.; Rayman, P.; Ireland, J.; Swaidani, S.; Li, G.; Bunting, K.D.; Rini, B.; Finke, J.H.; Cohen, P.A. Direct and differential suppression of myeloid-derived suppressor cell subsets by sunitinib is compartmentally constrained. *Cancer Res.* **2010**, *70*, 3526–3536. [CrossRef] [PubMed]
66. Geevarghese, A.; Herman, I.M. Pericyte-endothelial crosstalk: Implications and opportunities for advanced cellular therapies. *Transl. Res.* **2014**, *163*, 296–306. [CrossRef]
67. Pan, J.; Mestas, J.; Burdick, M.D.; Phillips, R.J.; Thomas, G.V.; Reckamp, K. Stromal derived factor-1 (SDF-1/CXCL12) and CXCR4 in renal cell carcinoma metastasis. *Mol. Cancer* **2006**, *5*, 56. [CrossRef] [PubMed]
68. Zagzag, D.; Krishnamachary, B.; Yee, H.; Okuyama, H.; Chiriboga, L.; Ali, M.A. Stromal cell-derived factor-1α and CXCR4 expression in hemangioblastoma and clear cell-renal cell carcinoma: Von Hippel-Lindau loss-of-function induces expression of a ligand and its receptor. *Cancer Res.* **2005**, *65*, 6178–6188. [CrossRef]
69. Xu, Y.; Lu, Y.; Song, J.; Dong, B.; Kong, W.; Xue, W. Cancer-associated fibroblasts promote renal cell carcinoma progression. *Tumor Biol.* **2015**, *36*, 3483–3488. [CrossRef]
70. Kakarla, S.; Song, X.T.; Gottschalk, S. Cancer-associated fibroblasts as targets for immunotherapy. *Immunotherapy* **2012**, *4*, 1129–1138. [CrossRef]
71. Errarte, P.; Guarch, R.; Pulido, R.; Blanco, L.; Nunes-Xavier, C.E.; Beitia, M.; Gil, J.; Angulo, J.C.; Lopez, J.L.; Larrinaga, G. The expression of fibroblast activation protein in clear cell renal cell carcinomas is associated with synchronous lymph node metastases. *PLoS ONE* **2016**, *11*, e0169105. [CrossRef]

72. Crawford, Y.; Kasman, I.; Yu, L.; Zhong, C.; Wu, X.; Modrusan, Z.; Kaminker, J.; Ferrara, N. PDGF-C mediates the angiogenic and tumorigenic properties of fibroblasts associated with tumors refractory to anti-VEGF treatment. *Cancer Cell* **2009**, *15*, 21–34. [CrossRef]
73. Bingle, L.; Brown, N.J.; Lewis, C.E. The role of tumour-associated macrophages in tumour progression: Implications for new anticancer therapies. *J. Pathol.* **2002**, *196*, 254–265. [CrossRef] [PubMed]
74. Krug, S.; Abbassi, R.; Griesmann, H.; Sipos, B.; Wiese, D.; Rexin, P.; Blank, A.; Perren, A.; Haybaeck, J.; Hüttelmaier, S. Therapeutic targeting of tumor-associated macrophages in pancreatic neuroendocrine tumors. *Int. J. Cancer.* **2018**, *143*, 1806–1816. [CrossRef] [PubMed]
75. Kalbasi, A.; Ribas, A. Tumour-intrinsic resistance to immune checkpoint blockade. *Nat. Rev. Immunol.* **2020**, *20*, 25–39. [CrossRef] [PubMed]
76. Restifo, N.P.; Esquivel, F.; Kawakami, Y.; Yewdell, J.W.; Mulé, J.J.; Rosenberg, S.A.; Bennink, J.R. Identification of human cancers deficient in antigen processing. *J. Exp. Med.* **1993**, *177*, 265–272. [CrossRef]
77. Platanias, L.C. Mechanisms of type-I- and type-II-interferon-mediated signalling. *Nat. Rev. Immunol.* **2005**, *5*, 375–386. [CrossRef]
78. Zaretsky, J.M.; Garcia-Diaz, A.; Shin, D.S.; Escuin-Ordinas, H.; Hugo, W.; Hu-Lieskovan, S.; Torrejon, D.Y.; Abril-Rodriguez, G.; Sandoval, S.; Barthly, L.; et al. Mutations associated with acquired resistance to PD-1 blockade in melanoma. *N. Engl. J. Med.* **2016**, *375*, 819–829. [CrossRef]
79. Spranger, S.; Bao, R.; Gajewski, T.F. Melanoma-intrinsic β-catenin signalling prevents anti-tumour immunity. *Nature* **2015**, *523*, 231–235. [CrossRef]
80. Sweis, R.F.; Spranger, S.; Bao, R.; Paner, G.P.; Stadler, W.M.; Steinberg, G.; Gajewski, T.F. Molecular drivers of the non-T-cell-inflamed tumor microenvironment in urothelial bladder cancer. *Cancer Immunol. Res.* **2016**, *4*, 563–568. [CrossRef]
81. Seiwert, T.Y.; Zuo, Z.; Keck, M.K.; Khattri, A.; Pedamallu, C.S.; Stricker, T.; Brown, C.; Pugh, T.J.; Stojanov, P.; Cho, J.; et al. Integrative and comparative genomic analysis of HPV-positive and HPV-negative head and neck squamous cell carcinomas. *Clin. Cancer Res.* **2015**, *21*, 632–641. [CrossRef] [PubMed]
82. Jiménez-Sánchez, A.; Memon, D.; Pourpe, S.; Veeraraghavan, H.; Li, Y.; Vargas, H.A.; Gill, M.B.; Park, K.J.; Zivanovic, O.; Konner, J.; et al. Heterogeneous tumor-immune microenvironments among differentially growing metastases in an ovarian cancer patient. *Cell* **2017**, *170*, 927–938.e20. [CrossRef] [PubMed]
83. Zhao, F.; Xiao, C.; Evans, K.S.; Theivanthiran, T.; DeVito, N.; Holtzhausen, A.; Liu, J.; Liu, X.; Boczkowski, D.; Nair, S.; et al. Paracrine Wnt5a-β-catenin signaling triggers a metabolic program that drives dendritic cell tolerization. *Immunity* **2018**, *48*, 147–160.e7. [CrossRef]
84. Zhan, T.; Rindtorff, N.; Boutros, M. Wnt signaling in cancer. *Oncogene* **2017**, *36*, 1461–1473. [CrossRef] [PubMed]
85. Boni, A.; Cogdill, A.P.; Dang, P.; Udayakumar, D.; Njauw, C.-N.J.; Sloss, C.M.; Ferrone, C.R.; Flaherty, K.T.; Lawrence, D.P.; Fisher, D.E.; et al. Selective BRAFV600E inhibition enhances T-cell recognition of melanoma without affecting lymphocyte function. *Cancer Res.* **2010**, *70*, 5213–5219. [CrossRef]
86. Ricketts, C.J.; De Cubas, A.A.; Fan, H.; Smith, C.C.; Lang, M.; Reznik, E.; Bowlby, R.; Gibb, E.A.; Akbani, R.; Beroukhim, R.; et al. The cancer genome atlas comprehensive molecular characterization of renal cell carcinoma. *Cell Rep.* **2018**, *23*, 313–326.e5. [CrossRef]
87. Peng, W.; Chen, J.Q.; Liu, C.; Malu, S.; Creasy, C.; Tetzlaff, M.T.; Xu, C.; McKenzie, J.A.; Zhang, C.; Liang, X.; et al. Loss of PTEN promotes resistance to T cell-mediated immunotherapy. *Cancer Discov.* **2016**, *6*, 202–216. [CrossRef]
88. Goel, S.; DeCristo, M.J.; Watt, A.C.; BrinJones, H.; Sceneay, J.; Li, B.B.; Khan, N.; Uberllacker, J.M.; Xie, S.; Metzger-Filho, O.; et al. CDK4/6 inhibition triggers anti-tumour immunity. *Nature* **2017**, *548*, 471–475. [CrossRef]
89. Jerby-Arnon, L.; Shah, P.; Cuoco, M.S.; Rodman, C.; Su, M.J.; Melms, J.C.; Leeson, R.; Kanodia, A.; Mei, S.; Lin, J.-R.; et al. A cancer cell program promotes T cell exclusion and resistance to checkpoint blockade. *Cell* **2018**, *175*, 984–997.e24. [CrossRef]
90. Deng, J.; Wang, E.S.; Jenkins, R.W.; Li, S.; Dries, R.; Yates, K.; Chhabra, S.; Huang, W.; Liu, H.; Aref, A.R.; et al. CDK4/6 inhibition augments antitumor immunity by enhancing T-cell activation. *Cancer Discov.* **2018**, *8*, 216–233. [CrossRef]
91. Wang, X.; Zhang, H.; Chen, X. Drug resistance and combating drug resistance in cancer. *Cancer Drug Resist* **2019**, *2*, 141–160. [CrossRef]
92. Sade-Feldman, M.; Jiao, Y.J.; Chen, J.H.; Rooney, M.S.; Barzily-Rokni, M.; Eliane, J.-P.; Bjorgaard, S.L.; Hammond, M.R.; Vitzthum, H.; Blackmon, S.M.; et al. Resistance to checkpoint blockade therapy through inactivation of antigen presentation. *Nat. Commun.* **2017**, *8*, 1136. [CrossRef]
93. Fridman, W.H.; Pagès, F.; Sautès-Fridman, C.; Galon, J. The immune contexture in human tumours: Impact on clinical outcome. *Nat. Rev. Cancer* **2012**, *12*, 298–306. [CrossRef]
94. Becht, E.; Giraldo, N.A.; Lacroix, L.; Buttard, B.; Elarouci, N.; Petitprez, F.; Selves, J.; Laurent-Puig, P.; Sautès-Fridman, C.; Fridman, W.H.; et al. Estimating the population abundance of tissue-infiltrating immune and stromal cell populations using gene expression. *Genome Biol.* **2016**, *17*, 218.
95. Giraldo, N.A.; Becht, E.; Pagès, F.; Skliris, G.; Verkarre, V.; Vano, Y.; Mejean, A.; Saint-Aubert, N.; Lacroix, L.; Natario, I.; et al. Orchestration and prognostic significance of immune checkpoints in the microenvironment of primary and metastatic renal cell cancer. *Clin. Cancer Res.* **2015**, *21*, 3031–3040. [CrossRef] [PubMed]

96. Choueiri, T.K.; Escudier, B.; Powles, T.; Tannir, N.M.; Mainwaring, P.N.; Rini, B.I.; Hammers, H.J.; Donskov, F.; Roth, B.J.; Peltola, K.; et al. METEOR investigators. Cabozantinib versus everolimus in advanced renal cell carcinoma (METEOR): Final results from a randomised, open-label, phase 3 trial. *Lancet Oncol.* **2016**, *17*, 917–927. [CrossRef]
97. Giraldo, N.A.; Becht, E.; Vano, Y.; Petitprez, F.; Lacroix, L.; Validire, P.; Sanchez-Salas, R.; Ingels, A.; Oudard, S.; Moatti, A.; et al. Tumor-infiltrating and peripheral blood T-cell immunophenotypes predict early relapse in localized clear cell renal cell carcinoma. *Clin. Cancer Res.* **2017**, *23*, 4416–4428.
98. McDermott, D.F.; Huseni, M.A.; Atkins, M.B.; Motzer, R.J.; Rini, B.I.; Escudier, B.; Fong, L.; Joseph, R.W.; Pal, S.K.; Reeves, J.A.; et al. Clinical activity and molecular correlates of response to atezolizumab alone or in combination with bevacizumab versus sunitinib in renal cell carcinoma. *Nat. Med.* **2018**, *6*, 749–757. [CrossRef] [PubMed]
99. Motzer, R.J.; Banchereau, R.; Hamidi, H.; Powles, T.; McDermott, D.; Atkins, M.B.; Escudier, B.; Liu, L.-F.; Leng, N.; Abbas, A.R.; et al. Molecular Subsets in Renal Cancer Determine Outcome to Checkpoint and Angiogenesis Blockade. *Cancer Cell* **2020**, *38*, 803–817.e4.
100. Seeber, A.; Klinglmair, G.; Fritz, J.; Steinkohl, F.; Zimmer, K.-C.; Aigner, F.; Horninger, W.; Gastl, G.; Zelger, B.; Brunner, A.; et al. High IDO-1 expression in tumor endothelial cells is associated with response to immunotherapy in metastatic renal cell carcinoma. *Cancer Sci.* **2018**, *109*, 1583–1591. [CrossRef]
101. Chanmee, T.; Ontong, P.; Konno, K.; Itano, N. Tumor-associated macrophages as major players in the tumor microenvironment. *Cancers* **2014**, *6*, 1670–1690. [CrossRef] [PubMed]
102. Mier, J.W. The tumor microenvironment in renal cell cancer. *Curr. Opin. Oncol.* **2019**, *31*, 194–199. [CrossRef]
103. Komohara, Y.; Hasita, H.; Ohnishi, K.; Fujiwara, Y.; Suzu, S.; Eto, M.; Takeya, M. Macrophage infiltration and its prognostic relevance in clear cell renal cell carcinoma. *Cancer Sci.* **2011**, *102*, 1424–1431. [CrossRef] [PubMed]
104. Rosser, E.C.; Mauri, C. Regulatory B cells: Origin, phenotype, and function. *Immunity* **2015**, *42*, 607–612. [CrossRef]
105. Sarvaria, A.; Madrigal, J.A.; Saudemont, A. B cell regulation in cancer and anti-tumor immunity. *Cell Mol. Immunol.* **2017**, *14*, 662–674. [CrossRef]
106. Helmink, B.A.; Reddy, S.M.; Gao, J.; Zhang, S.; Basar, R.; Thakur, R.; Yizhak, K.; Sade-Feldman, M.; Blando, J.; Han, G.; et al. B cells and tertiary lymphoid structures promote immunotherapy response. *Nature* **2020**, *577*, 549–555. [CrossRef]
107. Petitprez, F.; de Reyniès, A.; Keung, E.Z.; Chen, T.W.W.; Sun, C.M.; Calderaro, J.; Jeng, Y.-M.; Hsiao, L.-P.; Lacroix, L.; Bougoüin, A.; et al. B cells are associated with survival and immunotherapy response in sarcoma. *Nature* **2020**, *577*, 556–560. [CrossRef]
108. Finkin, S.; Yuan, D.; Stein, I.; Taniguchi, K.; Weber, A.; Unger, K.; Browning, J.L.; Goossens, N.; Nakagawa, S.; Gunasekaran, G.; et al. Ectopic lymphoid structures function as microniches for tumor progenitor cells in hepatocellular carcinoma. *Nat. Immunol.* **2015**, *16*, 1235–1244. [CrossRef]
109. Grivennikov, S.I.; Greten, F.R.; Karin, M. Immunity, inflammation, and cancer. *Cell* **2010**, *140*, 883–899. [CrossRef]
110. Garcia-Diaz, A.; Shin, D.S.; Moreno, B.H.; Saco, J.; Escuin-Ordinas, H.; Rodriguez, G.A.; Zaretsky, J.M.; Sun, L.; Hugo, W.; Wang, X.; et al. Interferon receptor signaling pathways regulating PD-L1 and PD-L2 expression. *Cell Rep.* **2017**, *19*, 1189–1201. [CrossRef]
111. Bui, J.D.; Schreiber, R.D. Cancer immunosurveillance, immunoediting and inflammation: Independent or interdependent processes? *Curr. Opin. Immunol.* **2007**, *19*, 203–208. [CrossRef]
112. Stubbs, M.; McSheehy, P.M.; Griffiths, J.R.; Bashford, C.L. Causes and consequences of tumour acidity and implications for treatment. *Mol. Med. Today* **2000**, *6*, 15–19. [CrossRef]
113. Sormendi, S.; Wielockx, B. Hypoxia pathway proteins as central mediators of metabolism in the tumor cells and their microenvironment. *Front Immunol.* **2018**, *9*, 40. [CrossRef] [PubMed]
114. Khan, K.A.; Kerbel, R.S. Improving immunotherapy outcomes with anti-angiogenic treatments and vice versa. *Nat. Rev. Clin. Oncol.* **2018**, *15*, 310–324. [CrossRef]
115. Garcia-Lora, A.; Algarra, I.; Garrido, F. MHC class I antigens, immune surveillance, and tumor immune escape. *J. Cell Physiol.* **2003**, *195*, 346–355. [CrossRef] [PubMed]
116. Tatli Dogan, H.; Kiran, M.; Bilgin, B.; Kiliçarslan, A.; Sendur, M.A.N.; Yalçin, B.; Ardiçoglu, A.; Atmaca, A.F.; Gumuskaya, B. Prognostic significance of the programmed death ligand 1 expression in clear cell renal cell carcinoma and correlation with the tumor microenvironment and hypoxia-inducible factor expression. *Diagn. Pathol.* **2018**, *13*, 60. [CrossRef]
117. Zhang, J.; Shi, Z.; Xu, X.; Yu, Z.; Mi, J. The influence of microenvironment on tumor immunotherapy. *FEBS J.* **2019**, *286*, 4160–4175. [CrossRef]
118. Romero-Garcia, S.; Moreno-Altamirano, M.M.B.; Prado-Garcia, H.; Sánchez-García, F.J. Lactate contribution to the tumor microenvironment: Mechanisms, effects on immune cells and therapeutic relevance. *Front Immunol.* **2016**, *7*, 52. [CrossRef]
119. Pan, D.; Kobayashi, A.; Jiang, P.; Ferrari de Andrade, L.; Tay, R.E.; Luoma, A.M.; Tsoucas, D.; Qiu, X.; Lim, K.; Rao, P.; et al. A major chromatin regulator determines resistance of tumor cells to T cell-mediated killing. *Science* **2018**, *359*, 770–775. [CrossRef]
120. Varela, I.; Tarpey, P.; Raine, K.; Huang, D.; Ong, C.K.; Stephens, P.; Davies, H.; Jones, D.; Lin, M.-L.; Teague, J.; et al. Exome sequencing identifies frequent mutation of the SWI/SNF complex gene PBRM1 in renal carcinoma. *Nature* **2011**, *469*, 539–542. [CrossRef] [PubMed]
121. Santoni, M.; Massari, F.; Amantini, C.; Nabissi, M.; Maines, F.; Burattini, L.; Berardi, R.; Santoni, G.; Montironi, R.; Tortora, G.; et al. Emerging role of tumor-associated macrophages as therapeutic targets in patients with metastatic renal cell carcinoma. *Cancer Immunol. Immunother.* **2013**, *62*, 1757–1768. [CrossRef] [PubMed]

122. Miao, D.; Margolis, C.A.; Gao, W.; Voss, M.H.; Li, W.; Martini, D.J.; Norton, C.; Bossé, D.; Wankowicz, S.M.; Cullen, D.; et al. Genomic correlates of response to immune checkpoint therapies in clear cell renal cell carcinoma. *Science* **2018**, *359*, 801–806. [CrossRef] [PubMed]
123. Braun, D.A.; Ishii, Y.; Walsh, A.M.; Van Allen, E.M.; Wu, C.J.; Shukla, S.A.; Choueiri, T.K. Clinical validation of PBRM1 alterations as a marker of immune checkpoint inhibitor response in renal cell carcinoma. *JAMA Oncol.* **2019**, *5*, 1631–1633. [CrossRef] [PubMed]
124. Aili, A.; Jie, W.; Lixiang, X.; Junjie, W. Mutational Analysis of PBRM1 and Significance of PBRM1 Mutation in Anti-PD-1 Immunotherapy of Clear Cell Renal Cell Carcinoma. *Front Oncol.* **2021**, *11*, 712765. [CrossRef] [PubMed]
125. Das, M.; Zhu, C.; Kuchroo, V.K. Tim-3 and its role in regulating anti-tumor immunity. *Immunol. Rev.* **2017**, *1*, 97–111. [CrossRef]
126. Acharya, N.; Sabatos-Peyton, C.; Carrizosa Anderson, A. Tim-3 finds its place in the cancer immunotherapy landscape. *J. Immunother. Cancer* **2020**, *8*, e000911. [CrossRef]
127. Granier, C.; Dariane, C.; Combe, P.; Verkarre, V.; Urien, S.; Badoual, C.; Roussel, H.; Mandavit, M.; Ravel, P.; Sibony, M.; et al. Tim-3 expression on tumor-infiltrating PD-1+CD8+ T cells correlates with poor clinical outcome in renal cell carcinoma. *Cancer Res.* **2017**, *77*, 1075–1082. [CrossRef]
128. Motzer, R.J.; Escudier, B.; McDermott, D.F.; George, S.; Hammers, H.J.; Srinivas, S.; Tykodi, S.S.; Sosman, J.A.; Procopio, G.; Plimack, E.R.; et al. Nivolumab versus Everolimus in Advanced Renal Cell Carcinoma. *N. Engl. J. Med.* **2015**, *373*, 1803–1813. [CrossRef]
129. Triebel, F.; Jitsukawa, S.; Baixeras, E.; Roman-Roman, S.; Genevee, C.; Viegas-Pequignot, E.; Hercend, T. LAG-3, a novel lymphocyte activation gene closely related to CD4. *J. Exp. Med.* **1990**, *171*, 1393–1405. [CrossRef]
130. Goldberg, M.V.; Drake, C.G. LAG-3 in Cancer Immunotherapy. *Curr. Top. Microbiol. Immunol.* **2011**, *344*, 269–278.
131. Sittig, S.P.; Kollgaard, T.; Gronbaek, K.; Idorn, M.; Hennenlotter, J.; Stenzl, A.; Gouttefangeas, C.; Thor Straten, P. Clonal expansion of renal cell carcinoma-infiltrating T lymphocytes. *Oncoimmunology* **2013**, *2*, e26014. [CrossRef]
132. Miao, W.; Qi, D.; Jiangtao, J.; Yuhan, W.; Yuting, L.; Qin, L. LAG3 and its emerging role in cancer immunotherapy. *Clin. Transl. Med.* **2021**, *3*, e365.
133. Long, L.; Xue, Z.; Fuchun, C.; Qi, P.; Phiphatwatchara, P.; Yuyang, Z.; Honglei, C. The promising immune checkpoint LAG-3: From tumor microenvironment to cancer immunotherapy. *Genes Cancer* **2018**, *9*, 176–189. [CrossRef] [PubMed]
134. Marhelava, K.; Pilch, Z.; Bajor, M.; Graczyk-Jarzynka, A.; Zagozdzon, R. Targeting negative and positive immune checkpoints with monoclonal antibodies in therapy of cancer. *Cancers* **2019**, *11*, 1756. [CrossRef]
135. Solomon, B.L.; Garrido-Laguna, I. Tigit: A novel immunotherapy target moving from bench to bedside. *Cancer Immunol. Immunother.* **2018**, *67*, 1659–1667. [CrossRef]
136. Brenner, W.; Farber, G.; Herget, T.; Lehr, H.A.; Hengstler, J.G.; Thuroff, J.W. Loss of tumor suppressor protein PTEN during renal carcinogenesis. *Int. J. Cancer* **2002**, *99*, 53–57. [CrossRef]
137. Makhov, P.B.; Golovine, K.; Kutikov, A.; Teper, E.; Canter, D.J.; Simhan, J.; Uzzo, R.G.; Kolenko, V.M. Modulation of Akt/mTOR Signaling Overcomes Sunitinib Resistance in Renal and Prostate Cancer Cells. *Mol. Cancer Ther.* **2012**, *11*, 1510–1517. [CrossRef] [PubMed]
138. Molina, A.M.; Feldman, D.R.; Voss, M.H.; Ginsberg, M.S.; Baum, M.S.; Brocks, D.R.; Fischer, P.M.; Trinos, M.J.; Patil, S.; Motzer, R.J. Phase 1 trial of everolimus plus sunitinib in patients with metastatic renal cell carcinoma. *Cancer* **2012**, *118*, 1868–1876. [CrossRef]
139. Allen, E.; Walters, I.B.; Hanahan, D. Brivanib, a dual FGF/VEGF inhibitor, is active both first and second line against mouse pancreatic neuroendocrine tumors developing adaptive/evasive resistance to VEGF inhibition. *Clin. Cancer Res.* **2011**, *17*, 5299–5310. [CrossRef] [PubMed]
140. Singh, H.; Brave, M.; Beaver, J.A.; Cheng, J.; Tang, S.; Zahalka, E.; Palmby, T.R.; Venugopal, R.; Song, P.; Liu, Q.; et al. U.S. Food and Drug Administration Approval: Cabozantinib for the Treatment of Advanced Renal Cell Carcinoma. *Clin. Cancer Res.* **2017**, *23*, 330–335. [CrossRef] [PubMed]
141. Powles, T.; Albiges, L.; Bex, A.; Grünwald, V.; Porta, C.; Procopio, G.; Schmidinger, M.; Suárez, C.; De Velasco, G.; On behalf of the Esmo Guidelines Committee. Esmo clinical practice guideline update on the use of immunotherapy in early stage and advanced renal cell carcinoma. *Ann. Oncol Off. J Eur. Soc. Med. Oncol.* **2021**, *32*, 1511–1519. [CrossRef]
142. Ciamporcero, E.; Miles, K.M.; Adelaiye, R.; Ramakrishnan, S.; Shen, L.; Ku, S.; Pizzimenti, S.; Sennino, B.; Barrera, G.; Pili, R. Combination strategy targeting VEGF and HGF/c-met in human renal cell carcinoma models. *Mol. Cancer Ther.* **2015**, *14*, 101–110. [CrossRef]
143. Pal, S.K.; Tangen, C.; Thompson, I.M., Jr.; Balzer-Haas, N.; George, D.J.; Heng, D.; Shuch, B.; Stein, M.; Tretiakova, M.; Humphrey, P.; et al. A comparison of sunitinib with cabozantinib, crizotinib, and savolitinib for treatment of advanced papillary renal cell carcinoma: A randomised, open-label, phase 2 trial. *Lancet* **2021**, *397*, 695–703. [CrossRef]
144. Atkins, M.B.; Gravis, G.; Drosik, K.; Demkow, T.; Tomczak, P.; Wong, S.S.; Michaelson, M.D.; Choueiri, T.K.; Wu, B.; Navale, L.; et al. Trebananib (AMG 386) in Combination with Sunitinib in Patients with Metastatic Renal Cell Cancer: An Open-Label, Multicenter, Phase II Study. *J. Clin. Oncol.* **2015**, *33*, 3431–3438. [CrossRef]
145. Huang, H.; Lai, J.Y.; Do, J.; Liu, D.; Li, L.; Del Rosario, J.; Doppalapudi, V.R.; Pirie-Shepherd, S.; Levin, N.; Bradshaw, C.; et al. Specifically targeting angiopoietin-2 inhibits angiogenesis, Tie2-expressing monocyte infiltration, and tumor growth. *Clin. Cancer Res.* **2011**, *17*, 1001–1011. [CrossRef]

146. Cao, R.; Zhang, Y. The functions of E(Z)/EZH2-mediated methylation of lysine 27 in histone H3. *Curr. Opin. Genet. Dev.* **2004**, *14*, 155–164. [CrossRef]
147. Italiano, A.; Soria, J.C.; Toulmonde, M.; Michot, J.M.; Lucchesi, C.; Varga, A.; Coindre, J.M.; Blakemore, S.J.; Clawson, A.; Suttle, B.; et al. Tazemetostat, an EZH2 inhibitor, in relapsed or refractory B-cell non-Hodgkin lymphoma and advanced solid tumours: A first-in-human, open-label, phase 1 study. *Lancet Oncol.* **2018**, *19*, 649–659. [CrossRef]
148. Morschhauser, F.; Tilly, H.; Chaidos, A.; McKay, P.; Phillips, T.; Assouline, S.; Batlevi, C.L.; Campbell, P.; Ribrag, V.; Damaj, G.L.; et al. Tazemetostat for patients with relapsed or refractory follicular lymphoma: An open-label, single-arm, multicentre, phase 2 trial. *Lancet Oncol.* **2020**, *21*, 1433–1442. [CrossRef]
149. Hoy, S.M. Tazemetostat: First Approval. *Drugs* **2020**, *80*, 513–521. [CrossRef] [PubMed]
150. Wu, S.; Huang, L.; Shen, R.; Bernard-Cacciarella, M.; Zhou, P.; Hu, C.; Di Benedetto, M.; Janin, A.; Bousquet, G.; Li, H.; et al. Drug resistance-related sunitinib sequestration in autophagolysosomes of endothelial cells. *Int. J. Oncol.* **2020**, *56*, 113–122. [CrossRef]
151. Wiedmer, T.; Blank, A.; Pantasis, S.; Normand, L.; Bill, R.; Krebs, P.; Tschan, M.P.; Miranoni, I.; Perren, A. Autophagy inhibition improves sunitinib efficacy in pancreatic neuroendocrine tumors via a lysosome-dependent mechanism. *Mol. Cancer Ther.* **2017**, *16*, 2502–2515. [CrossRef] [PubMed]
152. Franco, M.; Pàez-Ribes, M.; Cortez, E.; Casanovas, O.; Pietras, K. Use of a Mouse Model of Pancreatic Neuroendocrine Tumors to Find Pericyte Biomarkers of Resistance to Anti-angiogenic Therapy. *Horm. Metab. Res.* **2011**, *43*, 884–889. [CrossRef] [PubMed]
153. Mita, A.C.; Takimoto, C.H.; Mita, M.; Tolcher, A.; Sankhala, K.; Sarantopoulos, J.; Valdivieso, M.; Wood, L.; Rasmussen, E.; Sun, Y.N.; et al. Phase 1 study of AMG 386, a selective angiopoietin 1/2−neutralizing peptibody, in combination with chemotherapy in adults with advanced solid tumors. *Clin. Cancer Res.* **2010**, *16*, 3044–3056. [CrossRef]
154. Kreamer, K.M. Immune Checkpoint Blockade: A New Paradigm in Treating Advanced Cancer. *J. Adv. Pract. Oncol.* **2014**, *5*, 418–431.
155. Motzer, R.J.; Tannir, N.M.; McDermott, D.F.; Frontera, O.A.; Melichar, B.; Choueiri, T.K.; Plimack, E.R.; Barthélémy, P.; Porta, C.; George, S.; et al. Nivolumab plus Ipilimumab versus Sunitinib in Advanced Renal-Cell Carcinoma. *N. Engl. J. Med.* **2018**, *378*, 1277–1290. [CrossRef]
156. Rini, B.I.; Plimack, E.R.; Stus, V.; Gafanov, R.; Hawkins, R.; Nosov, D.; Pouliot, F.; Alekseev, B.; Soulières, D.; Melichar, B.; et al. Pembrolizumab plus Axitinib versus Sunitinib for Advanced Renal-Cell Carcinoma. *N. Engl. J. Med.* **2019**, *380*, 1116–1127. [CrossRef]
157. Motzer, R.J.; Penkov, K.; Haanen, J.; Rini, B.; Albiges, L.; Campbell, M.T.; Venugopal, B.; Kollmannsberger, C.; Negrier, S.; Uemura, M.; et al. Avelumab plus Axitinib versus Sunitinib for Advanced Renal-Cell Carcinoma. *N. Engl. J. Med.* **2019**, *380*, 1103–1115. [CrossRef]
158. He, Y.; Cao, J.; Zhao, C.; Li, X.; Zhou, C.; Hirsch, F.R. TIM-3, a promising target for cancer immunotherapy. *Oncol. Targets Ther.* **2018**, *11*, 7005–7009. [CrossRef]
159. Zelba, H.; Bedke, J.; Hennenlotter, J.; Mostböck, S.; Zettl, M.; Zichner, T.; Chandran, A.; Stenzl, A.; Rammensee, H.; Gouttefangeas, C. PD-1 and LAG-3 Dominate Checkpoint Receptor-Mediated T-cell Inhibition in Renal Cell Carcinoma. *Cancer. Immunol. Res.* **2019**, *7*, 1891–1899. [CrossRef]
160. Brignone, C.; Escudier, B.; Grygar, C.; Marcu, M.; Triebel, F. A phase I pharmacokinetic and biological correlative study of IMP321, a novel MHC class II agonist, in patients with advanced renal cell carcinoma. *Clin. Cancer Res.* **2009**, *15*, 6225–6231. [CrossRef]
161. Braun, D.A.; Bakouny, Z.; Hirsch, L.; Flippot, R.; Van Allen, E.M.; Wu, C.J.; Choueiri, T.K. Beyond conventional immune-checkpoint inhibition—Novel immunotherapies for renal cell carcinoma. *Nat. Rev. Clin. Oncol.* **2021**, *18*, 199–214. [CrossRef]
162. Mitchell, T.C.; Hamid, O.; Smith, D.C.; Bauer, T.M.; Wasser, J.S.; Olszanski, A.J.; Luke, J.J.; Balmanoukian, A.S.; Schmidt, E.V.; Zhao, Y.; et al. Epacadostat plus pembrolizumab in patients with advanced solid tumors: Phase I results from a multicenter, open-label phase I/II trial (ECHO-202/KEYNOTE-037). *J. Clin. Oncol.* **2018**, *36*, 3223–3230. [CrossRef]
163. Long, G.V.; Dummer, R.; Hamid, O.; Gajewski, T.F.; Caglevic, C.; Dalle, S.; Arance, A.; Carlino, M.S.; Grob, J.J.; Kim, T.M.; et al. Epacadostat plus pembrolizumab versus placebo plus pembrolizumab in patients with unresectable or metastatic melanoma (ECHO-301/KEYNOTE-252): A phase 3, randomised, double-blind study. *Lancet Oncol.* **2019**, *20*, 1083–1097. [CrossRef]
164. Corrales, L.; Glickman, L.H.; McWhirter, S.M.; Kanne, D.B.; Sivick, K.E.; Katibah, G.E.; Woo, S.R.; Lemmens, E.; Banda, T.; Leong, J.J.; et al. Direct activation of STING in the tumor microenvironment leads to potent and systemic tumor regression and immunity. *Cell Rep.* **2015**, *11*, 1018–1030. [CrossRef] [PubMed]
165. Poeck, H.; Besch, R.; Maihoefer, C.; Renn, M.; Tormo, D.; Morskaya, S.S.; Kirschnek, S.; Gaffal, E.; Landsberg, J.; Hellmuth, J.; et al. 5′-Triphosphate-siRNA: Turning gene silencing and Rig-I activation against melanoma. *Nat. Med.* **2008**, *14*, 1256–1263. [CrossRef]
166. Sullivan, R.J. Back to the future: Rethinking and retooling il2 in the immune checkpoint inhibitor era. *Cancer Discov.* **2019**, *9*, 694–695. [CrossRef]
167. Sharma, M.; Khong, H.; Fa'ak, F.; Bentebibel, S.E.; Janssen, L.; Chesson, B.C.; Creasy, C.A.; Forget, M.A.; Kahn, L.; Pazdrak, B.; et al. bempegaldesleukin selectively depletes intratumoral tregs and potentiates t cell-mediated cancer therapy. *Nat. Commun.* **2020**, *11*, 661. [CrossRef]
168. Vano, Y.A.; Rioux-Leclercq, N.; Dalban, C.; Sautes-Fridman, C.; Bougoüin, A.; Chaput, N.; Chouaib, S.; Beuselinck, B.; Chevreau, C.; Gross-Goupil, M.; et al. NIVOREN GETUG-AFU 26 translational study: Association of PD-1, AXL, and PBRM-1 with outcomes in patients (pts) with metastatic clear cell renal cell carcinoma (mccRCC) treated with nivolumab (N). *J. Clin. Oncol.* **2020**, *38*, 618. [CrossRef]

169. Cannarile, M.A.; Weisser, M.; Jacob, W.; Jegg, A.M.; Ries, C.H.; Rüttinger, D. Colony-stimulating factor 1 receptor (CSF1R) inhibitors in cancer therapy. *J. Immunother. Cancer* **2017**, *5*, 53. [CrossRef] [PubMed]
170. Blass, E.; Ott, P.A. Advances in the development of personalized neoantigen-based therapeutic cancer vaccines. *Nat. Rev. Clin. Oncol.* **2021**, *18*, 215–229. [CrossRef]
171. Graham, J.; Dudani, S.; Heng, D. Prognostication in kidney cancer: Recent advances and future directions. *J. Clin. Oncol.* **2018**, *36*, 3567–3573. [CrossRef]
172. Rodriguez-Vida, A.; Strijbos, M.; Hutson, T. Predictive and prognostic biomarkers of targeted agents and modern immunotherapy in renal cell carcinoma. *ESMO Open* **2016**, *1*, e00001. [CrossRef]
173. Templeton, A.J.; Knox, J.J.; Lin, X.; Simantov, R.; Xie, W.; Lawrence, N.; Broom, R.; Fay, A.P.; Rini, B.; Donskov, F.; et al. Change in neutrophil-to-lymphocyte ratio in response to targeted therapy for metastatic renal cell carcinoma as a prognosticator and biomarker of efficacy. *Eur. Urol.* **2016**, *70*, 358–364. [CrossRef]
174. Viers, B.R.; Houston Thompson, R.; Boorjian, S.A.; Boorjian, S.A.; Lohse, C.M.; Leibovich, B.C.; Tollefson, M.K. Preoperative neutrophil-lymphocyte ratio predicts death among patients with localized clear cell renal carcinoma undergoing nephrectomy. *Urol. Oncol.* **2014**, *32*, 1277–1284. [CrossRef]
175. Beuselinck, B.; Job, S.; Becht, E.; Karadimou, A.; Verkarre, V.; Couchy, G.; Giraldo, N.; Rioux-Leclercq, N.; Molinié, V.; Sibony, M.; et al. Molecular subtypes of clear cell renal cell carcinoma are associated with sunitinib response in the metastatic setting. *Clin. Cancer Res.* **2015**, *21*, 1329–1339. [CrossRef]
176. Jiang, T.; Zhou, C. The past, present and future of immunotherapy against tumor. *Transl. Lung Cancer Res.* **2015**, *4*, 253–264.
177. Rini, B.I.; Huseni, M.; Atkins, M.; McDermott, D.; Powles, T.; Escudier, B.; Banchereau, R.; Liu, L.-F.; Leng, N.; Fan, J.; et al. Molecular correlates differentiate response to atezolizumab (atezo) + bevacizumab (bev) vs sunitinib (sun): Results from a phase iii study (immotion151) in untreated metastatic renal cell carcinoma (mrcc). *Ann. Oncol.* **2018**, *29*, viii724–viii725. [CrossRef]
178. Rini, B. Vascular endothelial growth factor-targeted therapy in renal cell carcinoma: Current status and future directions. *Clin. Cancer Res.* **2007**, *13*, 1098–1106. [CrossRef]
179. Jubb, M.; Pham, T.; Hanby, A.; Frantz, G.; Peale, F.; Wu, T.; Koeppen, H.; Hillan, K. Expression of vascular endothelial growth factor, hypoxia inducible factor 1alpha, and carbonic anhydrase IX in human tumours. *J. Clin. Pathol.* **2004**, *57*, 504–512. [CrossRef]

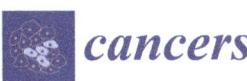

Review

The Role of Epigenetics in the Progression of Clear Cell Renal Cell Carcinoma and the Basis for Future Epigenetic Treatments

Javier C. Angulo [1,2,*], Claudia Manini [3], Jose I. López [4,5], Angel Pueyo [6,7], Begoña Colás [8] and Santiago Ropero [8]

1. Clinical Department, Faculty of Medical Sciences, European University of Madrid, 28005 Madrid, Spain
2. Department of Urology, University Hospital of Getafe, Getafe, 28907 Madrid, Spain
3. Department of Pathology, San Giovanni Bosco Hospital, 10154 Turin, Italy; claudia.manini@aslcittaditorino.it
4. Department of Pathology, Cruces University Hospital, 48903 Barakaldo, Spain; joseignacio.lopez@osakidetza.eus
5. BioCruces-Bizkaia Health Research Institute, 48903 Barakaldo, Spain
6. Foundation for Biomedical Research, Innovation of University Hospitals Infanta Leonor and South-East, 28003 Madrid, Spain; angel.pueyo@salud.madrid.org
7. Heath Science PhD Program, UCAM Universidad Católica San Antonio de Murcia, Guadalupe de Maciascoque, 30107 Murcia, Spain
8. Biochemistry and Molecular Biology Unit, Department of Systems Biology, University of Alcalá, 28805 Alcalá de Henares, Spain; begona.colas@uah.es (B.C.); santiago.ropero@uah.es (S.R.)
* Correspondence: javier.angulo@universidadeuropea.es

Citation: Angulo, J.C.; Manini, C.; López, J.I.; Pueyo, A.; Colás, B.; Ropero, S. The Role of Epigenetics in the Progression of Clear Cell Renal Cell Carcinoma and the Basis for Future Epigenetic Treatments. *Cancers* **2021**, *13*, 2071. https://doi.org/10.3390/cancers13092071

Academic Editor: Guido Martignoni

Received: 12 March 2021
Accepted: 23 April 2021
Published: 25 April 2021

Publisher's Note: MDPI stays neutral with regard to jurisdictional claims in published maps and institutional affiliations.

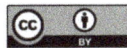

Copyright: © 2021 by the authors. Licensee MDPI, Basel, Switzerland. This article is an open access article distributed under the terms and conditions of the Creative Commons Attribution (CC BY) license (https://creativecommons.org/licenses/by/4.0/).

Simple Summary: The accumulated evidence on the role of epigenetic markers of prognosis in clear cell renal cell carcinoma (ccRCC) is reviewed, as well as state of the art on epigenetic treatments for this malignancy. Several epigenetic markers are likely candidates for clinical use, but still have not passed the test of prospective validation. Development of epigenetic therapies, either alone or in combination with tyrosine-kinase inhibitors of immune-checkpoint inhibitors, are still in their infancy.

Abstract: Clear cell renal cell carcinoma (ccRCC) is curable when diagnosed at an early stage, but when disease is non-confined it is the urologic cancer with worst prognosis. Antiangiogenic treatment and immune checkpoint inhibition therapy constitute a very promising combined therapy for advanced and metastatic disease. Many exploratory studies have identified epigenetic markers based on DNA methylation, histone modification, and ncRNA expression that epigenetically regulate gene expression in ccRCC. Additionally, epigenetic modifiers genes have been proposed as promising biomarkers for ccRCC. We review and discuss the current understanding of how epigenetic changes determine the main molecular pathways of ccRCC initiation and progression, and also its clinical implications. Despite the extensive research performed, candidate epigenetic biomarkers are not used in clinical practice for several reasons. However, the accumulated body of evidence of developing epigenetically-based biomarkers will likely allow the identification of ccRCC at a higher risk of progression. That will facilitate the establishment of firmer therapeutic decisions in a changing landscape and also monitor active surveillance in the aging population. What is more, a better knowledge of the activities of chromatin modifiers may serve to develop new therapeutic opportunities. Interesting clinical trials on epigenetic treatments for ccRCC associated with well established antiangiogenic treatments and immune checkpoint inhibitors are revisited.

Keywords: renal cell carcinoma; biomarker; DNA methylation; epigenetics

1. Current Management of Renal Cell Carcinoma

Renal cell carcinoma (RCC) is the seventh most common form of human neoplasm, with an incidence of 10 new cases per 100,000 inhabitants in Western Europe and United States. Its incidence is steadily rising due to increased incidental detection. Among the genitourinary tumors RCC is the one with highest mortality, with approximately 76% global 5-year survival rate, and accounts for 2% of global cancer deaths in the world [1]. Probably the main clinico-pathological parameters, that predict prognosis in this malignancy, are nuclear grade, tumor stage, cell type, tumor architecture, and tumor diameter [2]. However, Fuhrman grade, node involvement, number of different metastatic sites, and whether cancer-directed surgery is recommended and performed are the major factors involved in the prediction of prognosis in metastatic RCC [3].

Histological variants characterize different subtypes within RCC [4]. The most common is clear cell RCC (ccRCC) that accounts for a total 75% of cases. Papillary RCC (pRCC) is the second in terms of frequency, approximately 20%. Chromophobe RCC and its benign counterpart oncocytoma account each for approximately 5%. Other rarer tumors enter in the differential diagnosis of solid renal masses [5]. Both ccRCC and pRCC arise from the proximal tubule while chromophobe RCC (chRCC) has an origin in the distal part of the nephron. Each type has different morphology but also different genetics and behavior. Tumor grade has prognostic value for ccRCC. An individual tumor can have mixed histology and different subtypes can occasionally appear within the same kidney. Heterogeneity of RCC stands at the molecular, genomic, histopathological, and clinical levels [6,7]. It explains how appropriate tumor sampling is needed for a correct identification, and implies great difficulty for the development of accurate diagnostic and prognostic markers. In fact, among the many candidates investigated, no marker of ccRCC has reached the clinic today.

Sensitive and specific molecular markers for the diagnosis and monitoring of RCC are lacking [8,9]. Tumor heterogeneity of the disease, worsened by specific histological subtypes, also affect the search for accurate biomarkers [10]. Likely earlier detection and better clinical monitoring of this malignancy might help to improve its prognosis [11]. Compared to other subtypes, ccRCC has a more unfavorable prognosis. Although, it is curable when diagnosed early, no screening strategy is being used. Small renal masses are often detected by imaging studies performed for other reasons and tend to be treated by nephron-sparing surgery, although ablation or active surveillance when diagnosed in an elder population is increasingly used. In this clinical situation, imaging monitoring to evaluate clinical progression is mandatory in the absence of reliable molecular tumor marker of disease progression. Many candidates, including a number of epigenetic markers such as DNA methylation profiling, have been proposed both for screening and prognostic evaluation [12–19]. In fact, DNA methylation presents itself as a potentially strong biomarker to predict aggressive behavior and risk of tumor recurrence in patients with apparently less aggressive renal tumors [20].

Radical nephrectomy or partial nephrectomy, that imply total or partial removal of the kidney, are the main therapeutic basis of local and locally advanced disease [21]. Approximately 30% of the patients develop metastases, either synchronically or during follow-up, and for the last decades have been treated with adjuvant or palliative classical immunotherapy with interferon-α2b (IFN-α2b), high-dose interleukin-2 (IL-2), systemic targeted therapies including tyrosine kinase inhibitors (TKI) targeting the VEGF signaling axis (sorafenib, sunitinib, pazopanib, axitinib, lenvatinib, and cabozantinib) or mTOR inhibitors (everolimus and temsirolimus) or the anti-VEGF monoclonal antibody bevacizumab. First-line options for metastatic ccRCC included sunitinib, pazopanib or the combination bevacizumab plus interferon-α and second-line options were axitinib and cabozantinib. Despite all treatment efforts, advanced disease implies very low survival rates. Median duration of response was 9 months for the first-line setting and 6 months for the second-line. In the absence of toxicity most of these agents have been given sequentially until further disease progression. Cytoreductive nephrectomy was also advocated whenever possible in cases with metastatic onset to reduce the tumor burden and avoid further metastatic seed.

Many studies are currently evaluating the combination of anti-VEGF therapy with the new generation of immunotherapy agents T-cell immune checkpoint inhibitors (ICI), that include antibodies against programmed cell death protein ligand-1 (PDL1) avelumab and atezolizumab, antibodies against programmed cell death protein 1 (PD1) nivolumab and pembrolizumab, and the inhibitor of cytotoxic T-lymphocyte-associated protein 4

(CTLA-4) ipilimumab. Blockade of the PD1–PDL1 axis promotes T cell activation and immune killing of cancer cells. ICIs have very recently become first-line standards of care as improved survival for ipilimumab and nivolumab combined has been demonstrated in the intermediate and poor-risk group, while pembrolizumab plus axitinib combination is recommended, for both unfavorable and favorable disease. Cabozantinib remains a valid alternative for the intermediate and high-risk group. To summarize, in patients previously treated with TKIs that progress, nivolumab, cabozantinib, axitinib, or the combination of ipilimumab and nivolumab appear indicated; while in patients already treated with ICI, any VEGF-targeted therapy previously unused together with ICI therapy appears a valid option [22–25].

PDL1 immunohistochemical expression in tumor cells or in tumor-infiltrating mononuclear cells (TIMC) has been thoroughly evaluated as biomarkers for the prediction of ICI response in metastatic disease. However, PDL1 expression is not a good predictive marker and does not serve to assign the most convenient therapy. Response rates are better in PDL1 positive tumors, but PDL1 negative ones also respond [26]. It is important to note that the role of CTLA-4 expression in TIMC has been forgotten to evaluate response to ICI. Many issues are responsible for the failure to develop predictive biomarkers, to name dynamic expression, and the aforementioned heterogeneity within primary tumor, and between primary and metastases [27]. Seric levels of PDL1 could be a novel prognostic factor in ccRCC and also a predictor of response to TKI-based therapy [28]. It is a paradox that despite the fact that treatments for metastatic ccRCC are targeted, the approach for immunotherapy is far from being targeted.

Abnormal epigenetic patterns will give new opportunities to develop novel therapies in RCC. Some drugs targeting the epigenetic system are currently under investigation; however, strategies that combine therapies targeting epigenetic machinery with conventional therapies for this malignancy, either targeting tyrosine kinases, mTOR or immune checkpoints at different combinations are still at infancy. Maybe closer is the practical utility of epigenetic therapies to solve or delay therapy resistance in ccRCC, and also to identify the populations in which prolonged response to a certain therapy could be expected. Hopefully the introduction of biomarkers into clinical practice will allow personalized patient care for renal cancer [29,30].

2. Epigenetics of Clear Cell Renal Cell Carcinoma

Epigenetics studies the inheritable phenotype resulting from changes in gene expression without alteration of the DNA sequence. As such, cancer epigenetics deals with the inheritable but reversible changes associated with gene expression dysregulation that manifest in a pre-malignant phenotype with the genomic sequence unaltered. Interest in epigenetic alterations associated with ccRCC provides an optimal scenario in the search for new tumor markers in this malignancy, and also to develop new treatment strategies facilitated by the reversibility of epigenetic modifications. The main epigenetic mechanisms are DNA methylation, chromatin remodeling, post-translational histone modifications, short-noncoding RNAs, also known as microRNAs (miRNA), and long-noncoding RNAs (lncRNA) [31–33].

Interestingly, all the epigenetic modifications work together to regulate chromatin structure and gene expression. Disruption of the epigenetic homeostasis may derive from deregulation of epigenetic modifiers. That means altered epigenetic modifications can be explained by changes in expression and function of epigenetics writers, erasers, and readers. These changes can be due to genetic alterations, linking genetics, and epigenetics in carcinogenesis.

Translational epigenetic research is a growing field to identify and validate new markers leading to personalized medicine. Among the many epigenetic changes and signatures identified in RCC, aberrant promoter methylation of more than 200 genes have been reported and more than 120 miRNAs are deregulated [34]. According to several recent systematic reviews of diagnostic DNA methylation biomarkers in this disease, none of the biomarkers proposed exceeds level of evidence III, which means their clinical utility is limited [34,35]. Promising biomarkers should be validated not only in sample banks, but also in prospective clinical trials before their use can be generalized [29]. In every case after the publication of a potential biomarker, prospective cohort studies that increase the evidence are lacking. Additionally, more standardized methodology is needed to facilitate reproducibility, and that hinders clinical translation [35]. Bias in sample selection and handling, DNA methylation detection methods and genomic location of the assay can also bring confounding results. In addition, the selection of normal tissue for comparison with neoplasia can be problematic because aberrant promoter methylation is an early event in carcinogenesis allowing its detection in normal appearing tissue surrounding the tumor. Finally, inter-individual study comparison is most often lacking for further biomarker validation.

However, there is no doubt that DNA methylation and histone modification patterns have a crucial role in the regulation of global and local gene expression and may play an outstanding role both in carcinogenesis and tumor progression. Firstly, epigenetic deregulation can lead precursor cells to proliferate and block their differentiation as seems to occur in germ cell malignancies [36]. This is of primary importance in childhood renal kidney tumors like nephroblastoma [37]. Probably the most interesting epigenetic mechanism in ccRCC stands in common mutations in chromatin regulator genes that complement the inactivation of Von Hippel Lindau (*VHL*) tumor suppressor gene (TSG), and Hypoxia-inducible factors (HIF) pathway that allow tumor cell survival in a characteristic status of pseudo-hypoxia. *VHL* gene is frequently inactivated in sporadic ccRCC by mutation, loss of heterozygosity, or promoter hypermethylation [38]. In addition, several miRNAs have been associated with VHL-HIF pathway. In particular, downregulation of MIR-30c has been associated with loss of VHL in RCC [39]. However, little is known about the relationship between lncRNAs and VHL–HIF pathway. A study comparing lncRNA expression profile in VHL-wild type and VHL-mutant RCC cell lines and demonstrated that LncRNA-SARCC is differentially regulated in a VHL dependent manner in RCC cell lines and tumor samples [40].

Recent genome-wide sequencing studies have revealed a number of mutations of genes coding for epigenome modifiers and chromatin remodelers, like *PBRM1* (40%), *SETD2* (10%), *KDM5C* (10%), *KDM6A* (1%), and *BAP1* (10–15%). Most of the mutations of histone modifier genes described in ccRCC are truncating and inactivating mutations producing loss of functions [41,42]. Apart from *VHL* mutations these are among the most common somatic genetic abnormalities encountered in renal tumors [43,44]. Very interestingly, 90% of sporadic ccRCC are affected by a 50Mb deletion on chromosome 3p where not only *VHL* but also *PBRM1*, *BAP1*, and *SETD2* are located and act as a functional gene group [43]. The function of these epigenetic modifiers stands in DNA repair and maintenance of genomic integrity by regulating splicing and other processes like cytoskeletal regulation that also contribute to genomic stability. *KDM5D* and *KDM6C* located on the Y chromosome, are homologs of the X-lined genes *KDM5C* and *KDM6A*, and are often deleted in male patients with ccRCC [43]. Understanding how chromatin modifiers contribute to RCC tumorigenicity will serve to develop the basis for therapeutic interventions as well. Finally, it is important to recognize that epigenetic modifications work together and can also regulate one another, thus diversifying their function. This regulatory network has been defined as epigenetic crosstalk.

Epigenetic changes can be evaluated in samples obtained with minimal invasion (e.g., urine or plasma), and this represents an added attraction to introduce epigenetic studies in the clinic. Obtaining DNA non-invasively from renal cells in urine is an ideal scenario for epigenetically based detection of ccRCC. Additionally, DNA can be obtained from fresh tumor or paraffin-embedded tissue. Liquid biopsy from direct washing of fresh biopsies can be an optimal method as well, to evaluate epigenetic changes that would facilitate accurate detection, tumor subtype determination, and evaluation of prognosis as well [45].

More recently detection of RCC using plasma and urine cell-free DNA methylomes has also been confirmed [46,47].

The potential of renal cancer epigenomics has been investigated later than in other urologic malignancies, but the understanding of how genomics and epigenomics disturb biologic functions and determine intratumor heterogeneity will help to explain the complex reality of RCC and the differences in molecular cancer phenotypes [48]. The growing field of knowledge to determine the real impact of altered epigenetic patterns and their role in the diagnosis, monitoring, classification, prognosis, and treatment of kidney cancer is the main objective of this review.

2.1. Abnormal DNA Methylation

DNA methylation is the most widely studied epigenetic modification so far, and consists of the addition of a methyl group to the Cytosine within the CpG dinucleotide. This epigenetic modification is a reversible process regulated by writers, DNA methyl transferases (DNMT), erasers, and Ten-eleven translocation (TET). The maintenance of DNA methylation through replication is ensured by DNA (cytosine-5)-methyltransferase 1 (DNMT1) but de novo DNA methylation is mediated by DNMT3A and DNMT3B [49]. DNMTs transfer the methyl group from S-adenosyl methionine (SAM) to carbon-5 of the cytosine. The proportion of CpG dinucleotides in the human genome is lower than expected from the abundance of cytosine and guanine. The distribution of the CpGs is not uniform and concentrates in short areas, called CpG islands, located mainly in the promoter regions of approximately 60% of known genes [50]. Promoter DNA methylation is a mark of transcriptional repression, while gene body DNA methylation is generally associated with a permissive transcriptional state. This epigenetic modification is crucial in several physiologic functions, including X-chromosome inactivation, silencing of tissue specific genes, imprinting and genomic stability, and changes due to senescence. In normal cells, around 80% of CpGs are methylated, including repetitive genomic sequences and transposons but most of the CpG islands are unmethylated allowing gene expression when necessary, but this methylation pattern is altered in malignant transformation. Two major changes occur in cancer affecting DNA methylation: global DNA hypomethylation of the genome and aberrant hypermethylation of the promoter region of TSGs. Age and environmental changes also have a strong effect on DNA methylation. The methylation of a gene promoter causes gene silencing through a transcription failure.

DNA hypomethylation primarily affects repetitive sequences and pericentromeric regions that are methylated in normal cells. Loss of methylation at these elements in cancer may result in chromosomal instability and mutations [50,51]. In addition, the hypomethylation of CpG sites has been associated with the over-expression of oncogenes within cancer cells and with deregulation of proteins involved in the complex balance between methylation and the maintenance of the chromatin structure [50]. Hypermethylation of CpG islands located in the promoter regions of some TSGs prevents gene expression and, therefore, its protective role in the development of tumors. Gene silencing by promoter hypermethylation in cancer has been studied in depth and affects important functions for cell cycle, DNA repair, cell adhesion and invasion, apoptosis, miRNA expression, metabolism of carcinogens, and response to hormones. In particular, silencing of negative regulators of cell cycle (*RASSF1* and *KILLIN*), activation of Wnt pathway by suppression of Wnt antagonists (*SFRP1, SFRP2, SFRP5,* and *WIF-1*), TGF-β activation by promoter methylation of negative regulators (*GATA-3, GREM-1,* and *SMAD-6*) and silencing pro-apoptotic genes (*APAF-1*) are the most important mechanisms that explain why gene hypermethylation plays an important role in development and progression of RCC [33,52].

Characterizing methylation patterns and signatures in cancer is one of the bases for the desired personalized medicine in the search for biomarkers. First of all, unlike mutations and other genetic alterations, methylation always occurs in defined regions of DNA and can be precisely detected with resolution [53]. Secondly, every tumor type has a specific methylation profile, referred to as hypermethylome, somehow different from that of other neoplasia. Thirdly, methylation-specific PCR (MSP) derived methods enable a fast, simple method to detect methylated alleles of a certain gene in samples with low tumor content and even in biological fluids [54,55]. However, among the limitations to generalize application of epigenetic markers in RCC is also cell type specificity and the aforementioned heterogeneity of this malignancy [56].

2.1.1. DNA Methylation as Marker of RCC Diagnoses

Aberrant DNA methylation is an early event in carcinogenesis, thus DNA methylation biomarkers has been implemented for the diagnosis of a wide range of malignancies including prostate, colorectal, and pulmonary neoplasia [57]. Regarding RCC, LINE1 methylation levels in leukocyte DNA measured prior to cancer diagnosis has been identified as a biomarker of RCC risk among male smokers [58]. Diagnostic DNA methylation biomarkers, despite being very promising for RCC, have not reached clinical practice yet [35]. However, it is well known that some genes including *APC*, *BNC1*, *CDH1*, *ECAD*, *GSTP1*, *KTN19*, *IGFBP1*, *IGFBP3*, *MGMT*, *PTGS2*, *p14ARF*, *p16/CDKN2a*, *p16INK4a*, *RASSF1A*, *RARB2*, *SRFP*, *TIMP3*, *UCHL1*, and *VHL* are silenced in RCC by DNA methylation and this could be useful for the diagnosis of RCC in tumor tissue, serum, or urine samples, both in the familiar and sporadic forms [12,59–66]. Concordance between serum and tissue DNA hypermethylation profile has been proved, especially with grade and tumor stage [67].

2.1.2. DNA Methylation as Marker of RCC Subtyping

Classification of sporadic RCC into different histologic subtypes is allowed by multi-gene quantitative methylation profiling because DNA methylation signatures reveal cell ontogeny and establish differences between precursor cells in the nephron [18,68]. *VHL* methylation is restricted to ccRCC. *RASSF1A* and *SPINT2* are more frequently methylated in pRCC [63,69,70] while *COL1A1* and *IGFBP1* hypermethylation is more common in ccRCC [62,63]. *CDH1* methylation is significantly higher in ccRCC than in chRCC or oncocytoma [63], important discrimination due to the benign nature of oncocytoma. In fact, data from The Cancer Genome Atlas (TCGA) revealed that of all RCC subtypes, oncocytoma and chRCC are the most similar but, what is even more interesting, a signature of 30 hypermethylated genes distinguishes oncocytoma from chRCC [48,71] involved, among others, in Wnt, MAPK, and TGFβ signaling [48]. From a practical perspective the distinction between oncocytoma and ccRCC can be performed with very high sensitivity and specificity using a three-gene promoter methylation panel (*OXR1*, *MST1R*, and *HOXA9*) and this distinction could be very useful to allow unnecessary overtreatment if performed in preoperative biopsies before nephrectomy [14].

2.1.3. DNA Methylation as Marker of RCC Prognosis

Although classical histologic parameters are the most valuable tools to evaluate prognosis, nuclear grade and staging have some limitations to precisely predict the clinical outcome in RCC. DNA methylation-based classification is highly relevant for clinical management of RCC as it serves to identify the prognosis of different epigenetic subtypes. In fact, DNA methylation data can classify inherent tumor heterogeneity into specific-prognosis subgroups according to DNA methylation at promoter sites identified in The Cancer Genome Atlas (TCGA) network [72]. Integrated genomic and epigenomic analysis revealed significant correlations between the total number of genetic aberrations and total number of hypermethylated CpGs [73]. In recent years, several groups have used multi-omic data analysis to reveal groups of differentially methylated and expressed genes in surgically resected specimens of RCC or in the open data of ccRCC in TCGA (TCGA Research Network). The evidence generated confirms cluster analysis based on genome-wide promoter methylation serves to identify panels of methylated genes associated to ccRCC disease progression [17,34,72–83]. Some of these panels have been validated in an independent retrospective cohort and some have been incorporated into prognostic risk score models to enhance their prognostic biomarker effect [77,78]. However, none has been prospectively validated in multicenter studies [35]. Additionally, a methylated site signature useful for prediction of prognosis has been identified for pRCC, validated in the TCGA and GEO cohorts and incorporated in a nomogram that predicts an individual's risk of survival in pRCC [80]. Again, this panel has not yet been revalidated prospectively.

Some of the panels focus mainly on two or more genes for prognostic classification of ccRCC patients [17,74,81–83]. Other investigations evaluate tumor prognosis and progression based on analyzing the functional role of a particular gene and the likely mechanisms involved. In this sense, promoter CpG methylation of γ-catenin is considered an independent predictor for survival and disease progression [84]. Other hypermethylated genes associated with worse RCC disease-specific survival are: GATA Binding Protein 5 (*GATA5*), that codify for a DNA-binding transcription factor [85,86]; Gremlin 1 (*GREM1*), related to cytokine activity and bone morphogenic protein [87]; HIC ZBTB Transcriptional Repressor 1 (*HIC1*), related both to DNA-binding transcription factor activity and histone deacetylase binding [88]; Junction Plakoglobin (*JUP*), related to protein homodimerization activity and protein kinase binding [84]; neural EGFL like 1 (*NELL1*), linked to calcium ion binding [76]; Protocadherin 8 (*PCDH8*), also related to calcium ion binding [89]; Phosphatase and Tensin Homolog (*PTEN*), related to protein kinase binding [90]; Ras Association Domain Family Member 1 (*RASSF1A*) that encodes a protein similar to the RAS effector proteins [91,92]; sarcosine dehydrogenase (*SARDH*), associated to oxidoreductase activity [93]; and Secreted Frizzled Related Protein 1 (*SFRP1*), related to G protein-coupled receptor activity [94,95]. Very recently some methylated genes with prognostic value in pRCC have also been described [96].

2.2. Methyl-Binding Proteins

Methyl-binding proteins (MBP) are readers of DNA methylation. They bind to methylated CpG nucleotides and induce gene silencing by recruiting repressor complex containing histones deacetylates (HDAC) linking the DNA methylation with histone modifications [97]. The MBP family is composed of human proteins MBD1, MBD2, MBD3, MBD4, and MECP2. Each of them, with the exception of MBD3, is capable of binding specifically to methylated DNA. Among them MBD2 is the MBP with highest affinity for methylated DNA. MBD2 alters the structure of chromatin and mimics chromatin remodeling or modification factors, and may serve as transcriptional repressor or activator, depending on the cell context [98]. MBD2 upregulation has been reported in many different malignancies such as RCC and is associated to neoplastic progression, with potential as a biomarker and a therapeutic target [99].

2.3. Post-Translational Histone Modifications

Chromatin is a complex nucleoprotein structure formed by DNA, histones, and other proteins. The DNA is wrapped around an octamer of histones (2H2A, 2H2B, 2H3, and 2H4) that is the repeating unit of chromatin. The chemical modifications of amino acids in the external tail of histone molecules determines changes in the chromatin structure. Lysine residues can undergo methylation, acetylation, or ubiquitylation, while arginine residues can be methylated and the serine residues phosphorylated [100]. The best studied histone modifications are acetylation and methylation of lysine present at the N-terminal tails of histones H3 and H4. These histone modifications are reversible and result from the balance of two enzymatic activities: histone acetyltransferases (HAT) and histone deacetylases (HDAC) regulate histone acetylation, while histone methyltransferases (HMT) and histone demethylases (HDMT) regulate histone methylation. The combination of all histone modifications builds the histone code that regulates all chromatin functions [39,101,102] (Figure 1).

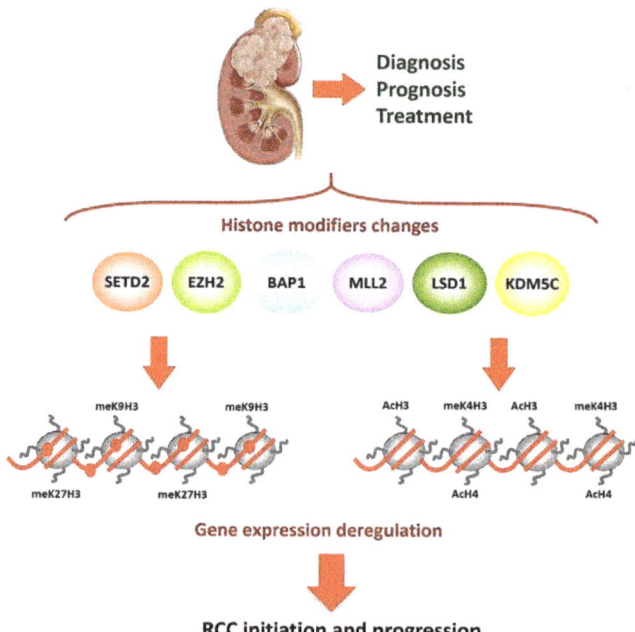

Figure 1. Summary of the altered histone modifiers genes in RCC. Histone modifiers changes induce gene expression deregulation and thus RCC initiation and progression. These alterations can be used as biomarkers for RCC diagnosis and prognosis. H3Ac, global acetylation of histone H3; meK9H3, methylated lys9 of Histone H3; meK27H3, methylated lys27 of Histone H3; meK4H3, methylated lys4 of Histone H3.

Post-translational histone modifications play a very important role in regulating, not only chromatin structure but also gene expression. Changes in the acetylation and methylation state of histone tails convert loosely packed regions with high transcriptional activity into densely packed ones with scarce activity. Acetylation is associated with a more open conformation and is related with active transcription. The effect of methylation depends on the residue affected and also on the degree of methylation; the methylation of H3K4, H3K36, and H3K79 activates transcription while methylation of H3K9, H3K27, and H4K20 produces repression [33,103].

Global histone modifications are likely markers of cancer prognosis in RCC [104]. Diminished H3K4me2 and H3K18Ac levels worsen prognosis [105] while acetylated histone H3 (H3Ac) immunostaining inversely correlates with staging, Fuhrman grade, and tumor progression [106]. Similarly, it has been suggested that H3K9Ac and H3K18Ac levels could monitor patients with RCC after surgery, but as far as we know these likely markers have not been confirmed in prospective validations [107,108]. H3K27 methylation levels also correlate with established clinical-pathological variables and survival in RCC [104]. Additionally, H3K27me1/-me2/-me3 staining is significantly more intense in pRCC than in ccRCC, and H3K27me3 levels are higher in oncocytoma than in RCC [104]. The monomethylation of histone H3 on lysine 27 (H3K27me1) plays key roles in the cellular processes, interacts with the DNA sequence of the miRNAs and regulates the transcription of miRNAs [109]. The enrichment analysis of molecular function shows H3K27me1-associated miRNAs are linked to RNA binding and protein binding involved in the transcription and translation regulation. As a result, the biological roles of the H3K27me1 appear closely related to miRNAs downstream [109].

Histone modifications alterations in cancer can be explained by changes in the activity or expression of histone modifiers and readers, and these changes could be valuable in cancer management. Different studies indicate that changes in histone modifications in RCC are related to hypoxia and the prognostic relevance of associated alterations. There is a strong relation between hypoxia and epigenetic regulation, especially histone modifications. One of the mechanisms involved in the epigenetic-altered landscape in RCC related to hypoxic effect is the regulation of Jumonji domain containing histone demethylases by the mediator of hypoxic response HIFα [110]. A number of genes that encode histone-modifying enzymes are mutated in ccRCC [41,111]. Inactivating mutations described for *SETD2* (H3K36 methyltransferase), *KDM5C* (H3K4 demethylase), *KMD6A* (H3K27 demethylase), *MLL2* (H3K4 methyltransferase), Polybromo 1 (*PBRM1*), BRCA1 Associated Protein-1 (*BAP1*) remain among the most interesting epigenetic mechanisms for ccRCC progression. This merits a brief description of the function of some of them.

SETD2, located at chromosome 3p near *VHL*, *BAP1*, and *PBRM1* genes, is inactivated in approximately 10% of RCCs which results in global reduction in the histone mark trimethylation of lysine 3 of histone H3 (H3K36me3) and a global loss of DNA methylation across the genome. This gene is involved in genome stability as trimethylation of H3K36 by *SETD2* is required for DNA repairing system through both homologous recombination repair and mismatch repair [112,113]. DNMT3B-mediated de novo DNA methylation occurs at the intron of genes marked with H3K36me3 but not those lacking H3K36me3.

Mutations in the switching defective/sucrose nonfermenting (SWI/SNF) chromatin remodeling complex gene *PBRM1* are identified in approximately 40% of ccRCC [114]. The SWI/SNF complex mobilizes nucleosome and modulates chromatin structure, thus affecting transcription, DNA repair, cell proliferation, and cell death. It is essentially a key regulator of gene expression and is associated with numerous transcription factors [115]. Inactivation of *PBRM1* causes enhanced cell proliferation and cell migration. It also regulates the expression of genes the products of which are involved in cell adhesion, like E-cadherin [116]. Thus, inactivation of the *PBRM1* TSG amplifies the HIF-response of *VHL* negative ccRCC [117,118]. *PBMR1* has been proposed as a tumor suppressor gene in ccRCC since its re-expression in ccRCC cell lines lacking *PBMR1* function decreased cell proliferation by upregulating genes involved in cell adhesion and apoptosis [116]. *PBRM1* is implicated in the regulation of gene expression through its bromodomains. In particular, *PBRM1* contains six bromodomains that bind acetylated histones, thus serving as a reader for H3K14Ac, and target SWI/SNF chromatin remodeler complex to DNA regulatory regions [119]. In addition, PBRM1 also binds to acetylated p53 and facilitates its binding to regulatory elements at the promoter genes regulated by p53 in ccRCC [120].

BAP1 is also located very close to *SETD2* and *PBRM1* genes and is mutated in more than 10% of ccRCCs. BAP1 forms a multiprotein complex with breast cancer type 1 (BRCA1) susceptibility protein to regulate DNA damage response and cell cycle control, but its exact function in ccRCC remains largely unknown [43].

Lysine Demethylase 6A (*KDM6A*) and Lysin Demethylase 5C (*KDM5C*) are X-linked histone demethylase-coding genes located near each other in Xp11. *KDM6A* codifies a protein that demethylases lysine 27 in histone 3 (H3K27) and is mutated in only 1% of ccRCCs, while *KDM5C* encodes H3K4 demethylase and its mutation is present in approximately 10% of ccRCCs [41,121]. In urothelial bladder cancer KDM6A-deficient cells depend on EZH2, a HMT that methylates lysine 27 on histone H3 (H3K27). Inhibition of EZH2 has been suggested as an effective therapeutic approach to *KDM6A*-mutated tumors [122]. *KDM5C* acts as TSG and its deficiency results in genomic instability and aggressive forms of ccRCC [123]. Interestingly both *KMD6A* and *KDM5C* are considered escape from X-inactivation tumor suppressor or EXIT genes. Their homologues on chromosome Y, *KDM6C*, and *KDM5D* are downregulated due to loss of chromosome Y in 40% of male patients with ccRCC [124]. This fact is most likely involved in male predominance of ccRCC.

Lysine-specific histone Demethylase 1A (LSD1 or KDM1A) can demethylate both lysine 4 and lysine 9 of histone H3 (H3K4me and H3K9me), thereby acting as a co-activator or a co-repressor, depending on the context. It has been found as a part of several histone deacetylase complexes, and silences genes by functioning as a histone demethylase. Conversely, it can also act as coactivator of androgen receptor (AR) dependent transcription and is regulated by AR activity in renal cells [125]. The mammalian homolog of LSD1, LSD2 has been associated with tumor stage and metastasis in ccRCC and, thus proposed as a biomarker for ccRCC progression. Moreover, LSD1 and LSD2 expression was correlated in metastatic ccRCC [126].

Enhancer of zeste homolog 2 (*EZH2*), as has been previously mentioned, codify for a HMT acting as a transcriptional repressor through regulating the methylation of histone H3 at lysine 27. Not much evidence exists regarding EZH2 in ccRCC but high tumor and initial reports suggested EZH2 level was associated with less aggressive tumor phenotypes and favorable prognosis [127]. However, more recent evidence has confirmed high EZH2 expression correlates with poor overall survival in RCC, especially in advanced disease by promoting VEGF expression and cell proliferation while inhibiting apoptosis [128,129]. In agreement with these data, EZH2 represses the expression of E-cadherin through increased levels of H3K27me3, promoting epithelial mesenchymal transition (EMT) and metastases [130].

These studies point out it is interesting to pay attention to the clinical significance of mutations in histone or chromatin modifiers. Mutations in *SETD2* and *KDM5C* are mutually exclusive, as are mutations of *PBRM1* and *BAP1* [43]. *BAP1* or *KDM5C* mutations in ccRCC associate with aggressive disease, high Fuhrman grade, and metastatic at presentation (Figure 1), that imply worse prognosis and instantaneous activation of mTOR signaling [117,131]. However, mTOR activation in *PBRM1* mutated tumors occurs after long latency periods. Additionally, the clinical significance of *SETD2* and *PBRM1* mutations is not well known [43,132,133].

2.4. miRNAs

miRNAs are small non-coding RNAs of approximately 22 nucleotides in length implicated in posttranscriptional regulation of gene expression. miRNAs regulate a wide spectrum of cellular processes acting as oncogene or as tumor suppressors of the genes they regulate [134]. A number of functional studies have revealed deregulated miRNA (either upregulation or downregulation) involved in cell cycle regulation, apoptosis, cell adhesion, and extracellular matrix or metabolism with a key role in RCC [111,135–137]. In this sense, miR-21 is silenced by promoter methylation in RCC, and its expression inhibits RCC growth through regulating LIVIN, a member of the inhibitor of apoptosis proteins [138].

Numerous reports suggest circulating miRNAs have the potential to be used as biomarkers in patients with RCC. However, findings are diverse, probably due to methodological differences and histological variations in the study cohorts. Initial studies evaluating the implications of serum miRNAs gave conflicting results [139,140]. Currently, the use of two or more miRNAs for diagnosis and molecular classification of RCC is well accepted, supporting miRNA signatures as clinical tools [141]. Most miRNAs are tandemly clustered and co-expression patterns for miR-8, miR-199, miR-506, and other families are downregulated in ccCRC [135].

Different miRNAs are deregulated in RCC. Upregulation of miR-1233 was observed but no prognostic implication could be proved [139]. miR-378 and miR-451 combined serve to identify cancer with 81% sensitivity and 83% specificity [142]. Similarly, miR-210 has 81% sensitivity and 79% specificity for RCC diagnosis [143]. Combining miR-155 upregulation and miR-141 downregulation improves discrimination of ccRCC [144]. However, the best combination reported in terms of diagnostic accuracy could be miR-141 and miR-200b, with 99% sensitivity and 100% specificity [145]. This panel also distinguished chRCC from oncocytoma with 90% sensitivity and 100% specificity [145].

Regarding the prognostic role of miRNAs, overexpression of miR-221 and miR-32 are predictors of RCC mortality [146,147]. Similarly, miR-30a-5p downregulation, probably due to aberrant promoter methylation, is common in ccRCC and can be evaluated both in tumor tissue and urine samples to predict metastatic dissemination and worse survival [148]. Members of the miR-200 family and miR-205 promote EMT and reduced transcription and expression of E-cadherin [149]. They are also induced by bone morphogenetic proteins, part of the TGFβ superfamily of proteins, that antagonizes EMT [150]. miR-454 accelerates RCC progression via suppressing methyl-CpG binding protein 2 (*MECP2*) expression, which may provide a novel potential target of RCC treatment in the future. MiR-454 inhibition and *MECP2* overexpression could both decrease the proliferative, migrative, and invasive abilities of RCC cells and also serve as an independent prognostic factor in RCC [151].

In summary, profiling miRNA in RCC preludes development of new tumor markers [141,151–153] but probably even more interesting is the fact that many miRNAs, such as miR-21, miR-155, miR-214, miR-31, and miR-146a, have been implicated in the regulation of immune and stromal cells, and in the modulation of the host immune response [154]. miRNA signatures may be implicated in radio and chemosensitivity and also to predict the response to TKI therapy [141]. Unfortunately, miRNAs occur in a wide spectrum of diseased and benign conditions and are far from being specific for ccRCC, and this limits the possibilities for their use in clinical practice.

2.5. lncRNAs

Long non-coding RNAs are a class of transcripts longer than 200 nucleotides that do not codify for proteins and are emerging as regulators of important cellular functions. Although their ultimate function is not very well known, several studies suggest they are involved in apoptosis, cell migration, and cell cycle, and play very critical roles in gene expression regulation, including gene transcription, post-transcriptional regulation, and epigenetic regulation. Differential expression of lncRNAs has been identified in RCC and normal renal tissue [155–157] but only a few of these lncRNAs have been studied in depth.

HOX transcript antisense intergenic RNA (HOTAIR) has been proposed as oncogene silencing several TSGs working together with EZH2 and H3K27 histone mark [158]. HOTAIR favors the metastatic process of RCC by upregulation of the histone demethylase KDM6B and its target gene *SNAI1* involved in EMT [159]. More interesting is the lncRNA H19 that is expressed only during embryogenesis, but re-expressed triggered by HIFα in neoplastic renal cells but not in normal kidneys. H19 is implicated, among others functions, in epithelial to mesenchymal transition (EMT) and mesenchymal to epithelial transition (MET) strongly suggesting an oncogenic role in RCC. In addition, H19 is overexpressed in tumor tissues and has been proposed as an independent predictor for the clinical outcome of RCC patients [160].

DNA methylation-deregulated and RNA m6A reader-cooperating (DMDRMR) is another lncRNA recently recognized to facilitate tumor growth and metastasis in ccRCC. DMDRMR binds insulin-like growth factor 2 mRNA-binding protein 3 (IGF2BP3) to stabilize target genes, including the cell cycle kinase CDK4 and several extracellular matrix components (*LAMA5*, *COL6A1*, and *FN1*) [161]. The cooperation between DMDRMR and IGF2BP3 regulates target genes in an m6A-dependent manner and may represent a potential diagnostic, prognostic, and likely therapeutic target in ccRCC.

Another lncRNA important in RCC is KCNQ1 downstream neighbor (KCNQ1DN), downregulated both in neoplastic tissue and cell lines. In vivo experiments with nude mice showed that KCNQ1DN overexpression repressed both the growth of xenograft tumors and the expression of the oncogen *c-Myc*, thus representing a novel target for future therapeutic options in RCC [96]. Reduced expression of KCNQ1DN is also observed in Wilms' tumor [162].

2.6. RNA Methylation

Recent studies also show that RNA methylation serves to epigenetically regulate biological functions. The N6-methyladenosine (m6A) RNA methylation is the most frequent, abundant, and conserved form of RNA methylation reported both in messenger

RNAs and lncRNAs. Other well-characterized RNA modifications are 5-methylcytosine (m5C), N7-methylguanosine (m7G), and pseudo-uridine [163,164]. Genome wide changes in gene expression have been reported due to reversible changes in m6A methylation [165]. Same as DNA methylation or histone modifications, m6A methylation is regulated by several methyltransferases, demethylases, and other RNA binding proteins. Methyltransferases involved in the generation of the m6A modification of RNA are m6A writers, while demethylases causing m6A removal are termed m6A eraser. Many RNA binding proteins, including IGF2BP1, IGF2BP2, IGF2BP3, YTHDF1, YTHDF2, YTHDF3, YTHDC1, YTHDC2, HNRNPC, HNRNPA2B1, and RBMX, act as m6A readers, and this regulatory process plays a critical role in stem cell differentiation, development and tumor progression [166,167]. The body of evidence regarding RNA methylation in RCC is still scarce but the expression of some m6A RNA methylation regulatory genes (*IGF2BP3*, *KIAA1429*, and *HNRNPC*) have been recently described as independent predictors of prognosis in pRCC [168]. Other studies point out the expression of RNA methylation modifiers as biomarkers of RCC subtyping. VIRMA and YTHDC2 mRNA expression levels were lower in chRCC and pRCC compared to ccRCC [169].

3. Epigenetic-Based Therapeutic Opportunities in ccRCC

Development of epigenetic therapies has been under extensive clinical investigation for the last two decades and may become a promising strategy to restore silenced gene expression both in malignant and non-malignant disease [149,170,171]. The rationale of an epigenetic treatment should consist in reprogramming the pattern of gene expression in cancer cells to result in the induction of apoptosis or in the loss of cell capacity for uncontrolled proliferation and tumor growth, also making cancer more susceptible to conventional therapies [172]. Epigenetic therapy targets three different protein categories: writers, enzymes that establish epigenetic marks; erasers, enzymes that remove epigenetic marks; readers, proteins that recognize epigenetics modifications, and, when recruited to these marks, bring in other protein complexes to exert the desired function.

In the last decades, most of the studies have focused on the use of writers (DNMTs, HATs, and HMTs) and erasers (TET, HDACs, and HDMs) as therapeutics targets, but in recent years a number of studies show the potential use of epigenetic readers as new therapeutic targets. This group of proteins include the bromodomain-containing family of proteins that recognize acetylated lysine residues, the chromodomain-containing proteins that bind to methylated histones, and MBDs, mentioned previously, that bind to methylated DNA [171,173].

Until now DNMT and HDACs inhibitors have been approved by the US FDA for the treatment of hematologic malignancies and myelodysplastic syndromes. These and other drugs with the capacity to inhibit DNMT (decitabine, zacitidine, and guadecitabine) or HDAC (vorinostat, panobinostat, romidepsin, entinostat, belinostat, and AR-42) are being investigated in solid malignancies for their potential to reactivate the expression of silenced TSGs [170,171,174]. There are great expectations for the therapeutic potential and pharmacologic development of these and other agents in early clinical studies in urologic cancer, and more specifically in RCC [149,175]. The role of nutritional interventions affecting epigenetic changes has also been taken into account in breast and prostate cancers [176], but not so far in RCC. The development of new drug alternative for ccRCC has been very promising in the last decades but we can say epigenetic therapy for kidney cancer remains in its infancy.

Future development combination therapies may follow the lead of hematologic malignancies and investigate epigenetic treatments in cases in which current antiangiogenic treatments or immunotherapies (mainly TKIs or ICIs) have failed. However, currently, only phase I/II clinical trials on single-agent or combined therapies for RCC have been completed and the response rate observed is poor and disappointing, with only few patients simply reaching stable disease (Table 1).

Table 1. Epigenetic treatments alone or in combination with other treatments used in clinical trials conducted on patients with metastatic or unresectable renal cell carcinoma, or in advanced solid tumors including renal cell carcinoma (clinicaltrials.gov, accessed on 1 March 2021). HDAC: Histone deacetylase; DNMT: DNA methyltransferase. Ref.: reference number as cited in the text.

Epigenetic Drug	Combined Therapy	Phase	Trial Registry	Ref.
HDAC Inhibition				
Vorinostat	-	II	NCT00278395	-
Vorinostat	Isotretinoin	I/II	NCT00324740	-
Vorinostat	Bevacizumab	I/II	NCT00324870	[177]
Vorinostat	Sirolimus	I	NCT01087554	[178]
Vorinostat	Ridaforolimus	I	-	[179]
Vorinostat	Pembrolizumab	I	NCT02619253	-
Panobinostat	Sorafenib	I	NCT01005797	-
Panobinostat	-	II	NCT00550277	[180]
Panobinostat	Everolimus	I/II	NCT01582009	[181]
Entinostat	Isotretinoin	I	-	[182]
Entinostat	IL-2	I/II	NCT01038778	[183]
Entinostat	IL-2	I/II	NCT03501381	-
Entinostat	Atezolizumab plus Bevacizumab	I/II	NCT03024437	-
Entinostat	Nivolumab plus Ipilimumab	II	NCT03552380	-
Depsipeptide	-	II	-	[184]
Romidepsin	-	I	NCT01638533	-
Romidepsin	-	II	NCT00106613	[185]
Belinostat	-	I	NCT00413075	[186]
DNMT Inhibition				
Azacytidine	IFN-α	I	NCT00217542	-
Azacytidine	Valproic Acid	I	-	[187]
Azacytidine	Bevacizumab	I/II	NCT00934440	-
Decitabine	-	I	-	[188]
Decitabine	IL-2	I	-	[189]
Decitabine	IFN-α	II	NCT00561912	-
Decitabine	Anti-PD-1	I/II	NCT02961101	-
Decitabine	MBG453	I	NCT02608268	-
Decitabine	Oxaliplatin	II	NCT04049344	-
Oligonucleotide MG98	-	I/II	NCT00003890	[190]
Oligonucleotide MG98	IFN-α	I/II	-	[191]
Other Therapeutic Strategies				
miRNA MRX34	-	I	NCT01829971	-
Oligonucleotide GTI-2040	Capecitabine	I/II	NCT00056173	[192]
Oligonucleotide Oblimersen	IFN-α	II	NCT00059813	[193]

3.1. DNMT Inhibition Alone or in Combination with Other Therapies

DNMT inhibitors (DNMTi) are cytidine analogues that block the DNMT activity when incorporated into DNA and also induce their degradation. So, DNMTi produce passive DNA demethylation and induce the expression of genes that have been silenced by promoter DNA methylation, thus reactivating silenced TSGs in cancer. The exposure of different tumor cells to low doses of DNMTi cause apoptosis, reduced cell cycle activity, and decreased stem cell function [194].

Azacytidine (Dacogen®) and decitabine (Vidaza®) are approved by the FDA for the treatment of hematologic malignancies and myelodysplastic syndromes. Guadecitabine (SGI-110), a next-generation hypomethylating agent, is also used in patients with relapsed or refractory acute myeloid leukemia with acceptable efficacy and tolerability profile [195]. Additionally, a phase III trial to evaluate guadecitabine as second-line in patients with myelodysplastic syndromes or chronic myelomonocytic leukemia previously treated with hypomethylating agents is being conducted (EudraCT 2015-005257-12). A rational design of new combination strategies to further exploit the epigenetic mode of action of these two drugs in different areas of clinical oncology was proposed, especially in combination approaches with other anticancer strategies [196].

3.1.1. Azacytidine (5-Azacytidine)

Epigenetic therapy is a promising potential therapy for solid tumors. Integrative expression and methylation data analysis of 63 cancer cell lines (breast, colorectal, and ovarian) after treatment with the DNMTi azacytidine demonstrated significant enrichment for immunomodulatory pathways. These results suggest the possibility of a broad immune stimulatory role for DNA demethylating drugs in solid malignancies [197]. On the other hand, suppressed cell proliferation (>50% reduction in colony formation assay) with azacytidine therapy was detected, both in cell lines with VHL promoter methylation and also in some RCC cell lines without *VHL* TSG methylation, thus suggesting that multiple methylated TSGs might determine the response to demethylating therapies [198].

A phase I trial enrolled 55 patients with advanced neoplastic disease, that included two patients with RCC, to evaluate the combination of azacytidine subcutaneously administered with oral valproic acid. One patient with RCC presented a stable disease for 6 months with a significant increase in histone acetylation. Grade 1 and 2 toxicities were reported [187]. Another phase I trial was performed to evaluate the side effects and best dose of recombinant interferon alfa-2b together with azacytidine for patients with stage III or stage IV melanoma or stage IV kidney cancer that cannot be removed by surgery (NCT00217542). Results have not been published. A phase II trial was specifically intended to evaluate low dose decitabine plus interferon alfa-2b in advanced renal cell carcinoma (NCT00561912) but was terminated early due to slow accrual and unavailable treatment agent. Another study evaluated the effectiveness of azacytidine and bevacizumab in advanced RCC (NCT00934440) with the intention to identify the maximum tolerable dose and assess toxicity. Overall, three different doses were evaluated for each drug. Dose for azacytidine ranged between 35 and 75 mg/m^2/day for 7 days. All patients presented adverse effects of different degree. Time to progression registered was 5.6 months. Results have not been published.

3.1.2. Decitabine (5-Aza-2′-Deoxycytidine)

Preclinical evidence with the DNMTi decitabine is abundant in renal cancer cell lines. Decitabine inhibits the proliferation of RCC cells via G2/M cell cycle arrest by suppressing p38-NF-κB activity [199]. It also induces apoptosis by regulating the Wnt/β-catenin signal pathway through re-expression of *sFRP2* gene [200]. Additionally, combined treatment with decitabine and valproic acid, a HDAC inhibitor, synergistically inhibits cell growth and migration in ccRCC cell lines [201]. These evidences support targeting DNA methylation with decitabine to treat advanced RCC.

Monotherapy with decitabine was investigated in a phase I study at different doses from 2.5 to 20 mg/m^2 on days 1–5 in 31 patients with refractory malignancies, including three patients with RCC. Decreased DNA methylation after treatment was evidenced both in tumor and in peripheral blood mononuclear cells. Decitabine also decreased DNMT1 and induced tumor apoptosis [188].

Another phase I trial which evaluated sequential low-dose decitabine plus high-dose IL-2 presented some interesting results in modulating the toxicity and anti-tumor activity of immunotherapy in melanoma, but not in RCC. In this study decitabine caused grade 4 neutropenia lasting more than a week in most patients, and a trend toward a higher incidence of toxicity with increasing decitabine doses was evidenced [189]. The combination of low-dose decitabine with IFNα2b was also evaluated in advanced RCC (NCT00561912), but results have not been reported.

Resistance of RCC to the apoptosis-inducing effects of IFNs was postulated to result from epigenetic silencing of genes by DNA methylation [202]. Decitabine and selective depletion of DNMT1 by phosphorothioate oligonucleotide antisense were used to reverse silencing, in cells resistant to apoptosis induction by IFNα2 and IFNβ. The proapoptotic tumor suppressor *RASSF1A* was reactivated by DNMT1 inhibitors in the cell lines investigated and this was associated with demethylation of its promoter region [203].

The combination of anticancer agents and epigenetic drugs sustains a novel therapeutic strategy. The effectivity rate of chemotherapy for RCC is very low and the high expression of certain drug transporters in the kidney, like the human organic cation transporter OCT2, is partly responsible for this multidrug resistance. Combined treatment using the DNMT inhibitor decitabine and the HDAC inhibitor vorinostat significantly increased the expression of OCT2 in RCC cell lines, which sensitized these cells to oxaliplatin [204]. In this sense, a phase II trial with decitabine combined with oxaliplatin in patients with advanced RCC (NCT04049344) is currently recruiting patients in Zhejiang Cancer Hospital, with the intention of evaluating whether decitabine sensitizes RCC cells to oxaliplatin.

3.1.3. MG98

Another inhibitor of DNMT, the antisense oligodeoxynucleotide MG98 was intravenously administered at a dose of 360 mg/m^2 twice weekly for three consecutive weeks out of four in 17 patients with advanced RCC receiving a median of two cycles with no objective responses. Mild hematologic toxicity, elevation of transaminases, fatigue, fever, and nausea were observed [190]. Despite the disappointing results, MG98 was investigated in combination with IFNα2b in patients with advanced RCC [191]. Another phase-II trial explored two schedules of MG98 with IFNα2b and described frequent disease stabilization and partial response in one case [205].

3.2. HDAC Inhibition Alone or in Combination with Other Therapies

HDAC inhibitors (HDACi) are approved for cutaneous T-cell lymphoma and peripheral T-cell lymphoma. They have dose and compound dependent pleiotropic effects. They induce epigenetic effects either through histone acetylation or by influencing the acetylation status of nonhistone or non-nuclear proteins. A synergy between DNA demethylation and histone deacetylase inhibition has been confirmed to re-express genes silenced in cancer cells [206]. However, from the clinical perspective, some compounds have followed a more productive clinical investigation than others, but today none is approved to treat ccRCC.

3.2.1. Vorinostat

Clinical trials with HDACi in RCC have given mixed results. A phase I trial evaluated the anti-tumor activity of vorinostat (SAHA) as oral agent in 14 patients with advanced RCC (NCT00278395) and showed toxicity in 50% of the cases and 14% serious adverse events. Another study (NCT00324870) evaluated oral vorinostat with becacizumab and observed 18% response rate, mainly partial responses, with an acceptable toxicity and a median overall survival of 13.9 months, thus suggesting clinical activity [177].

A phase I study of sorafenib and vorinostat in patients with advanced solid tumors with expanded cohorts in RCC and non-small cell lung cancer (NSCLC) used oral vorinostat 200–400 mg to establish the recommended phase II dose (NCT00635791). Although tolerable in other tumor types, sorafenib associated to vorinostat was not found tolerable without dose reductions or delays in RCC and NSCLC patients. No complete response was seen but minor responses were observed in RCC [207]. Another dose-limiting toxicity trial with vorinostat plus isotretinoin (NCT00324740) was also performed in 12 patients with recurrent or advanced RCC, of which 33% suffered well tolerated adverse effects, mainly anorexia and weight loss.

Since AKT activation is a possible mechanism of resistance to mTOR inhibitors, adding vorinostat (or another HDACi) was proposed as a route to circumvent AKT-mediated resistance to mTOR inhibitors in experimental studies performed on synovial sarcoma cells [208]. The combination of sirolimus and vorinostat has yielded preliminary anticancer activity in patients with refractory Hodgkin lymphoma, perivascular epithelioid tumor, and hepatocellular carcinoma [178]. Based on these findings another study explored the combination of HDAC and mTOR inhibition in RCC and other solid malignancies. In total, 13 patients with RCC (10 ccRCC and 3 pRCC) were treated with vorinostat and ridaforolimus. Using a dose escalation design, various dose combinations were tested concurrently in separate cohorts. Dosing was limited by thrombocytopenia. Two patients, both with papillary RCC, maintained stable response 54 and 80 weeks, respectively [179]. Additionally, a phase I study with dose finding and extension cohorts using pembrolizumab and vorinostat in patients with advanced or metastatic RCC, urothelial cancer or prostate cancer (NCT02619253) has concluded recruitment, but results are under evaluation.

3.2.2. Panobinostat

Preclinical studies with the pan-deacetylase inhibitor panobinostat (LBH589) have shown induced cell cycle arrest and apoptosis in renal cancer cells and a reduction in tumor size using xenografts mice models [209]. A phase II study was performed to evaluate the activity of panobinostat in refractory renal carcinoma (NCT00550277). In total, 20 patients with advanced ccRCC who had received previous therapy with at least one angiogenesis inhibitor and one mTORi were treated with panobinostat 45 mg orally, twice a week, and evaluated every 2 months. Panobinostat was generally well-tolerated but 30% experienced serious adverse effects. There were no objective responses and all patients progressed or stopped treatment within the first 4 months [180].

A synergistic activity of dual HDAC and mTOR inhibition was confirmed in Hodgkin lymphoma and multiple myeloma cell lines [210,211]. A phase I, dose-finding trial for everolimus combined with panobinostat in advanced ccRCC was performed (NCT01582009). Overall, 21 patients completed this trial which was recently published. Oral everolimus 5 mg daily and panobinostat 10 mg 3 times weekly (weeks 1 and 2) given in 21-day cycles was the maximum tolerated dose. Improved clinical outcomes were not demonstrated as the median time to disease progression was 4.1 months [181].

Synergistic effects have been observed in the combination of TKi, such as imatinib, dasatinib, or sorafenib, with an array of HDACi including vorinostat, romidepsin, or panobinostat [212]. As an example, combination therapy with panobinostat and sorafenib proved to significantly decrease vessel density and tumor volume, and also to increase survival in hepatocellular carcinoma xenografts [213]. Regarding RCC, a phase I study of panobinostat in combination with sorafenib in soft tissue, renal and lung cancers (NCT01005797) was started in 2009 and, with a long history of changes and latest version submitted on 2017, its findings have not yet been reported.

3.2.3. Entinostat (MS-275)

Entinostat reverts retinoid resistance by reverting Retinoic acid receptor β2 (RARβ2) epigenetic silencing in a human RCC model and has a synergistic anti-tumor activity in combination with 13-cis-retinoic acid compared with single agents, suggesting that the combination of HDACi and retinoids represents a novel therapeutic approach for RCC [214]. This observation led to a phase I study with entinostat in combination with 13-cis-retinoic acid in patients with metastatic or advanced solid tumors or lymphomas (NCT00098891). The combination was reasonably well tolerated and the recommended doses were 4 mg/m^2 once weekly for entinostat and 1 mg/kg/day for 13-cis-retinoic acid. However, no tumor response was evidenced [182].

There are two very interesting trials that are evaluating the combination of entinostat with IL-2. Both are active trials that hopefully will be completed by 2024. One is a phase I/II trial that studies the side effects and best dose of entinostat when given together with IL-2 and the clinical evolution of metastatic RCC with this regime (NCT01038778) [183]. The other is also a phase I/II multicenter, randomized, open label study between high dose IL-2 (3 courses of high dose interleukin 600,000 units/kg administered IV every 8 h on Days 1–5 and Days 15–19, maximum 28 doses) vs. high dose IL-2 (same dose) plus entinostat (5 mg orally given every 2 weeks starting on day 14) in ccRCC (NCT03501381).

These trials have been prolonged because the clinical management with high-dose IL-2 has been abandoned with the advent of antiangiogenic and immune-checkpoint inhibiting drugs.

Consequently, two new trials that evaluate entinostat in combination with more actual therapies for ccRCC are currently open. One of these trials, still recruiting patients, evaluates the combination of atezolizumab with entinostat and bevacizumab in patients with advanced RCC (NCT03024437). This study will assess the immunomodulatory activity of entinostat in patients receiving the PD-L1 inhibitor atezolizumab. Additionally, the combination with bevacizumab provides an effective VEGF inhibition to potentiate the immune response and anti-tumor effect induced by atezolizumab [25]. The overall hypothesis is that entinostat will increase the immune response and anti-tumor effect induced by the PD-L1 inhibition by suppressing Treg function, based on the hypothesis that low dose HDACi will have a suppressive function on Tregs but not on effector T-cells. The dose of entinostat starts with 1 mg and is escalated up to 5 mg. The proposed dose and schedule for atezolizumab and bevacizumab follows the standard of the phase III study IMmotion151 (NCT0242082) [215].

The other active clinical trial on the association between HDACi and ICI investigates entinostat with nivolumab plus ipilimumab in previously treated RCC (NCT03552380). This is a phase II, open-label, safety, pharmacodynamic and efficacy study radiologically assessed for patients with metastatic RCC who have progressed on ipilimumab plus nivolumab regimen. The trial starts with a dose finding study for oral entinostat. Following the first 4 cycles of multiple combination treatment ipilimumab will be discontinued, and treatment with entinostat and nivolumab continued until disease progression or prohibitive toxicity. Anti-tumor activity is being assessed every 6 weeks.

3.2.4. Other HDACi

Other compounds with HDACi activity have been investigated and, although selected for preclinical investigation, their pharmacological development has not been completed. Depsipeptide, a cyclic peptide, was isolated from Chrombacterium violaceum during a screening program for anti-oncogene agents. It exerts potent anti-tumor activity against human tumor cell lines and xenografts [216]. A phase II study was performed in patients with metastatic RCC but showed insufficient activity and investigation was abandoned [184].

Romidepsin (FK228) also showed anti-proliferative activity in vitro against multiple mouse and human tumor cell lines and in vivo in human tumor xenograft models [185], but an exploratory phase II trial evaluating its activity and tolerability in patients with metastatic RCC progressive following or during immunotherapy (NCT00106613) was undertaken but results have not been communicated.

Belinostat (PXD101) is another HDACi that has been investigated in patients with advanced refractory solid tumors including mainly colorectal cancer. Stable disease was observed in 39% of the patients included and, among them in 1 of 6 patients with RCC [186]. However, no further investigation has been performed with this compound in RCC.

AR-42 is another HDACi currently investigated in patients with multiple myeloma and T- and B-cell lymphomas [217]. Inhibition of pancreatic cancer cells by regulating p53 expression, inducing cell cycle arrest, particularly at the G2/M stage, and activating multiple apoptosis pathways has been demonstrated [218]. Combined AR-42 and pazopanib have been investigated in advanced sarcoma and RCC (NCT02795819). Of 6 patients recruited, 4 were evaluated for response, and stabilization of disease was confirmed in 2; however, the trial was interrupted because of unacceptable toxicity.

3.3. Other Epigenetic Therapies

A more targeted epigenetic therapy based on strategies other than demethylation and histone deacetylase inhibition has been sought after for decades. The strategies investigated include silence miRNAs that are overexpressed, such as, for example anti-mRNA oligonucleotides, miRNA-mask antisense oligonucleotides, and miRNA sponges to restore the expression of miRNAs that are downregulated. Some studies point out the use of miRNAs as therapeutics and several clinical trials are currently trying miRNA molecules [219]. However, specific delivery of these miRNA-based therapies is challenging, if not impossible. The only therapy of this kind investigated today for RCC was MRX34. MRX34 miRNA mimics the tumor suppressor miRNA34 and was tested in a phase I clinical trial for advanced or metastatic RCC and other cancers. Unfortunately, the trial was abandoned early because of serious immunologic adverse events (NCT01829971).

Oblimersen (G3139) is a phosphorothioate antisense oligonucleotide used for chronic lymphocytic leukemia and for advanced melanoma. It targets the sequence around translation initiation of the bcl-2 mRNA inhibiting its translation, resulting in decreased levels of the bcl-2 protein, an apoptotic inhibitor expressed in some types of cancer and linked to tumor drug resistance. Therefore, this target has the potential to enhance the efficacy of standard cytotoxic chemotherapy. In RCC cells, oblimersen induced a specific downregulation of Bcl-2, mainly through a Fas-dependent pathway, and was considered a potential therapy for metastatic RCC in combination with IFN-α [220]. However, a phase II study with oblimersen and IFN-α in metastatic RCC revealed oblimersen did not appear sufficiently active to warrant further development in advanced RCC [193].

GTI-2040 is another antisense agent that targets the small subunit component of human ribonucleotide reductase and displays potent anti-tumor activity against different neoplasia [221]. A synergistic effect with IFN-α for apoptosis and decreased proliferation was suggested [192]. However, a phase I/II study of GTI-2040 and capecitabine in patients with RCC gave very disappointing results [222].

Tazemetostat (EPZ-6438), a EZH2 selective inhibitor, was approved for the treatment of advanced epithelioid sarcoma and its effect in enhancing the therapeutic response to 5-fluorouracil in colorectal cancers has been recently confirmed [223]. Other EZH2 inhibitors are now under clinical evaluation and offer alternative approaches to target this HMT [224]. lncRNAs are also a promising source to develop new target therapies in the future. Many deregulated lncRNA interact with EZH2 to silence TSGs and to induce EMT. As a result, inhibitors of EZH2 and consequently H3K27 methylation remain a very interesting opportunity to develop future RCC therapies [149].

Another opportunity of epigenetic therapy stands in the phenomenon of synthetic lethality that describes a relationship between two genes, the loss of which is incompatible with cell survival. So, contrary to gain-of-function mutations in oncogenes, loss-of-function mutations in TSGs are even more challenging to approach from the therapeutical perspective. Loss-of function mutations in chromatin modifiers has several theoretical applications. For example, loss of *SETD2* becomes synthetically lethal with loss of mitotic inhibitor protein kinase Wee1 [113], loss of *BAP1* is synthetically lethal with simultaneous inhibition of EZH2 or PRC2 [225], and a third mechanism is loss of *PBRM1*, ARID1A, and some components of the SWI/SNF complex, together with inhibition of EZH2 [44,226]. Additionally, *PBRM1* loss promotes immunogenicity in RCC by activation of IFN-responsive genes and probably also confers sensitivity to immune checkpoint inhibitors [44]. Hopefully future developments can take advantage of the improved knowledge in epigenetic modifiers activity in ccRCC to support new therapeutic approaches.

3.4. Caveats and Limitations of Epigenetic Therapy

Targeting the epigenome appears an attractive treatment option for RCC because the epigenetic dysregulation of this neoplasia is very extensive and affects many different signaling pathways and tumor hallmarks. The classical concept of an epigenetic therapy centers on the restoration of a neoplastic epigenetic pattern to a normal one. However, the initial therapeutic experience with the drugs available today has been certainly disappointing.

Epigenetic therapy has a robust preclinical base, but many problems remain and need be solved before its generalization. The most important limitation is the lack of selectivity because epigenetic events are ubiquitously distributed across normal and cancer cells. Cancer cells can be sensitive to this regulation, but normal cells have the ability to compensate for these epigenetic changes [227]. Besides, demethylating agents not only restore the expression of genes that have been aberrantly silenced during tumor progression, but also activate genes that are normally repressed by promoter DNA methylation. Another limitation is the need to determine the most important epigenetic alterations for a particular neoplasia. In fact, results of epigenetic therapy in hematologic malignancies are impressive, but not in solid tumors. In addition, all the clinical trials performed are early clinical phase studies, and the number of patients treated with epigenetic therapies and the length of these treatments has been very limited, making difficult the evaluation of long-term safety and real-practice clinical efficacy.

The issue that ccRCC is subject to extensive intra-tumoral heterogeneity is an evident drawback for the development of diagnostic and therapeutic strategies and remains a challenge in modern oncology [10,228]. Multi-regional sequencing has confirmed that renal tumors often harbor different sub-clones that can differ in their spectra of mutations in different epigenetic regulatory tumor suppressor genes. These findings suggest that new therapeutic strategies targeting gene dosage and epigenetic modification should be considered for improved personalized cancer medicine [229]. Single-cell technology and multisite tumor sampling could represent an opportunity to overcome this obstacle [230,231].

The modern paradigm of treatment for metastatic RCC is based on antiangiogenic therapy and combined immune modulation. A realistic potential application of epigenetic therapy today would be to reverse the resistance to treatment with antiangiogenic drugs once they became unresponsive [232,233]. Another promising possibility in treating advanced ccRCC would be the combination of epigenetic drugs and modern immunotherapy using antibodies that block programmed cell death protein 1 (PD1) and its ligands [234]. It would be desirable that epigenetics-based treatments could re-sensitize the host immune response to immunotherapies and restore immunogenicity enforcing the expression of tumor associated antigens, checkpoint ligands in tumor cells, and antigen-processing machinery components [235]. Recent data show that *PBRM1* loss is associated with a less immunogenic tumor microenvironment and upregulated angiogenesis [236]. PBRM1 deficient RenCa subcutaneous tumors in mice are more resistant to ICI, and a retrospective analysis of the IMmotion150 trial also suggests that *PBRM1* mutation reduces benefit from immune checkpoint blockade [151,215].

Nevertheless, the role of PBRM1 mutations in ccRCC in relation to the immune microenvironment is not totally clear. PBRM1 loss of function may alter global tumor-cell expression profiles and influence responsiveness to ICI. Recent studies show truncating mutations in PBRM1 increase the clinical benefit of ICI therapy in patients with metastatic ccRCC [237,238]. PBRM1 alterations have also been clinically validated as marker of ICI responsiveness in RCC but the effect on response and survival is modest and has been mainly observed in the subset of patients who received prior antiangiogenic therapy [239]. The value of PBRM1 mutations in the first-line ICI setting needs further investigation.

The position and results achieved by standard therapies in metastatic ccRCC based on TKIs, m-TORIs, and ICIs, alone or in combination, cannot be easily achieved by other novel therapies. So, epigenetic treatments, via several signaling mechanisms involving both tumor cells and host immune cells, might enhance the efficacy of immune checkpoint therapy in RCC [240]. The combination of epigenetic therapy and immunotherapy is being intensively investigated, and novel trials will be needed to elucidate this role as adjunctive therapy. Epigenetic inhibitors are able to reverse or overcome immune resistance to immunotherapy treatment through upregulation of chemokine expression, antigen processing and presentation machinery, and immune checkpoint molecules [241]. As such, the rationale is that the epigenetic modifiers can be used to prime and sensitize T cells to immunotherapy. Administering "epitherapy" in conjunction with ICI could decrease T-cell exhaustion and avoid immunotherapy resistance.

Additionally, genetic alterations in histone modifier genes in RCC could not only be responsible for the pathogenesis of the disease but also represent potential biomarkers of response to immunotherapies [242]. In this sense, despite the initial failure of epigenetic treatments to reach the clinic, epigenetic therapy is currently a promising strategy for anti-cancer treatment and for development of new ccRCC tumor markers. However, optimized modern epigenetic treatment options, possibly in combination with other treatments, still remain to be discovered.

4. Conclusions

Epigenetic studies have provided a large body of evidence regarding hypermethylated genes, histone-modifying enzymes or miRNAs and new challenges at bench side of patients with RCC. Less invasive diagnosis, histologic subtyping, clinical monitoring of the disease and prognostic evaluation will surely benefit from this increased epigenetic knowledge. However, despite the evidence accumulated, no pure epigenetic biomarker has completed evaluation in phase III studies or is commercially available for clinical use in ccRCC. Prospective multicenter validation is needed before a novel generation of biomarkers become accessible and have the potential to make great strides in personalized medicine. Additionally, early clinical trials have been conducted to evaluate epigenetic therapies for RCC, either alone or in combination with other therapies including IFN-α2b, IL-2, anti-VEGF, TKIs, and mTOR inhibitors. Newer clinical trials are ongoing to investigate the combination of epigenetic treatments with the ICIs pembrolizumab and atezolizumab. There is no doubt that the study of renal cancer epigenetics is still in a formative stage and its application to develop new therapeutic strategies is no more than promising.

Author Contributions: Conceptualization, J.C.A., J.I.L. and S.R.; Data curation, J.C.A., C.M., J.I.L., A.P., B.C. and S.R.; Formal analysis, J.C.A., C.M., J.I.L., B.C. and S.R.; Funding acquisition, S.R.; Supervision, S.R.; Writing—original draft, J.C.A. and S.R.; Writing—review and editing, J.C.A., C.M., J.I.L., A.P., B.C. and S.R. All authors have read and agreed to the published version of the manuscript.

Funding: The study was funded by Grants from the Instituto de Salud Carlos III (PI16/00594, PI19/00213) and co-funded by the European Regional Development Fund (ERDF).

Institutional Review Board Statement: The present study including all its experiments comply with current Spanish and European Union legal regulations. No data from patients were used.

Informed Consent Statement: Informed consent was not needed.

Data Availability Statement: Full data will be available from the Corresponding Author upon reasonable request.

Conflicts of Interest: The authors declare no conflict of interest. The funders had no role in the design of the study; in the collection, analyses, or interpretation of data; in the writing of the manuscript, or in the decision to publish the results.

References

1. Padala, S.A.; Barsouk, A.; Thandra, K.C.; Saginala, K.; Mohammed, A.; Vakiti, A.; Rawla, P.; Barsouk, A. Epidemiology of Renal Cell Carcinoma. *World J. Oncol.* **2020**, *11*, 79–87. [CrossRef]
2. Bot, F.J.; Godschalk, J.C.J.; Krishnadath, K.K.; Van Der Kwast, T.H.; Bosman, F.T.; But, F.J.; Der Van Kwast, T.H.M. Prognostic factors in renal-cell carcinoma: Immunohistochemical detection of p53 protein versus clinico-pathological parameters. *Int. J. Cancer* **1994**, *57*, 634–637. [CrossRef]
3. Zheng, W.; Zhu, W.; Yu, S.; Li, K.; Ding, Y.; Wu, Q.; Tang, Q.; Zhao, Q.; Lu, C.; Guo, C. Development and validation of a nomogram to predict overall survival for patients with metastatic renal cell carcinoma. *BMC Cancer* **2020**, *20*, 1066. [CrossRef] [PubMed]
4. Trpkov, K.; Hes, O.; Williamson, S.R.; Adeniran, A.J.; Agaimy, A.; Alaghehbandan, R.; Amin, M.B.; Argani, P.; Chen, Y.-B.; Cheng, L.; et al. New developments in existing WHO entities and evolving molecular concepts: The Genitourinary Pathology Society (GUPS) update on renal neoplasia. *Mod. Pathol.* **2021**, 1–33. [CrossRef]
5. Srigley, J.R.; Delahunt, B.; Eble, J.N.; Egevad, L.; Epstein, J.I.; Grignon, D.; Hes, O.; Moch, H.; Montironi, R.; Tickoo, S.K.; et al. The International Society of Urological Pathology (ISUP) Vancouver classification of renal neoplasia. *Am. J. Surg. Pathol.* **2013**, *37*, 1469–1489. [CrossRef]
6. Maher, E.R. Genomics and epigenomics of renal cell carcinoma. *Semin. Cancer Biol.* **2013**, *23*, 10–17. [CrossRef]
7. Moch, H. An overview of renal cell cancer: Pathology and genetics. *Semin. Cancer Biol.* **2013**, *23*, 3–9. [CrossRef] [PubMed]
8. Costa-Pinheiro, P.; Montezuma, D.; Henrique, R.; Jerónimo, C. Diagnostic and prognostic epigenetic biomarkers in cancer. *Epigenomics* **2015**, *7*, 1003–1015. [CrossRef]

9. Solano-Iturri, J.D.; Errarte, P.; Etxezarraga, M.C.; Echevarria, E.; Angulo, J.; López, J.I.; Larrinaga, G. Altered Tissue and Plasma Levels of Fibroblast Activation Protein-α (FAP) in Renal Tumours. *Cancers* **2020**, *12*, 3393. [CrossRef]
10. López, J.I. Intratumor heterogeneity in clear cell renal cell carcinoma: A review for the practicing pathologist. *APMIS* **2016**, *124*, 153–159. [CrossRef]
11. Rydzanicz, M.; Wrzesiński, T.; Bluyssen, H.A.; Wesoły, J. Genomics and epigenomics of clear cell renal cell carcinoma: Recent developments and potential applications. *Cancer Lett.* **2013**, *341*, 111–126. [CrossRef] [PubMed]
12. Onay, H.; Pehlivan, S.; Koyuncuoglu, M.; Kirkali, Z.; Özkinay, F. Multigene Methylation Analysis of Conventional Renal Cell Carcinoma. *Urol. Int.* **2009**, *83*, 107–112. [CrossRef]
13. Lasseigne, B.N.; Burwell, T.C.; Patil, M.A.; Absher, D.M.; Brooks, J.D.; Myers, R.M. DNA methylation profiling reveals novel diagnostic biomarkers in renal cell carcinoma. *BMC Med.* **2014**, *12*, 235. [CrossRef]
14. Pires-Luís, A.S.; Costa-Pinheiro, P.; Ferreira, M.J.; Antunes, L.; Lobo, F.; Oliveira, J.; Henrique, R.; Jerónimo, C. Identification of clear cell renal cell carcinoma and oncocytoma using a three-gene promoter methylation panel. *J. Transl. Med.* **2017**, *15*, 149. [CrossRef] [PubMed]
15. Lasseigne, B.N.; Brooks, J.D. The Role of DNA Methylation in Renal Cell Carcinoma. *Mol. Diagn. Ther.* **2018**, *22*, 431–442. [CrossRef]
16. Ellinger, J.; Müller, S.C.; Dietrich, D. Epigenetic biomarkers in the blood of patients with urological malignancies. *Expert Rev. Mol. Diagn.* **2015**, *15*, 505–516. [CrossRef] [PubMed]
17. Wei, J.-H.; Haddad, A.; Wu, K.-J.; Zhao, H.-W.; Kapur, P.; Zhang, Z.-L.; Zhao, L.-Y.; Chen, Z.-H.; Zhou, Y.-Y.; Zhou, J.-C.; et al. A CpG-methylation-based assay to predict survival in clear cell renal cell carcinoma. *Nat. Commun.* **2015**, *6*, 8699. [CrossRef]
18. Malouf, G.G.; Su, X.; Zhang, J.; Creighton, C.J.; Ho, T.H.; Lu, Y.; Raynal, N.J.-M.; Karam, J.A.; Tamboli, P.; Allanick, F.; et al. DNA Methylation Signature Reveals Cell Ontogeny of Renal Cell Carcinomas. *Clin. Cancer Res.* **2016**, *22*, 6236–6246. [CrossRef]
19. Angulo, J.C.; López, J.I.; Ropero, S. DNA Methylation and Urological Cancer, a Step Towards Personalized Medicine: Current and Future Prospects. *Mol. Diagn. Ther.* **2016**, *20*, 531–549. [CrossRef] [PubMed]
20. El Khoury, L.Y.; Fu, S.; Hlady, R.A.; Wagner, R.T.; Wang, L.; Eckel-Passow, J.E.; Castle, E.P.; Stanton, M.L.; Thompson, R.H.; Parker, A.S.; et al. Identification of DNA methylation signatures associated with poor outcome in lower-risk Stage, Size, Grade and Necrosis (SSIGN) score clear cell renal cell cancer. *Clin. Epigenetics* **2021**, *13*, 1–16. [CrossRef]
21. Mir, M.C.; Derweesh, I.; Porpiglia, F.; Zargar, H.; Mottrie, A.; Autorino, R. Partial Nephrectomy Versus Radical Nephrectomy for Clinical T1b and T2 Renal Tumors: A Systematic Review and Meta-analysis of Comparative Studies. *Eur. Urol.* **2017**, *71*, 606–617. [CrossRef]
22. Albiges, L.; Powles, T.; Staehler, M.; Bensalah, K.; Giles, R.H.; Hora, M.; Kuczyk, M.A.; Lam, T.B.; Ljungberg, B.; Marconi, L.; et al. Updated European Association of Urology Guidelines on Renal Cell Carcinoma: Immune Checkpoint Inhibition Is the New Backbone in First-line Treatment of Metastatic Clear-cell Renal Cell Carcinoma. *Eur. Urol.* **2019**, *76*, 151–156. [CrossRef]
23. Jonasch, E. NCCN Guidelines Updates: Management of Metastatic Kidney Cancer. *J. Natl. Compr. Cancer Netw.* **2019**, *17*, 587–589.
24. Motzer, R.J.; Penkov, K.; Haanen, J.; Rini, B.; Albiges, L.; Campbell, M.T.; Venugopal, B.; Kollmannsberger, C.; Negrier, S.; Uemura, M. Avelumab plus Axitinib versus Sunitinib for Advanced Renal-Cell Carcinoma. *N. Engl. J. Med.* **2019**, *380*, 1103–1115. [CrossRef]
25. Angulo, J.C.; Shapiro, O. The Changing Therapeutic Landscape of Metastatic Renal Cancer. *Cancers* **2019**, *11*, 1227. [CrossRef] [PubMed]
26. Khagi, Y.; Kurzrock, R.; Patel, S.P. Next generation predictive biomarkers for immune checkpoint inhibition. *Cancer Metastasis Rev.* **2017**, *36*, 179–190. [CrossRef] [PubMed]
27. Simonaggio, A.; Epaillard, N.; Pobel, C.; Moreira, M.; Oudard, S.; Vano, Y.-A. Tumor Microenvironment Features as Predictive Biomarkers of Response to Immune Checkpoint Inhibitors (ICI) in Metastatic Clear Cell Renal Cell Carcinoma (mccRCC). *Cancers* **2021**, *13*, 231. [CrossRef]
28. Larrinaga, G.; Solano-Iturri, J.D.; Errarte, P.; Unda, M.; Loizaga-Iriarte, A.; Pérez-Fernández, A.; Echevarría, E.; Asumendi, A.; Manini, C.; Angulo, J.C.; et al. Soluble PD-L1 Is an Independent Prognostic Factor in Clear Cell Renal Cell Carcinoma. *Cancers* **2021**, *13*, 667. [CrossRef] [PubMed]
29. Vasudev, N.S.; Selby, P.J.; Banks, R.E. Renal cancer biomarkers: The promise of personalized care. *BMC Med.* **2012**, *10*, 112. [CrossRef]
30. Hsieh, J.J.; Chen, D.; Wang, P.I.; Marker, M.; Redzematovic, A.; Chen, Y.-B.; Selcuklu, S.D.; Weinhold, N.; Bouvier, N.; Huberman, K.H.; et al. Genomic Biomarkers of a Randomized Trial Comparing First-line Everolimus and Sunitinib in Patients with Metastatic Renal Cell Carcinoma. *Eur. Urol.* **2017**, *71*, 405–414. [CrossRef]
31. Taby, R.; Issa, J.-P.J. Cancer Epigenetics. *CA Cancer J. Clin.* **2010**, *60*, 376–392. [CrossRef]
32. Valdés-Mora, F.; Clark, S.J. Prostate cancer epigenetic biomarkers: Next-generation technologies. *Oncogene* **2015**, *34*, 1609–1618. [CrossRef]
33. Xing, T.; He, H. Epigenomics of clear cell renal cell carcinoma: Mechanisms and potential use in molecular pathology. *Chin. J. Cancer Res.* **2016**, *28*, 80–91. [PubMed]
34. Joosten, S.C.; Deckers, I.A.; Aarts, M.J.; Hoeben, A.; Van Roermund, J.G.; Smits, K.M.; Melotte, V.; Van Engeland, M.; Tjan-Heijnen, V.C. Prognostic DNA methylation markers for renal cell carcinoma: A systematic review. *Epigenomics* **2017**, *9*, 1243–1257. [CrossRef] [PubMed]

35. Lommen, K.; Vaes, N.; Aarts, M.J.; van Roermund, J.G.; Schouten, L.J.; Oosterwijk, E.; Melotte, V.; Tjan-Heijnen, V.C.; van Engeland, M.; Smits, K.M. Diagnostic DNA Methylation Biomarkers for Renal Cell Carcinoma: A Systematic Review. *Eur. Urol. Oncol.* **2021**, *4*, 215–226. [CrossRef]
36. Schulz, W.A.; Sørensen, K.D. Epigenetics of Urological Cancers. *Int. J. Mol. Sci.* **2019**, *20*, 4775. [CrossRef]
37. Wang, J.; Wang, L.; Zhang, D.; Fan, Y.; Jia, Z.; Qin, P.; Yu, J.; Zheng, S.; Yang, F. Identification of potential serum biomarkers for Wilms tumor after excluding confounding effects of common systemic inflammatory factors. *Mol. Biol. Rep.* **2012**, *39*, 5095–5104. [CrossRef] [PubMed]
38. Kim, H.S.; Kim, J.H.; Jang, H.J.; Han, B.; Zang, D.Y. Clinicopathologic Significance of VHL Gene Alteration in Clear-Cell Renal Cell Carcinoma: An Updated Meta-Analysis and Review. *Int. J. Mol. Sci.* **2018**, *19*, 2529. [CrossRef]
39. Huang, J.; Yao, X.; Zhang, J.; Dong, B.; Chen, Q.; Xue, W.; Liu, D.; Huang, Y. Hypoxia-induced downregulation of miR-30c promotes epithelial-mesenchymal transition in human renal cell carcinoma. *Cancer Sci.* **2013**, *104*, 1609–1617. [CrossRef]
40. Zhai, W.; Sun, Y.; Jiang, M.; Wang, M.; Gasiewicz, T.A.; Zheng, J. Differential regulation of LncRNA-SARCC suppresses VHL-mutant RCC cell proliferation yet promotes VHL-normal RCC cell proliferation via modulating androgen receptor/HIF-2α/C-MYC axis under hypoxia. *Oncogene* **2016**, *35*, 4866–4880. [CrossRef] [PubMed]
41. Dalgliesh, G.L.; Furge, K.; Greenman, C.; Chen, L.; Bignell, G.; Butler, A.; Davies, H.; Edkins, S.; Hardy, C.; Latimer, C.; et al. Systematic sequencing of renal carcinoma reveals inactivation of histone modifying genes. *Nature* **2010**, *463*, 360–363. [CrossRef]
42. Thévenin, A.; Ein-Dor, L.; Ozery-Flato, M.; Shamir, R. Functional gene groups are concentrated within chromosomes, among chromosomes and in the nuclear space of the human genome. *Nucleic Acids Res.* **2014**, *42*, 9854–9861. [CrossRef]
43. Mehdi, A.; Riazalhosseini, Y. Epigenome Aberrations: Emerging Driving Factors of the Clear Cell Renal Cell Carcinoma. *Int. J. Mol. Sci.* **2017**, *18*, 1774. [CrossRef]
44. De Cubas, A.A.; Rathmell, W.K. Epigenetic modifiers: Activities in renal cell carcinoma. *Nat. Rev. Urol.* **2018**, *15*, 599–614. [CrossRef] [PubMed]
45. Nalejska, E.; Mączyńska, E.; Lewandowska, M.A. Prognostic and Predictive Biomarkers: Tools in Personalized Oncology. *Mol. Diagn. Ther.* **2014**, *18*, 273–284. [CrossRef] [PubMed]
46. Skrypkina, I.; Tsyba, L.; Onyshchenko, K.; Morderer, D.; Kashparova, O.; Nikolaienko, O.; Panasenko, G.; Vozianov, S.; Romanenko, A.; Rynditch, A. Concentration and Methylation of Cell-Free DNA from Blood Plasma as Diagnostic Markers of Renal Cancer. *Dis. Markers* **2016**, *2016*, 3693096. [CrossRef]
47. Nuzzo, P.V.; Berchuck, J.E.; Korthauer, K.; Spisak, S.; Nassar, A.H.; Alaiwi, S.A.; Chakravarthy, A.; Shen, S.Y.; Bakouny, Z.; Boccardo, F.; et al. Detection of renal cell carcinoma using plasma and urine cell-free DNA methylomes. *Nat. Med.* **2020**, *26*, 1041–1043. [CrossRef]
48. Slater, A.A.; Alokail, M.; Gentle, D.; Yao, M.; Kovacs, G.; Maher, E.R.; Latif, F. DNA methylation profiling distinguishes histological subtypes of renal cell carcinoma. *Epigenetics* **2013**, *8*, 252–267. [CrossRef] [PubMed]
49. Goll, M.G.; Bestor, T.H. Eukaryotic cytosine methyltransferases. *Annu. Rev. Biochem.* **2005**, *74*, 481–514. [CrossRef]
50. Esteller, M. Epigenetics in Cancer. *N. Engl. J. Med.* **2008**, *358*, 1148–1159. [CrossRef] [PubMed]
51. Esteller, M. Cancer epigenomics: DNA methylomes and histone-modification maps. *Nat. Rev. Genet.* **2007**, *8*, 286–298. [CrossRef]
52. Shenoy, N.; Vallumsetla, N.; Zou, Y.; Galeas, J.N.; Shrivastava, M.; Hu, C.; Susztak, K.; Verma, A. Role of DNA methylation in renal cell carcinoma. *J. Hematol. Oncol.* **2015**, *8*, 88. [CrossRef] [PubMed]
53. Jones, P.A. Functions of DNA methylation: Islands, start sites, gene bodies and beyond. *Nat. Rev. Genet.* **2012**, *13*, 484–492. [CrossRef] [PubMed]
54. Frommer, M.; McDonald, L.E.; Millar, D.S.; Collis, C.M.; Watt, F.; Grigg, G.W.; Molloy, P.L.; Paul, C.L. A genomic sequencing protocol that yields a positive display of 5-methylcytosine residues in individual DNA strands. *Proc. Natl. Acad. Sci. USA* **1992**, *89*, 1827–1831. [CrossRef] [PubMed]
55. Herman, J.G.; Graff, J.R.; Myöhänen, S.; Nelkin, B.D.; Baylin, S.B. Methylation-specific PCR: A novel PCR assay for methylation status of CpG islands. *Proc. Natl. Acad. Sci. USA* **1996**, *93*, 9821–9826. [CrossRef] [PubMed]
56. Hoffman, A.M.; Cairns, P. Epigenetics of kidney cancer and bladder cancer. *Epigenomics* **2011**, *3*, 19–34. [CrossRef]
57. Koch, A.; Joosten, S.C.; Feng, Z.; De Ruijter, T.C.; Draht, M.X.; Melotte, V.; Smits, K.M.; Veeck, J.; Herman, J.G.; Van Neste, L.; et al. Analysis of DNA methylation in cancer: Location revisited. *Nat. Rev. Clin. Oncol.* **2018**, *15*, 459–466. [CrossRef] [PubMed]
58. Karami, S.; Andreotti, G.; Liao, L.M.; Pfeiffer, R.M.; Weinstein, S.J.; Purdue, M.P.; Hofmann, J.N.; Albanes, D.; Männistö, S.; Moore, L.E. LINE1 methylation levels in pre-diagnostic leukocyte DNA and future renal cell carcinoma risk. *Epigenetics* **2015**, *10*, 282–292. [CrossRef]
59. Herman, J.G.; Latif, F.; Weng, Y.; Lerman, M.I.; Zbar, B.; Liu, S.; Samid, D.; Duan, D.S.; Gnarra, J.R.; Linehan, W.M. Silencing of the VHL tumor-suppressor gene by DNA methylation in renal carcinoma. *Proc. Natl. Acad. Sci. USA* **1994**, *91*, 9700–9704. [CrossRef]
60. Battagli, C.; Uzzo, R.G.; Dulaimi, E.; De Caceres, I.I.; Krassenstein, R.; Al-Saleem, T.; E Greenberg, R.; Cairns, P. Promoter hypermethylation of tumor suppressor genes in urine from kidney cancer patients. *Cancer Res.* **2003**, *63*, 8695–8699.
61. Hoque, M.O.; Begum, S.; Topaloglu, O.; Jeronimo, C.; Mambo, E.; Westra, W.H.; Califano, J.A.; Sidransky, D. Quantitative Detection of Promoter Hypermethylation of Multiple Genes in the Tumor, Urine, and Serum DNA of Patients with Renal Cancer. *Cancer Res.* **2004**, *64*, 5511–5517. [CrossRef] [PubMed]
62. Ibanez de Caceres, I.; Dulaimi, E.; Hoffman, A.M.; Al-Saleem, T.; Uzzo, R.G.; Cairns, P. Identification of novel target genes by an epigenetic reactivation screen of renal cancer. *Cancer Res.* **2006**, *66*, 5021–5028. [CrossRef] [PubMed]

63. Costa, V.L.; Henrique, R.; Ribeiro, F.R.; Pinto, M.; Oliveira, J.; Lobo, F.; Teixeira, M.R.; Jerónimo, C. Quantitative promoter methylation analysis of multiple cancer-related genes in renal cell tumors. *BMC Cancer* **2007**, *7*, 133. [CrossRef] [PubMed]
64. Peters, I.; Rehmet, K.; Wilke, N.; A Kuczyk, M.; Hennenlotter, J.; Eilers, T.; Machtens, S.; Jonas, U.; Serth, J. RASSF1A promoter methylation and expression analysis in normal and neoplastic kidney indicates a role in early tumorigenesis. *Mol. Cancer* **2007**, *6*, 49. [CrossRef]
65. Morris, M.R.; Ricketts, C.J.; Gentle, D.; McRonald, F.; Carli, N.; Khalili, H.; Brown, M.; Kishida, T.; Yao, M.; Banks, R.E.; et al. Genome-wide methylation analysis identifies epigenetically inactivated candidate tumour suppressor genes in renal cell carcinoma. *Oncogene* **2011**, *30*, 1390–1401. [CrossRef]
66. Hauser, S.; Zahalka, T.; Fechner, G.; Müller, S.C.; Ellinger, J. Serum DNA hypermethylation in patients with kidney cancer: Results of a prospective study. *Anticancer. Res.* **2013**, *33*, 4651–4656.
67. Urakami, S.; Shiina, H.; Enokida, H.; Hirata, H.; Kawamoto, K.; Kawakami, T.; Kikuno, N.; Tanaka, Y.; Majid, S.; Nakagawa, M.; et al. Wnt Antagonist Family Genes as Biomarkers for Diagnosis, Staging, and Prognosis of Renal Cell Carcinoma Using Tumor and Serum DNA. *Clin. Cancer Res.* **2006**, *12*, 6989–6997. [CrossRef]
68. Gonzalgo, M.L.; Yegnasubramanian, S.; Yan, G.; Rogers, C.G.; Nicol, T.L.; Nelson, W.G.; Pavlovich, C.P. Molecular Profiling and Classification of Sporadic Renal Cell Carcinoma by Quantitative Methylation Analysis. *Clin. Cancer Res.* **2004**, *10*, 7276–7283. [CrossRef]
69. Morris, M.R.; Gentle, D.; Abdulrahman, M.; Maina, E.N.; Gupta, K.; Banks, R.E.; Wiesener, M.S.; Kishida, T.; Yao, M.; Teh, B.; et al. Tumor Suppressor Activity and Epigenetic Inactivation of Hepatocyte Growth Factor Activator Inhibitor Type 2/SPINT2 in Papillary and Clear Cell Renal Cell Carcinoma. *Cancer Res.* **2005**, *65*, 4598–4606. [CrossRef]
70. McRonald, F.E.; Morris, M.R.; Gentle, D.; Winchester, L.; Baban, D.; Ragoussis, J.; Clarke, N.W.; Brown, M.D.; Kishida, T.; Yao, M.; et al. CpG methylation profiling in VHL related and VHL unrelated renal cell carcinoma. *Mol. Cancer* **2009**, *8*, 31. [CrossRef]
71. Brennan, K.; Metzner, T.J.; Kao, C.-S.; Massie, C.E.; Stewart, G.D.; Haile, R.W.; Brooks, J.D.; Hitchins, M.P.; Leppert, J.T.; Gevaert, O. Development of a DNA Methylation–Based Diagnostic Signature to Distinguish Benign Oncocytoma From Renal Cell Carcinoma. *JCO Precis. Oncol.* **2020**, *4*, 1141–1151. [CrossRef] [PubMed]
72. Chen, W.; Zhuang, J.; Wang, P.P.; Jiang, J.; Lin, C.; Zeng, P.; Liang, Y.; Zhang, X.; Dai, Y.; Diao, H. DNA methylation-based classification and identification of renal cell carcinoma prognosis-subgroups. *Cancer Cell Int.* **2019**, *19*, 185. [CrossRef]
73. Evelönn, E.A.; Landfors, M.; Haider, Z.; Köhn, L.; Ljungberg, B.; Roos, G.; Degerman, S. DNA methylation associates with survival in non-metastatic clear cell renal cell carcinoma. *BMC Cancer* **2019**, *19*, 65. [CrossRef]
74. Van Vlodrop, I.J.H.; Joosten, S.C.; De Meyer, T.; Smits, K.M.; Van Neste, L.; Melotte, V.; Baldewijns, M.M.L.L.; Schouten, L.J.; van den Brandt, P.A.; Jeschke, J.; et al. A Four-Gene Promoter Methylation Marker Panel Consisting of GREM1, NEURL, LAD1, and NEFH Predicts Survival of Clear Cell Renal Cell Cancer Patients. *Clin. Cancer Res.* **2017**, *23*, 2006–2018. [CrossRef] [PubMed]
75. Ricketts, C.J.; De Cubas, A.A.; Fan, H.; Smith, C.C.; Lang, M.; Reznik, E.; Bowlby, R.; Gibb, E.A.; Akbani, R.; Beroukhim, R.; et al. The Cancer Genome Atlas Comprehensive Molecular Characterization of Renal Cell Carcinoma. *Cell Rep.* **2018**, *23*, 3698. [CrossRef]
76. Peters, I.; Dubrowinskaja, N.; Hennenlotter, J.; Antonopoulos, W.I.; Von Klot, C.A.; Tezval, H.; Stenzl, A.; Kuczyk, M.A.; Serth, J. DNA methylation of neural EGFL like 1 (NELL1) is associated with advanced disease and the metastatic state of renal cell cancer patients. *Oncol. Rep.* **2018**, *40*, 3861–3868. [CrossRef]
77. Hu, F.; Zeng, W.; Liu, X. A Gene Signature of Survival Prediction for Kidney Renal Cell Carcinoma by Multi-Omic Data Analysis. *Int. J. Mol. Sci.* **2019**, *20*, 5720. [CrossRef] [PubMed]
78. Peng, Q.; Zhou, Y.; Jin, L.; Cao, C.; Gao, C.; Zhou, J.; Yang, D.; Zhu, J. Development and validation of an integrative methylation signature and nomogram for predicting survival in clear cell renal cell carcinoma. *Transl. Androl. Urol.* **2020**, *9*, 1082–1098. [CrossRef] [PubMed]
79. Wang, Y.; Chen, L.; Ju, L.; Qian, K.; Wang, X.; Xiao, Y.; Wang, G. Epigenetic signature predicts overall survival clear cell renal cell carcinoma. *Cancer Cell Int.* **2020**, *20*, 564. [CrossRef]
80. Wang, J.; Zhang, Q.; Zhu, Q.; Liu, C.; Nan, X.; Wang, F.; Fang, L.; Liu, J.; Xie, C.; Fu, S.; et al. Identification of methylation-driven genes related to prognosis in clear-cell renal cell carcinoma. *J. Cell. Physiol.* **2019**, *235*, 1296–1308. [CrossRef]
81. Kang, H.W.; Park, H.; Seo, S.P.; Byun, Y.J.; Piao, X.-M.; Kim, S.M.; Kim, W.T.; Yun, S.-J.; Jang, W.; Shon, H.S.; et al. Methylation Signature for Prediction of Progression Free Survival in Surgically Treated Clear Cell Renal Cell Carcinoma. *J. Korean Med. Sci.* **2019**, *34*, e144. [CrossRef]
82. Shi, S.; Ye, S.; Wu, X.; Xu, M.; Zhuo, R.; Liao, Q.; Xi, Y. A Two-DNA Methylation Signature to Improve Prognosis Prediction of Clear Cell Renal Cell Carcinoma. *Yonsei Med. J.* **2019**, *60*, 1013–1020. [CrossRef]
83. Kim, Y.; Jang, W.; Piao, X.; Yoon, H.; Byun, Y.J.; Kim, J.S.; Kim, S.M.; Lee, S.K.; Seo, S.P.; Kang, H.W.; et al. ZNF492 and GPR149 methylation patterns as prognostic markers for clear cell renal cell carcinoma: Array-based DNA methylation profiling. *Oncol. Rep.* **2019**, *42*, 453–460. [CrossRef]
84. Breault, J.E.; Shiina, H.; Igawa, M.; Ribeiro-Filho, L.A.; Deguchi, M.; Enokida, H.; Urakami, S.; Terashima, M.; Nakagawa, M.; Kane, C.J.; et al. Methylation of the gamma-catenin gene is associated with poor prognosis of renal cell carcinoma. *Clin. Cancer Res.* **2005**, *11*, 557–564. [PubMed]

85. Peters, I.; Eggers, H.; Atschekzei, F.; Hennenlotter, J.; Waalkes, S.; Tränkenschuh, W.; Großhennig, A.; Merseburger, A.S.; Stenzl, A.; Kuczyk, M.A.; et al. GATA5CpG island methylation in renal cell cancer: A potential biomarker for metastasis and disease progression. *BJU Int.* **2012**, *110*, E144–E152. [CrossRef] [PubMed]
86. Peters, I.; Gebauer, K.; Dubrowinskaja, N.; Atschekzei, F.; Kramer, M.W.; Hennenlotter, J.; Tezval, H.; Abbas, M.; Scherer, R.; Merseburger, A.S.; et al. GATA5 CpG island hypermethylation is an independent predictor for poor clinical outcome in renal cell carcinoma. *Oncol. Rep.* **2014**, *31*, 1523–1530. [CrossRef]
87. Van Vlodrop, I.J.H.; Baldewijns, M.M.L.; Smits, K.M.; Schouten, L.J.; van Neste, L.; Van Criekinge, W.; van Poppel, H.; Lerut, E.; Schuebel, K.E.; Ahuja, N.; et al. Prognostic significance of Gremlin1 (GREM1) promoter CpG island hypermethylation in clear cell renal cell carcinoma. *Am. J. Pathol.* **2010**, *176*, 575–584. [CrossRef] [PubMed]
88. Eggers, H.; Steffens, S.; Grosshennig, A.; Becker, J.U.; Hennenlotter, J.; Stenzl, A.; Merseburger, A.S.; Serth, J. Prognostic and diagnostic relevance of hypermethylated in cancer 1 (HIC1) CpG island methylation in renal cell carcinoma. *Int. J. Oncol.* **2012**, *40*, 1650–1658. [CrossRef]
89. Lin, Y.-L.; Wang, Y.-L.; Fu, X.-L.; Ma, J.-G. Aberrant Methylation of PCDH8 is a Potential Prognostic Biomarker for Patients with Clear Cell Renal Cell Carcinoma. *Med. Sci. Monit.* **2014**, *20*, 2380–2385. [CrossRef]
90. Kim, H.L.; Seligson, D.; Liu, X.; Janzen, N.; Bui, M.H.; Yu, H.; Shi, T.; Belldegrun, A.S.; Horvath, S.; Figlin, R.A. Using tumor markers to predict the survival of patients with metastatic renal cell carcinoma. *J. Urol.* **2005**, *173*, 1496–1501. [CrossRef]
91. Kawai, Y.; Sakano, S.; Suehiro, Y.; Okada, T.; Korenaga, Y.; Hara, T.; Naito, K.; Matsuyama, H.; Hinoda, Y. Methylation level of the RASSF1A promoter is an independent prognostic factor for clear-cell renal cell carcinoma. *Ann. Oncol.* **2010**, *21*, 1612–1617. [CrossRef] [PubMed]
92. Klacz, J.; Wierzbicki, P.M.; Wronska, A.; Rybarczyk, A.; Stanislawowski, M.; Slebioda, T.; Olejniczak, A.; Matuszewski, M.; Kmiec, Z. Decreased expression of RASSF1A tumor suppressor gene is associated with worse prognosis in clear cell renal cell carcinoma. *Int. J. Oncol.* **2016**, *48*, 55–66. [CrossRef] [PubMed]
93. Mazdak, M.; Tezval, H.; Callauch, J.C.; Dubrowinskaja, N.; Peters, I.; Bokemeyer, C.; Hennenlotter, J.; Stenzl, A.; Kuczyk, M.A.; Serth, J. DNA methylation of sarcosine dehydrogenase (SARDH) loci as a prognosticator for renal cell carcinoma. *Oncol. Rep.* **2019**, *42*, 2159–2168. [CrossRef] [PubMed]
94. Atschekzei, F.; Hennenlotter, J.; Jänisch, S.; Großhennig, A.; Tränkenschuh, W.; Waalkes, S.; Peters, I.; Dörk, T.; Merseburger, A.S.; Stenzl, A.; et al. SFRP1CpG island methylation locus is associated with renal cell cancer susceptibility and disease recurrence. *Epigenetics* **2012**, *7*, 447–457. [CrossRef] [PubMed]
95. Ricketts, C.J.; Hill, V.K.; Linehan, W.M. Tumor-Specific Hypermethylation of Epigenetic Biomarkers, Including SFRP1, Predicts for Poorer Survival in Patients from the TCGA Kidney Renal Clear Cell Carcinoma (KIRC) Project. *PLoS ONE* **2014**, *9*, e85621. [CrossRef]
96. Yang, M.; Hlady, R.A.; Zhou, D.; Ho, T.H.; Robertson, K.D. In silico DNA methylation analysis identifies potential prognostic biomarkers in type 2 papillary renal cell carcinoma. *Cancer Med.* **2019**, *8*, 5760–5768. [CrossRef] [PubMed]
97. Parry, L.; Clarke, A.R. The roles of the methyl-CpG binding proteins in cancer. *Genes Cancer* **2011**, *2*, 618–630. [CrossRef]
98. Mahmood, N.; Rabbani, S.A. DNA Methylation Readers and Cancer: Mechanistic and Therapeutic Applications. *Front. Oncol.* **2019**, *9*, 489. [CrossRef]
99. Li, L.; Li, N.; Liu, N.; Huo, F.; Zheng, J. MBD2 Correlates with a Poor Prognosis and Tumor Progression in Renal Cell Carcinoma. *Oncotargets Ther.* **2020**, *13*, 10001–10012. [CrossRef]
100. Felsenfeld, G.; Groudine, M. Controlling the double helix. *Nature* **2003**, *421*, 448–453. [CrossRef] [PubMed]
101. Ropero, S.; Esteller, M. The role of histone deacetylases (HDACs) in human cancer. *Mol. Oncol.* **2007**, *1*, 19–25. [CrossRef] [PubMed]
102. Larkin, J.; Goh, X.Y.; Vetter, M.; Pickering, L.; Swanton, C. Epigenetic regulation in RCC: Opportunities for therapeutic intervention? *Nat. Rev. Urol.* **2012**, *9*, 147–155. [CrossRef]
103. Ramakrishnan, S.; Ellis, L.; Pili, R. Histone modifications: Implications in renal cell carcinoma. *Epigenomics* **2013**, *5*, 453–462. [CrossRef]
104. Rogenhofer, S.; Kahl, P.; Mertens, C.; Hauser, S.; Hartmann, W.; Büttner, R.; Müller, S.C.; Von Ruecker, A.; Ellinger, J. Global histone H3 lysine 27 (H3K27) methylation levels and their prognostic relevance in renal cell carcinoma. *BJU Int.* **2012**, *109*, 459–465. [CrossRef]
105. Seligson, D.B.; Horvath, S.; McBrian, M.A.; Mah, V.; Yu, H.; Tze, S.; Wang, Q.; Chia, D.; Goodglick, L.; Kurdistani, S.K. Global Levels of Histone Modifications Predict Prognosis in Different Cancers. *Am. J. Pathol.* **2009**, *174*, 1619–1628. [CrossRef] [PubMed]
106. Ellinger, J.; Kahl, P.; Mertens, C.; Rogenhofer, S.; Hauser, S.; Hartmann, W.; Bastian, P.J.; Büttner, R.; Müller, S.C.; von Ruecker, A. Prognostic relevance of global histone H3 lysine 4 (H3K4) methylation in renal cell carcinoma. *Int. J. Cancer* **2010**, *127*, 2360–2366. [CrossRef] [PubMed]
107. Minardi, D.; Lucarini, G.; Filosa, A.; Milanese, G.; Zizzi, A.; Di Primio, R.; Montironi, R.; Muzzonigro, G. Prognostic role of global DNA-methylation and histone acetylation in pT1a clear cell renal carcinoma in partial nephrectomy specimens. *J. Cell. Mol. Med.* **2009**, *13*, 2115–2121. [CrossRef]
108. Mosashvilli, D.; Kahl, P.; Mertens, C.; Holzapfel, S.; Rogenhofer, S.; Hauser, S.; Büttner, R.; Von Ruecker, A.; Müller, S.C.; Ellinger, J. Global histone acetylation levels: Prognostic relevance in patients with renal cell carcinoma. *Cancer Sci.* **2010**, *101*, 2664–2669. [CrossRef]

109. Huang, G.; Zhang, G.; Yu, Z. Computational prediction and analysis of histone H3k27me1-associated miRNAs. *Biochim. Biophys. Acta BBA Proteins Proteom.* **2021**, *1869*, 140539. [CrossRef]
110. Pollard, P.J.; Loenarz, C.; Mole, D.R.; McDonough, M.A.; Gleadle, J.M.; Schofield, C.J.; Ratcliffe, P.J. Regulation of Jumonji-domain-containing histone demethylases by hypoxia-inducible factor (HIF)-1α. *Biochem. J.* **2008**, *416*, 387–394. [CrossRef]
111. Henrique, R.; Luís, A.S.; Jerónimo, C. The Epigenetics of Renal Cell Tumors: From Biology to Biomarkers. *Front. Genet.* **2012**, *3*, 94. [CrossRef] [PubMed]
112. Li, F.; Mao, G.; Tong, D.; Huang, J.; Gu, L.; Yang, W.; Li, G.-M. The Histone Mark H3K36me3 Regulates Human DNA Mismatch Repair through Its Interaction with MutSα. *Cell* **2013**, *153*, 590–600. [CrossRef]
113. Pfister, S.X.; Ahrabi, S.; Zalmas, L.-P.; Sarkar, S.; Aymard, F.; Bachrati, C.Z.; Helleday, T.; Legube, G.; La Thangue, N.B.; Porter, A.C.; et al. SETD2-Dependent Histone H3K36 Trimethylation Is Required for Homologous Recombination Repair and Genome Stability. *Cell Rep.* **2014**, *7*, 2006–2018. [CrossRef] [PubMed]
114. Valera, V.A.; Walter, B.A.; Linehan, W.M.; Merino, M.J. Regulatory Effects of microRNA-92 (miR-92) on VHL Gene Expression and the Hypoxic Activation of miR-210 in Clear Cell Renal Cell Carcinoma. *J. Cancer* **2011**, *2*, 515–526. [CrossRef] [PubMed]
115. Reisman, D.; Glaros, S.; Thompson, E.A. The SWI/SNF complex and cancer. *Oncogene* **2009**, *28*, 1653–1668. [CrossRef] [PubMed]
116. Chowdhury, B.; Porter, E.G.; Stewart, J.C.; Ferreira, C.R.; Schipma, M.J.; Dykhuizen, E.C. PBRM1 Regulates the Expression of Genes Involved in Metabolism and Cell Adhesion in Renal Clear Cell Carcinoma. *PLoS ONE* **2016**, *11*, e0153718. [CrossRef] [PubMed]
117. Kapur, P.; Peña-Llopis, S.; Christie, A.; Zhrebker, L.; Pavía-Jiménez, A.; Rathmell, W.K.; Xie, X.-J.; Brugarolas, J. Effects on survival of BAP1 and PBRM1 mutations in sporadic clear-cell renal-cell carcinoma: A retrospective analysis with independent validation. *Lancet Oncol.* **2013**, *14*, 159–167. [CrossRef]
118. Gao, W.; Li, W.; Xiao, T.; Liu, X.L.; Kaelin, W.C. Inactivation of the PBRM1 tumor suppressor gene amplifies the HIF-response in VHL-/- clear cell renal carcinoma. *Proc. Natl. Acad. Sci. USA* **2017**, *114*, 1027–1032. [CrossRef] [PubMed]
119. Porter, E.G.; Dykhuizen, E.C. Individual Bromodomains of Polybromo-1 Contribute to Chromatin Association and Tumor Suppression in Clear Cell Renal Carcinoma. *J. Biol. Chem.* **2017**, *292*, 2601–2610. [CrossRef] [PubMed]
120. Cai, W.; Su, L.; Liao, L.; Liu, Z.Z.; Langbein, L.; Dulaimi, E.; Testa, J.R.; Uzzo, R.G.; Zhong, Z.; Jiang, W.; et al. PBRM1 acts as a p53 lysine-acetylation reader to suppress renal tumor growth. *Nat. Commun.* **2019**, *10*, 5800. [CrossRef]
121. Barski, A.; Cuddapah, S.; Cui, K.; Roh, T.-Y.; Schones, D.E.; Wang, Z.; Wei, G.; Chepelev, I.; Zhao, K. High-Resolution Profiling of Histone Methylations in the Human Genome. *Cell* **2007**, *129*, 823–837. [CrossRef]
122. Ler, L.D.; Ghosh, S.; Chai, X.; Thike, A.A.; Heng, H.L.; Siew, E.Y.; Dey, S.; Koh, L.K.; Lim, J.Q.; Lim, W.K.; et al. Loss of tumor suppressor KDM6A amplifies PRC2-regulated transcriptional repression in bladder cancer and can be targeted through inhibition of EZH2. *Sci. Transl. Med.* **2017**, *9*, eaai8312. [CrossRef]
123. Rondinelli, B.; Rosano, D.; Antonini, E.; Frenquelli, M.; Montanini, L.; Huang, D.; Segalla, S.; Yoshihara, K.; Amin, S.B.; Lazarevič, D.; et al. Histone demethylase JARID1C inactivation triggers genomic instability in sporadic renal cancer. *J. Clin. Investig.* **2016**, *126*, 4387. [CrossRef]
124. Arseneault, M.; Monlong, J.; Vasudev, N.S.; Laskar, R.S.; Safisamghabadi, M.; Harnden, P.; Egevad, L.; Nourbehesht, N.; Panichnantakul, P.; Holcatova, I.; et al. Loss of chromosome Y leads to down regulation of KDM5D and KDM6C epigenetic modifiers in clear cell renal cell carcinoma. *Sci. Rep.* **2017**, *7*, 44876. [CrossRef]
125. Lee, K.-H.; Kim, B.-C.; Jeong, S.-H.; Jeong, C.W.; Ku, J.H.; Kwak, C.; Kim, H.H. Histone Demethylase LSD1 Regulates Kidney Cancer Progression by Modulating Androgen Receptor Activity. *Int. J. Mol. Sci.* **2020**, *21*, 6089. [CrossRef] [PubMed]
126. Kumar, A.; Kumari, N.; Nallabelli, N.; Sharma, U.; Rai, A.; Singh, S.K.; Kakkar, N.; Prasad, R. Expression profile of H3K4 demethylases with their clinical and pathological correlation in patients with clear cell renal cell carcinoma. *Gene* **2020**, *739*, 144498. [CrossRef] [PubMed]
127. Hinz, S.; Weikert, S.; Magheli, A.; Hoffmann, M.; Engers, R.; Miller, K.; Kempkensteffen, C. Expression Profile of the Polycomb Group Protein Enhancer of Zeste Homologue 2 and its Prognostic Relevance in Renal Cell Carcinoma. *J. Urol.* **2009**, *182*, 2920–2925. [CrossRef]
128. Liu, L.; Xu, Z.; Zhong, L.; Wang, H.; Jiang, S.; Long, Q.; Xu, J.; Guo, J. Prognostic Value of EZH2 Expression and Activity in Renal Cell Carcinoma: A Prospective Study. *PLoS ONE* **2013**, *8*, e81484. [CrossRef]
129. Xu, Z.Q.; Zhang, L.; Gao, B.S.; Wan, Y.G.; Zhang, X.H.; Chen, B.; Wang, Y.T.; Sun, N.; Fu, Y.W. EZH2 promotes tumor progression by increasing VEGF expression in clear cell renal cell carcinoma. *Clin. Transl. Oncol.* **2015**, *17*, 41–49. [CrossRef] [PubMed]
130. Liu, L.; Xu, Z.; Zhong, L.; Wang, H.; Jiang, S.; Long, Q.; Xu, J.; Guo, J. Enhancer of zeste homolog 2 (EZH2) promotes tumour cell migration and invasion via epigenetic repression of E-cadherin in renal cell carcinoma. *BJU Int.* **2016**, *117*, 351–362. [CrossRef]
131. Peña-Llopis, S.; Vega-Rubín-de-Celis, S.; Liao, A.; Leng, N.; Pavía-Jiménez, A.; Wang, S.; Yamasaki, T.; Zhrebker, L.; Sivanand, S.; Spence, P.; et al. BAP1 loss defines a new class of renal cell carcinoma. *Nat. Genet.* **2012**, *44*, 751–759. [CrossRef] [PubMed]
132. Hakimi, A.A.; Ostrovnaya, I.; Reva, B.; Schultz, N.; Chen, Y.-B.; Gonen, M.; Liu, H.; Takeda, S.; Voss, M.H.; Tickoo, S.K.; et al. Adverse Outcomes in Clear Cell Renal Cell Carcinoma with Mutations of 3p21 Epigenetic Regulators BAP1 and SETD2: A Report by MSKCC and the KIRC TCGA Research Network. *Clin. Cancer Res.* **2013**, *19*, 3259–3267. [CrossRef] [PubMed]
133. Hakimi, A.A.; Chen, Y.-B.; Wren, J.; Gonen, M.; Abdel-Wahab, O.; Heguy, A.; Liu, H.; Takeda, S.; Tickoo, S.K.; Reuter, V.E.; et al. Clinical and Pathologic Impact of Select Chromatin-modulating Tumor Suppressors in Clear Cell Renal Cell Carcinoma. *Eur. Urol.* **2013**, *63*, 848–854. [CrossRef]

134. Outeiro-Pinho, G.; Barros-Silva, D.; Correia, M.P.; Henrique, R.; Jerónimo, C. Renal Cell Tumors: Uncovering the Biomarker Potential of ncRNAs. *Cancers* **2020**, *12*, 2214. [CrossRef]
135. Zhou, L.; Chen, J.; Li, Z.; Li, X.; Hu, X.; Huang, Y.; Zhao, X.; Liang, C.; Wang, Y.; Sun, L.; et al. Integrated Profiling of MicroRNAs and mRNAs: MicroRNAs Located on Xq27.3 Associate with Clear Cell Renal Cell Carcinoma. *PLoS ONE* **2010**, *5*, e15224. [CrossRef] [PubMed]
136. Liu, H.; Brannon, A.R.; Reddy, A.R.; Alexe, G.; Seiler, M.W.; Arreola, A.; Oza, J.H.; Yao, M.; Juan, D.; Liou, L.S.; et al. Identifying mRNA targets of microRNA dysregulated in cancer: With application to clear cell Renal Cell Carcinoma. *BMC Syst. Biol.* **2010**, *4*, 51. [CrossRef]
137. Liu, W.; Zabirnyk, O.; Wang, H.; Shiao, Y.-H.; Nickerson, M.L.; Khalil, S.; Anderson, L.M.; O Perantoni, A.; Phang, J.M. miR-23b targets proline oxidase, a novel tumor suppressor protein in renal cancer. *Oncogene* **2010**, *29*, 4914–4924. [CrossRef]
138. Xu, H.; Wu, S.; Shen, X.; Shi, Z.; Wu, D.; Yuan, Y.; Jiang, W.; Wang, Q.; Ke, Q.; Mao, Q.; et al. Methylation-mediated miR-214 regulates proliferation and drug sensitivity of renal cell carcinoma cells through targeting LIVIN. *J. Cell. Mol. Med.* **2020**, *24*, 6410–6425. [CrossRef]
139. Wulfken, L.M.; Moritz, R.; Ohlmann, C.; Holdenrieder, S.; Jung, V.; Becker, F.; Herrmann, E.; Walgenbach-Brünagel, G.; Von Ruecker, A.; Müller, S.C.; et al. MicroRNAs in Renal Cell Carcinoma: Diagnostic Implications of Serum miR-1233 Levels. *PLoS ONE* **2011**, *6*, e25787. [CrossRef]
140. Hauser, S.; Wulfken, L.M.; Holdenrieder, S.; Moritz, R.; Ohlmann, C.-H.; Jung, V.; Becker, F.; Herrmann, E.; Walgenbach-Brünagel, G.; Von Ruecker, A.; et al. Analysis of serum microRNAs (miR-26a-2*, miR-191, miR-337-3p and miR-378) as potential biomarkers in renal cell carcinoma. *Cancer Epidemiol.* **2012**, *36*, 391–394. [CrossRef]
141. Tsiakanikas, P.; Giaginis, C.; Kontos, C.K.; Scorilas, A. Clinical utility of microRNAs in renal cell carcinoma: Current evidence and future perspectives. *Expert Rev. Mol. Diagn.* **2018**, *18*, 981–991. [CrossRef] [PubMed]
142. Redova, M.; Poprach, A.; Nekvindova, J.; Iliev, R.; Radova, L.; Lakomy, R.; Svoboda, M.; Vyzula, R.; Slaby, O. Circulating miR-378 and miR-451 in serum are potential biomarkers for renal cell carcinoma. *J. Transl. Med.* **2012**, *10*, 55. [CrossRef]
143. Zhao, A.; Li, G.; Péoc'H, M.; Genin, C.; Gigante, M. Serum miR-210 as a novel biomarker for molecular diagnosis of clear cell renal cell carcinoma. *Exp. Mol. Pathol.* **2013**, *94*, 115–120. [CrossRef] [PubMed]
144. Jung, M.; Mollenkopf, H.-J.; Grimm, C.; Wagner, I.; Albrecht, M.; Waller, T.; Pilarsky, C.; Johannsen, M.; Stephan, C.; Lehrach, H.; et al. MicroRNA profiling of clear cell renal cell cancer identifies a robust signature to define renal malignancy. *J. Cell. Mol. Med.* **2009**, *13*, 3918–3928. [CrossRef] [PubMed]
145. Silva-Santos, R.M.; Costapinheiro, P.; De Luis, A.; Antunes, L.; Lobo, F.D.A.; De Oliveira, J.M.P.F.; Henrique, R.D.S.; Jeronimo, C. MicroRNA profile: A promising ancillary tool for accurate renal cell tumour diagnosis. *Br. J. Cancer* **2013**, *109*, 2646–2653. [CrossRef]
146. Petillo, D.; Kort, E.J.; Anema, J.; Furge, K.A.; Yang, X.J.; Teh, B.T. MicroRNA profiling of human kidney cancer subtypes. *Int. J. Oncol.* **2009**, *35*, 109–114. [CrossRef]
147. Teixeira, A.L.; Ferreira, M.; Silva, J.; Gomes, M.; Dias, F.; Santos, J.I.; Maurício, J.; Lobo, F.; Medeiros, R. Higher circulating expression levels of miR-221 associated with poor overall survival in renal cell carcinoma patients. *Tumor Biol.* **2014**, *35*, 4057–4066. [CrossRef]
148. Outeiro-Pinho, G.; Barros-Silva, D.; Aznar, E.; Sousa, A.-I.; Vieira-Coimbra, M.; Oliveira, J.; Gonçalves, C.S.; Costa, B.M.; Junker, K.; Henrique, R.; et al. MicroRNA-30a-5pme: A novel diagnostic and prognostic biomarker for clear cell renal cell carcinoma in tissue and urine samples. *J. Exp. Clin. Cancer Res.* **2020**, *39*, 98. [CrossRef]
149. Joosten, S.C.; Smits, K.M.; Aarts, M.J.; Melotte, V.; Koch, A.; Tjan-Heijnen, V.C.; Van Engeland, M. Epigenetics in renal cell cancer: Mechanisms and clinical applications. *Nat. Rev. Urol.* **2018**, *15*, 430–451. [CrossRef]
150. Mitsui, Y.; Hirata, H.; Arichi, N.; Hiraki, M.; Yasumoto, H.; Chang, I.; Fukuhara, S.; Yamamura, S.; Shahryari, V.; Deng, G.; et al. Inactivation of bone morphogenetic protein 2 may predict clinical outcome and poor overall survival for renal cell carcinoma through epigenetic pathways. *Oncotarget* **2015**, *6*, 9577–9591. [CrossRef]
151. Liu, H.; Liu, Q.-L.; Zhai, T.-S.; Lu, J.; Dong, Y.-Z.; Xu, Y.-F. Silencing miR-454 suppresses cell proliferation, migration and invasion via directly targeting MECP2 in renal cell carcinoma. *Am. J. Transl. Res.* **2020**, *12*, 4277–4289.
152. White, N.M.A.; Khella, H.W.Z.; Grigull, J.; Adzovic, S.; Youssef, Y.M.; Honey, R.J.; Stewart, R.; Pace, K.T.; Bjarnason, G.A.; Jewett, M.A.S.; et al. miRNA profiling in metastatic renal cell carcinoma reveals a tumour-suppressor effect for miR-215. *Br. J. Cancer* **2011**, *105*, 1741–1749. [CrossRef] [PubMed]
153. Lawrie, C.H.; Larrea, E.; Larrinaga, G.; Goicoechea, I.; Arestin, M.; Fernandez-Mercado, M.; Hes, O.; Cáceres, F.; Manterola, L.; López, J.I. Targeted next-generation sequencing and non-coding RNA expression analysis of clear cell papillary renal cell carcinoma suggests distinct pathological mechanisms from other renal tumour subtypes. *J. Pathol.* **2014**, *232*, 32–42. [CrossRef]
154. Liu, M.; Zhou, J.; Chen, Z.; Cheng, A.S.-L. Understanding the epigenetic regulation of tumours and their microenvironments: Opportunities and problems for epigenetic therapy. *J. Pathol.* **2017**, *241*, 10–24. [CrossRef] [PubMed]
155. Yu, G.; Yao, W.; Wang, J.; Ma, X.; Xiao, W.; Li, H.; Xia, D.; Yang, Y.; Deng, K.; Xiao, H.; et al. LncRNAs Expression Signatures of Renal Clear Cell Carcinoma Revealed by Microarray. *PLoS ONE* **2012**, *7*, e42377. [CrossRef] [PubMed]
156. Qin, C.; Han, Z.; Qian, J.; Bao, M.; Li, P.; Ju, X.; Zhang, S.; Zhang, L.; Li, S.; Cao, Q.; et al. Expression Pattern of Long Non-Coding RNAs in Renal Cell Carcinoma Revealed by Microarray. *PLoS ONE* **2014**, *9*, e99372. [CrossRef]

157. Blondeau, J.J.; Deng, M.; Syring, I.; Schrödter, S.; Schmidt, D.; Perner, S.; Müller, S.C.; Ellinger, J. Identification of novel long non-coding RNAs in clear cell renal cell carcinoma. *Clin. Epigenetics* **2015**, *7*, 10. [CrossRef] [PubMed]
158. Wu, Y.; Liu, J.; Zheng, Y.; You, L.; Kuang, D.; Liu, T. Suppressed expression of long non-coding RNA HOTAIR inhibits proliferation and tumourigenicity of renal carcinoma cells. *Tumor Biol.* **2014**, *35*, 11887–11894. [CrossRef] [PubMed]
159. Xia, M.; Yao, L.; Zhang, Q.; Wang, F.; Mei, H.; Guo, X.; Huang, W. Long noncoding RNA HOTAIR promotes metastasis of renal cell carcinoma by up-regulating histone H3K27 demethylase JMJD3. *Oncotarget* **2017**, *8*, 19795–19802. [CrossRef] [PubMed]
160. Raveh, E.; Matouk, I.J.; Gilon, M.; Hochberg, A. The H19 Long non-coding RNA in cancer initiation, progression and metastasis—A proposed unifying theory. *Mol. Cancer* **2015**, *14*, 184. [CrossRef] [PubMed]
161. Gu, Y.; Niu, S.; Wang, Y.; Duan, L.; Pan, Y.; Tong, Z.; Zhang, X.; Yang, Z.; Peng, B.; Wang, X.; et al. DMDRMR-Mediated Regulation of m6A-Modified CDK4 by m6A Reader IGF2BP3 Drives ccRCC Progression. *Cancer Res.* **2020**, *81*, 923–934. [CrossRef]
162. Xin, Z.; Soejima, H.; Higashimoto, K.; Yatsuki, H.; Zhu, X.; Satoh, Y.; Masaki, Z.; Kaneko, Y.; Jinno, Y.; Fukuzawa, R.; et al. A Novel Imprinted Gene, KCNQ1DN, within the WT2 Critical Region of Human Chromosome 11p15.5 and Its Reduced Expression in Wilms' Tumors. *J. Biochem.* **2000**, *128*, 847–853. [CrossRef]
163. Roundtree, I.A.; Evans, M.E.; Pan, T.; He, C. Dynamic RNA Modifications in Gene Expression Regulation. *Cell* **2017**, *169*, 1187–1200. [CrossRef] [PubMed]
164. Enroth, C.; Poulsen, L.D.; Iversen, S.; Kirpekar, F.; Albrechtsen, A.; Vinther, J. Detection of internal N7-methylguanosine (m7G) RNA modifications by mutational profiling sequencing. *Nucleic Acids Res.* **2019**, *47*, e126. [CrossRef] [PubMed]
165. Fu, Y.; Dominissini, D.; Rechavi, G.; He, C. Gene expression regulation mediated through reversible m^{6}A RNA methylation. *Nat. Rev. Genet.* **2014**, *15*, 293–306. [CrossRef] [PubMed]
166. Yang, Y.; Hsu, P.J.; Chen, Y.S.; Yang, Y.G. Dynamic transcriptomic m6A decoration: Writers, erasers, readers and functions in RNA metabolism. *Cell Res.* **2018**, *28*, 616–624. [CrossRef]
167. Li, Y.; Xiao, J.; Bai, J.; Tian, Y.; Qu, Y.; Chen, X.; Wang, Q.; Li, X.; Zhang, Y.; Xu, J. Molecular characterization and clinical relevance of m6A regulators across 33 cancer types. *Mol. Cancer* **2019**, *18*, 137. [CrossRef] [PubMed]
168. Sun, Z.; Jing, C.; Xiao, C.; Li, T.; Wang, Y. Prognostic risk signature based on the expression of three m6A RNA methylation regulatory genes in kidney renal papillary cell carcinoma. *Aging* **2020**, *12*, 22078–22094. [CrossRef]
169. Lobo, J.; Barros-Silva, D.; Henrique, R.; Jerónimo, C. The Emerging Role of Epitranscriptomics in Cancer: Focus on Urological Tumors. *Genes* **2018**, *9*, 552. [CrossRef]
170. Yoo, C.B.; Jones, P.A. Epigenetic therapy of cancer: Past, present and future. *Nat. Rev. Drug Discov.* **2006**, *5*, 37–50. [CrossRef] [PubMed]
171. Arrowsmith, C.H.; Bountra, C.; Fish, P.V.; Lee, K.; Schapira, M. Epigenetic protein families: A new frontier for drug discovery. *Nat. Rev. Drug Discov.* **2012**, *11*, 384–400. [CrossRef] [PubMed]
172. Issa, J.-P.J.; Kantarjian, H.M. Targeting DNA Methylation. *Clin. Cancer Res.* **2009**, *15*, 3938–3946. [CrossRef] [PubMed]
173. Chi, P.; Allis, C.D.; Wang, G.G. Covalent histone modifications—Miswritten, misinterpreted and mis-erased in human cancers. *Nat. Rev. Cancer* **2010**, *10*, 457–469. [CrossRef]
174. Marques-Magalhães, Â.; Graca, I.; Henrique, R.; Jerónimo, C. Targeting DNA Methyltranferases in Urological Tumors. *Front. Pharmacol.* **2018**, *9*, 366. [CrossRef] [PubMed]
175. Faleiro, I.; Leão, R.; Binnie, A.; De Mello, R.A.; Maia, A.-T.; Castelo-Branco, P. Epigenetic therapy in urologic cancers: An update on clinical trials. *Oncotarget* **2017**, *8*, 12484–12500. [CrossRef]
176. Wu, Y.; Sarkissyan, M.; Vadgama, J.V. Epigenetics in Breast and Prostate Cancer. *Methods Mol. Biol.* **2015**, *1238*, 425–466. [CrossRef]
177. Pili, R.; Liu, G.; Chintala, S.; Verheul, H.; Rehman, S.; Attwood, K.; Lodge, M.A.; Wahl, R.; Martin, J.I.; Miles, K.M.; et al. Combination of the histone deacetylase inhibitor vorinostat with bevacizumab in patients with clear-cell renal cell carcinoma: A multicentre, single-arm phase I/II clinical trial. *Br. J. Cancer* **2017**, *116*, 874–883. [CrossRef] [PubMed]
178. Park, H.; Garrido-Laguna, I.; Naing, A.; Fu, S.; Falchook, G.S.; Piha-Paul, S.A.; Wheler, J.J.; Hong, D.S.; Tsimberidou, A.M.; Subbiah, V.; et al. Phase I dose-escalation study of the mTOR inhibitor sirolimus and the HDAC inhibitor vorinostat in patients with advanced malignancy. *Oncotarget* **2016**, *7*, 67521–67531. [CrossRef] [PubMed]
179. Zibelman, M.; Wong, Y.-N.; Devarajan, K.; Malizzia, L.; Corrigan, A.; Olszanski, A.J.; Denlinger, C.S.; Roethke, S.K.; Tetzlaff, C.H.; Plimack, E.R. Phase I study of the mTOR inhibitor ridaforolimus and the HDAC inhibitor vorinostat in advanced renal cell carcinoma and other solid tumors. *Investig. New Drugs* **2015**, *33*, 1040–1047. [CrossRef]
180. Hainsworth, J.D.; Infante, J.R.; Spigel, D.R.; Arrowsmith, E.R.; Boccia, R.V.; Burris, H.A. A phase II trial of panobinostat, a histone deacetylase inhibitor, in the treatment of patients with refractory metastatic renal cell carcinoma. *Cancer Investig.* **2011**, *29*, 451–455. [CrossRef]
181. Wood, A.; George, S.; Adra, N.; Chintala, S.; Damayanti, N.; Pili, R. Phase I study of the mTOR inhibitor everolimus in combination with the histone deacetylase inhibitor panobinostat in patients with advanced clear cell renal cell carcinoma. *Investig. New Drugs* **2020**, *38*, 1108–1116. [CrossRef]
182. Pili, R.; Salumbides, B.; Zhao, M.; Altiok, S.; Qian, D.; Zwiebel, J.; Carducci, M.A.; Rudek, M.A. Phase I study of the histone deacetylase inhibitor entinostat in combination with 13-cis retinoic acid in patients with solid tumours. *Br. J. Cancer* **2012**, *106*, 77–84. [CrossRef] [PubMed]

183. Pili, R.; Quinn, D.I.; Hammers, H.J.; Monk, P.; George, S.; Dorff, T.B.; Olencki, T.; Shen, L.; Orillion, A.; LaMonica, D.; et al. Immunomodulation by Entinostat in Renal Cell Carcinoma Patients Receiving High-Dose Interleukin 2: A Multicenter, Single-Arm, Phase I/II Trial (NCI-CTEP#7870). *Clin. Cancer Res.* **2017**, *23*, 7199–7208. [CrossRef]
184. Stadler, W.M.; Margolin, K.; Ferber, S.; McCulloch, W.; Thompson, J.A. A Phase II Study of Depsipeptide in Refractory Metastatic Renal Cell Cancer. *Clin. Genitourin. Cancer* **2006**, *5*, 57–60. [CrossRef] [PubMed]
185. Whitehead, R.P.; Rankin, C.; Hoff, H.M.G.; Gold, P.J.; Billingsley, K.G.; Chapman, R.A.; Wong, L.; Ward, J.H.; Abbruzzese, J.L.; Blanke, C.D. Phase II Trial of depsipeptide (NSC-630176) in previously treated colorectal cancer patients with advanced disease: A Southwest Oncology Group Study (S0336). *Investig. New Drugs* **2009**, *27*, 469–475. [CrossRef] [PubMed]
186. Steele, N.L.; Plumb, J.A.; Vidal, L.; Tjørnelund, J.; Knoblauch, P.; Rasmussen, A.; Ooi, C.E.; Buhl-Jensen, P.; Brown, R.; Evans, T.J.; et al. A Phase 1 Pharmacokinetic and Pharmacodynamic Study of the Histone Deacetylase Inhibitor Belinostat in Patients with Advanced Solid Tumors. *Clin. Cancer Res.* **2008**, *14*, 804–810. [CrossRef] [PubMed]
187. Braiteh, F.; Soriano, A.O.; Garcia-Manero, G.; Hong, D.; Johnson, M.M.; Silva, L.D.P.; Yang, H.; Alexander, S.; Wolff, J.; Kurzrock, R. Phase I Study of Epigenetic Modulation with 5-Azacytidine and Valproic Acid in Patients with Advanced Cancers. *Clin. Cancer Res.* **2008**, *14*, 6296–6301. [CrossRef] [PubMed]
188. Stewart, D.J.; Issa, J.-P.; Kurzrock, R.; Nunez, M.I.; Jelinek, J.; Hong, D.; Oki, Y.; Guo, Z.; Gupta, S.; Wistuba, I.I. Decitabine Effect on Tumor Global DNA Methylation and Other Parameters in a Phase I Trial in Refractory Solid Tumors and Lymphomas. *Clin. Cancer Res.* **2009**, *15*, 3881–3888. [CrossRef]
189. Gollob, J.A.; Sciambi, C.J.; Peterson, B.L.; Richmond, T.; Thoreson, M.; Moran, K.; Dressman, H.K.; Jelinek, J.; Issa, J.-P.J. Phase I Trial of Sequential Low-Dose 5-Aza-2′-Deoxycytidine Plus High-Dose Intravenous Bolus Interleukin-2 in Patients with Melanoma or Renal Cell Carcinoma. *Clin. Cancer Res.* **2006**, *12*, 4619–4627. [CrossRef]
190. Winquist, E.; Knox, J.; Ayoub, J.-P.; Wood, L.; Wainman, N.; Reid, G.K.; Pearce, L.; Shah, A.; Eisenhauer, E. Phase II trial of DNA methyltransferase 1 inhibition with the antisense oligonucleotide MG98 in patients with metastatic renal carcinoma: A National Cancer Institute of Canada Clinical Trials Group investigational new drug study. *Investig. New Drugs* **2006**, *24*, 159–167. [CrossRef]
191. Amato, R.J. Inhibition of DNA Methylation by Antisense Oligonucleotide MG98 as Cancer Therapy. *Clin. Genitourin. Cancer* **2007**, *5*, 422–426. [CrossRef]
192. Vassilakos, A.; Lee, Y.; Viau, S.; Feng, N.; Jin, H.; Chai, V.; Wang, M.; Avolio, T.; Wright, J.; Young, A.; et al. GTI-2040 displays cooperative anti-tumor activity when combined with interferon α against human renal carcinoma xenografts. *Int. J. Oncol.* **2009**, *34*, 33–42. [CrossRef]
193. Margolin, K.; Synold, T.W.; Lara, P.; Frankel, P.; Lacey, S.F.; Quinn, D.I.; Baratta, T.; Dutcher, J.P.; Xi, B.; Diamond, D.J.; et al. Oblimersen and α-interferon in metastatic renal cancer: A phase II study of the California Cancer Consortium. *J. Cancer Res. Clin. Oncol.* **2007**, *133*, 705–711. [CrossRef]
194. Tsai, H.-C.; Li, H.; Van Neste, L.; Cai, Y.; Robert, C.; Rassool, F.V.; Shin, J.J.; Harbom, K.M.; Beaty, R.; Pappou, E.; et al. Transient Low Doses of DNA-Demethylating Agents Exert Durable Antitumor Effects on Hematological and Epithelial Tumor Cells. *Cancer Cell* **2012**, *21*, 430–446. [CrossRef]
195. Roboz, G.J.; Kantarjian, H.M.; Yee, K.W.L.; Kropf, P.L.; O'Connell, C.L.; Griffiths, E.A.; Stock, W.; Daver, N.G.; Jabbour, E.; Ritchie, E.K.; et al. Dose, schedule, safety, and efficacy of guadecitabine in relapsed or refractory acute myeloid leukemia. *Cancer* **2018**, *124*, 325–334. [CrossRef]
196. Venturelli, S.; Berger, A.; Weiland, T.; Essmann, F.; Waibel, M.; Nuebling, T.; Häcker, S.; Schenk, M.; Schulze-Osthoff, K.; Salih, H.R.; et al. Differential Induction of Apoptosis and Senescence by the DNA Methyltransferase Inhibitors 5-Azacytidine and 5-Aza-2′-Deoxycytidine in Solid Tumor Cells. *Mol. Cancer Ther.* **2013**, *12*, 2226–2236. [CrossRef] [PubMed]
197. Li, H.; Chiappinelli, K.B.; Guzzetta, A.A.; Easwaran, H.; Yen, R.-W.C.; Vatapalli, R.; Topper, M.J.; Luo, J.; Connolly, R.M.; Azad, N.S.; et al. Immune regulation by low doses of the DNA methyltransferase inhibitor 5-azacitidine in common human epithelial cancers. *Oncotarget* **2014**, *5*, 587–598. [CrossRef] [PubMed]
198. Ricketts, C.J.; Morris, M.R.; Gentle, D.; Shuib, S.; Brown, M.; Clarke, N.; Wei, W.; Nathan, P.; Latif, F.; Maher, E.R. Methylation profiling and evaluation of demethylating therapy in renal cell carcinoma. *Clin. Epigenetics* **2013**, *5*, 16. [CrossRef] [PubMed]
199. Shang, D.; Han, T.; Xu, X.; Liu, Y. Decitabine induces G2/M cell cycle arrest by suppressing p38/NF-κB signaling in human renal clear cell carcinoma. *Int. J. Clin. Exp. Pathol.* **2015**, *8*, 11140–11148. [PubMed]
200. Konac, E.; Varol, N.; Yilmaz, A.; Menevse, S.; Sozen, S. DNA methyltransferase inhibitor-mediated apoptosis in the Wnt/β-catenin signal pathway in a renal cell carcinoma cell line. *Exp. Biol. Med. Maywood* **2013**, *238*, 1009–1016. [CrossRef]
201. Xi, W.; Chen, X.; Sun, J.; Wang, W.; Huo, Y.; Zheng, G.; Wu, J.; Li, Y.; Yang, A.; Wang, T. Combined Treatment with Valproic Acid and 5-Aza-2′-Deoxycytidine Synergistically Inhibits Human Clear Cell Renal Cell Carcinoma Growth and Migration. *Med Sci. Monit.* **2018**, *24*, 1034–1043. [CrossRef]
202. Reu, F.J.; Bae, S.I.; Cherkassky, L.; Leaman, D.W.; Lindner, D.; Beaulieu, N.; MacLeod, A.R.; Borden, E.C. Overcoming Resistance to Interferon-Induced Apoptosis of Renal Carcinoma and Melanoma Cells by DNA Demethylation. *J. Clin. Oncol.* **2006**, *24*, 3771–3779. [CrossRef]
203. Reu, F.J.; Leaman, D.W.; Maitra, R.R.; Bae, S.I.; Cherkassky, L.; Fox, M.W.; Rempinski, D.R.; Beaulieu, N.; MacLeod, A.R.; Borden, E.C. Expression of RASSF1A, an epigenetically silenced tumor suppressor, overcomes resistance to apoptosis induction by interferons. *Cancer Res.* **2006**, *66*, 2785–2793. [CrossRef] [PubMed]

204. Zhu, Q.; Yu, L.; Qin, Z.; Chen, L.; Hu, H.; Zheng, X.; Zeng, S. Regulation of OCT2 transcriptional repression by histone acetylation in renal cell carcinoma. *Epigenetics* 2019, *14*, 791–803. [CrossRef] [PubMed]
205. Amato, R.J.; Stephenson, J.; Hotte, S.; Nemunaitis, J.; Bélanger, K.; Reid, G.; Martell, R.E. MG98, a Second-Generation DNMT1 Inhibitor, in the Treatment of Advanced Renal Cell Carcinoma. *Cancer Investig.* 2012, *30*, 415–421. [CrossRef] [PubMed]
206. Cameron, E.E.; Bachman, K.E.; Myöhänen, S.; Herman, J.G.; Baylin, S.B. Synergy of demethylation and histone deacetylase inhibition in the re-expression of genes silenced in cancer. *Nat. Genet.* 1999, *21*, 103–107. [CrossRef]
207. Dasari, A.; Gore, L.; Messersmith, W.A.; Diab, S.; Jimeno, A.; Weekes, C.D.; Lewis, K.D.; Drabkin, H.A.; Flaig, T.W.; Camidge, D.R. A phase I study of sorafenib and vorinostat in patients with advanced solid tumors with expanded cohorts in renal cell carcinoma and non-small cell lung cancer. *Investig. New Drugs* 2013, *31*, 115–125. [CrossRef]
208. Morgan, S.S.; Cranmer, L.D. Vorinostat synergizes with ridaforolimus and abrogates the ridaforolimus-induced activation of AKT in synovial sarcoma cells. *BMC Res. Notes* 2014, *7*, 812. [CrossRef]
209. Cha, T.-L.; Chuang, M.-J.; Wu, S.-T.; Sun, G.-H.; Chang, S.-Y.; Yu, D.-S.; Huang, S.-M.; Huan, S.K.-H.; Cheng, T.-C.; Chen, T.-T.; et al. Dual Degradation of Aurora A and B Kinases by the Histone Deacetylase Inhibitor LBH589 Induces G2-M Arrest and Apoptosis of Renal Cancer Cells. *Clin. Cancer Res.* 2009, *15*, 840–850. [CrossRef]
210. Lemoine, M.; Derenzini, E.; Buglio, D.; Medeiros, L.J.; Davis, R.E.; Zhang, J.; Ji, Y.; Younes, A. The pan-deacetylase inhibitor panobinostat induces cell death and synergizes with everolimus in Hodgkin lymphoma cell lines. *Blood* 2012, *119*, 4017–4025. [CrossRef]
211. Beider, K.; Bitner, H.; Voevoda-Dimenshtein, V.; Rosenberg, E.; Sirovsky, Y.; Magen, H.; Canaani, J.; Ostrovsky, O.; Shilo, N.; Shimoni, A.; et al. The mTOR inhibitor everolimus overcomes CXCR4-mediated resistance to histone deacetylase inhibitor panobinostat through inhibition of p21 and mitotic regulators. *Biochem. Pharmacol.* 2019, *168*, 412–428. [CrossRef]
212. Ling, Y.; Liu, J.; Qian, J.; Meng, C.; Guo, J.; Gao, W.; Xiong, B.; Ling, C.; Zhang, Y. Recent Advances in Multi-target Drugs Targeting Protein Kinases and Histone Deacetylases in Cancer Therapy. *Curr. Med. Chem.* 2020, *27*, 7264–7288. [CrossRef]
213. Lachenmayer, A.; Toffanin, S.; Cabellos, L.; Alsinet, C.; Hoshida, Y.; Villanueva, A.; Minguez, B.; Tsai, H.-W.; Ward, S.C.; Thung, S.; et al. Combination therapy for hepatocellular carcinoma: Additive preclinical efficacy of the HDAC inhibitor panobinostat with sorafenib. *J. Hepatol.* 2012, *56*, 1343–1350. [CrossRef] [PubMed]
214. Wang, X.F.; Qian, D.Z.; Ren, M.; Kato, Y.; Wei, Y.; Zhang, L.; Fansler, Z.; Clark, D.; Nakanishi, O.; Pili, R. Epigenetic modulation of retinoic acid receptor beta2 by the histone deacetylase inhibitor MS-275 in human renal cell carcinoma. *Clin. Cancer Res.* 2005, *11*, 3535–3542. [CrossRef]
215. Rini, B.I.; Powles, T.; Atkins, M.B.; Escudier, B.; McDermott, D.F.; Suarez, C.; Bracarda, S.; Stadler, W.M.; Donskov, F.; Lee, J.L.; et al. Atezolizumab plus bevacizumab versus sunitinib in patients with previously untreated metastatic renal cell carcinoma (IMmotion151): A multicentre, open-label, phase 3, randomised controlled trial. *Lancet* 2019, *393*, 2404–2415. [CrossRef]
216. Chan, K.K.; Bakhtiar, R.; Jiang, C. Depsipeptide (FR901228, NSC-630176) pharmacokinetics in the rat by LC/MS/MS. *Investig. New Drugs* 1997, *15*, 195–206. [CrossRef]
217. Sborov, D.W.; Canella, A.; Hade, E.M.; Mo, X.; Khountham, S.; Wang, J.; Ni, W.; Poi, M.; Coss, C.; Liu, Z.; et al. A phase 1 trial of the HDAC inhibitor AR-42 in patients with multiple myeloma and T- and B-cell lymphomas. *Leuk. Lymphoma* 2017, *58*, 2310–2318. [CrossRef] [PubMed]
218. Chen, Y.-J.; Wang, W.-H.; Wu, W.-Y.; Hsu, C.-C.; Wei, L.-R.; Wang, S.-F.; Hsu, Y.-W.; Liaw, C.-C.; Tsai, W.-C. Novel histone deacetylase inhibitor AR-42 exhibits antitumor activity in pancreatic cancer cells by affecting multiple biochemical pathways. *PLoS ONE* 2017, *12*, e0183368. [CrossRef] [PubMed]
219. Chakraborty, C.; Sharma, A.R.; Sharma, G.; Lee, S.-S. Therapeutic advances of miRNAs: A preclinical and clinical update. *J. Adv. Res.* 2020, *28*, 127–138. [CrossRef] [PubMed]
220. Kelly, J.D.; Dai, J.; Eschwege, P.; Goldberg, J.S.; Duggan, B.P.; Williamson, K.E.; Bander, N.H.; Nanus, D.M. Downregulation of Bcl-2 sensitises interferon-resistant renal cancer cells to Fas. *Br. J. Cancer* 2004, *91*, 164–170. [CrossRef]
221. Lee, Y.; Vassilakos, A.; Feng, N.; Lam, V.; Xie, H.; Wang, M.; Jin, H.; Xiong, K.; Liu, C.; Wright, J.; et al. GTI-2040, an antisense agent targeting the small subunit component (R2) of human ribonucleotide reductase, shows potent antitumor activity against a variety of tumors. *Cancer Res.* 2003, *63*, 2802–2811.
222. Stadler, W.M.; Desai, A.A.; Quinn, D.I.; Bukowski, R.; Poiesz, B.; Kardinal, C.G.; Lewis, N.; Makalinao, A.; Murray, P.; Torti, F.M. A Phase I/II study of GTI-2040 and capecitabine in patients with renal cell carcinoma. *Cancer Chemother. Pharmacol.* 2008, *61*, 689–694. [CrossRef]
223. Tan, X.; Zhang, Z.; Liu, P.; Yao, H.; Shen, L.; Tong, J.-S. Inhibition of EZH2 enhances the therapeutic effect of 5-FU via PUMA upregulation in colorectal cancer. *Cell Death Dis.* 2020, *11*, 1061. [CrossRef] [PubMed]
224. Dockerill, M.; Gregson, C.; Donovan, D.H.O. Targeting PRC2 for the treatment of cancer: An updated patent review (2016–2020). *Expert Opin. Ther. Pat.* 2021, *31*, 1–17. [CrossRef] [PubMed]
225. LaFave, L.M.; Béguelin, W.; Koche, R.P.; Teater, M.; Spitzer, B.; Chramiec, A.; Papalexi, E.; Keller, M.D.; Hricik, T.; Konstantinoff, K.; et al. Loss of BAP1 function leads to EZH2-dependent transformation. *Nat. Med.* 2015, *21*, 1344–1349. [CrossRef] [PubMed]
226. Kim, K.H.; Kim, W.; Howard, T.P.; Vazquez, F.; Tsherniak, A.; Wu, J.N.; Wang, W.; Haswell, J.R.; Walensky, L.D.; Hahn, W.C.; et al. SWI/SNF-mutant cancers depend on catalytic and non-catalytic activity of EZH2. *Nat. Med.* 2015, *21*, 1491–1496. [CrossRef]
227. Cheng, Y.; He, C.; Wang, M.; Ma, X.; Mo, F.; Yang, S.; Han, J.; Wei, X. Targeting epigenetic regulators for cancer therapy: Mechanisms and advances in clinical trials. *Signal Transduct. Target. Ther.* 2019, *4*, 62. [CrossRef]

228. López, J.I.; Pulido, R.; Cortés, J.M.; Angulo, J.C.; Lawrie, C.H. Potential impact of PD-L1 (SP-142) immunohistochemical heterogeneity in clear cell renal cell carcinoma immunotherapy. *Pathol. Res. Pract.* **2018**, *214*, 1110–1114. [CrossRef]
229. Liu, S.; Yang, Z.; Li, G.; Li, C.; Luo, Y.; Gong, Q.; Wu, X.; Li, T.; Zhang, Z.; Xing, B.; et al. Multi-omics Analysis of Primary Cell Culture Models Reveals Genetic and Epigenetic Basis of Intratumoral Phenotypic Diversity. *Genom. Proteom. Bioinform.* **2019**, *17*, 576–589. [CrossRef]
230. Ortega, M.A.; Poirion, O.; Zhu, X.; Huang, S.; Wolfgruber, T.K.; Sebra, R.; Garmire, L.X. Using single-cell multiple omics approaches to resolve tumor heterogeneity. *Clin. Transl. Med.* **2017**, *6*, 46. [CrossRef]
231. López-Fernández, E.; López, J.I. The Impact of Tumor Eco-Evolution in Renal Cell Carcinoma Sampling. *Cancers* **2018**, *10*, 485. [CrossRef]
232. Zhao, T.; Bao, Y.; Gan, X.; Wang, J.; Chen, Q.; Dai, Z.; Liu, B.; Wang, A.; Sun, S.; Yang, F.; et al. DNA methylation-regulated QPCT promotes sunitinib resistance by increasing HRAS stability in renal cell carcinoma. *Theranostics* **2019**, *9*, 6175–6190. [CrossRef]
233. Xiong, Z.; Yuan, C.; Shi, J.; Xiong, W.; Huang, Y.; Xiao, W.; Yang, H.; Chen, K.; Zhang, X. Restoring the epigenetically silenced PCK2 suppresses renal cell carcinoma progression and increases sensitivity to sunitinib by promoting endoplasmic reticulum stress. *Theranostics* **2020**, *10*, 11444–11461. [CrossRef] [PubMed]
234. Lobo, J.; Jerónimo, C.; Henrique, R. Targeting the Immune system and Epigenetic Landscape of Urological Tumors. *Int. J. Mol. Sci.* **2020**, *21*, 829. [CrossRef]
235. Dunn, J.; Rao, S. Epigenetics and immunotherapy: The current state of play. *Mol. Immunol.* **2017**, *87*, 227–239. [CrossRef] [PubMed]
236. Liu, X.-D.; Kong, W.; Peterson, C.B.; McGrail, D.J.; Hoang, A.; Zhang, X.; Lam, T.; Pilie, P.G.; Zhu, H.; Beckermann, K.E.; et al. PBRM1 loss defines a nonimmunogenic tumor phenotype associated with checkpoint inhibitor resistance in renal carcinoma. *Nat. Commun.* **2020**, *11*, 2135. [CrossRef] [PubMed]
237. Miao, D.; Margolis, C.A.; Gao, W.; Voss, M.H.; Li, W.; Martini, D.J.; Norton, C.; Bossé, D.; Wankowicz, S.M.; Cullen, D.; et al. Genomic correlates of response to immune checkpoint therapies in clear cell renal cell carcinoma. *Science* **2018**, *359*, 801–806. [CrossRef]
238. Bi, K.; He, M.X.; Bakouny, Z.; Kanodia, A.; Napolitano, S.; Wu, J.; Grimaldi, G.; Braun, D.A.; Cuoco, M.S.; Mayorga, A.; et al. Tumor and immune reprogramming during immunotherapy in advanced renal cell carcinoma. *Cancer Cell* **2021**. [CrossRef] [PubMed]
239. Braun, D.A.; Ishii, Y.; Walsh, A.M.; Van Allen, E.M.; Wu, C.J.; Shukla, S.A.; Choueiri, T.K. Clinical Validation of PBRM1 Alterations as a Marker of Immune Checkpoint Inhibitor Response in Renal Cell Carcinoma. *JAMA Oncol.* **2019**, *5*, 1631–1633. [CrossRef] [PubMed]
240. Chiappinelli, K.B.; Zahnow, C.A.; Ahuja, N.; Baylin, S.B. Combining Epigenetic and Immunotherapy to Combat Cancer. *Cancer Res.* **2016**, *76*, 1683–1689. [CrossRef] [PubMed]
241. McGoverne, I.; Dunn, J.; Batham, J.; Tu, W.J.; Chrisp, J.; Rao, S. Epitherapy and immune checkpoint blockade: Using epigenetic reinvigoration of exhausted and dysfunctional T cells to reimburse immunotherapy response. *BMC Immunol.* **2020**, *21*, 22. [CrossRef]
242. Goldsamt, A.; Damayanti, N.P.; De Nigris, F.; Pili, R. Epigenetic dysregulation in advanced kidney cancer: Opportunities for therapeutic interventions. *Cancer J.* **2020**, *26*, 399–406. [CrossRef]

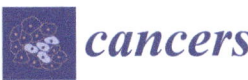

Review

Updates on Immunotherapy and Immune Landscape in Renal Clear Cell Carcinoma

Myung-Chul Kim [1,2], Zeng Jin [1,2], Ryan Kolb [1,2], Nicholas Borcherding [3], Jonathan Alexander Chatzkel [4], Sara Moscovita Falzarano [1,2] and Weizhou Zhang [1,2,*]

1 Department of Pathology, Immunology and Laboratory Medicine, University of Florida, Gainesville, FL 32610, USA; my.kim@ufl.edu (M.-C.K.); Zengjin@ufl.edu (Z.J.); Ryankolb@ufl.edu (R.K.); sfalzarano@ufl.edu (S.M.F.)
2 UF Health Cancer Center, University of Florida, Gainesville, FL 32610, USA
3 Department of Pathology and Immunology, Washington University, St. Louis, MO 63110, USA; borcherding.n@wustl.edu
4 Department of Medicine Hematology and Oncology Division, University of Florida, Gainesville, FL 32610, USA; Jonathan.Chatzkel@medicine.ufl.edu
* Correspondence: zhangw@ufl.edu; Tel.: +1-352-273-6748

Simple Summary: Clear cell renal cell carcinomas (ccRCC) have several distinct immunological features, including a high degree of immune infiltration and relatively low mutational burdens, the resistance to cytotoxic chemotherapy, and relative sensitivity to anti-angiogenic therapy and immunotherapies. Immune checkpoint inhibitor (ICI) therapy has become standard care in the treatment of ccRCC, but a better understanding of the molecular and cellular characteristics of ccRCC is needed to truly optimize the use of ICI therapy. With a focus on cancer immunology, we summarize the clinical trials of ICIs in ccRCC, the molecular and cellular correlates of these clinical trials, and the single-cell RNA sequencing studies to provide a comprehensive overview of the immune landscape within the ccRCC tumor microenvironment, in particular in the context of ICI therapy. We will discuss potential molecular and cellular biomarkers that can be used to predict therapeutic responses in ccRCC patients.

Abstract: Several clinicopathological features of clear cell renal cell carcinomas (ccRCC) contribute to make an "atypical" cancer, including resistance to chemotherapy, sensitivity to anti-angiogenesis therapy and ICIs despite a low mutational burden, and CD8[+] T cell infiltration being the predictor for poor prognosis–normally CD8[+] T cell infiltration is a good prognostic factor in cancer patients. These "atypical" features have brought researchers to investigate the molecular and immunological mechanisms that lead to the increased T cell infiltrates despite relatively low molecular burdens, as well as to decipher the immune landscape that leads to better response to ICIs. In the present study, we summarize the past and ongoing pivotal clinical trials of immunotherapies for ccRCC, emphasizing the potential molecular and cellular mechanisms that lead to the success or failure of ICI therapy. Single-cell analysis of ccRCC has provided a more thorough and detailed understanding of the tumor immune microenvironment and has facilitated the discovery of molecular biomarkers from the tumor-infiltrating immune cells. We herein will focus on the discussion of some major immune cells, including T cells and tumor-associated macrophages (TAM) in ccRCC. We will further provide some perspectives of using molecular and cellular biomarkers derived from these immune cell types to potentially improve the response rate to ICIs in ccRCC patients.

Keywords: single-cell RNA sequencing; immune landscape; cancer immunotherapy; clear cell renal cell carcinoma

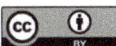

1. Introduction

Renal cell carcinomas (RCC) arise from the renal epithelium and account for more than 90% of cancers occurring in the kidney [1]. There are about 76,000 new cases annually in the U.S. and 403,000 worldwide, accounting for about 3% of all cancers [2,3].

About 70% of patients with RCC have localized tumors at the time of diagnosis, and 12% of the cancer patients have metastatic tumors [4]. Approximately 50% of patients with localized RCC ultimately develop metastatic disease, and the 5-year survival rate of patients with metastatic RCC is approximately 14% [1,5,6]. In general, about 25% to 50% of patients with primary RCC experience recurrence following nephrectomy after five years [7]. RCC is histologically classified into subtypes, of which clear cell RCC (ccRCC) is the most common–accounting for more than 80% of RCCs, followed by papillary RCC and chromophobe RCC [1,4]. ccRCC is characterized by the abundance of glycogen and lipids in the cytosol [1,4]. Most patients with ccRCC show chromosomal 3p loss and genomic mutations in the *Von Hippel-Lindau Tumor Suppressor* (*VHL*) allele [8], followed by secondary loss of multiple tumor suppressor genes, including *PBRM1*, *SETD2*, *BAP1*, and/or *KDM5C* [9]. The VHL inactivation stabilizes hypoxia-inducible factors (HIFs) in ccRCC, including HIF1α and HIF2α [10]. The activation of HIFs leads to transcriptional activation of numerous HIF target genes, including vascular endothelial growth factor (*VEGF*), which is one of the major known mechanisms responsible for high angiogenesis and inflammatory response in the ccRCC tumor microenvironment [10,11].

Tyrosine kinase inhibitors (TKIs) are representative first-line anti-angiogenic targeted therapies to inhibit VEGF and its receptor (VEGFR) signaling in patients with metastatic ccRCC. These TKIs are effective, with a limited number of patients showing complete remission of ccRCC [12]. Generally, however, these targeted therapies are only palliative, and the utility of this therapy is frequently limited by drug resistance [13].

The Food and Drug Administration (FDA) approved the use of nivolumab (anti-PD-1) for patients with RCC in 2015. Since then, numerous clinical trials have demonstrated the safety and efficacy of a variety of immune checkpoint inhibitors (ICI) for RCC patients [14,15]. Spontaneous immune activation is thought to contribute to the regression of 1 to 7% of ccRCC patients [16–19]. Early clinical trials enhancing T cell proliferation through high-dose interleukin 2 (IL-2) achieved up to 20% of therapeutic response [20]. ICI monotherapy showed 25 to 42% response rates in ccRCC patients [15,21]. In studies evaluating ICI in combination with anti-VEGF or TKIs as a first-line therapy, it significantly improved the clinical outcome in patients with ccRCC, showing an objective response rate (ORR) of 50 to 59%, including 4 to 12% complete response (CR) rates, depending on experimental settings [21–25]. Meanwhile, phase III clinical trials investigating ICI in combination with TKIs reported 48% to 82% of treatment-related adverse events with grade 3 or higher [22,23,25–27]. Safety evaluation reveals that the combinatorial therapy does not appear to present significantly higher toxicities compared with sunitinib monotherapy [28]. Patients with metastatic ccRCC reported better health-related quality of life given the combination treatment compared to sunitinib [29,30].

Genetic [31–38], molecular [21,22,25,38–40], and clinicopathological characteristics [38,41–44] of ccRCC have not been able to fully predict clinical outcomes and prognosis of patients. RCC has distinct immunological characteristics in regard to pathogenesis and treatment, distinguishing it from other types of cancer that respond to ICI therapy. RCC harbors a relatively low mutational burden, which is expected to produce low neoantigens for antigen presentation, a situation that is often associated with a poor response to ICI therapy. Counterintuitively, RCC is known to be highly immunogenic, resulting in the infiltration of immune cells, including CD8$^+$ T cells [45,46] with high cytotoxic activity [45,47]. Unlike most solid tumors, where the infiltration of CD8$^+$ T cells is normally associated with a good prognosis [44], increased CD8$^+$ T cell infiltration is not associated with prognosis in some studies [35,43,48,49] and actually predicted a poor prognosis in other studies [41–43]. Moreover, certain types of mutations that are associated with increased tumor antigen presentation and CD8$^+$ T cell infiltration in most solid tumors, such as missense mutations, are not correlated with T cell infiltration in RCC [45,47,50]. The expression of immune checkpoints, such as programmed cell death protein 1 (PD-1) and programmed death-ligand 1 (PD-L1), have not been convincingly shown to predict clinical response to ICI in RCC [21,22,25,38–40]. Meanwhile, new characteristics have been uncovered as potential factors that enable the prediction of clinical response to ICI. For example, human endogenous lentivirus virus expression or defective antigen presentation may be a key factor for poor response to ICI in ccRCC patients [38,45]. Taken together, current basic, translational, and clinical research underscores the need to further investigate the tumor immune microenvironment in ccRCC to predict patient outcomes, to identify patients who are likely to respond to immunotherapy, and/or to determine new immunotherapy modalities to treat patients who are not responsive to current ICI therapy.

Single-cell RNA sequencing (scRNAseq) technology dissects the dynamic and heterogeneous tumor microenvironment by characterizing the transcriptome and genome at the single-cell level, providing a prominent method for painting a detailed picture of the immune landscape when studying cancer immunology [51,52]. Integrating various components of scRNAseq transcriptome into multi-omics measurements provides a better understanding of cell identity, fate, and function in the context of both normal biology and pathology [52,53]. The application of scRNAseq to renal parenchyma or kidney cancer is just at its inception and is helping provide a clearer understanding of cell of origin, tumor and immune cell heterogeneity, immune-suppressive microenvironment, therapeutic response, and ultimately prediction of prognosis [54–62].

Here, we summarize the landmark clinical trials for immunotherapy applied to ccRCC and translational scRNAseq research focusing on ccRCC, which is the most immunogenic subtype among RCC subtypes [56]. This review provides translational evidence and potential targets that can be utilized to improve cancer immunotherapy.

2. Immunotherapeutic Updates of ccRCC

2.1. Cytokine-Based Immunotherapy

IL-2 is a cytokine that modulates immunity and tolerance by acting on lymphoid cells, including $CD8^+$ T cells, as a growth factor and activator [63]. The activation of $CD8^+$ T cells facilitates the tumor-killing effect through the recognition of neoantigens presented by the tumor cells [63]. The FDA approved the usage of high-dose IL-2 (600,000 IU/kg) in metastatic RCC in 1992 based on the pooled results of several phase II studies [64,65], representing the first FDA-approved immunotherapy for RCC. These pooled results showed a 14% overall ORR, with 5% of patients having a CR and 9% having a partial response (PR). An even higher dose of IL-2 (720,000 IU/kg) was administered to metastatic RCC patients, yielding a 20% ORR and 9% CR [66]. Similar results supporting the efficacy of a higher dose of IL-2 have been reported [64,67]; and intriguingly, the favorable response of high dose IL-2 was associated with PD-L1 expression, regardless of the patients' clinical classification [68]. High-dose IL-2 is clinically administered with intensive care requiring an inpatient hospital stay but with a subset of responders who have extremely durable responses. Several studies have determined the efficacy of interferon-α 2a (IFNα2a) and found anti-tumor effects on patients with advanced ccRCC with an ORR of 6% to 10% [69–71]. The ORRs of the two cytokines are in general low in ccRCC patients, and the major hurdle for their clinical use also lies in the significant toxicities affecting multiple major organs [72,73].

2.2. Tyrosine Kinase and mTOR Inhibitors

Following IL-2 therapy, clinical treatment of ccRCC moved more towards the use of tyrosine kinase inhibitors (TKIs) targeting VEGFA/VEGFR pathway and neoangiogenesis, including sunitinib, sorafenib, and cabozantinib for treating ccRCC patients [74–76]. In 2006, sunitinib was introduced to treat metastatic RCC patients as the first-line therapy after the phase III trial showed that patients with sunitinib treatment had a significantly longer PFS, compared to those who were treated with IFNα [76]. Sorafenib was another classical TKI approved as second-line therapy for patients who had disease progression following conventional therapy for ccRCC. Treatment with sorafenib significantly prolonged the PFS in advanced ccRCC patients when compared to placebo [75]. In subsequent years, more

TKI inhibitors with higher potency and more specificity, including pazopanib, cabozantinib, axitinib, and lenvatinib, were added to the treatment options for RCC patients [74,77–80].

Temsirolimus and everolimus are two inhibitors for the mammalian target of rapamycin (mTOR) that have been approved for treating RCC patients. mTOR is a highly conserved protein kinase that regulates HIFs-related metabolism and proliferation of ccRCC cells via the PI3K and Akt pathways [81–83]. In 2007, FDA approved treatment with temsirolimus following a phase III clinical trial in patients with metastatic RCC [84]. Patients receiving temsirolimus alone experienced longer overall survival (OS) and PFS than those who received IFNα alone. Everolimus was approved by FDA in 2009 for patients who failed sunitinib and sorafenib treatment [85], after showing clinical efficacy in patients who failed to respond to these therapies. Although numerous clinical trials and studies as described above have demonstrated the superior efficacy of TKIs to previous cytokine-based therapy, most ccRCC patients will develop acquired resistance within one year [86].

2.3. Immune Checkpoint Inhibitors

Currently, immune checkpoint blocking agents, including antibodies that inhibit PD-1, PD-L1, and cytotoxic T-lymphocyte-associated protein 4 (CTLA-4), are being successfully investigated and applied to the patients with ccRCC.

The first clinical trial of ICIs in ccRCC was conducted in 2007, attesting to the effect of CTLA-4 blockade in patients with metastatic RCC [87]. The phase II study included patients receiving either 3 mg/kg followed by 1 mg/kg or only 3 mg/kg of ipilimumab (anti-CTLA-4) for 3 weeks. One of the 21 patients with a lower dose and five of 40 patients with a higher dose had partial responses. There is a significant correlation between patients with autoimmune events and tumor regression, suggesting that the reinvigoration of CD8$^+$ T cells promotes the tumor-killing effect. However, due to limited efficacy, the use of ipilimumab as monotherapy for RCC was halted.

A second clinical trial of ICIs in patients with ccRCC attested to the effect of PD-1 blockade on patients with ccRCC, with an ORR of 27% (9 out 33 patients) [14]. In this later phase II study, patients with metastatic ccRCC previously treated with anti-VEGF therapy were administrated 0.3, 2, or 10 mg/kg nivolumab (anti-PD-1). The median PFS was 2.7 months, 4.0 months, and 4.2 months respectively. The OS was 18.2 months, 25.5 months, and 24.7 months respectively [88]. In CheckMate 025, a phase III study, patients previously treated with anti-angiogenic therapy received either 3 mg of nivolumab or 10 mg of everolimus [15,89]. Although progression-free survival showed no difference between the two treatments, the OS for nivolumab was 25.0 months compared to 19.6 months for everolimus (p = 0.002) [89]. Also, the nivolumab-treated group showed a greater response rate (25% compared to 5% in the everolimus-treated group). Extended follow-up confirmed the superior efficacy of nivolumab over everolimus.

The first combination therapy was initiated in 2012, attesting to the efficacy of nivolumab with sunitinib, pazopanib, or ipilimumab [90,91]. Patients treated with nivolumab plus sunitinib showed a 55% ORR and median PFS of 12.7 months. For the group treated with nivolumab plus pazopanib, the ORR was 45% and PFS was 7.2 months. The nivolumab plus ipilimumab treatment was divided into two dose regimens: patients received either 3 mg/kg of nivolumab and 1 mg/kg of ipilimumab or 1 mg/kg of nivolumab and 3 mg/kg of ipilimumab. Both treatment regimens had an ORR of about 40% and a 2-year OS of 68%. The nivolumab group showed a lower rate of adverse events (38.3%) compared to the ipilimumab group (61.7%). In the phase III CheckMate 214 trial, the combination of nivolumab with ipilimumab was tested against sunitinib alone [21,27,92]. According to the criterion from the International Metastatic RCC Database Consortium (IMDC), intermediate and poor-risk patients receiving nivolumab + ipilimumab had a survival rate of 75% at 18-months compared to a 60% survival rate at 18 months for sunitinib. The ORR was 42% for the group treated with nivolumab plus ipilimumab, compared to 27% for the group treated with sunitinib. The CR was 9% and 1% in the combination and monotherapy, respectively. In the follow-up study, the nivolumab plus ipilimumab combination had a superior OS to the sunitinib therapy within the intermediate and poor-risk and intent to treat patients.

Because anti-VEGF treatment was found to have immunomodulatory effects on different types of immune cells, including myeloid cells and regulatory T cells (Treg) [93–96], clinical trials with the combination of ICIs and anti-VEGF agents were investigated in RCC. In an open-label phase III trial (Keynote 426), 861 patients with previously untreated advanced ccRCC were assigned to either axitinib plus pembrolizumab (anti-PD-1) or sunitinib alone group [25,97,98]. The 1-year survival rate was 89.9% for the combination group compared to 78.3% for the sunitinib alone. The median PFS for the combination treatment was also significantly higher than the sunitinib alone group (15.1 months vs. 11.1 months). The ORR was 59.3% and 35.7%, respectively. The study revealed that patients treated with axitinib plus pembrolizumab demonstrated a better response in all three IMDC risk groups, regardless of PD-L1 expression. Another clinical trial (Clear/Keynote 581) confirmed the superior efficacy of the combination of pembrolizumab (anti-PD-1) plus lenvatinib—a TKI targeting RET, KIT, PDGFR, and VEGFRs—over everolimus [26]. In this phase III trial, 1069 untreated patients with ccRCC were assigned to pembrolizumab plus lenvatinib, lenvatinib plus everolimus, or sunitinib at a 1:1:1 ratio. The ORR was 71%, 53.5%, and 36.1%, and the median PFS was 23.9 months, 14.7 months, and 9.2 months for the experimental arms of pembrolizumab plus lenvatinib, lenvatinib plus everolimus, and sunitinib, respectively. Encouraging results were also obtained in the CheckMate 9ER trial where 651 untreated patients with advanced ccRCC were assigned to treatment with either Nivolumab (240 mg every 2 weeks) plus cabozantinib (40 mg once daily)—a TKI targeting AXL, RET, MET, TIE-2, and VEGFRs—or sunitinib (50 mg once daily for 4 weeks of each 6-week cycle) [22,99]. This phase III study showed that the combination significantly improved PFS and OS as compared to sunitinib alone. At 18.1 months of median follow-up, patients who received the combination had a median of 16.6 months of PFS with a 55.7% ORR, whereas those who received sunitinib alone had a median PFS of 8.3 months and a 27.1% ORR. At 12 months, the probability of OS was higher in the combination arm (85.7%) compared to those in the control arm (75.6%). The clinical benefit of the nivolumab and cabozantinib over sunitinib was observed regardless of PD-L1 expression.

The JAVELIN Renal 101 trial compared the combination of avelumab (anti-PD-L1) plus axitinib with sunitinib alone [23,100,101]. Patients with PD-L1 positive tumors (as defined by $\geq$1% of immune cells immunohistochemistry (IHC)-staining positive within the tested tumor area) showed a median PFS of 13.8 months for the combination therapy compared to 7.2 months for the sunitinib alone. The ORR was 55.2% and 25.5%, respectively. This study showed that avelumab plus axitinib could be an effective therapy for patients with PD-L1 positive ccRCC. However, the follow-up study on biomarker analysis revealed that the expression of PD-L1 was not correlated with a better response and PFS in patients receiving avelumab plus axitinib [33]. Another approved combination therapy for metastatic RCC is atezolizumab (anti-PD-L1) with bevacizumab—a monoclonal antibody targeting VEGFA. In the phase III study (IMmotion 151), patients were randomly assigned to atezolizumab with bevacizumab or sunitinib alone [24,30]. The median PFS survival was 11.2 and 7.7 months for the PD-L1 positive population (as defined by $\geq$1% of immune cells IHC-staining positive within the tested tumor area), tested with atezolizumab plus bevacizumab or sunitinib alone, respectively. There was a difference in OS, but the patients experienced fewer treatment-related adverse events.

Altogether, based on clinical trials and publications, the clinical benefit of immune checkpoint inhibitors and their combination with anti-angiogenic agents is evident in both untreated and treated patients with advanced ccRCC. Clinically relevant results from the phase III clinical trials are summarized in Table 1.

Table 1. Updated phase III clinical trials investigating immunotherapies for advanced ccRCC.

Study Name	Identifier	Agent	Target	Total	ORR	TRAE 3+	Citations
CheckMate 025 *	NCT01668784	Nivolumab	PD-1	821	23%	19%	[15,89]
CheckMate 214	NCT02231749	Nivolumab Ipilimumab	PD-1 CTLA-4	1096	39.1%	47.9%	[21,27,102]
IMmotion 151	NCT02420821	Atezolizumab Bevacizumab	PD-L1 VEGF	915	37%	40%	[24,30]
JAVELIN Renal 101	NCT02684006	Avelumab Axitinib	PD-L1 RTK	886	52.5%	71.2%	[23,101,103]
CLEAR	NCT02811861	Pembrolizumab Lenvatinib	PD-1 RTK	1069	71%	82.4%	[26]
Keynote 426	NCT02853331	Pembrolizumab Axitinib	PD-1 RTK	861	60.4%	66.4%	[25,97,98]
CheckMate 9ER	NCT03141177	Nivolumab Cabozantinib	PD-1 RTK	651	56.6%	75.3%	[22]

* This study used Everolimus as a control arm. Other studies used Sunitinib as a control arm. Abbreviation: ORR; objective response rate, TRAE; treatment-related adverse event, RTK; receptor tyrosine kinase.

2.4. Ongoing Clinical Trials

Table 2 summarizes the ongoing phase III clinical trials that cover a wide range of critical issues, including the efficacy of newly developed ICIs, the role of immune checkpoint in the previously established experimental arms, the efficacy of ICI as adjuvant therapy on the rate of recurrence following nephrectomy [104–106], and the effect of salvage ICI following progression on ICI treatment [107]. In addition, other studies are also testing the role of small molecules inhibitors in combination immunotherapy [108], the effect of IL-2 in combination with ICI [109], the efficacy of ICI on brain metastasis [110], and the optimal sequence of ICIs [111].

Briefly, the COSMIC-313 study is now being conducted to evaluate the efficacy of cabozantinib in combination with nivolumab and ipilimumab as the first therapy using a triplet. The study is designed to determine whether the addition of cabozantinib leads to clinical benefit over the combination of the ICIs as far as patient's PFS and OS. PDIGREE is another clinical trial investigating the therapeutic role of cabozantinib in patients who have completed receiving nivolumab and ipilimumab therapy. PIVOT-09 is being conducted to examine the effect of bempegaldesleukin (IL-2 agonist) in combination with nivolumab versus either sunitinib or cabozantinib, and this clinical trial will compare the ORR and OS in an intermediate or poor-risk group of untreated ccRCC patients.

Another study (NCT04736706) will determine the efficacy, safety, and the specific role of belzutifan (HIF-2 inhibitor) [115] and quavonlimab (anti-CTLA-4) in combination with pembrolizumab and lenvatinib. Clinical trials of RAMPART, CheckMate 914, IMmotion010, and NCT03055013, will determine the post-surgical clinical benefit of ICIs (anti-PD1/PD-L1 and/or anti-CTLA-4) versus active monitoring in patients with partial or total nephrectomy. NCT04510597 will study the role of cytoreductive nephrectomy in combination with systemic ICI in ccRCC patients. CheckMate-67T is being conducted to study the efficacy, safety, and tolerability of nivolumab when patients are given the ICI subcutaneously. NCT04157985 will determine the optimal treatment duration of anti-PD-1 and PD-L1 therapies.

In summary, clinical evidence is sufficient to demonstrate that ccRCC is highly immunogenic and has great potential for durable response to immunotherapy. The next step is to solve the riddle of why only some patients have clinical benefits during ICI treatment, while others show intrinsic or acquired resistance to ICIs and ensuing disease progression and poor prognosis. Various molecular features of ccRCC obtained from bulk multi-omics approaches cannot precisely predict patients' prognosis and clinical response to ICI, at least in part due to the substantial heterogeneity in immune cell contents in ccRCC. scRNAseq is the most comprehensive tool to study immune cells at the genome-wide and single-cell levels in order to uncover immune cell heterogeneity. Using scRNAseq to define the complex ccRCC immune microenvironment offers unique opportunity to elucidate potential mechanisms and/or markers for response to ICI therapy, as well as possible targets for improving response rates to ICIs.

Table 2. Ongoing phase III clinical trials investigating immunotherapies for advanced ccRCC.

Study Name	Identifier	Agent	Target	Control
COSMIC-313	NCT03937219 [108]	Nivolumab Ipilimumab Cabozantinib	PD-1 CTLA-4 RTK	Nivolumab and Ipilimumab
na	NCT03729245 [109]	Bempegaldesleukin Nivolumab	IL-2 agonist PD-1	Sunitinib Cabozantinib
Keynote 564	NCT03142334 [105]	Pembrolizumab	PD-1	Placebo
Contact 03	NCT04338269 [107]	Atezolizumab Cabozantinib	PD-L1 RTK	Cabozantinib
IMmotion 010	NCT03024996 [106]	Atezolizumab	PD-L1	Placebo following nephrectomy
PDIGREE	NCT03793166 [111]	Nivolumab Cabozantinib	PD-1 RTK	Nivolumab following Nivolumab and Ipilimumab
CheckMate 914	NCT03138512 [104]	Nivolumab Ipilimumab	PD-1 CTLA-4	Placebo following nephrectomy
PROSPER	NCT03055013 [112]	Nivolumab	PD-1	Monitoring after nephrectomy
CheckMate 920	NCT02982954 [113]	Nivolumab Ipilimumab	PD-1 CTLA-4	This clinical trial examines the safety of ICI in RCC patients with either brain metastasis or Karnofsky Performance Status 50–60%
na	NCT04736706	Pembrolizumab Quavonlimab Lenvatinib Belzutifan	PD-1 CTLA-4 RTK HIF2	Pembrolizumab and lenvatinib
na	NCT04523272	TQB2450 Anlotinib	PD-L1 RTK	Sunitinib
na	NCT04394975	Toripalimab Axitinib	PD-1 RTK	Sunitinib
na	NCT03873402	Nivolumab Ipilimumab	PD-1 CTLA-4	Nivolumab
RAMPART	NCT03288532 [114]	Durvalumab Tremelimumab	PD-1 CTLA-4	Monitoring after nephrectomy
CheckMate 67T	NCT04810078	Nivolumab	PD-1	This clinical trial examines the safety and efficacy of subcutaneous Nivolumab injection
PROBE	NCT04510597	Nivolumab Pembrolizumab Axitinib Avelumab	PD-1 PD-1 RTK PD-L1	This clinical trial examines the efficacy of cytoreductive nephrectomy in combination with ICI
na	NCT04157985	Nivolumab Pembrolizumab Ipilimumab Atezolizumab	PD-1 PD-1 CTLA-4 PD-L1	This clinical trial examines the length of treatment with ICI.

Abbreviation: ICI; immune checkpoint inhibitor, RTK; receptor tyrosine kinase, na; not applicable.

3. Single-Cell Genomics to Study the Tumor Microenvironment

Single-cell genomics determines the genetic, epigenetic, or chromatin structure information at the single cell level with optimized next-generation sequencing (NGS) technologies. scRNAseq has become a potent tool to provide a higher resolution of the transcriptome for individual cells. scRNAseq can be used to study the cellular heterogeneity for given tissues to identify a rare and novel cell population that would not be detected by conventional methods, to determine cell state transitions affected by intrinsic and extrinsic stimuli, to understand differential genes/pathway alterations between cell populations, and to explore the clonal status of T or B cells when combined with T or B cell receptor sequencing, etc. [116,117]

Here we summarize published studies adopting scRNAseq technology with a focus on cancer immunology of ccRCC (Table 3). We will introduce some basic concepts and common processes of scRNAseq technology, including scRNAseq library preparation and common computational analyses. In detail, single-cell analysis technologies, including scRNAseq, and their applications in cancer immunology have been previously reviewed in detail [51,117]. Different scRNAseq library preparation methods have been reviewed [118,119]. Current studies applying scRNAseq technology to RCC have largely adopted a droplet-based platform provided by 10× Genomics. As such, we mainly focus on a droplet-based microfluidic system for scRNAseq library preparation.

Table 3. scRNAseq studies identifying and characterizing immune environment associated with ccRCC progression and response to ICI.

Patient Number	Control Group	Experimental Group	Cell Number	Platform	Citation
3	PB	ccRCC	25,688	10× Genomics droplet-based	[58]
11	ANT	ccRCC	163,905	10× Genomics droplet-based	[61]
9	ANT	ccRCC	29,131	10× Genomics droplet-based	[56]
13	ANT	Advance stages of ccRCC	164,722	10× Genomics droplet-based	[60]
8	Primary and metastatic ccRCC (LN), ICI-untreated	Primary and metastatic ccRCC (LN, lung, abdomen), ICI-treated	34,326	10× Genomics droplet-based	[59]
6	ANT and primary ccRCC, ICI-untreated	PB, ANT, and multi-regions of primary and metastatic ccRCC (LN), ICI-treated	167,283	10× Genomics droplet-based	[55]
2	PB and multi-regions of primary ccRCC, ICI-untreated	PB and multi-regions of primary and metastatic ccRCC (adrenal gland, bone, nephrectomy bed), ICI-treated	26,456	10× Genomics droplet-based	[38]

Abbreviation: scRNAseq; single-cell RNA sequencing, ICI; immune checkpoint inhibitor, LN; lymph node, ccRCC; clear cell renal cell carcinoma, PB; peripheral blood, ANT; adjacent non-tumor tissue.

3.1. Basic Concept and Experiment-Related Workflow of Microfluidic-Based scRNAseq

Microfluidic droplet-based scRNAseq has been used as one of the useful platforms to study single-cells in cancer immunology [118–120]. The droplet-based microfluidic system does not necessarily need cell sorting but needs high viability cells for preserving molecular states and reads either 3′ or 5′ end of the transcripts with barcoding and unique molecular identifier (UMI) tagging [118–120]. Droplet-based scRNAseq is characterized by high cellular resolution, low amplification noise, and high cost-effectiveness for the transcriptome quantification of large numbers of cells [118–120]. Also, it is more suitable for the identification of diverse cell types and measurement of gene expression changes between conditions [118–120].

The microfluidic system automates parallel sample partitioning and captures the single cells into individual oil droplets containing uniquely barcoded beads called Gel Beads-In Emulsions (GEM) [118,120]. Poly(A) tail at the 3′ end of RNA extracted from a single-cell in an individual GEM is bound to millions of the barcoded oligonucleotides with high capture efficiency and reverse transcribed to the first strand of DNA. Subsequently, a second strand synthesizing process and a PCR amplifying process are conducted to generate analysis-ready transcriptomes on a cell-by-cell basis from the complementary DNA (cDNA) libraries [120]. Illumina sequencer is widely used for library sequencing, including published ccRCC scRNAseq studies. The directed 5′ or 3′ chemistry allows for 98 base pair sequencing, limiting the mutational analysis of sequences. Cell Ranger from 10× Genomics, one of the frequently used computational pipelines for handling raw data files, provides wrapper functions that support the packages required for the raw data pre-processing pipeline [118].

After data pre-processing, including quality control, sequence alignment, and quantification of the raw sequence, a gene expression matrix is generated from the reads mapped to exon regions with high mapping quality. R toolkit Seurat has been used for the data processing, generating the Seurat object as an input file for subsequent processes [121]. Bioconductor-based workflow and Scanpy are also popular toolkits for R and python users, respectively [122,123]. Data analysis and visualization follow a standard preprocessing workflow that includes selection and filtration of cells based on quality control, data normalization and scaling, and the detection of highly variable features. The highly variable features are used for principal component analysis (PCA). After the data pre-processing steps, a high-dimensional molecular profile for individual cells is computationally classified into distinct cell populations [117,121]. Individual cells are clustered based on distances of components and visualized by non-linear dimensionality reduction techniques, such as t-distributed stochastic neighbor embedding (t-SNE) [124] or uniform manifold approximation and projection (UMAP) [125]. Although analysis varies depending on the study design, one can conduct main analyses with complementary computational techniques, such as cell composition, cell state transitions, differential gene expression, pathway analysis, cell-fate trajectories, molecular interactions, and cellular interactions [118].

3.2. ScRNAseq in ccRCC

The tumor microenvironment of ccRCC is extremely heterogeneous in its molecular and immune phenotypes [11,58,126–128]. As discussed above, means of predicting response to ICI therapy in other solid tumors have not proven clinically useful in RCC. Single-cell proteomics, as implemented by flow cytometry, mass cytometry, or multiplexed immunohistochemistry, has identified cell composition and potential cell types that generate and maintain the immune suppressive microenvironment of RCC [43,46,61]. Although these single-cell analysis technologies are useful and informative, they are inherently limited by the available number of pre-selected antibodies, resulting in the identification of only anticipated cell types [117]. The deconvolution method using bulk RNA-seq can be used to estimate immune cell composition, but this method is nowhere close to fully reflecting the heterogeneous immune composition of any tissues [127,128]. Evaluation of proliferation of CD8$^+$ T cells by Ki-67 positivity has been indicated as a favorable prognostic factor [42], however, this has been contradicted by recent studies with scRNAseq results [58–60].

Currently, scRNAseq, which is not limited by the determining markers, has dissected tumor heterogeneity in multiple types of human solid cancers [51]. In ccRCC, a few studies with scRNAseq have just begun to investigate immune cell heterogeneity, immune pathogenesis, and response to immunotherapy [54–62]. Analyzing tumor-infiltrating immune cells by scRNAseq, especially focusing on T cell exhaustion, suppressive TAMs, and inhibitory cell to cell interactions has shown to have clinical prognostic and predictive value regarding clinical outcomes and the response to immunotherapy. Thus, it needs to provide evidence of the substantial potential of scRNAseq to give insights into some of the current issues regarding RCC immunotherapy. In this review, we highlight scRNAseq studies that report key events associated with the immune environment, ccRCC progression, and response to immunotherapy. Scheme and detailed information concerning scRNAseq studies applied to ccRCC is summarized in Figure 1 and Table 3.

To define the tumor-specific change in the infiltration of immune cells, our group [58] generated droplet-based scRNAseq and single-cell T cell receptor sequencing (scTCRseq) libraries and studied 25,688 cells from matched blood and primary. Tumor samples originating from 3 untreated patients diagnosed with different grades of ccRCC. We also integrated the scRNAseq data with a previous scRNAseq dataset containing 11,367 cells derived from normal renal parenchyma and blood. The study examined immune events and cell state transitions associated with a tumor-specific environment. There was a significant increase in the population of CD8$^+$ T cells and macrophages in ccRCC but a decrease in the population of CD4$^+$ T cells and B cells, compared to blood and non-tumor tissues. While infiltrating tumor tissue, CD8$^+$ T cells showed a transcriptional continuum from naïve to activation, but eventual exhaustion with highly expanded clonotypes. A small subset of tumor-infiltrating CD8$^+$ T cells were characterized by preferential cytokine signaling and associated with a favorable response to anti-PD1 therapy. In general, tumor-infiltrating CD4$^+$ T cells showed a transcriptional continuum toward more activated states, such as high cytolytic and interferon activities, as previously described [60]. Meanwhile, distinct subsets of TAMs characterized by the gene expression associated with either chemo/cytokines, apolipoproteins, or DC-like, showed high plasticity between pro- and anti-inflammatory phenotypes. Using machine-learning training with the Cancer Genome Atlas (TCGA) RCC cohort, we developed unique gene signatures defining either a subset of proliferative CD8$^+$ T cells or a subset of DC-like TAMs. Both scRNAseq signatures had a prognostic value of predicting a poorer prognosis in the OS of patients with ccRCC. Using external mass cytometry data [46], we also confirmed the existence of the proliferative CD8$^+$ T subset as a PD1$^+$Ki-67^{hi} phenotype in ccRCC. Supporting the scRNAseq-based prognostic model, the PD1$^+$Ki-67^{hi} CD8$^+$ T cells are highly enriched with co-stimulatory proteins and immune checkpoints, such as ICOS, 4-1BB, TIM-3, CTLA-4, HLA-DR, and CD38.

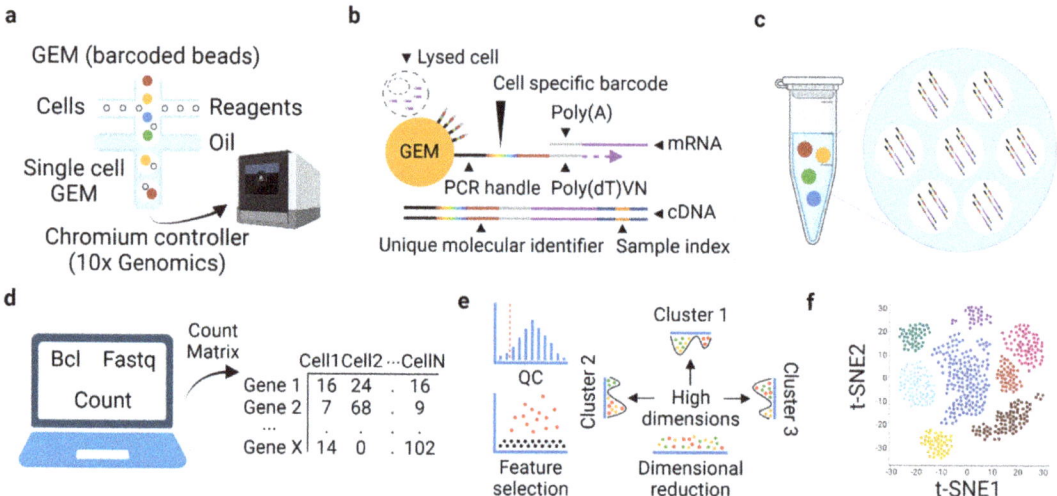

Figure 1. Scheme of droplet-based scRNAseq and standard bioinformatics pipeline. (**a**) Single cells are loaded to a microfluidic system and encapsulated to an oil droplet to generate single-cell GEM. (**b**) RNA released from the lysed single-cell is captured by barcoded oligonucleotides and reverse transcribed to the first and second strands of DNA. (**c**) PCR amplifying process is conducted to generate cDNA library, which is sequenced by Illumina sequencer. (**d**) Cell Ranger from 10× Genomics provides raw data pre-processing pipeline, resulting in the generation of a gene expression matrix. (**e**) Standard pre-processing steps for scRNAseq data. Low-quality cells are removed. Highly variable features are selected and used for principal component analysis. A high-dimensional molecular profile for individual cells is computationally classified into distinct cell populations. (**f**) Individual cells are visualized by non-linear dimensionality reduction techniques, such as t-SNE. Abbreviation: GEM; Gel Beads-In Emulsions, t-SNE; t-distributed stochastic neighbor embedding, cDNA; complementary DNA.

Zhang et al. [56] identified the peculiar immune environment and pathogenesis of ccRCC. The study analyzed 29,131 cells derived from adjacent non-tumor tissues and primary ccRCCs from 9 patients. In addition to identifying the putative cell of origin for ccRCC, the study evaluated the potential source of immune infiltration to ccRCC and the prognostic value of distinct cell populations. Supporting the previous scRNAseq study applied to ccRCC [57], a subset of proximal tubular cells and neoplastic epithelial cells were predicted to recruit immune cells to tumor site via IFN response, including especially secretion of serine protease C1s. This is further supported by a positive correlation between the degree of TAM fraction and the C1S gene expression in bulk RNA-seq, scRNAseq, and TCGA RCC datasets. Two different subsets of TAMs, defined by chemokine/cytokine- versus lysosome-related genes, had dichotomous prognostic values of predicting OS within the same TCGA RCC cohort. Using bulk RNA-seq obtained from metastatic ccRCC patients who were treated with TKI followed by anti-PD1 therapy, the study defined genes associated with clinical benefit. Notably, endothelial cells and pericytes predominantly expressed the genes negatively associated with the response, and genes associated with clinical benefit were primarily expressed among T cells. In TCGA ccRCC dataset, however, treatment-naïve patients with a high fraction of endothelial cells in localized ccRCC were predicted to have better OS. Patients with a high estimated fraction (>90th percentile) of either tumor-infiltrating CD8$^+$ T cells or plasmalemma vesicle associated protein (PLVAP)$^+$ endothelial cells were separately present in the scatter plot, suggesting mutual exclusivity of the two cell types concerning clinical outcome in the ccRCC environment.

Obradovic et al. [61] also identified and characterized the tumor-specific immune environment of ccRCC using scRNAseq data. The study studied 163,905 cells isolated from adjacent non-tumor tissues and primary, non-metastatic ccRCC from six untreated patients. Moving beyond mRNA expression, the study applied a specific algorithm, called VIPER, to scRNAseq data and inferred single-cell protein activity. Of note, the VIPER-based protein activity inference turned out to significantly overcome challenges of scRNAseq, including recovery of transcriptome dynamics masked by dropouts up to 70% to 80%, and thus was able to precisely predict single-cell protein activity. This was also validated by using flow cytometry and an external CITE-seq dataset. The integrated analysis enabled the identification of potentially targetable novel master regulatory proteins in a rare population that would have been undetectable by gene expression-based analysis. VIPER analysis led to the identification of ccRCC-infiltrating exhausted CD8$^+$ T cells, Treg, TAMs, and CD45$^-$ cell types with a high resolution. The protein activity of the C1Q family of proteins, APOE, and TREM-2 was significantly upregulated in macrophages in tumors compared to non-tumor tissues. VIPER was also successful in obtaining the inferred protein activity from bulk RNA-seq data derived from untreated ccRCC surgical resections. In two independent cohorts, the VIPER-applied protein signature of tumor-specific macrophages was not only preferentially enriched in patients who underwent post-surgical ccRCC recurrence but also significantly associated with the shorter time-to-recurrence in the Kaplan–Meier curve. The representative leading-edge proteins among TAM-defining markers were APOE and TREM-2. Using multiplexed immunohistochemistry, C1Q$^+$TREM-2$^+$ TAMs were found to be tumor-specific and C1Q$^+$TREM-2$^+$APOE$^+$ TAMs located significantly nearer the tumor cells than triple-negative TAMs. The proximity was also strengthened by the analysis of ligand-receptor interaction between tumor cells and APO$^+$ TAMs. The frequency of either C1Q$^+$ or TREM-2$^+$ TAMs was higher in tumor slide sections from patients with recurrence than those with non-recurrence. Clinically, the density of C1Q$^+$ TAMs above a certain threshold of 0.01 was significantly associated with ccRCC recurrence.

To define the change in the infiltration of immune cells with advancing ccRCC, Braun et al. [60] generated droplet-based scRNAseq and scTCRseq libraries and analyzed 164,722 cells isolated from blood, adjacent non-tumor tissues, and different stages of primary and metastatic ccRCC from 13 untreated patients. As RCC progressed from early to locally advanced and metastatic diseases, there was a consistent increase in the frequency of terminally exhausted CD8$^+$ T cells, Treg, CD14$^+$ monocytes, and immune suppressive M2-like TAMs, and a general decrease in the frequency of cytotoxic CD8$^+$ T cells, central memory CD4$^+$ T cells, and inflammatory M1-like TAMs. Pseudotime analysis coupled with gene signature also confirmed the progressive dysfunction and exhaustion of tumor-infiltrating CD8$^+$ T cells with advancing ccRCC. Likewise, the trajectory analysis showed preferential enrichment of pro-inflammatory and anti-inflammatory scRNAseq signatures in earlier-stage and metastatic-stage ccRCC, respectively. Ligand-receptor interactions were inferred to tumor-infiltrating immune cells. Intriguingly, while a majority of non-exhausted T cells in earlier-stage ccRCC were predicted to have few interactions, terminally exhausted CD8$^+$ T cells in advanced ccRCC were inferred to have numerous ligand-receptor pairs within the myeloid populations, including TAMs. With metastatic ccRCC samples, the inhibitory interaction between two populations was further supported by the multiplexed immunofluorescence-based spatial proximity and upregulated expression of ligands and their cognate receptors. Using multiple external ccRCC datasets [46,129,130], the authors also showed a significant increase in the proportion of terminally exhausted CD8$^+$ T cells and M2-like TAMs and the gene signature score defining the inhibitory interaction with the advancing ccRCC stage. The high expression of the gene signature was specifically associated with poor prognosis in the OS of patients with late-stage ccRCC. Meanwhile, the gene signature did not have prognostic value for predicting PFS and immune response to anti-PD1 therapy or mTOR inhibitor. On the other hand, scTCRseq results showed a significant decrease in the TCR diversity with advancing ccRCC stage, and there was a high proportion of terminally exhausted CD8$^+$ T cells with low TCR diversity in metastatic ccRCC. Contrary to the previous finding [62], the shared clonotypes were preferentially detected in tumors rather than non-tumor tissues.

To identify potential immune populations that drive the response to ICI, Krishna et al. [55] collected 167,283 cells from blood, adjacent non-tumor tissue, metastatic lymph node, and multiple regions of primary ccRCC from 2 untreated and 4 treated patients with ICI. Then, the authors generated droplet-based scRNAseq and scTCRseq libraries. First of all, multiregional sampling confirmed extensive heterogeneity within and between patients, highlighting the vulnerability of applying bulk RNA-seq-derived signatures to tumor region sampling bias. Mapping the immune environment of ccRCC identified diverse immune cell types, such as five well-defined CD8$^+$ T clusters and 4 clusters of TAMs characterized by HLA or ISG expression. Next, the authors co-analyzed scRNAseq and pathologic review, and identified that tissue-resident CD8$^+$ T cells, as well as CD4$^+$ T cells and NK cells, were heavily infiltrated in tumor regions associated with tumor regression or CR to ICI. Conversely, in tumor regions associated with resistance to ICI, a high proportion of HLA$^+$ TAMs were identified with a scarcity of T cells. Following ICI treatment, the tissue-resident CD8$^+$ T cells from the complete responders were found to solely undergo clonal expansion with unique TCR clonotypes, but the resistant non-responders also had the clonal expansion of the CD8$^+$ T subset. To estimate potential immune populations underlying ccRCC patient prognosis and response to ICI and TKIs, various clinical signatures, such as T effector, angiogenesis, and myeloid inflammation, were applied to multiple external ccRCC cohorts [37,78,128]. Results indicated that effector T cells and angiogenic myeloid cells had the potential to elicit a favorable response to anti-PD-L1 and TKI arms. Also, the scRNAseq signature of ISG^{high} TAMs was highly associated with angiogenesis in the TKI arm. In the end, the study validated the scRNAseq signatures that are highly specific for tissue-resident CD8$^+$ T cells or ISG^{high} TAMs, and applied them to IMmotion 150/151 (anti-PD-L1 plus anti-VEGF or TKI), JAVELIN Renal 101 (anti-PD-L1 plus TKI) ccRCC cohorts. Importantly, high levels of the tissue-resident CD8$^+$ T signature were significantly associated with improved PFS and better response in anti-PD-L1 and TKI arms. Autologously, the ISG^{high} TAMs signature was significantly associated with improved PFS in the TKI arm. However, both signatures did not predict clinical outcomes from the TCGA ccRCC dataset.

In a similar study of four anti-PD-1-treated patients and three untreated patients with primary and metastatic ccRCC, Bi et al. [59] generated a droplet-based scRNAseq library and analyzed 34,326 cells. The study started off applying progenitor or terminally exhausted signature to the scRNAseq immune subsets and identified 4-1BB^{low}CD8$^+$ T cells that resembled the progenitor exhausted population, which is known to persist long term, respond to anti-PD1 therapy, and ultimately differentiate into the terminally exhausted population in melanoma [131]. Following ICI treatment, the 4-1BB^{low}CD8$^+$ T cells were found to upregulate the expression of effector and co-stimulatory molecules, including GRANZYME A (GZMA) and FAS LIGAND (FASLG), and highly enriched with terminally exhausted signature. This result was also supported by the high enrichment score of 4-1BB-low signature in PD1-exposed CD8$^+$ T cells from the CheckMate 009 cohort. Similarly, ICI treatment rendered all distinct subsets of TAMs more M1-like and pro-inflammatory in responder patients, at least in part, as induced by IFN secreted from CD8$^+$ T cells. At the same time, however, the ICI-exposed 4-1BB^{low}CD8$^+$ T cells and TAMs also showed systemic and dramatic upregulation of immune checkpoint and evasion genes, suggesting progressive and eventual acquisition of ICI resistance. Two subsets of cancer cells identified were found to transcriptionally shift toward a pro-inflammatory state during ICI. Patients who had a high score of the gene signature that defined renal morphogenic and angiogenic cancer population showed the ICI-specific clinical benefit regarding OS in the CheckMate 025 cohort (anti-PD1 arm). Supporting different cell populations in a complex cross-talk in ccRCC environment, numerous ligand-receptor pairs, including IFNγ-producing CD8$^+$ T cells and type 2 IFN receptor on TAMs, were inferred and further supported by expression signatures and estimated immune cell fractions adapted from CheckMate 009 cohort.

Very recently, Au et al. [38] scrutinized key determinants that are responsible for clinical response in metastatic ccRCC patients before and after nivolumab treatment. Again, various tumor molecular features of ccRCC, including single mutations, copy number alterations, insertion-and-deletions, mutational burden, and neoantigen load, were not associated with favorable anti-PD-1 response. Of note, however, ccRCC-specific expression of human endogenous retrovirus was found to be associated with lack of response to nivolumab. In addition, it has been suggested that defects in antigen presentation, despite a high number of mutations resulting from defective DNA mismatch repair, might be a potential factor underlying poor response to ICI. Authors generated droplet-based scRNAseq and scTCRseq libraries and analyzed a total of 25,456 IgG4+ (anti-PD-1 antibody-bound) and IgG4- CD3 T cells isolated from a responder and a non-responder during nivolumab monotherapy. scRNA-seq showed that anti-PD-1 treatment renders nivolumab-bound ccRCC-infiltrating CD8$^+$ T cells immunologically activated in both responder and non-responder. Paired analysis of scRNAseq and scTCRseq found that nivolumab treatment induces clonal expansion of pre-existing CD8$^+$ T cells, and only the responder had clonal hyper-expansion of the nivolumab-bound CD8$^+$ T cells (as defined by more than 200 clones with the same complementary determining region 3 sequence). The expanded nivolumab-bound CD8$^+$ T cells had higher expression of GZMK gene in the responder than the non-responder. scRNAseq, flow cytometry, and multiplexed IHC confirmed the higher expression of GZMB and TCF7 in the nivolumab-bound CD8+ T cells from responders. Using previously published ccRCC-specific scRNA/scTCRseq datasets, they further validated their findings. As a result, expanded TCRs in responders but not the non-responders had higher expression of genes involved in T cell activation and co-stimulatory markers, including GZMK and 4-1BB. It should also be noted that nivolumab treatment not only reinvigorated CD8$^+$ T cells in the responder, but also caused T cell exhaustion and dysfunction, suggesting simultaneous development of resistance as consistent with the previous finding [59]. Finally, bulk and scTCRseq analysis before and after treatment demonstrated that responders have clonal expansion of pre-existing and novel TCRs from the nivolumab-bound CD8$^+$ T cells. However, non-responders had an overall paucity of expanded pre-existing TCRs, rather showing clonal replacement of expanded TCRs. The novel expanded T cell clones after nivolumab treatment were not associated with clinical response.

Meanwhile, several studies have also been reported using droplet-based scRNAseq technology to provide insight into normal and ccRCC immunobiology. Yu et al. [54] studied the inter-tumoral heterogeneity using bilateral ccRCC samples within a patient and identified the high similarity of the gene expression between the immune cells in the bilateral ccRCC. Liao et al. [132] mapped the atlas of single-cells that normally reside in healthy renal tissues, providing the reference data for normal renal cell biology and kidney disease. Besides the major analysis that identifies cancer cell identity, Young et al. [57] highlighted the VEGF signaling circuit in the ccRCC environment. The study identified that TAMs, as well as ccRCC cells, were a further source of VEGF, and VEGFR was highly expressed in ascending vasa recta endothelial cells. Using multiple types of human cancers, including ccRCC, Wu et al. [62] showed that expanded clonotypes from effector-like CD8$^+$ T cells were simultaneously detected in the tumor, non-tumor tissues, and peripheral blood. In particular, further evidence indicated that peripherally expanded T cells with ICI treatments were directly linked to tumor infiltration and eliciting an immune response, rather than reinvigorating the already exhausted T cells in the tumor environment. This study also identified distinct subsets of immune cells with a focus on T cells in ccRCC, but did not fully characterize tumor microenvironment. Kim et al. [133] compared and analyzed scRNAseq data generated from tumor cells isolated from the patient's metastatic ccRCC and the paired primary and metastatic ccRCC derived from the patient-derived xenograft (PDX) model. The study verified the current patient's drug refractoriness, identified candidate signaling pathways and drugs, and validated the predicted drug sensitivity using in vitro and in vivo assays, suggesting the clinical applicability of scRNAseq and combined mouse model to screen optimal choice of TKIs.

3.3. Major Immune Cell Types Associated with Poor Prognosis and Resistance to ICIs

The paradox where high infiltration of $CD8^+$ T cells is not linked to favorable prognosis and response to ICI in patients with ccRCC stems from the existence of exhausted and/or dysfunctional T cells. Indeed, the exhaustive status is shown to limit the actual effector function of the ccRCC-infiltrating $CD8^+$ T cells [58–60]. The exhaustive phenotype of the T cells is being overlapped by several groups, as characterized by upregulation of PD-1, LAG-3, TIM-3, CTLA-4, TOX, and CD39 [36,46,55,58,59,61]. scRNAseq studies identified the association between the exhausted and/or dysfunctional $CD8^+$ T cells and disease progression and/or resistance to ICI in patients with ccRCC. Supporting this, the exhausted T cells are unlikely to be fully reversed and reinvigorated by ICI during ccRCC treatments as suggested in other cancers [134–138].

The skewed polarization of TAMs toward M2-like or anti-inflammatory properties is a common feature of advanced ccRCC. Some TAM phenotypes have been reported to decrease the overall immune temperature of the ccRCC. For example, TAMs characterized by high expression of HLA are shown to promote resistance to ICI [55]. A subset of TAMs characterized by a high level of immune regulatory genes, such as APOE, C1Q, and TREM-2, has been commonly identified in the human ccRCC and RENCA model [55,58,60,61,139]. This subset is shown to be associated with a poor prognosis of ccRCC patients due to disease recurrence [61]. Complement activation and/or metabolic reprogramming can be key events associated with TAMs that shape the immunosuppressive tumor microenvironment of ccRCC [55,58,60,61,139].

Computational analysis using a repository of curated receptors, ligands, and their interactions enabled the identification of interactions between malignant and non-malignant cells in ccRCC [140,141]. There are multiple interactions reported between terminally exhausted $CD8^+$ T cells, M2-like/anti-inflammatory TAMs, and ccRCC cells via numerous pairs of ligands and their cognate receptors (Figure 2) [55,56,59–61]. The inhibitory circuit becomes significant as the disease progresses, which promotes an immune-suppressive tumor microenvironment. The signature related to these interactions is found to predict a worse overall prognosis but not a response to ICI of ccRCC patients [59]. Following ICI treatment, immune checkpoint and evasion genes, such as LGALS9 and NECTIN2 expressed on tumor cells as well as TAMs, may play a role in the acquired ICI resistance [59].

Treg cells are one of the important immune-suppressive cell types. Tumor-infiltrating Treg cells are highly immunosuppressive to effector cells. Most scRNAseq datasets have a relatively low abundance of Treg cells for ccRCC, one of the reasons that Treg cells are much less focused from the aforementioned scRNAseq datasets. scRNAseq analysis has identified the increase in the frequency of the tumor-infiltrating Treg cells with advancing ccRCC [60]. Patients showing CR to ICI have low Treg infiltration by scRNAseq [55]. We have particularly focused on tumor-infiltrating Treg cells from our own ccRCC dataset [58]. Comparing tumor-infiltrating versus blood Treg cells, we identified some common shared signature genes of tumor-infiltrating Treg cells, including some genes whose protein products are targetable such as CD177 and BCL2L1 (encoding BCL-X_L). Tumor-infiltrating Treg cells exhibit certain heterogeneity including two distinct populations, with one population showing strong suppressive capacity. We developed a unique tumor-infiltrating Treg cell signature with the prognostic value superior to some known Treg signatures [142]. The clinical importance of tumor-infiltrating Treg cells has been correlated with poor prognosis and response to immune perturbation in other studies as well [45,95,143]. A study observed that anti-PD-1 therapy induces hyper-progression with clonal expansion of tumor-infiltrating Treg cells with upregulation of some genes, including CD177 and BCL2L1 in a leukemic patient [144], the two genes we found to be elevated specifically in tumor-infiltrating Treg cells. CD177 is a surface protein and may modulate the immune suppressive function and maintain homeostasis of tumor-infiltrating Treg cells in ccRCC [142]. We have demonstrated that CD177$^+$ tumor-infiltrating Treg cells are hyper-suppressive to effector T cells and anti-CD177 antibody is able to block the suppressive function of CD177$^+$ tumor-infiltrating Treg cells. Our group has been actively developing other ways of targeting human tumor-infiltrating Treg cells to induce the degradation of BCL-X$_L$ using proteolysis-targeting chimera (PROTAC), which seems very effective for inducing anticancer immunity [145]. Taken together, Treg cells are a potential cell type that can be targeted for cancer immunotherapy.

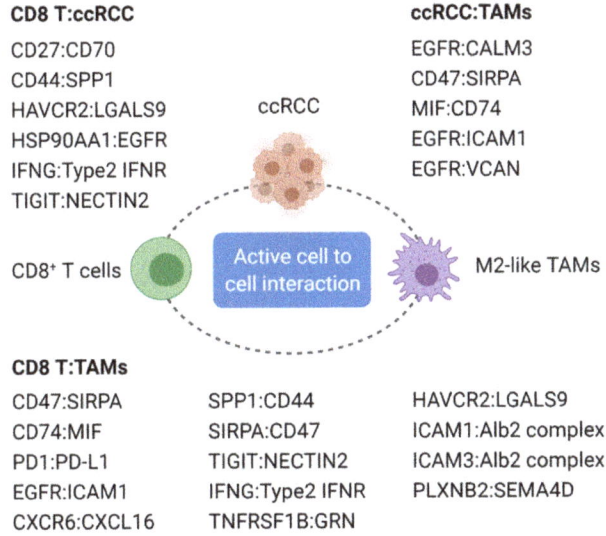

Figure 2. Ligand and receptor pairs potentially associated with ccRCC progression and resistance to ICI. A potential list of ligand and receptor pairs that are predicted by in silico analysis and commonly identified by published ccRCC scRNAseq studies are present. The cell to cell interaction via ligand and receptor pair has not been validated at the functional level. Abbreviation: ccRCC; clear cell renal cell carcinoma, TAMs; tumor-associated macrophages.

3.4. Limitations and Challenges in scRNAseq Technology

Accumulating scRNAseq studies have provided a tremendous amount of critical information that can help to solve the current issues, such as low efficacy and resistance to ICI in patients with ccRCC. Nevertheless, there are limitations and challenges in this scRNAseq technology. In general, the sample sizes are small due to the cost associated with scRNAseq. It is of the utmost importance to prepare freshly isolated single cells for the successful generation of the cDNA library [51]. Single-cell suspension with less than 70% of cell viability is not recommended for library preparation. A highly collaborative work setting is needed for prompt sample preparation and processing to secure cell viability. There is a high economic burden and upfront cost because drop-based scRNAseq platforms require expensive hardware and preparatory kits. Cell hashing and multiplexing technology where oligo-tagged antibodies against ubiquitously expressed surface proteins uniquely label cells from biologically different samples are expected to decrease costs [146]. Processing of the raw data to generate analyzable data form, scRNAseq data requires computing systems with high memory capacity. For example, the 10× Genomics Cell Ranger requires 64 gigabytes of RAM, up to 1.5 terabytes of disk space, and a Linux-based system. Newer alignment tools, such as Alven [147] or kallisto-bustools [148], cut these system requirements by an order of magnitude. The bioinformatic analysis of scRNAseq data is still challenging; in-depth analysis of the data requires experience in coding, which can be a barrier of entry for laboratories. There is still no standard guideline for processing workflow from quality control to determining resolution and dimensionality [149].

In addition to limitations concerning the bottlenecks in implementation, there are also challenges associated with scRNAseq technology. scRNAseq is invariably limited by the dropout phenomenon where up to 93% of the count matrix can be zeros [149,150]. From the immune perspective, this dropout effect, coupled with the use of a highly-variable gene approach, makes annotating cell types and discovering small immune populations difficult [151]. A certain type of immune cells can be more susceptible to dropout. Indeed, there is a preferential dropout of transcription factors and cytokines, making $CD4^+$ T cell annotation difficult [61,152]. Application of a specific algorithm to scRNAseq data to infer protein activity [61] or impute RNA values [153], at least in part, may overcome the dropout. In addition, changes in the generation of cDNA, e.g., through the adoption of the second-strand synthesis option, may also be advantageous in the recovery of cytokine and transcription factor expression [152]. Single-cell sequencing requires the generation of single-cell suspensions, leading to induction of specific genetic programs and loss of spatial information [154]. Platforms for spatial scRNAseq are emerging and will offer insights into cell-to-cell communications [155]. Unlike flow cytometry with established markers for antigen experience or cellular ontogeny, the scRNAseq toolkits are not as well-stocked. In terms of the latter, scRNAseq-based lineage tracing, using cellular tagging or mitochondrial variations, may offer a chance to look at the compartment-specific immune response [156,157]. The chemistry used to generate the cDNA libraries in scRNAseq utilize short 5′ or 3′ reads, limiting the assessment of mutational status, single-nucleotide polymorphisms, or alternative splicing, such as CD45RA versus CD45RO isoforms, which all play a role in the immune response. Recent improvements in scRNAseq chemistry may reduce this issue by generating longer cDNA sequences [158].

4. Perspectives and Clinical Implications

4.1. Consensus in Nomenclature

There is no doubt that utilizing scRNAseq technology to clinical samples enables the better dissection of tumor microenvironment of ccRCC or other cancers, providing insight into various types of immune cells that are critical for either shaping immune-suppressive environment or driving a favorable immune response following ICI. The big picture of immune cell composition can be painted at a much higher resolution than what traditional bulk RNAseq or flow cytometry have been provided, along with the gene expression data of individual immune cells. As we discussed about different studies related to the nomenclature of distinct cell subsets, it becomes evident that the field is far away from achieving consensus based on signature gene expression. As ccRCC enters the immunotherapy era, elevation in tumor-infiltrating $CD8^+$ T cells, though they have been known as a bad prognosis before immunotherapy became the standard frontline treatment, provides an immune-hot microenvironment for ICI to work. Although most studies borrowed signatures based on melanoma studies to determine the nature of CD8 clusters, different studies used different nomenclatures. A similar situation applies to other major immune cell types including $CD4^+$ T cells and macrophages. Based on publications and after carefully comparing different populations, $CD8^+$ T cells from ccRCC have the three major populations as in melanomas, including the naïve like, cytotoxic, and dysfunctional [159], as well as a relative consensus on the proliferative and tissue-resident memory (TRM) populations. Apparently, the dysfunctional group consists of a series of populations at different and likely continuous functional stages that could be the potential targets of ICIs, with a 4-1BB^{low} cluster showing feature of progenitor exhausted phenotype and can be expanded by ICIs for cancer cell killing [55,59]. This 4-1BB^{low} CD8$^+$ T could be a similar population identified in another study as TRM as both populations exhibit the expression of intermediate immune checkpoints, effector/activation molecules and likely CD44 and CD103 [55,59] that are used to define TRM cells. A clear understanding of these populations should be based on the integration of these datasets and will be able to direct the prediction of patients who may benefit from ICIs.

TAMs are another major focus on ccRCC studies with 2–5 sub-clusters from different studies. The nomenclature for TAMs can be misleading since quite a few studies still used M1-like and M2-like names to define the subtle difference of their M1 or M2 signatures. Nearly all studies did not show a distinct separation of M1- versus M2-like TAMs that rather secrete M1 and/or M2 cytokines at various levels. Several studies used the marker genes such as HLA, interferon signaling genes (ISG), other lead genes or cluster numbers to define and imply functional differences. It is clear that TAMs are very important in the pathogenesis of ccRCC and can be the major predictor for the sensitivity to ICIs. The clearer designation of different TAM clusters is important for using these TAM-related signatures for clinical predictions.

4.2. ScRNAseq Reveals Mechanisms of Immune Activation

The major action of ICIs in melanoma is to rejuvenate pre-existing exhausted CD8$^+$ T cells, a well-accepted mechanism of action for ICI-based cancer immunotherapy. Recent development in the field identified a potential novel mechanism by ICI-induced clonal replacement, i.e. the replacement of old CD8$^+$ T cell clones with new clones from blood or adjacent normal tissues. Clonal expansion of ccRCC-infiltrating non-exhausted CD8$^+$ T cells and/or de novo introduction of peripherally expanded CD8$^+$ T cells to tumor site can be a more convincing and potential mechanism underlying the immune response to ICI than the widely presumed reinvigoration of the pre-existing exhausted CD8$^+$ T cells [44,55,62,135,137,138,160,161]. In agreement with this notion, a recent study [38] clearly demonstrated that the diversity of pre-existing CD8$^+$ T cell clones, likely those similar to 4-1BB^{low} or TRM populations identified from other studies [55,59], are critical for eliciting the favorable response within nivolumab-treated ccRCC patients. Nivolumab maintains and expands these pre-existing CD8 T cell clones to elicit an effective anti-tumor immune response. In non-responders, clonal expansion of exhausted CD8$^+$ T cells [55] and expanded CD8$^+$ T cells with novel TCRs are not associated with clinical response to nivolumab in ccRCC patients [38]. This novel mechanism of action makes it critical to identify the diversity of pre-existing CD8$^+$ T cell clones within tumor microenvironment and to set up a threshold using deep learning to predict patient responses to ICIs. Figure 3 illustrates the current concept of immunotherapy driving clinical response to ICI in patients with ccRCC.

The presence of distinct subsets of immune suppressive and/or pro-angiogenic TAMs is believed to lead to ccRCC progression and inhibit the immune response to ICI. Potential mechanisms of action include inhibitory cell-to-cell communications, modulation of complement activation and/or metabolic reprogramming [55,56,58–61,139]. Machine-learning based algorithm has the capacity to identify the potential cell-cell interactions and TAMs process many interactions with cancer cells and other immune cells (Figure 2) to facilitate cancer progression in late stage of ccRCC patients by either directly promoting angiogenesis and/or cancer cell aggressiveness, or by indirectly inducing a more immune-suppressive network. Currently there is no effective treatment to eliminate or inhibit these TAMs, but scRNAseq-based research has defined certain populations that can be shaped by ICIs in responders where ICIs induce a more M1-like responses at the same time upregulating several immune checkpoints such as VSIR, VSIG4, PD-L2, and SIGLEC10 [59]. The function of these immune checkpoints is yet-to-be validated whether they can induce ICI resistance, but if confirmed, following treatment regimens should involve in antibodies targeting those novel checkpoints.

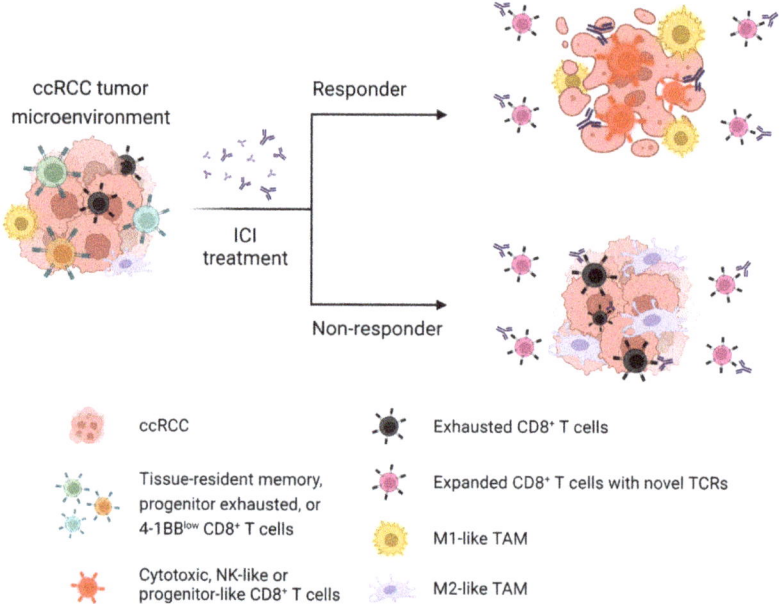

Figure 3. Current concept of immunotherapy driving clinical response to ICI in patients with ccRCC. Pre-existing CD8+ T cell clones phenotyped by CD69+ZNF683+ TRM, progenitor exhausted, or 4-1BB^{low} are considered to have a critical role in favorable response to ICI in ccRCC patients. In responders, ICI-bound expanded CD8+ T cells exhibit cytotoxic, NK-like, or progenitor-like phenotypes. In contrast, non-responders had no clonal expansion of the tumor-reactive CD8+ T cell clones. In both responders and non-responders, pre-existing exhausted T cells are clonally expanded following ICI treatment. In ccRCC, clonal expansion of CD8+ T cells with novel TCRs are not associated with clinical response to ICI. Following ICI treatment, TAMs shift toward M1-like or pro-inflammatory phenotype in responders, whereas non-responders have skewed polarization of TAMs toward M2-like or anti-inflammatory phenotype in ccRCC tumor microenvironment. CD69, ZNF683, and CD103 are commonly expressed in CD8+ TRM cells. 4-1BB^{low} CD8+ T cells are highly enriched with progenitor exhausted signature. The tumor-reactive effector-like CD8+ T cells commonly express GZMA, GZMB, GZMK, PRF1, IFNG, NKG7, CCL3, CCL5, and CXCL13 genes, as well as co-inhibitory receptors, such as PD-1, TIM-3, LAG3, and TIGIT genes. Terminally exhausted phenotype is characterized by high expression of PD-1, LAG-3, TIM-3, CTLA-4, TOX, and CD39. M1-like TAMs are highly enriched with signatures of interferon signaling, antigen presentation, and proteasome function. M2-like TAMs are commonly characterized by high expression of HLA, APOE, C1QA, and TREM-2. Abbreviation: ccRCC; clear cell renal cell carcinoma, ICI; immune checkpoint inhibitor, TAMs; tumor-associated macrophages, NK; natural killer, TCR; T cell receptor.

Another complexity comes from the interactions between essential components within ccRCC involving cancer cells, immune cells and others. An oversimplified version is shown in Figure 2 where many ligand/receptor pairs exist and can potentially induce complex cellular interactions. How can we use the identified and known information to extract the dominant signaling pair that can be interrupted? For example, as many as 14 pairs of interaction are identified between CD8+ T cells and TAMs including PD-1/PD-L1 pair that may dominate the immune-suppressive responses within responders treated with anti-PD-1/PD-L1 antibodies. The question is whether we can develop testing and bioinformatics pipeline for clinical treatment selections rather than treating all patients with the same drugs that are known to have relatively low responses rate.

4.3. Conclusions Remarks

Current scRNAseq studies have been limited by the small patient cohorts and the lack of experimental validations at functional levels. Can therapeutic intervention cause the hypothesized immune modulation in TME within patients' tumors? Future work will be required to longitudinally address the characteristics of highly effective T cells against ccRCC in different perspectives, such as stem cell-like, metabolic, transcriptional, and epigenetic states [44]. The standardization of experimental methods, such as scRNAseq studies pooling clinical trials and in vitro or in vivo preclinical perturbation models will be required to address the effect of blocking immune checkpoints or key inhibitory molecules on the reinvigoration of exhausted T cell function, replacement of exhausted T cells by non-exhausted effector T cells, or shifting anti-inflammatory TAMs to pro-inflammatory ones [133,138,139]. Multi-omics approaches to the ccRCC environment, including spatial transcriptomics and proteomics, may reveal new gene signatures and molecular targets that reflect a functional immune niche or escape [44]. Further studies are warranted to evaluate other, less-characterized cell types, such as antigen-presenting cells or regulatory T cells, to identify novel therapeutic targets that address immune dysfunction in ccRCC [33,40,43,55,59,60,139,162–164].

Author Contributions: Conceptualization, M.-C.K. and W.Z.; writing—original draft preparation, M.-C.K. and Z.J.; writing—review and editing, M.-C.K., R.K., N.B., J.A.C., S.M.F. and W.Z.; supervision, W.Z.; project administration, W.Z.; funding acquisition, W.Z. All authors have read and agreed to the published version of the manuscript.

Funding: The work was partially supported by NIH grants CA200673 (W.Z.), CA203834 (W.Z.), CA260239 (W.Z.), DOD/CDMRP grants BC180227 and BC200100 (W.Z.). W.Z. was also supported by an endowment fund from the Dr. and Mrs. James Robert Spenser Family.

Conflicts of Interest: The authors declare no conflict of interest.

References

1. Hsieh, J.J.; Purdue, M.P.; Signoretti, S.; Swanton, C.; Albiges, L.; Schmidinger, M.; Heng, D.Y.; Larkin, J.; Ficarra, V. Renal cell carcinoma. *Nat. Rev. Dis. Primers* **2017**, *3*, 1–19. [CrossRef] [PubMed]
2. Siegel, R.L.; Miller, K.D.; Fuchs, H.E.; Jemal, A. Cancer statistics, 2021. *CA A Cancer J. Clin.* **2021**, *71*, 7–33. [CrossRef] [PubMed]
3. Bray, F.; Ferlay, J.; Soerjomataram, I.; Siegel, R.L.; Torre, L.A.; Jemal, A. Global cancer statistics 2018: GLOBOCAN estimates of incidence and mortality worldwide for 36 cancers in 185 countries. *CA A Cancer J. Clin.* **2018**, *68*, 394–424. [CrossRef] [PubMed]
4. Rini, B.I.; Campbell, S.C.; Escudier, B. Renal cell carcinoma. *Lancet* **2009**, *373*, 1119–1132. [CrossRef]
5. Chow, W.-H.; Dong, L.M.; Devesa, S.S. Epidemiology and risk factors for kidney cancer. *Nat. Rev. Urol.* **2010**, *7*, 245–257. [CrossRef]
6. Gong, J.; Maia, M.C.; Dizman, N.; Govindarajan, A.; Pal, S.K. Metastasis in renal cell carcinoma: Biology and implications for therapy. *Asian J. Urol.* **2016**, *3*, 286–292. [CrossRef]
7. Janzen, N.K.; Kim, H.L.; Figlin, R.A.; Belldegrun, A.S. Surveillance after radical or partial nephrectomy for localized renal cell carcinoma and management of recurrent disease. *Urol. Clin.* **2003**, *30*, 843–852. [CrossRef]
8. Nickerson, M.L.; Jaeger, E.; Shi, Y.; Durocher, J.A.; Mahurkar, S.; Zaridze, D.; Matveev, V.; Janout, V.; Kollarova, H.; Bencko, V. Improved identification of von Hippel-Lindau gene alterations in clear cell renal tumors. *Clin. Cancer Res.* **2008**, *14*, 4726–4734. [CrossRef]
9. Sato, Y.; Yoshizato, T.; Shiraishi, Y.; Maekawa, S.; Okuno, Y.; Kamura, T.; Shimamura, T.; Sato-Otsubo, A.; Nagae, G.; Suzuki, H. Integrated molecular analysis of clear-cell renal cell carcinoma. *Nat. Genet.* **2013**, *45*, 860–867. [CrossRef]
10. Kaelin, W.G., Jr. Von hippel-lindau disease. *Annu. Rev. Pathol. Mech. Dis.* **2007**, *2*, 145–173. [CrossRef]
11. Vuong, L.; Kotecha, R.R.; Voss, M.H.; Hakimi, A.A. Tumor microenvironment dynamics in clear-cell renal cell carcinoma. *Cancer Discov.* **2019**, *9*, 1349–1357. [CrossRef] [PubMed]
12. Albiges, L.; Oudard, S.; Negrier, S.; Caty, A.; Gravis, G.; Joly, F.; Duclos, B.; Geoffrois, L.; Rolland, F.; Guillot, A. Complete remission with tyrosine kinase inhibitors in renal cell carcinoma. *J. Clin. Oncol.* **2012**, *30*, 482–487. [CrossRef] [PubMed]
13. Buczek, M.; Escudier, B.; Bartnik, E.; Szczylik, C.; Czarnecka, A. Resistance to tyrosine kinase inhibitors in clear cell renal cell carcinoma: From the patient's bed to molecular mechanisms. *Biochim. Biophys. Acta-Rev. Cancer* **2014**, *1845*, 31–41. [CrossRef] [PubMed]
14. Topalian, S.L.; Hodi, F.S.; Brahmer, J.R.; Gettinger, S.N.; Smith, D.C.; McDermott, D.F.; Powderly, J.D.; Carvajal, R.D.; Sosman, J.A.; Atkins, M.B. Safety, activity, and immune correlates of anti–PD-1 antibody in cancer. *N. Engl. J. Med.* **2012**, *366*, 2443–2454. [CrossRef]

15. Motzer, R.J.; Escudier, B.; McDermott, D.F.; George, S.; Hammers, H.J.; Srinivas, S.; Tykodi, S.S.; Sosman, J.A.; Procopio, G.; Plimack, E.R. Nivolumab versus everolimus in advanced renal-cell carcinoma. *N. Engl. J. Med.* **2015**, *373*, 1803–1813. [CrossRef] [PubMed]
16. Challis, G.; Stam, H. The spontaneous regression of cancer: A review of cases from 1900 to 1987. *Acta Oncol.* **1990**, *29*, 545–550. [CrossRef]
17. Everson, T.C.; Cole, W.H. Spontaneous regression of cancer: Preliminary report. *Ann. Surg.* **1956**, *144*, 366. [CrossRef]
18. Snow, R.M.; Schellhammer, P.F. Spontaneous regression of metastatic renal cell carcinoma. *Urology* **1982**, *20*, 177–181. [CrossRef]
19. Janiszewska, A.D.; Poletajew, S.; Wasiutyński, A. Spontaneous regression of renal cell carcinoma. *Contemp. Oncol.* **2013**, *17*, 123. [CrossRef]
20. Rosenberg, S.A. IL-2: The first effective immunotherapy for human cancer. *J. Immunol.* **2014**, *192*, 5451–5458. [CrossRef]
21. Motzer, R.J.; Tannir, N.M.; McDermott, D.F.; Frontera, O.A.; Melichar, B.; Choueiri, T.K.; Plimack, E.R.; Barthélémy, P.; Porta, C.; George, S. Nivolumab plus ipilimumab versus sunitinib in advanced renal-cell carcinoma. *N. Engl. J. Med.* **2018**, *378*, 1277–1290. [CrossRef] [PubMed]
22. Choueiri, T.K.; Powles, T.; Burotto, M.; Escudier, B.; Bourlon, M.T.; Zurawski, B.; Oyervides Juárez, V.M.; Hsieh, J.J.; Basso, U.; Shah, A.Y. Nivolumab plus cabozantinib versus sunitinib for advanced renal-cell carcinoma. *N. Engl. J. Med.* **2021**, *384*, 829–841. [CrossRef] [PubMed]
23. Motzer, R.; Penkov, K.; Haanen, J.; Rini, B.; Albiges, L.; Campbell, M.T.; Venugopal, B.; Kollmannsberger, C.; Negrier, S.; Uemura, M. Avelumab plus axitinib versus sunitinib for advanced renal-cell carcinoma. *N. Engl. J. Med.* **2019**, *380*, 1103–1115. [CrossRef] [PubMed]
24. Rini, B.I.; Powles, T.; Atkins, M.B.; Escudier, B.; McDermott, D.F.; Suarez, C.; Bracarda, S.; Stadler, W.M.; Donskov, F.; Lee, J.L. Atezolizumab plus bevacizumab versus sunitinib in patients with previously untreated metastatic renal cell carcinoma (IMmotion151): A multicentre, open-label, phase 3, randomised controlled trial. *Lancet* **2019**, *393*, 2404–2415. [CrossRef]
25. Rini, B.I.; Plimack, E.R.; Stus, V.; Gafanov, R.; Hawkins, R.; Nosov, D.; Pouliot, F.; Alekseev, B.; Soulières, D.; Melichar, B. Pembrolizumab plus axitinib versus sunitinib for advanced renal-cell carcinoma. *N. Engl. J. Med.* **2019**, *380*, 1116–1127. [CrossRef]
26. Motzer, R.; Alekseev, B.; Rha, S.-Y.; Porta, C.; Eto, M.; Powles, T.; Grünwald, V.; Hutson, T.E.; Kopyltsov, E.; Méndez-Vidal, M.J. Lenvatinib plus pembrolizumab or everolimus for advanced renal cell carcinoma. *N. Engl. J. Med.* **2021**, *384*, 1289–1300. [CrossRef]
27. Motzer, R.J.; Rini, B.I.; McDermott, D.F.; Frontera, O.A.; Hammers, H.J.; Carducci, M.A.; Salman, P.; Escudier, B.; Beuselinck, B.; Amin, A. Nivolumab plus ipilimumab versus sunitinib in first-line treatment for advanced renal cell carcinoma: Extended follow-up of efficacy and safety results from a randomised, controlled, phase 3 trial. *Lancet Oncol.* **2019**, *20*, 1370–1385. [CrossRef]
28. Massari, F.; Mollica, V.; Rizzo, A.; Cosmai, L.; Rizzo, M.; Porta, C. Safety evaluation of immune-based combinations in patients with advanced renal cell carcinoma: A systematic review and meta-analysis. *Expert. Opin. Drug. Saf.* **2020**, *19*, 1329–1338. [CrossRef]
29. Cella, D.; Grünwald, V.; Escudier, B.; Hammers, H.J.; George, S.; Nathan, P.; Grimm, M.O.; Rini, B.I.; Doan, J.; Ivanescu, C.; et al. Patient-reported outcomes of patients with advanced renal cell carcinoma treated with nivolumab plus ipilimumab versus sunitinib (CheckMate 214): A randomised, phase 3 trial. *Lancet Oncol.* **2019**, *20*, 297–310. [CrossRef]
30. Atkins, M.B.; Rini, B.I.; Motzer, R.J.; Powles, T.; McDermott, D.F.; Suarez, C.; Bracarda, S.; Stadler, W.M.; Donskov, F.; Gurney, H. Patient-reported outcomes from the phase III Randomized IMmotion151 Trial: Atezolizumab + Bevacizumab versus sunitinib in treatment-naive metastatic renal cell carcinoma. *Clin. Cancer Res.* **2020**, *26*, 2506–2514.
31. Motzer, R.J.; Banchereau, R.; Hamidi, H.; Powles, T.; McDermott, D.; Atkins, M.B.; Escudier, B.; Liu, L.-F.; Leng, N.; Abbas, A.R. Molecular subsets in renal cancer determine outcome to checkpoint and angiogenesis blockade. *Cancer Cell* **2020**, *38*, 803–817.e804. [CrossRef] [PubMed]
32. Abou Alaiwi, S.; Nassar, A.H.; Xie, W.; Bakouny, Z.; Berchuck, J.E.; Braun, D.A.; Baca, S.C.; Nuzzo, P.V.; Flippot, R.; Mouhieddine, T.H. Mammalian SWI/SNF complex genomic alterations and immune checkpoint blockade in solid tumors. *Cancer Immunol. Res.* **2020**, *8*, 1075. [CrossRef] [PubMed]
33. Motzer, R.J.; Robbins, P.B.; Powles, T.; Albiges, L.; Haanen, J.B.; Larkin, J.; Mu, X.J.; Ching, K.A.; Uemura, M.; Pal, S.K. Avelumab plus axitinib versus sunitinib in advanced renal cell carcinoma: Biomarker analysis of the phase 3 JAVELIN Renal 101 trial. *Nat. Med.* **2020**, *26*, 1733–1741. [CrossRef] [PubMed]
34. Miao, D.; Margolis, C.A.; Gao, W.; Voss, M.H.; Li, W.; Martini, D.J.; Norton, C.; Bossé, D.; Wankowicz, S.M.; Cullen, D. Genomic correlates of response to immune checkpoint therapies in clear cell renal cell carcinoma. *Science* **2018**, *359*, 801–806. [CrossRef]
35. Braun, D.A.; Hou, Y.; Bakouny, Z.; Ficial, M.; Sant'Angelo, M.; Forman, J.; Ross-Macdonald, P.; Berger, A.C.; Jegede, O.A.; Elagina, L. Interplay of somatic alterations and immune infiltration modulates response to PD-1 blockade in advanced clear cell renal cell carcinoma. *Nat. Med.* **2020**, *26*, 909–918. [CrossRef] [PubMed]
36. Braun, D.A.; Ishii, Y.; Walsh, A.M.; Van Allen, E.M.; Wu, C.J.; Shukla, S.A.; Choueiri, T.K. Clinical validation of PBRM1 alterations as a marker of immune checkpoint inhibitor response in renal cell carcinoma. *JAMA Oncol.* **2019**, *5*, 1631–1633. [CrossRef] [PubMed]
37. McDermott, D.F.; Huseni, M.A.; Atkins, M.B.; Motzer, R.J.; Rini, B.I.; Escudier, B.; Fong, L.; Joseph, R.W.; Pal, S.K.; Reeves, J.A. Clinical activity and molecular correlates of response to atezolizumab alone or in combination with bevacizumab versus sunitinib in renal cell carcinoma. *Nat. Med.* **2018**, *24*, 749–757. [CrossRef]

38. Au, L.; Hatipoglu, E.; Robert de Massy, M.; Litchfield, K.; Beattie, G.; Rowan, A.; Schnidrig, D.; Thompson, R.; Byrne, F.; Horswell, S.; et al. Determinants of anti-PD-1 response and resistance in clear cell renal cell carcinoma. *Cancer Cell* **2021**, *39*, 1497–1518.e1411. [CrossRef]
39. Erlmeier, F.; Weichert, W.; Schrader, A.J.; Autenrieth, M.; Hartmann, A.; Steffens, S.; Ivanyi, P. Prognostic impact of PD-1 and its ligands in renal cell carcinoma. *Med. Oncol.* **2017**, *34*, 99. [CrossRef]
40. Labriola, M.K.; Zhu, J.; Gupta, R.; McCall, S.; Jackson, J.; Kong, E.F.; White, J.R.; Cerqueira, G.; Gerding, K.; Simmons, J.K. Characterization of tumor mutation burden, PD-L1 and DNA repair genes to assess relationship to immune checkpoint inhibitors response in metastatic renal cell carcinoma. *J. Immunother. Cancer* **2020**, *8*, e000319. [CrossRef]
41. Fridman, W.H.; Zitvogel, L.; Sautès–Fridman, C.; Kroemer, G. The immune contexture in cancer prognosis and treatment. *Nat. Rev. Clin. Oncol.* **2017**, *14*, 717–734. [CrossRef] [PubMed]
42. Nakano, O.; Sato, M.; Naito, Y.; Suzuki, K.; Orikasa, S.; Aizawa, M.; Suzuki, Y.; Shintaku, I.; Nagura, H.; Ohtani, H. Proliferative activity of intratumoral CD8+ T-lymphocytes as a prognostic factor in human renal cell carcinoma: Clinicopathologic demonstration of antitumor immunity. *Cancer Res.* **2001**, *61*, 5132–5136. [PubMed]
43. Murakami, T.; Tanaka, N.; Takamatsu, K.; Hakozaki, K.; Fukumoto, K.; Masuda, T.; Mikami, S.; Shinojima, T.; Kakimi, K.; Tsunoda, T. Multiplexed single-cell pathology reveals the association of CD8 T-cell heterogeneity with prognostic outcomes in renal cell carcinoma. *Cancer Immunol. Immunother.* **2021**, *70*, 3001–3013. [CrossRef] [PubMed]
44. Jansen, C.S.; Prokhnevska, N.; Master, V.A.; Sanda, M.G.; Carlisle, J.W.; Bilen, M.A.; Cardenas, M.; Wilkinson, S.; Lake, R.; Sowalsky, A.G. An intra-tumoral niche maintains and differentiates stem-like CD8 T cells. *Nature* **2019**, *576*, 465–470. [CrossRef]
45. Şenbabaoğlu, Y.; Gejman, R.S.; Winer, A.G.; Liu, M.; Van Allen, E.M.; de Velasco, G.; Miao, D.; Ostrovnaya, I.; Drill, E.; Luna, A. Tumor immune microenvironment characterization in clear cell renal cell carcinoma identifies prognostic and immunotherapeutically relevant messenger RNA signatures. *Genome Biol.* **2016**, *17*, 231. [CrossRef]
46. Chevrier, S.; Levine, J.H.; Zanotelli, V.R.T.; Silina, K.; Schulz, D.; Bacac, M.; Ries, C.H.; Ailles, L.; Jewett, M.A.S.; Moch, H. An immune atlas of clear cell renal cell carcinoma. *Cell* **2017**, *169*, 736–749.e718. [CrossRef]
47. Rooney, M.S.; Shukla, S.A.; Wu, C.J.; Getz, G.; Hacohen, N. Molecular and genetic properties of tumors associated with local immune cytolytic activity. *Cell* **2015**, *160*, 48–61. [CrossRef]
48. Patel, H.D.; Puligandla, M.; Shuch, B.M.; Leibovich, B.C.; Kapoor, A.; Master, V.A.; Drake, C.G.; Heng, D.Y.; Lara, P.N.; Choueiri, T.K. The future of perioperative therapy in advanced renal cell carcinoma: How can we PROSPER? *Future Oncol.* **2019**, *15*, 1683–1695. [CrossRef]
49. Baine, M.K.; Turcu, G.; Zito, C.R.; Adeniran, A.J.; Camp, R.L.; Chen, L.; Kluger, H.M.; Jilaveanu, L.B. Characterization of tumor infiltrating lymphocytes in paired primary and metastatic renal cell carcinoma specimens. *Oncotarget* **2015**, *6*, 24990. [CrossRef]
50. Matsushita, H.; Vesely, M.D.; Koboldt, D.C.; Rickert, C.G.; Uppaluri, R.; Magrini, V.J.; Arthur, C.D.; White, J.M.; Chen, Y.-S.; Shea, L.K. Cancer exome analysis reveals a T-cell-dependent mechanism of cancer immunoediting. *Nature* **2012**, *482*, 400–404. [CrossRef]
51. Sun, G.; Li, Z.; Rong, D.; Zhang, H.; Shi, X.; Yang, W.; Zheng, W.; Sun, G.; Wu, F.; Cao, H. Single-cell RNA sequencing in cancer: Applications, advances, and emerging challenges. *Mol. Ther. Oncolytics* **2021**, *21*, 183–206. [CrossRef] [PubMed]
52. Papalexi, E.; Satija, R. Single-cell RNA sequencing to explore immune cell heterogeneity. *Nat. Rev. Immunol.* **2018**, *18*, 35–45. [CrossRef] [PubMed]
53. Kelsey, G.; Stegle, O.; Reik, W. Single-cell epigenomics: Recording the past and predicting the future. *Science* **2017**, *358*, 69–75. [CrossRef] [PubMed]
54. Yu, Z.; Lu, W.; Su, C.; Lv, Y.; Ye, Y.; Guo, B.; Liu, D.; Yan, H.; Mi, H.; Li, T. Single-cell RNA-seq identification of the cellular molecular characteristics of sporadic bilateral clear cell renal cell carcinoma. *Front. Oncol.* **2021**, *11*, 1825. [CrossRef] [PubMed]
55. Krishna, C.; DiNatale, R.G.; Kuo, F.; Srivastava, R.M.; Vuong, L.; Chowell, D.; Gupta, S.; Vanderbilt, C.; Purohit, T.A.; Liu, M. Single-cell sequencing links multiregional immune landscapes and tissue-resident T cells in ccRCC to tumor topology and therapy efficacy. *Cancer Cell* **2021**, *39*, 662–677.e666. [CrossRef] [PubMed]
56. Zhang, Y.; Narayanan, S.P.; Mannan, R.; Raskind, G.; Wang, X.; Vats, P.; Su, F.; Hosseini, N.; Cao, X.; Kumar-Sinha, C. Single-cell analyses of renal cell cancers reveal insights into tumor microenvironment, cell of origin, and therapy response. *Proc. Natl. Acad. Sci. USA* **2021**, *118*, e2103240118. [CrossRef]
57. Young, M.D.; Mitchell, T.J.; Braga, F.A.V.; Tran, M.G.; Stewart, B.J.; Ferdinand, J.R.; Collord, G.; Botting, R.A.; Popescu, D.-M.; Loudon, K.W. Single-cell transcriptomes from human kidneys reveal the cellular identity of renal tumors. *Science* **2018**, *361*, 594–599. [CrossRef] [PubMed]
58. Borcherding, N.; Vishwakarma, A.; Voigt, A.P.; Bellizzi, A.; Kaplan, J.; Nepple, K.; Salem, A.K.; Jenkins, R.W.; Zakharia, Y.; Zhang, W. Mapping the immune environment in clear cell renal carcinoma by single-cell genomics. *Commun. Biol.* **2021**, *4*, 1–11. [CrossRef]
59. Bi, K.; He, M.X.; Bakouny, Z.; Kanodia, A.; Napolitano, S.; Wu, J.; Grimaldi, G.; Braun, D.A.; Cuoco, M.S.; Mayorga, A. Tumor and immune reprogramming during immunotherapy in advanced renal cell carcinoma. *Cancer Cell* **2021**, *39*, 649–661.e645. [CrossRef]
60. Braun, D.A.; Street, K.; Burke, K.P.; Cookmeyer, D.L.; Denize, T.; Pedersen, C.B.; Gohil, S.H.; Schindler, N.; Pomerance, L.; Hirsch, L. Progressive immune dysfunction with advancing disease stage in renal cell carcinoma. *Cancer Cell* **2021**, *39*, 632–648.e638. [CrossRef]

61. Obradovic, A.; Chowdhury, N.; Haake, S.M.; Ager, C.; Wang, V.; Vlahos, L.; Guo, X.V.; Aggen, D.H.; Rathmell, W.K.; Jonasch, E. Single-cell protein activity analysis identifies recurrence-associated renal tumor macrophages. *Cell* **2021**, *184*, 2988–3005.e2916. [CrossRef] [PubMed]
62. Wu, T.D.; Madireddi, S.; de Almeida, P.E.; Banchereau, R.; Chen, Y.-J.J.; Chitre, A.S.; Chiang, E.Y.; Iftikhar, H.; O'Gorman, W.E.; Au-Yeung, A. Peripheral T cell expansion predicts tumour infiltration and clinical response. *Nature* **2020**, *579*, 274–278. [CrossRef] [PubMed]
63. Malek, T.R. The biology of interleukin-2. *Annu. Rev. Immunol.* **2008**, *26*, 453–479. [CrossRef] [PubMed]
64. Fisher, R.I.; Rosenberg, S.A.; Fyfe, G. Long-term survival update for high-dose recombinant interleukin-2 in patients with renal cell carcinoma. *Cancer J. Sci. Am.* **2000**, *6*, S55–S57.
65. Fyfe, G.; Fisher, R.I.; Rosenberg, S.A.; Sznol, M.; Parkinson, D.R.; Louie, A.C. Results of treatment of 255 patients with metastatic renal cell carcinoma who received high-dose recombinant interleukin-2 therapy. *J. Clin. Oncol.* **1995**, *13*, 688–696. [CrossRef]
66. Klapper, J.A.; Downey, S.G.; Smith, F.O.; Yang, J.C.; Hughes, M.S.; Kammula, U.S.; Sherry, R.M.; Royal, R.E.; Steinberg, S.M.; Rosenberg, S. High-dose interleukin-2 for the treatment of metastatic renal cell carcinoma: A retrospective analysis of response and survival in patients treated in the surgery branch at the National Cancer Institute between 1986 and 2006. *Cancer* **2008**, *113*, 293–301. [CrossRef]
67. McDermott, D.F.; Regan, M.M.; Clark, J.I.; Flaherty, L.E.; Weiss, G.R.; Logan, T.F.; Kirkwood, J.M.; Gordon, M.S.; Sosman, J.A.; Ernstoff, M.S. Randomized phase III trial of high-dose interleukin-2 versus subcutaneous interleukin-2 and interferon in patients with metastatic renal cell carcinoma. *J. Clin. Oncol.* **2005**, *23*, 133–141. [CrossRef]
68. McDermott, D.F.; Cheng, S.-C.; Signoretti, S.; Margolin, K.A.; Clark, J.I.; Sosman, J.A.; Dutcher, J.P.; Logan, T.F.; Curti, B.D.; Ernstoff, M.S. The high-dose aldesleukin "select" trial: A trial to prospectively validate predictive models of response to treatment in patients with metastatic renal cell carcinoma. *Clin. Cancer Res.* **2015**, *21*, 561–568. [CrossRef]
69. Minasian, L.M.; Motzer, R.J.; Gluck, L.; Mazumdar, M.; Vlamis, V.; Krown, S.E. Interferon alfa-2a in advanced renal cell carcinoma: Treatment results and survival in 159 patients with long-term follow-up. *J. Clin. Oncol.* **1993**, *11*, 1368–1375. [CrossRef]
70. Negrier, S.; Escudier, B.; Lasset, C.; Douillard, J.-Y.; Savary, J.; Chevreau, C.; Ravaud, A.; Mercatello, A.; Peny, J.; Mousseau, M. Recombinant human interleukin-2, recombinant human interferon alfa-2a, or both in metastatic renal-cell carcinoma. *N. Engl. J. Med.* **1998**, *338*, 1272–1278. [CrossRef]
71. Motzer, R.J.; Murphy, B.A.; Bacik, J.; Schwartz, L.H.; Nanus, D.M.; Mariani, T.; Loehrer, P.; Wilding, G.; Fairclough, D.L.; Cella, D. Phase III trial of interferon alfa-2a with or without 13-cis-retinoic acid for patients with advanced renal cell carcinoma. *J. Clin. Oncol.* **2000**, *18*, 2972–2980. [CrossRef]
72. Dutcher, J. Current status of interleukin-2 therapy for metastatic renal cell carcinoma and metastatic melanoma. *Oncology* **2002**, *16*, 4–10. [PubMed]
73. Motzer, R.J.; Bacik, J.; Murphy, B.A.; Russo, P.; Mazumdar, M. Interferon-alfa as a comparative treatment for clinical trials of new therapies against advanced renal cell carcinoma. *J. Clin. Oncol.* **2002**, *20*, 289–296. [CrossRef] [PubMed]
74. Choueiri, T.K.; Hessel, C.; Halabi, S.; Sanford, B.; Michaelson, M.D.; Hahn, O.; Walsh, M.; Olencki, T.; Picus, J.; Small, E.J. Cabozantinib versus sunitinib as initial therapy for metastatic renal cell carcinoma of intermediate or poor risk (Alliance A031203 CABOSUN randomised trial): Progression-free survival by independent review and overall survival update. *Eur. J. Cancer* **2018**, *94*, 115–125. [CrossRef] [PubMed]
75. Escudier, B.; Eisen, T.; Stadler, W.M.; Szczylik, C.; Oudard, S.; Siebels, M.; Negrier, S.; Chevreau, C.; Solska, E.; Desai, A.A. Sorafenib in advanced clear-cell renal-cell carcinoma. *N. Engl. J. Med.* **2007**, *356*, 125–134. [CrossRef]
76. Gore, M.E.; Szczylik, C.; Porta, C.; Bracarda, S.; Bjarnason, G.A.; Oudard, S.; Hariharan, S.; Lee, S.-H.; Haanen, J.; Castellano, D. Safety and efficacy of sunitinib for metastatic renal-cell carcinoma: An expanded-access trial. *Lancet Oncol.* **2009**, *10*, 757–763. [CrossRef]
77. Hutson, T.E.; Lesovoy, V.; Al-Shukri, S.; Stus, V.P.; Lipatov, O.N.; Bair, A.H.; Rosbrook, B.; Chen, C.; Kim, S.; Vogelzang, N.J. Axitinib versus sorafenib as first-line therapy in patients with metastatic renal-cell carcinoma: A randomised open-label phase 3 trial. *Lancet Oncol.* **2013**, *14*, 1287–1294. [CrossRef]
78. Motzer, R.J.; Hutson, T.E.; Cella, D.; Reeves, J.; Hawkins, R.; Guo, J.; Nathan, P.; Staehler, M.; de Souza, P.; Merchan, J.R. Pazopanib versus sunitinib in metastatic renal-cell carcinoma. *N. Engl. J. Med.* **2013**, *369*, 722–731. [CrossRef]
79. Choueiri, T.K.; Halabi, S.; Sanford, B.L.; Hahn, O.; Michaelson, M.D.; Walsh, M.K.; Feldman, D.R.; Olencki, T.; Picus, J.; Small, E.J. Cabozantinib versus sunitinib as initial targeted therapy for patients with metastatic renal cell carcinoma of poor or intermediate risk: The alliance A031203 CABOSUN trial. *J. Clin. Oncol.* **2017**, *35*, 591. [CrossRef]
80. Motzer, R.J.; Hutson, T.E.; Glen, H.; Michaelson, M.D.; Molina, A.; Eisen, T.; Jassem, J.; Zolnierek, J.; Maroto, J.P.; Mellado, B. Lenvatinib, everolimus, and the combination in patients with metastatic renal cell carcinoma: A randomised, phase 2, open-label, multicentre trial. *Lancet Oncol.* **2015**, *16*, 1473–1482. [CrossRef]
81. Hudson, C.C.; Liu, M.; Chiang, G.G.; Otterness, D.M.; Loomis, D.C.; Kaper, F.; Giaccia, A.J.; Abraham, R.T. Regulation of hypoxia-inducible factor 1α expression and function by the mammalian target of rapamycin. *Mol. Cell. Biol.* **2002**, *22*, 7004–7014. [CrossRef] [PubMed]
82. Toschi, A.; Edelstein, J.; Rockwell, P.; Ohh, M.; Foster, D. HIFα expression in VHL-deficient renal cancer cells is dependent on phospholipase D. *Oncogene* **2008**, *27*, 2746–2753. [CrossRef]

83. Thomas, G.V.; Tran, C.; Mellinghoff, I.K.; Welsbie, D.S.; Chan, E.; Fueger, B.; Czernin, J.; Sawyers, C.L. Hypoxia-inducible factor determines sensitivity to inhibitors of mTOR in kidney cancer. *Nat. Med.* **2006**, *12*, 122–127. [CrossRef] [PubMed]
84. Hudes, G.; Carducci, M.; Tomczak, P.; Dutcher, J.; Figlin, R.; Kapoor, A.; Staroslawska, E.; Sosman, J.; McDermott, D.; Bodrogi, I. Temsirolimus, interferon alfa, or both for advanced renal-cell carcinoma. *N. Engl. J. Med.* **2007**, *356*, 2271–2281. [CrossRef] [PubMed]
85. Motzer, R.J.; Escudier, B.; Oudard, S.; Hutson, T.E.; Porta, C.; Bracarda, S.; Grünwald, V.; Thompson, J.A.; Figlin, R.A.; Hollaender, N. Efficacy of everolimus in advanced renal cell carcinoma: A double-blind, randomised, placebo-controlled phase III trial. *Lancet* **2008**, *372*, 449–456. [CrossRef]
86. Mollica, V.; Di Nunno, V.; Gatto, L.; Santoni, M.; Scarpelli, M.; Cimadamore, A.; Lopez-Beltran, A.; Cheng, L.; Battelli, N.; Montironi, R. Resistance to systemic agents in renal cell carcinoma predict and overcome genomic strategies adopted by tumor. *Cancers* **2019**, *11*, 830. [CrossRef]
87. Yang, J.C.; Hughes, M.; Kammula, U.; Royal, R.; Sherry, R.M.; Topalian, S.L.; Suri, K.B.; Levy, C.; Allen, T.; Mavroukakis, S. Ipilimumab (anti-CTLA4 antibody) causes regression of metastatic renal cell cancer associated with enteritis and hypophysitis. *J. Immunother.* **2007**, *30*, 825. [CrossRef]
88. Motzer, R.J.; Rini, B.I.; McDermott, D.F.; Redman, B.G.; Kuzel, T.M.; Harrison, M.R.; Vaishampayan, U.N.; Drabkin, H.A.; George, S.; Logan, T.F. Nivolumab for metastatic renal cell carcinoma: Results of a randomized phase II trial. *J. Clin. Oncol.* **2015**, *33*, 1430. [CrossRef]
89. Motzer, R.J.; Escudier, B.; George, S.; Hammers, H.J.; Srinivas, S.; Tykodi, S.S.; Sosman, J.A.; Plimack, E.R.; Procopio, G.; McDermott, D.F. Nivolumab versus everolimus in patients with advanced renal cell carcinoma: Updated results with long-term follow-up of the randomized, open-label, phase 3 CheckMate 025 trial. *Cancer* **2020**, *126*, 4156–4167. [CrossRef]
90. Amin, A.; Plimack, E.R.; Ernstoff, M.S.; Lewis, L.D.; Bauer, T.M.; McDermott, D.F.; Carducci, M.; Kollmannsberger, C.; Rini, B.I.; Heng, D.Y. Safety and efficacy of nivolumab in combination with sunitinib or pazopanib in advanced or metastatic renal cell carcinoma: The CheckMate 016 study. *J. Immunother. Cancer* **2018**, *6*, 109. [CrossRef]
91. Hammers, H.J.; Plimack, E.R.; Infante, J.R.; Rini, B.I.; McDermott, D.F.; Lewis, L.D.; Voss, M.H.; Sharma, P.; Pal, S.K.; Razak, A.R.A. Safety and efficacy of nivolumab in combination with ipilimumab in metastatic renal cell carcinoma: The CheckMate 016 study. *J. Clin. Oncol.* **2017**, *35*, 3851. [CrossRef]
92. Motzer, R.J.; Escudier, B.; McDermott, D.F.; Frontera, O.A.; Melichar, B.; Powles, T.; Donskov, F.; Plimack, E.R.; Barthélemy, P.; Hammers, H.J. Survival outcomes and independent response assessment with nivolumab plus ipilimumab versus sunitinib in patients with advanced renal cell carcinoma: 42-month follow-up of a randomized phase 3 clinical trial. *J. Immunother. Cancer* **2020**, *8*, e000891. [CrossRef]
93. Griffioen, A.W. Anti-angiogenesis: Making the tumor vulnerable to the immune system. *Cancer Immunol. Immunother.* **2008**, *57*, 1553–1558. [CrossRef] [PubMed]
94. Kusmartsev, S.; Eruslanov, E.; Kübler, H.; Tseng, T.; Sakai, Y.; Su, Z.; Kaliberov, S.; Heiser, A.; Rosser, C.; Dahm, P. Oxidative stress regulates expression of VEGFR1 in myeloid cells: Link to tumor-induced immune suppression in renal cell carcinoma. *J. Immunol.* **2008**, *181*, 346–353. [CrossRef] [PubMed]
95. Adotevi, O.; Pere, H.; Ravel, P.; Haicheur, N.; Badoual, C.; Merillon, N.; Medioni, J.; Peyrard, S.; Roncelin, S.; Verkarre, V. A decrease of regulatory T cells correlates with overall survival after sunitinib-based antiangiogenic therapy in metastatic renal cancer patients. *J. Immunother.* **2010**, *33*, 991–998. [CrossRef]
96. Hirsch, L.; Flippot, R.; Escudier, B.; Albiges, L. Immunomodulatory roles of VEGF pathway inhibitors in renal cell carcinoma. *Drugs* **2020**, *80*, 1169–1181. [CrossRef] [PubMed]
97. Powles, T.; Plimack, E.R.; Soulières, D.; Waddell, T.; Stus, V.; Gafanov, R.; Nosov, D.; Pouliot, F.; Melichar, B.; Vynnychenko, I. Pembrolizumab plus axitinib versus sunitinib monotherapy as first-line treatment of advanced renal cell carcinoma (KEYNOTE-426): Extended follow-up from a randomised, open-label, phase 3 trial. *Lancet Oncol.* **2020**, *21*, 1563–1573. [CrossRef]
98. Rini, B.I.; Plimack, E.R.; Stus, V.; Waddell, T.; Gafanov, R.; Pouliot, F.; Nosov, D.; Melichar, B.; Soulieres, D.; Borchiellini, D. Pembrolizumab (pembro) plus axitinib (axi) versus sunitinib as first-line therapy for advanced clear cell renal cell carcinoma (ccRCC): Results from 42-month follow-up of KEYNOTE-426. *J. Clin. Oncol.* **2021**, *39*, 4500. [CrossRef]
99. Motzer, R.J.; Choueiri, T.K.; Powles, T.; Burotto, M.; Bourlon, M.T.; Hsieh, J.J.; Maruzzo, M.; Shah, A.Y.; Suarez, C.; Barrios, C.H. Nivolumab+ cabozantinib (NIVO+ CABO) versus sunitinib (SUN) for advanced renal cell carcinoma (aRCC): Outcomes by sarcomatoid histology and updated trial results with extended follow-up of CheckMate 9ER. *J. Clin. Oncol.* **2021**, *39*, 308. [CrossRef]
100. Haanen, J.B.; Larkin, J.; Choueiri, T.K.; Albiges, L.; Rini, B.I.; Atkins, M.B.; Schmidinger, M.; Penkov, K.; Thomaidou, D.; Wang, J. Efficacy of avelumab+ axitinib (A+ Ax) versus sunitinib (S) by IMDC risk group in advanced renal cell carcinoma (aRCC): Extended follow-up results from JAVELIN Renal 101. *J. Clin. Oncol.* **2021**, *39*, 4574. [CrossRef]
101. Choueiri, T.; Motzer, R.; Rini, B.; Haanen, J.; Campbell, M.; Venugopal, B.; Kollmannsberger, C.; Gravis-Mescam, G.; Uemura, M.; Lee, J. Updated efficacy results from the JAVELIN Renal 101 trial: First-line avelumab plus axitinib versus sunitinib in patients with advanced renal cell carcinoma. *Ann. Oncol.* **2020**, *31*, 1030–1039. [CrossRef] [PubMed]
102. Albiges, L.; Tannir, N.M.; Burotto, M.; McDermott, D.; Plimack, E.R.; Barthélemy, P.; Porta, C.; Powles, T.; Donskov, F.; George, S. Nivolumab plus ipilimumab versus sunitinib for first-line treatment of advanced renal cell carcinoma: Extended 4-year follow-up of the phase III CheckMate 214 trial. *ESMO Open* **2020**, *5*, e001079. [CrossRef]

103. Tomita, Y.; Motzer, R.J.; Choueiri, T.K.; Rini, B.I.; Miyake, H.; Oya, M.; Albiges, L.; Fujii, Y.; Umeyama, Y.; Wang, J. Efficacy of avelumab plus axitinib (A+ Ax) versus sunitinib (S) by number of IMDC risk factors and tumor sites at baseline in advanced renal cell carcinoma (aRCC): Extended follow-up results from JAVELIN Renal 101. *J. Clin. Oncol.* **2021**, *39*, 302. [CrossRef]
104. Bex, A.; Russo, P.; Tomita, Y.; Grünwald, V.; Ramirez, L.-M.; McHenry, B.M.; Motzer, R.J. A phase III, randomized, placebo-controlled trial of nivolumab or nivolumab plus ipilimumab in patients with localized renal cell carcinoma at high-risk of relapse after radical or partial nephrectomy (CheckMate 914). *J. Clin. Oncol.* **2020**, *38*, TPS5099. [CrossRef]
105. Choueiri, T.K.; Quinn, D.I.; Zhang, T.; Gurney, H.; Doshi, G.K.; Cobb, P.W.; Parnis, F.; Lee, J.-L.; Park, S.H.; Semenov, A. KEYNOTE-564: A phase 3, randomized, double blind, trial of pembrolizumab in the adjuvant treatment of renal cell carcinoma. *J. Clin. Oncol.* **2018**, *36*, TPS4599. [CrossRef]
106. Uzzo, R.; Bex, A.; Rini, B.I.; Albiges, L.; Suarez, C.; Donaldson, F.; Asakawa, T.; Schiff, C.; Pal, S.K. A phase III study of atezolizumab (atezo) vs. placebo as adjuvant therapy in renal cell carcinoma (RCC) patients (pts) at high risk of recurrence following resection (IMmotion010). *J. Clin. Oncol.* **2017**, *35*, TPS4598. [CrossRef]
107. Pal, S.K.; Albiges, L.; Suarez Rodriguez, C.; Liu, B.; Doss, J.; Khurana, S.; Scheffold, C.; Voss, M.H.; Choueiri, T.K. CONTACT-03: Randomized, open-label phase III study of atezolizumab plus cabozantinib versus cabozantinib monotherapy following progression on/after immune checkpoint inhibitor (ICI) treatment in patients with advanced/metastatic renal cell carcinoma. *J. Clin. Oncol.* **2021**, *39*, TPS370. [CrossRef]
108. Choueiri, T.K.; Albiges, L.; Powles, T.; Scheffold, C.; Wang, F.; Motzer, R.J. A phase III study (COSMIC-313) of cabozantinib (C) in combination with nivolumab (N) and ipilimumab (I) in patients (pts) with previously untreated advanced renal cell carcinoma (aRCC) of intermediate or poor risk. *J. Clin. Oncol.* **2020**, *38*, TPS767. [CrossRef]
109. Tannir, N.M.; Agarwal, N.; Pal, S.K.; Cho, D.C.; Formiga, M.; Guo, J.; George, D.J.; Tagliaferri, M.A.; Singel, S.M.; O'Keeffe, B.A. PIVOT-09: A phase III randomized open-label study of bempegaldesleukin (NKTR-214) plus nivolumab versus sunitinib or cabozantinib (investigator's choice) in patients with previously untreated advanced renal cell carcinoma (RCC). *J. Clin. Oncol.* **2020**, *38*, TPS763. [CrossRef]
110. Emamekhoo, H.; Olsen, M.; Carthon, B.C.; Drakaki, A.; Percent, I.J.; Molina, A.M.; Cho, D.C.; Bendell, J.C.; Gordan, L.N.; Rezazadeh Kalebasty, A. Safety and efficacy of nivolumab plus ipilimumab (NIVO+ IPI) in patients with advanced renal cell carcinoma (aRCC) with brain metastases: Interim analysis of CheckMate 920. *J. Clin. Oncol.* **2019**, *37*, 4517. [CrossRef]
111. Zhang, T.; Ballman, K.V.; Choudhury, A.D.; Chen, R.C.; Watt, C.; Wen, Y.; Zemla, T.; Emamekhoo, H.; Gupta, S.; Morris, M.J. PDIGREE: An adaptive phase 3 trial of PD-inhibitor nivolumab and ipilimumab (IPI-NIVO) with VEGF TKI cabozantinib (CABO) in metastatic untreated renal cell cancer (Alliance A031704). *J. Clin. Oncol.* **2019**, *39*, TPS366. [CrossRef]
112. Harshman, L.C.; Puligandla, M.; Haas, N.B.; Allaf, M.; Drake, C.G.; McDermott, D.F.; Signoretti, S.; Cella, D.; Gupta, R.T.; Shuch, B.M. PROSPER: A phase III randomized study comparing perioperative nivolumab (nivo) versus observation in patients with localized renal cell carcinoma (RCC) undergoing nephrectomy (ECOG-ACRIN 8143). *J. Clin. Oncol.* **2019**, *37*, TPS684. [CrossRef]
113. Tykodi, S.S.; Gordan, L.N.; Alter, R.S.; Arrowsmith, E.; Harrison, M.R.; Percent, I.J.; Singal, R.; Van Veldhuizen, P.J.; George, D.J.; Hutson, T.E. Nivolumab plus ipilimumab in patients with advanced non-clear cell renal cell carcinoma (nccRCC): Safety and efficacy from CheckMate 920. *J. Clin. Oncol.* **2021**, *39*, 309. [CrossRef]
114. Oza, B.; Frangou, E.; Smith, B.; Bryant, H.; Kaplan, R.; Choodari-Oskooei, B.; Powles, T.; Stewart, G.D.; Albiges, L.; Bex, A.; et al. RAMPART: A phase III multi-arm multi-stage trial of adjuvant checkpoint inhibitors in patients with resected primary renal cell carcinoma (RCC) at high or intermediate risk of relapse. *Contemp. Clin. Trials* **2021**, *108*, 106482. [CrossRef] [PubMed]
115. Choueiri, T.K.; Kaelin, W.G. Targeting the HIF2–VEGF axis in renal cell carcinoma. *Nat. Med.* **2020**, *26*, 1519–1530. [CrossRef]
116. Kolodziejczyk, A.A.; Kim, J.K.; Svensson, V.; Marioni, J.C.; Teichmann, S.A. The technology and biology of single-cell RNA sequencing. *Mol. Cell* **2015**, *58*, 610–620. [CrossRef]
117. Davis-Marcisak, E.F.; Deshpande, A.; Stein-O'Brien, G.L.; Ho, W.J.; Laheru, D.; Jaffee, E.M.; Fertig, E.J.; Kagohara, L.T. From bench to bedside: Single-cell analysis for cancer immunotherapy. *Cancer Cell* **2021**, *39*, 1062–1080. [CrossRef]
118. Zheng, G.X.; Terry, J.M.; Belgrader, P.; Ryvkin, P.; Bent, Z.W.; Wilson, R.; Ziraldo, S.B.; Wheeler, T.D.; McDermott, G.P.; Zhu, J. Massively parallel digital transcriptional profiling of single cells. *Nat. Commun.* **2017**, *8*, 14049. [CrossRef]
119. Ziegenhain, C.; Vieth, B.; Parekh, S.; Reinius, B.; Guillaumet-Adkins, A.; Smets, M.; Leonhardt, H.; Heyn, H.; Hellmann, I.; Enard, W. Comparative analysis of single-cell RNA sequencing methods. *Mol. Cell* **2017**, *65*, 631–643.e634. [CrossRef]
120. Hwang, B.; Lee, J.H.; Bang, D. Single-cell RNA sequencing technologies and bioinformatics pipelines. *Exp. Mol. Med.* **2018**, *50*, 319. [CrossRef]
121. Satija, R.; Farrell, J.A.; Gennert, D.; Schier, A.F.; Regev, A. Spatial reconstruction of single-cell gene expression data. *Nat. Biotechnol.* **2015**, *33*, 495–502. [CrossRef]
122. Amezquita, R.A.; Lun, A.T.; Becht, E.; Carey, V.J.; Carpp, L.N.; Geistlinger, L.; Marini, F.; Rue-Albrecht, K.; Risso, D.; Soneson, C. Orchestrating single-cell analysis with Bioconductor. *Nat. Methods* **2020**, *17*, 137–145. [CrossRef] [PubMed]
123. Wolf, F.A.; Angerer, P.; Theis, F.J. SCANPY: Large-scale single-cell gene expression data analysis. *Genome Biol.* **2018**, *19*, 1–5. [CrossRef]
124. Van der Maaten, L.; Hinton, G. Visualizing data using t-SNE. *J. Mach. Learn. Res.* **2008**, *9*, 2579–2605.
125. McInnes, L.; Healy, J.; Melville, J. Umap: Uniform manifold approximation and projection for dimension reduction. *arXiv* **2018**, arXiv:1802.03426.

126. Beksac, A.T.; Paulucci, D.J.; Blum, K.A.; Yadav, S.S.; Sfakianos, J.P.; Badani, K.K. Heterogeneity in renal cell carcinoma. *Oncol. Semin. Orig. Investig.* **2017**, *35*, 507–515. [CrossRef] [PubMed]
127. van den Heuvel, C.N.; van Ewijk, A.; Zeelen, C.; de Bitter, T.; Huynen, M.; Mulders, P.; Oosterwijk, E.; Leenders, W.P. Molecular profiling of druggable targets in clear cell renal cell carcinoma through targeted RNA sequencing. *Front. Oncol.* **2019**, *9*, 117. [CrossRef]
128. Network, C.G.A.R. Comprehensive molecular characterization of clear cell renal cell carcinoma. *Nature* **2013**, *499*, 43.
129. Liu, J.; Lichtenberg, T.; Hoadley, K.A.; Poisson, L.M.; Lazar, A.J.; Cherniack, A.D.; Kovatich, A.J.; Benz, C.C.; Levine, D.A.; Lee, A.V. An integrated TCGA pan-cancer clinical data resource to drive high-quality survival outcome analytics. *Cell* **2018**, *173*, 400–416.e411. [CrossRef]
130. Ricketts, C.J.; De Cubas, A.A.; Fan, H.; Smith, C.C.; Lang, M.; Reznik, E.; Bowlby, R.; Gibb, E.A.; Akbani, R.; Beroukhim, R. The cancer genome atlas comprehensive molecular characterization of renal cell carcinoma. *Cell Rep.* **2018**, *23*, 313–326.e315. [CrossRef]
131. Miller, B.C.; Sen, D.R.; Al Abosy, R.; Bi, K.; Virkud, Y.V.; LaFleur, M.W.; Yates, K.B.; Lako, A.; Felt, K.; Naik, G.S. Subsets of exhausted CD8+ T cells differentially mediate tumor control and respond to checkpoint blockade. *Nat. Immunol.* **2019**, *20*, 326–336. [CrossRef]
132. Liao, J.; Yu, Z.; Chen, Y.; Bao, M.; Zou, C.; Zhang, H.; Liu, D.; Li, T.; Zhang, Q.; Li, J. Single-cell RNA sequencing of human kidney. *Sci. Data* **2020**, *7*, 1–9. [CrossRef] [PubMed]
133. Kim, K.-T.; Lee, H.W.; Lee, H.-O.; Song, H.J.; Shin, S.; Kim, H.; Shin, Y.; Nam, D.-H.; Jeong, B.C.; Kirsch, D.G. Application of single-cell RNA sequencing in optimizing a combinatorial therapeutic strategy in metastatic renal cell carcinoma. *Genome Biol.* **2016**, *17*, 80. [CrossRef]
134. Ghoneim, H.E.; Fan, Y.; Moustaki, A.; Abdelsamed, H.A.; Dash, P.; Dogra, P.; Carter, R.; Awad, W.; Neale, G.; Thomas, P.G. De novo epigenetic programs inhibit PD-1 blockade-mediated T cell rejuvenation. *Cell* **2017**, *170*, 142–157.e119. [CrossRef] [PubMed]
135. Scott, A.C.; Dündar, F.; Zumbo, P.; Chandran, S.S.; Klebanoff, C.A.; Shakiba, M.; Trivedi, P.; Menocal, L.; Appleby, H.; Camara, S. TOX is a critical regulator of tumour-specific T cell differentiation. *Nature* **2019**, *571*, 270–274. [CrossRef]
136. Pauken, K.E.; Sammons, M.A.; Odorizzi, P.M.; Manne, S.; Godec, J.; Khan, O.; Drake, A.M.; Chen, Z.; Sen, D.R.; Kurachi, M. Epigenetic stability of exhausted T cells limits durability of reinvigoration by PD-1 blockade. *Science* **2016**, *354*, 1160–1165. [CrossRef] [PubMed]
137. Khan, O.; Giles, J.R.; McDonald, S.; Manne, S.; Ngiow, S.F.; Patel, K.P.; Werner, M.T.; Huang, A.C.; Alexander, K.A.; Wu, J.E. TOX transcriptionally and epigenetically programs CD8+ T cell exhaustion. *Nature* **2019**, *571*, 211–218. [CrossRef] [PubMed]
138. Qi, Y.; Xia, Y.; Lin, Z.; Qu, Y.; Qi, Y.; Chen, Y.; Zhou, Q.; Zeng, H.; Wang, J.; Chang, Y. Tumor-infiltrating CD39+ CD8+ T cells determine poor prognosis and immune evasion in clear cell renal cell carcinoma patients. *Cancer Immunol. Immunother.* **2020**, *69*, 1565–1576. [CrossRef]
139. Aggen, D.H.; Ager, C.R.; Obradovic, A.Z.; Chowdhury, N.; Ghasemzadeh, A.; Mao, W.; Chaimowitz, M.G.; Lopez-Bujanda, Z.A.; Spina, C.S.; Hawley, J.E. Blocking IL1 beta promotes tumor regression and remodeling of the myeloid compartment in a renal cell carcinoma model: Multidimensional analyses. *Clin. Cancer Res.* **2021**, *27*, 608–621. [CrossRef]
140. Efremova, M.; Vento-Tormo, M.; Teichmann, S.A.; Vento-Tormo, R. CellPhoneDB: Inferring cell–cell communication from combined expression of multi-subunit ligand–receptor complexes. *Nat. Protoc.* **2020**, *15*, 1484–1506. [CrossRef]
141. Lizio, M.; Abugessaisa, I.; Noguchi, S.; Kondo, A.; Hasegawa, A.; Hon, C.C.; De Hoon, M.; Severin, J.; Oki, S.; Hayashizaki, Y. Update of the FANTOM web resource: Expansion to provide additional transcriptome atlases. *Nucleic Acids Res.* **2019**, *47*, D752–D758. [CrossRef]
142. Kim, M.C.; Borcherding, N.; Ahmed, K.K.; Voigt, A.P.; Vishwakarma, A.; Kolb, R.; Kluz, P.N.; Pandey, G.; De, U.; Drashansky, T.; et al. CD177 modulates the function and homeostasis of tumor-infiltrating regulatory T cells. *Nat Commun.* **2021**, *12*, 5764. [CrossRef] [PubMed]
143. Jensen, H.K.; Donskov, F.; Nordsmark, M.; Marcussen, N.; von der Maase, H. Increased intratumoral FOXP3-positive regulatory immune cells during interleukin-2 treatment in metastatic renal cell carcinoma. *Clin. Cancer Res.* **2009**, *15*, 1052–1058. [CrossRef] [PubMed]
144. Rauch, D.A.; Conlon, K.C.; Janakiram, M.; Brammer, J.E.; Harding, J.C.; Ye, B.H.; Zang, X.; Ren, X.; Olson, S.; Cheng, X. Rapid progression of adult T-cell leukemia/lymphoma as tumor-infiltrating Tregs after PD-1 blockade. *Blood J. Am. Soc. Hematol.* **2019**, *134*, 1406–1414. [CrossRef] [PubMed]
145. Kolb, R.; De, U.; Khan, S.; Luo, Y.; Kim, M.-C.; Yu, H.; Wu, C.; Mo, J.; Zhang, X.; Zhang, P. Proteolysis-targeting chimera against BCL-X L destroys tumor-infiltrating regulatory T cells. *Nat. Commun.* **2021**, *12*, 1–9.
146. Stoeckius, M.; Zheng, S.; Houck-Loomis, B.; Hao, S.; Yeung, B.Z.; Mauck, W.M., 3rd; Smibert, P.; Satija, R. Cell Hashing with barcoded antibodies enables multiplexing and doublet detection for single cell genomics. *Genome Biol.* **2018**, *19*, 224. [CrossRef] [PubMed]
147. Srivastava, A.; Malik, L.; Smith, T.; Sudbery, I.; Patro, R. Alevin efficiently estimates accurate gene abundances from dscRNA-seq data. *Genome Biol.* **2019**, *20*, 65. [CrossRef]
148. Melsted, P.; Booeshaghi, A.S.; Liu, L.; Gao, F.; Lu, L.; Min, K.H.J.; da Veiga Beltrame, E.; Hjörleifsson, K.E.; Gehring, J.; Pachter, L. Modular, efficient and constant-memory single-cell RNA-seq preprocessing. *Nat. Biotechnol.* **2021**, *39*, 813–818. [CrossRef]

149. Lähnemann, D.; Köster, J.; Szczurek, E.; McCarthy, D.J.; Hicks, S.C.; Robinson, M.D.; Vallejos, C.A.; Campbell, K.R.; Beerenwinkel, N.; Mahfouz, A.; et al. Eleven grand challenges in single-cell data science. *Genome Biol.* **2020**, *21*, 31. [CrossRef]
150. Qiu, P. Embracing the dropouts in single-cell RNA-seq analysis. *Nat. Commun.* **2020**, *11*, 1169. [CrossRef]
151. Kharchenko, P.V. The triumphs and limitations of computational methods for scRNA-seq. *Nat. Methods* **2021**, *18*, 723–732. [CrossRef]
152. Hughes, T.K.; Wadsworth, M.H., 2nd; Gierahn, T.M.; Do, T.; Weiss, D.; Andrade, P.R.; Ma, F.; de Andrade Silva, B.J.; Shao, S.; Tsoi, L.C.; et al. Second-Strand Synthesis-Based Massively Parallel scRNA-Seq Reveals Cellular States and Molecular Features of Human Inflammatory Skin Pathologies. *Immunity* **2020**, *53*, 878–894.e877. [CrossRef] [PubMed]
153. Hou, W.; Ji, Z.; Ji, H.; Hicks, S.C. A systematic evaluation of single-cell RNA-sequencing imputation methods. *Genome Biol.* **2020**, *21*, 218. [CrossRef] [PubMed]
154. van den Brink, S.C.; Sage, F.; Vértesy, Á.; Spanjaard, B.; Peterson-Maduro, J.; Baron, C.S.; Robin, C.; Van Oudenaarden, A. Single-cell sequencing reveals dissociation-induced gene expression in tissue subpopulations. *Nat. Methods* **2017**, *14*, 935–936. [CrossRef] [PubMed]
155. Cang, Z.; Nie, Q. Inferring spatial and signaling relationships between cells from single cell transcriptomic data. *Nat. Commun.* **2020**, *11*, 2084. [CrossRef]
156. Lareau, C.A.; Ludwig, L.S.; Muus, C.; Gohil, S.H.; Zhao, T.; Chiang, Z.; Pelka, K.; Verboon, J.M.; Luo, W.; Christian, E.; et al. Massively parallel single-cell mitochondrial DNA genotyping and chromatin profiling. *Nat. Biotechnol.* **2021**, *39*, 451–461. [CrossRef]
157. VanHorn, S.; Morris, S.A. Next-Generation Lineage Tracing and Fate Mapping to Interrogate Development. *Dev. Cell.* **2021**, *56*, 7–21. [CrossRef]
158. Singh, M.; Al-Eryani, G.; Carswell, S.; Ferguson, J.M.; Blackburn, J.; Barton, K.; Roden, D.; Luciani, F.; Giang Phan, T.; Junankar, S.; et al. High-throughput targeted long-read single cell sequencing reveals the clonal and transcriptional landscape of lymphocytes. *Nat. Commun.* **2019**, *10*, 3120. [CrossRef]
159. van der Leun, A.M.; Thommen, D.S.; Schumacher, T.N. CD8(+) T cell states in human cancer: Insights from single-cell analysis. *Nat. Rev. Cancer* **2020**, *20*, 218–232. [CrossRef]
160. Sade-Feldman, M.; Yizhak, K.; Bjorgaard, S.L.; Ray, J.P.; de Boer, C.G.; Jenkins, R.W.; Lieb, D.J.; Chen, J.H.; Frederick, D.T.; Barzily-Rokni, M. Defining T cell states associated with response to checkpoint immunotherapy in melanoma. *Cell* **2018**, *175*, 998–1013.e1020. [CrossRef]
161. Yost, K.E.; Satpathy, A.T.; Wells, D.K.; Qi, Y.; Wang, C.; Kageyama, R.; McNamara, K.L.; Granja, J.M.; Sarin, K.Y.; Brown, R.A. Clonal replacement of tumor-specific T cells following PD-1 blockade. *Nat. Med.* **2019**, *25*, 1251–1259. [CrossRef] [PubMed]
162. Giraldo, N.A.; Becht, E.; Vano, Y.; Petitprez, F.; Lacroix, L.; Validire, P.; Sanchez-Salas, R.; Ingels, A.; Oudard, S.; Moatti, A. Tumor-infiltrating and peripheral blood T-cell immunophenotypes predict early relapse in localized clear cell renal cell carcinoma. *Clin. Cancer Res.* **2017**, *23*, 4416–4428. [CrossRef] [PubMed]
163. Noessner, E.; Brech, D.; Mendler, A.N.; Masouris, I.; Schlenker, R.; Prinz, P.U. Intratumoral alterations of dendritic-cell differentiation and CD8+ T-cell anergy are immune escape mechanisms of clear cell renal cell carcinoma. *Oncoimmunology* **2012**, *1*, 1451–1453. [CrossRef] [PubMed]
164. Atkins, D.; Ferrone, S.; Schmahl, G.E.; Störkel, S.; Seliger, B. Down-regulation of HLA class I antigen processing molecules: An immune escape mechanism of renal cell carcinoma? *J. Urol.* **2004**, *171*, 885–889. [CrossRef] [PubMed]

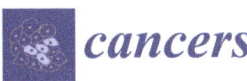

Article

Integrated mRNA and miRNA Transcriptomic Analyses Reveals Divergent Mechanisms of Sunitinib Resistance in Clear Cell Renal Cell Carcinoma (ccRCC)

María Armesto [1], Maitane Marquez [1], María Arestin [1], Peio Errarte [2], Ane Rubio [1], Lorea Manterola [1], Jose I. López [3,4] and Charles H. Lawrie [1,5,6,*]

1. Molecular Oncology Group, Biodonostia Research Institute, 20014 San Sebastián, Spain; maria.armesto@biodonostia.org (M.A.); maitane.marquez@biodonostia.org (M.M.); maria.arestin@biodonostia.org (M.A.); ane.rubio2@gmail.com (A.R.); lmcareaga@gmail.com (L.M.)
2. Onena Medicines S.L., 20014 San Sebastián, Spain; Peio@onenameds.com
3. Department of Pathology, Cruces University Hospital, 48903 Barakaldo, Spain; joseignacio.lopez@osakidetza.eus
4. Biomarkers in Cancer Unit, Biocruces Research Institute, 48903 Barakaldo, Spain
5. IKERBASQUE, Basque Foundation for Science, 48011 Bilbao, Spain
6. Radcliffe Department of Medicine, University of Oxford, Oxford OX3 9BQ, UK
* Correspondence: charles.lawrie@biodonostia.org; Tel.: +34-943-006-138

Simple Summary: Clear cell renal cell carcinoma (ccRCC) is a frequent cancer that causes more than 100,000 deaths every year. Treatment with drugs that target enzymes that help tumours grow such as sunitinib have greatly improved the prospects for ccRCC patients, however a large proportion of patients become resistant. We created sunitinib resistant cell lines and identified consequent changes in gene (and miRNA) expression by microarray analyses. Using this approach, we identified different pathways of resistance suggesting that tumour cells have many ways to overcome sunitinib treatment. We were able to overcome resistance in cells by inhibiting a protein, PD-L1, that is targeted by many immunotherapeutics currently in use for ccRCC patients suggesting a combination of immunotherapy and sunitinib may benefit patients. In addition, we identified miRNAs that are common to multiple resistance mechanisms suggesting they may be useful targets for future studies.

Abstract: The anti-angiogenic therapy sunitinib remains the standard first-line treatment for metastatic clear cell renal cell carcinoma (ccRCC). However, acquired resistance develops in nearly all responsive patients and represents a major source of treatment failure. We used an integrated miRNA and mRNA transcriptomic approach to identify miRNA:target gene interactions involved in sunitinib resistance. Through the generation of stably resistant clones in three ccRCC cell lines (786-O, A498 and Caki-1), we identified non-overlapping miRNA:target gene networks, suggesting divergent mechanisms of sunitinib resistance. Surprisingly, even though the genes involved in these networks were different, they shared targeting by multiple members of the *miR-17~92* cluster. In 786-O cells, targeted genes were related to hypoxia/angiogenic pathways, whereas, in Caki-1 cells, they were related to inflammatory/proliferation pathways. The immunotherapy target PD-L1 was consistently up-regulated in resistant cells, and we demonstrated that the silencing of this gene resulted in an increase in sensitivity to sunitinib treatment only in 786-O-resistant cells, suggesting that some ccRCC patients might benefit from combination therapy with PD-L1 checkpoint inhibitors. In summary, we demonstrate that, although there are clearly divergent mechanisms of sunitinib resistance in ccRCC subtypes, the commonality of miRNAs in multiple pathways could be targeted to overcome sunitinib resistance.

Keywords: renal cancer; sunitinib; resistance; miRNA; transcriptome; pathway analysis; clear cell renal cell carcinoma

1. Introduction

Renal carcinomas are one of the most common types of cancer in the Western world, accounting for ~3% of adult tumours or more than 200,000 new cases each year [1]. Clear cell renal cell carcinoma (ccRCC) represents 80–90% of renal carcinomas and accounts for more than 100,000 deaths worldwide each year [2–5]. Nearly a third of patients present with locally advanced and/or metastatic disease that typically shows limited responsiveness to traditional therapies such as chemotherapy, radiotherapy, or cytokine therapy [6]. Moreover, ccRCC is a highly vascularized cancer that is frequently associated with mutations in the von Hippel–Lindau (VHL) gene that promotes the angiogenic pathway and can be further subclassified into those with proangiogenic and proinflammatory tumours [7].

The antiangiogenic therapy sunitinib (Sutent™) is currently the standard first-line treatment for metastatic ccRCC (mccRCC) [8,9]. Sunitinib is a small molecule inhibitor of multiple receptor tyrosine kinases (RTKs), including vascular endothelial growth factor receptor (VEFGR), platelet-derived growth factor receptors (PDGFR), fms-related tyrosine kinase 3 (FLT3), stem cell growth factor receptor KIT, and RET [10,11]. However, despite the clear improvements for ccRCC patients receiving this treatment, the clinical benefit of sunitinib on progression-free-survival (PFS) is limited, as more than half of patients do not respond to initial therapy, and of those that do, nearly all develop resistance after ~24 months [12,13]. Therefore, there is an urgent need for a better understanding of the molecular basis of sunitinib resistance in order to identify biomarkers of resistance that will allow for the detection of nonresponsive ccRCC patients that could benefit from up-front alternative treatment regimens, as well as developing new tools that could improve the treatment response in responsive patients.

Although many publications have investigated the molecular basis of sunitinib resistance [14–19], and several have considered the role of microRNAs (miRNAs) [20–27], only a few have taken an integrated genomic approach to identify miRNA-target gene interactions that can give functional insights into resistance mechanisms [28,29]. Therefore, we used generated multiple sunitinib-resistant clones in primary tumour ccRCC cell lines that are VHL-defective (786-O and A498) and the metastatic, VHL-functional, Caki-1 cell line. Changes in the expression of both miRNAs and genes were elucidated in the resistant clones by microarray analysis and differentially expressed genes that were targeted by differentially expressed miRNAs were identified by network analysis (Figure 1). These results were confirmed by both mRNA and protein levels and the immunotherapy target PD-L1 was identified as being up-regulated in resistant cell lines. Silencing of PD-L1 was demonstrated to restore the sensitivity of resistant 786-O cells.

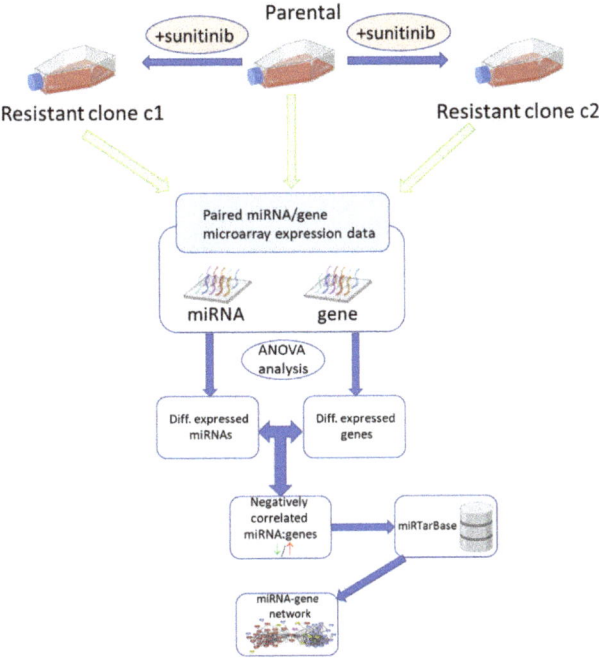

Figure 1. Schematic diagram of experimental workflow for the identification of miRNA:gene interactions involved in sunitinib resistance.

2. Results

2.1. Generating In Vitro Models of Sunitinib Resistance

Sunitinib-resistant 786-O, A498, and Caki-1 clones were generated by serial passage in increasing concentrations of sunitinib until 10 µM was reached. Two independent resistant clones were developed for each cell line and the IC_{50} of each clone was calculated by MTT assay (Figures S1–S3 and Table 1).

Table 1. IC_{50} values of parental and sunitinib-resistant clones c1 and c2 generated from 786-O, A498, and Caki-1 cell lines as measured by MTT assay.

		IC_{50} Value		
Cell Line	**Biological Replicate**	**Parental**	**Clone c1 (*p*-Value)**	**Clone c2 (*p*-Value)**
786-O	A	5.7	17.32	13.54
	B	11.39	23.3	20.07
	C	6.7	20.4	12.8
	Average	7.93	20.34 **	15.47 *
A498	A	10.48	11.92	14.36
	B	7.682	12.42	16.04
	C	7.18	12.01	10.54
	Average	8.44	12.12 *	13.64 *
Caki-1	A	9.5	16.8	18
	B	9	14.6	17.3
	C	12.2	16.2	14.7
	Average	10.2	15.87 **	16.67 *

Values of biological triplicates are indicated by letters A–C. The dose response curves used to generate the IC_{50} values can be found in Figures S1–S3. *p*-values were calculated by an independent t-test and significance denoted by * $p < 0.05$, ** $p < 0.01$.

As can be seen from Table 1, the average IC_{50} value of the sunitinib-resistant clones c1 and c2 were significantly higher than their respective parental control cell lines.

2.2. Non-Coding RNA and Gene Expression in Sunitinib-Resistant Cells

In order to look at which miRNAs and genes were involved in the resistant phenotype of the cell lines, we carried out microarray analyses. Unsupervised cluster analysis demonstrated that the miRNA expression profile of the resistant cell lines differed from that of the parental control cell lines in all three cell lines (Figure 2A–D). Moreover, there was a clear difference in miRNA expression between c1 and c2 in cell lines, suggesting different mechanisms of resistance, although this difference was most pronounced in Caki-1 cells.

Using ANOVA analysis, we identified 253 differentially expressed miRNAs between resistant 786-O clone c1 and the parental control, of which 184 were up-regulated and 69 were down-regulated. There were 234 miRNAs differentially expressed miRNAs between clone c2 and parental control; 182 were up-regulated and 52 were down-regulated. Over 60% (184/303) of each of these differentially expressed miRNAs were common to both clone c1 and clone c2 (Figure 2A,B; Table S1). In A498 cells, we identified 102 differentially expressed miRNAs between clone c1 and the parental control, of which 68 were up-regulated and 34 were down-regulated. For clone c2, 107 miRNAs were differentially expressed when compared with the parental; 61 were up-regulated and 46 were down-regulated. Nearly 32% (51/158) of these miRNAs were commonly dysregulated in the two clones (Figure 2C; Table S2). In the Caki-1 cell line, we identified 678 differentially expressed miRNAs between clone c1 and the parental control, of which 324 were up-regulated and 354 were down-regulated. For the clone c2, 514 miRNAs were differentially expressed when compared with the parental; 245 were upregulated and 269 were downregulated. Nearly 30% (273/919) of these miRNAs were commonly dysregulated in the two clones (Figure 2D; Table S3).

In addition to miRNA analyses, we carried out gene expression analysis on the same samples using Affymetrix Clariom D microarrays. Unsupervised cluster analysis of gene probes (intensity > 50) showed a similar relationship between samples as with the miRNAs (Figure 2E–H). In other words, there was a distinct gene profile between the parental control cell lines and the resistant cell lines, and the two resistant clones, c1 and c2, had distinct gene expression profiles. Similar to miRNA expression, these differences were most pronounced in Caki-1 cells. There were 4869 gene probes identified as being differentially expressed ($p < 0.05$; >2 or <−2-fold) between 786-O c1 and parental cells, 2608 of which encoded for annotated genes (1913 up-regulated and 695 down-regulated). In clone c2, there were 3994 differentially expressed genes, of which 2029 encoded for annotated genes (1397 up-regulated and 632 down-regulated). There were 1383 genes in common (43% of 3254) (Figure 2E,F; Table S4). For A498 cells, 3019 probes were identified as being differentially expressed between c1 and parental cells, of which 1523 encoded for annotated genes; 972 of these were up-regulated and 551 were down-regulated. There were 2953 probes differentially expressed between c2 and parental cells, of which 1411 encoded genes were comprised of 806 up-regulated and 605 down-regulated genes. There were 621 of 2313 (27%) genes that were commonly dysregulated in both clones (Figure 2G; Table S5). In the Caki-1 cell line, there were 7059 genes differentially expressed between c1 and parental cells, of which 2905 were annotated (883 up-regulated, 2022 down-regulated). For clone c2, 6201 genes were differentially expressed, 2370 of which were annotated (1153 up-regulated, 1217 down-regulated). A total of 990 genes (23%) were common between c1 and c2 (Figure 2H; Table S6).

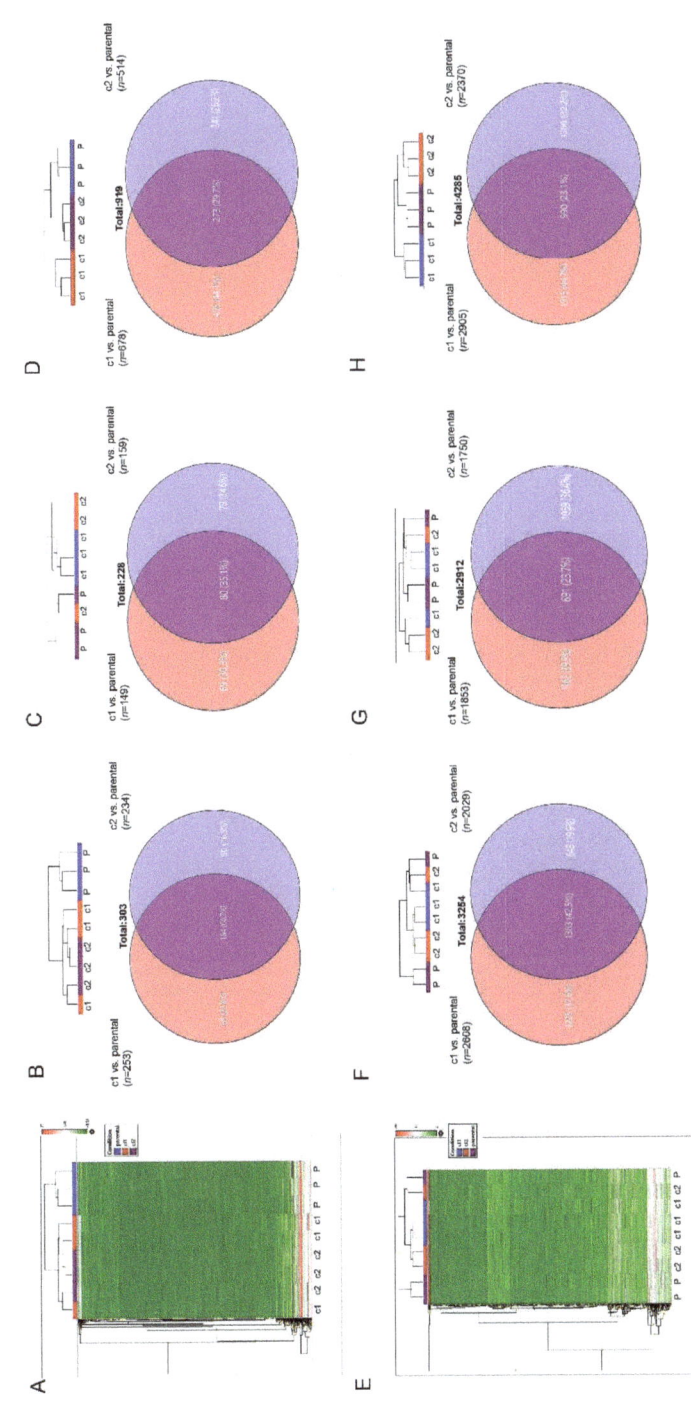

Figure 2. Microarray analysis of gene and miRNA expression in resistant and parental control cell lines: (**A**) Representative unsupervised cluster analysis of miRNA expression (786-O cells). (**B**–**D**) (Top) Dendrogram of unsupervised cluster analysis showing relationship between samples at level of miRNA expression; (Bottom) Venn diagram depicting differentially expressed miRNAs in resistant clones relative to parental control cells. (**B**) 786-O cells, (**C**) A498 cells, (**D**) Caki-1 cells. (**E**) Representative unsupervised cluster analysis of gene expression (786-O cells). (**F**–**H**) (Top) Dendrogram of unsupervised cluster analysis showing relationship between samples at level of gene expression; (Bottom) Venn diagram depicting differentially expressed genes in resistant clones relative to parental control cells. (**F**) 786-O cells, (**G**) A498 cells, (**H**) Caki-1 cells. The original heatmap analyses are shown in Figure S4. Differentially expressed miRNAs and genes that are common between the resistant clones are listed in (Tables S1–S6).

2.3. Interaction Network Analysis between Differentially Expressed Genes and miRNAs

In order to identify which of the differentially expressed genes were regulated by miRNAs, we mapped the differentially expressed miRNA and gene expression data sets for each resistant clone to a network containing experimentally validated miRNA-gene target interactions (n = 3502) that were obtained from the miRTarBase database [30]. For the 786-O c1 cells, 545 (19%) of differentially expressed genes and miRNAs mapped to this network from 253 and 2608 differentially expressed miRNAs and genes, respectively (n = 2861), and 453 (20%) from the 234 and 2029 differentially expressed miRNA and genes from c2 (n = 2263). In the A498 cell line, out of the 1625 differentially expressed genes and miRNAs for c1 (102 miRNAs and 1523 genes), 338 (21%) mapped to the miRNA:gene interaction network, whereas, for c2, 313 (21%) of the 1518 genes and miRNAs (n = 107 and 1411, respectively) were present in the network. For Caki-1, out of the 3583 differentially expressed genes and miRNAs in c1 (n = 678 and 2905, respectively), 696 (19%) were mapped to the interaction network, and in c2 there were 577 (20%) of 2884 (514 and 2370 miRNAs and genes, respectively).

The mapped differentially expressed miRNAs and genes were separated into miRNAs that were up-regulated and genes that were down-regulated and vice versa. These lists were used to create networks from miRNA:genes that were common to both c1 and c2 clones (Figures 1 and 3). For 786-O cells, for example, there were 76 gene:miRNA interactions, 71 interactions involving 18 down-regulated miRNAs with 53 different genes, and 5 interactions with 5 up-regulated miRNAs with four different genes (Figure 3A; Table 2). For A498, there was only one commonly up-regulated miRNA (*miR-34c-5p*) that targeted two genes, and one down-regulated miRNA (*miR-145-5p*) that targeted four genes—a total of six miRNA:gene interactions (Figure 3B; Table 2). For the Caki-1 cell line, there were 26 miRNA:gene interactions, three up-regulated miRNA targeting six genes, and 12 down-regulated miRNAs targeting twelve different genes (Figure 3C; Table 2). Only two genes (*ITGB3* and *TNFAIP3*) were in common between the cell lines (i.e., 786-O and Caki-1).

Table 2. List of differentially expressed genes (in both clones) targeted by differentially expressed miRNAs (in both clones) in sunitinib-resistant ccRCC cell lines.

Cell	miRNA/Gene	miRNA	Target Gene(s)
786-0	↑/↓	hsa-miR-663a	CDKN1A
	↑/↓	hsa-miR-572	CDKN1A
	↑/↓	hsa-miR-638	PTEN
	↑/↓	hsa-miR-612	SP1
	↑/↓	hsa-miR-212-3p	RFXAP
	↓/↑	hsa-miR-106a-5p	SIRPA, MMP2, HIF1A
	↓/↑	hsa-miR-30d-5p	KPNB1, BNIP3L, BECN1
	↓/↑	hsa-miR-140-3p	ATP6AP2, FN1
	↓/↑	hsa-miR-26b-5p	PTGS2, ST8SIA4
	↓/↑	hsa-miR-17-5p	MMP2, SIRPA, GPR137B, EPAS1, VLDLR, HIF1A
	↓/↑	hsa-miR-200a-3p	WASF3, CD274
	↓/↑	hsa-miR-200b-3p	LOX, FN1, CD274, WASF3, MSN, FERMT2, FSCN1, RAB23
	↓/↑	hsa-miR-210-3p	HIF1A, BDNF, NCAM1, EHD2, TFRC
	↓/↑	hsa-miR-328-3p	PTPRJ, MMP16
	↓/↑	hsa-miR-34a-5p	BECN1, VAMP2, FUT8, INHBB, NOTCH2, MAGEA2, MAGEA3, L1CAM, AXL, PAM, SYT1, CD274
	↓/↑	hsa-miR-21-5p	BASP1, RECK, NFIB, SATB1, RHOB, PIAS3, DUSP10, LRP6
	↓/↑	hsa-miR-146a-5p	L1CAM, NOTCH2, PTGS2, HOXD10, RAC1
	↓/↑	hsa-miR-20a-5p	SIRPA, EPAS1, KIF26B, CRIM1, HIF1A, TSG101
	↓/↑	hsa-miR-17-3p	ITGA5, ITGB3
	↓/↑	hsa-miR-99a-5p	SMARCA5
	↓/↑	hsa-miR-18a-5p	PIAS3, TNFAIP3, HIF1A, TBPL1
	↓/↑	hsa-miR-25-5p	PRKCZ

Table 2. *Cont.*

Cell	miRNA/Gene	miRNA	Target Gene(s)
A498	↑/↓	hsa-miR-34c-5p	ITPR1, HNF4A
	↓/↑	hsa-miR-145-5p	ITGB8, CTGFL, VPS51, EGFR
Caki-1	↑/↓	hsa-miR-148b-3p	SLC2A1
	↑/↓	hsa-miR-192-5p	ITGB3, ITGAV, CAV1, WNK1
	↑/↓	hsa-miR-29b-3p	DNMT3B
	↓/↑	hsa-miR-138-5p	CCND1
	↓/↑	hsa-miR-193b-3p	CCND1, AKR1C2
	↓/↑	hsa-miR-92a-5p	KLF2
	↓/↑	hsa-miR-296-3p	ICAM1
	↓/↑	hsa-miR-106b-5p	BMP2, RND3, CCND1
	↓/↑	hsa-miR-106b-3p	BMP2
	↓/↑	hsa-miR-130b-3p	IRF1
	↓/↑	hsa-miR-708-5p	CCND1
	↓/↑	hsa-miR-18a-5p	TNFAIP3, CTGF
	↓/↑	hsa-miR-17-5p	CCND1, BMP2, TCEAL1, RND3
	↓/↑	hsa-miR-1180-3p	TCEAL1
	↓/↑	hsa-miR-550a-5p	CPEB4

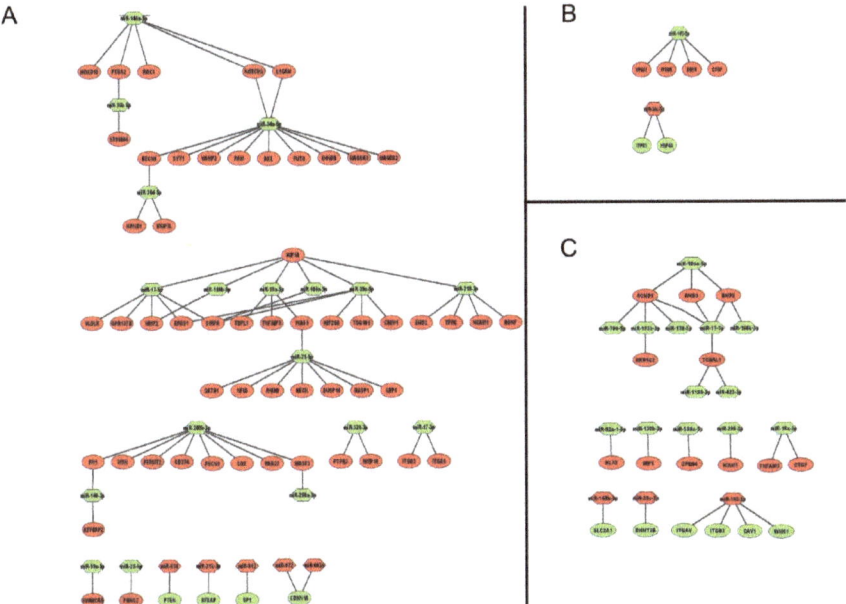

Figure 3. miRNA-gene network analysis in (**A**) 786-O, (**B**) A498, and (**C**) Caki-1 cells. Ellipsoidal nodes represent target genes and hexagonal nodes miRNAs, red colour denotes colour denotes upregulation and green downregulation.

On the basis of their role in the sunitinib-resistance miRNA-gene interaction networks, we selected eleven miRNAs and seven genes for further analysis by qRT-PCR. miRNAs *miR-18a-5p, miR-17-5p, miR-106a-5p, miR-34a-5p, miR-146-5p, miR-200a-3p, miR-210-3p, miR-21-5p, miR-15a-5p, miR-638,* and *miR-29b-3p* were measured in the cell lines by qRT-PCR (Figure **??**A–K respectively). As can be seen from these results, levels of multiple members of the *miR-17~92* cluster (i.e., *miR-18-5p, miR- miR-17-5p,* and *miR-106-5p* (Figure **??**A–C respectively)) were significantly down-regulated in all of the resistant clones relative to the parental cell lines in 786-O, A498, and Caki-1 cells. Similarly, we observed significant down-regulation of *miR-34a-5p* in resistant clones of all the three cell lines (Figure **??**D). *miR-146-5p* was down-regulated in both clones of 786-O and Caki-1, and clone c2 of A498 was up-regulated more than 15-fold in c1 of A498 cells (Figure **??**E). *miR-200a-3p* was significantly down-regulated in both 786-O and Caki-1 cells but not A498 cells where this miRNA was up-regulated in resistant cells (Figure ??F). Caki-1 and A498 cells showed significant down-regulation of *miR-210-3p* in resistant clones, whereas this miRNA was up-regulated in 786-O cells (Figure ??G). *miR-21-5p* was up-regulated in A498 and Caki-1 cells but down-regulated in 786-O cells (Figure ??H). In contrast to the aforementioned miRNAs, *miR-15a-5p*, *miR-638*, and *miR-29b-3p* differed in expression between different resistant clones. For example, *miR-15a-5p* was up-regulated in c1 but not c2 in both 786-O and Caki-1 cells but up-regulated in both A498 clones (Figure ??I). For *miR-638*, both resistant clones of 786-O cells, as well as c1 of Caki-1 and c2 of A498 cells, were up-regulated compared to parental cells, whereas c2 of Caki-1 and c1 of A498 cells were down-regulated (Figure ??J). *miR-29b-3p* was down-regulated in both clones of 786-O and A498, but only c2 of Caki-1 cells while c1 was up-regulated compared to the parental Caki-1 cells (Figure ??K).

Of the nine genes that were measured by qRT-PCR, only *CD274* (encoding for PD-L1 protein) displayed a consistent expression pattern (i.e., up-regulated) in all three cell lines with both resistant clones (Figure 5A). *HIF1A* was up-regulated in both c1 and c2 of 786-O and Caki-1 cells, as well as c2 of A498, but down-regulated in c1 of A498 (Figure 5B). The closely related gene *EPAS1* (encoding for HIF2α protein) was also up-regulated in both clones of Caki-1 (and c1 of A498), but down-regulated in 786-O-resistant clones and c2 of A498 cells (Figure 5C). A similar pattern was observed for *CCND1*, *NOTCH2*, and *TNFAIP3*, which were also down-regulated in resistant clones of 786-O cells but up-regulated in both Caki-1 and A498-resistant clones (Figure 5D, 5E and 5F, respectively). In contrast, levels of *L1CAM* were up-regulated in both resistant clones of 786-O and Caki-1 cells but only up-regulated in c1 of A498 cells (Figure 5G). Levels of *PTEN* were down-regulated in 786-O cells and c1 of A498 cells but up-regulated in Caki-1 cells and c2 of A498 cells (Figure 5H). Levels of *EGFR* were similarly down-regulated in 786-O and A498-resistant clones but down-regulated in 786-O-resistant clones (Figure 5I).

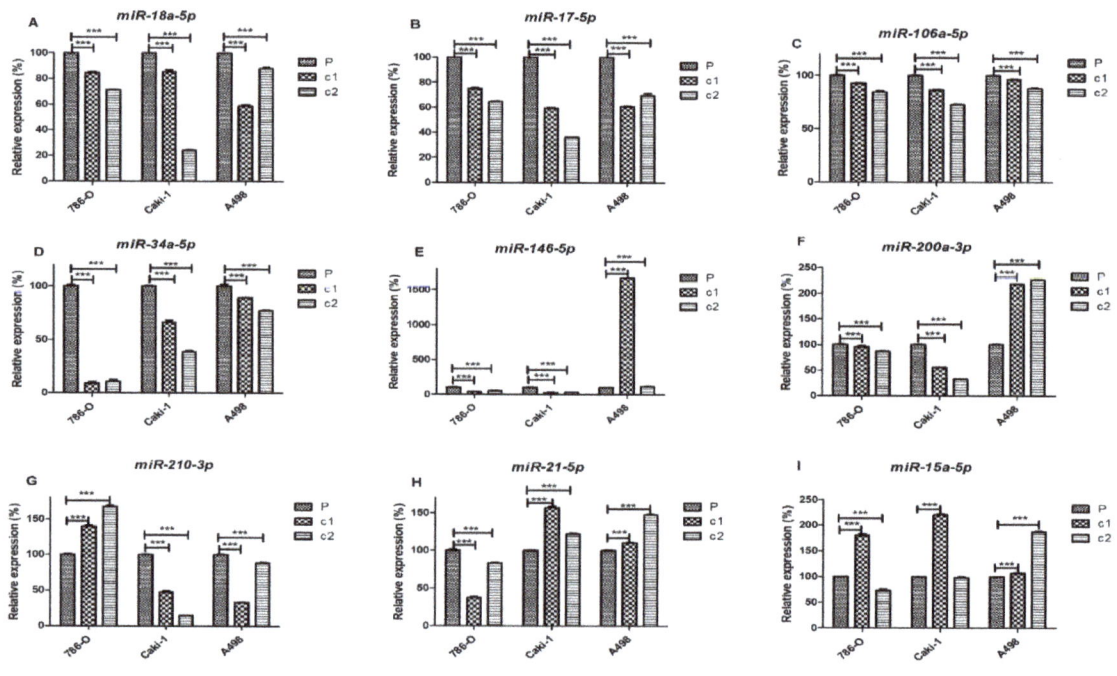

Figure 4. *Cont.*

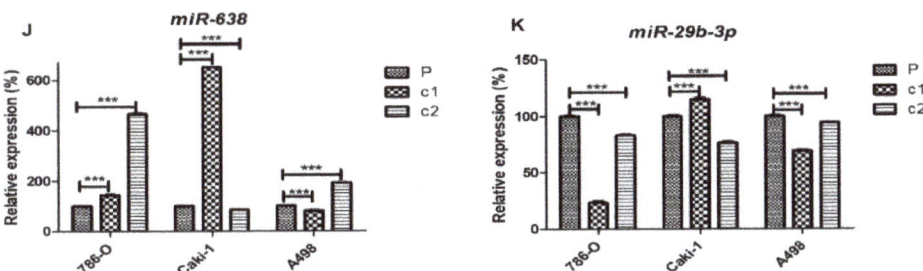

Figure 4. miRNA expression in resistant clones and parental samples of 786-O, Caki-1, and A498 cell lines: The levels of (**A**) *miR-18a-5p*, (**B**) *miR-17-5p*, (**C**) *miR-106-5p*, (**D**) *miR-34a-5p*, (**E**) *miR-146-5p*, (**F**) *miR-200a-3p*, (**G**) *miR-210-3p*, (**H**) *miR-21-5p*, (**I**) *miR-15a-5p* (**J**) *miR-638*, and (**K**) *miR-29b-3p* in both clones and parental cells were measured by qRT-PCR using *snoRNU48* as a reference gene. Expression is shown relative to parental expression. Experiments were performed in biological and technical triplicate. The significance of comparisons are denoted by *** $p < 0.001$.

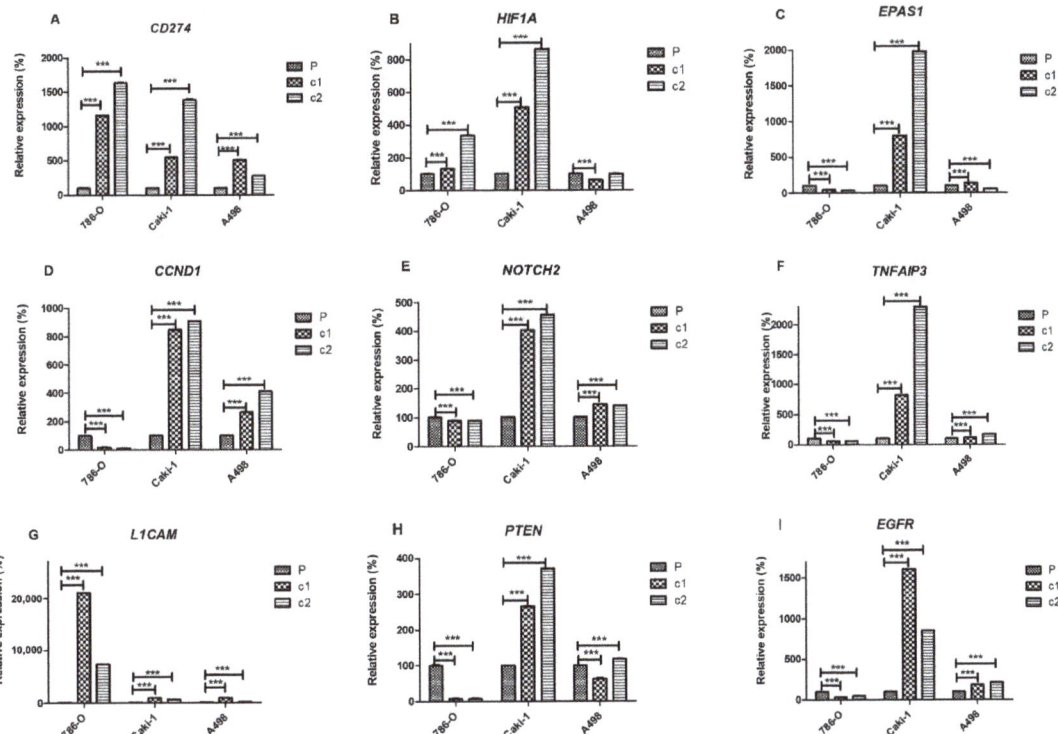

Figure 5. Gene expression in resistant clones and parental cells of 786-O, Caki-1, and A498 cell lines. Levels of (**A**) *CD274*, (**B**) *HIF1A*, (**C**) *EPAS1*, (**D**) *CCND1*, (**E**) *NOTCH2*, (**F**) *TNFAIP3*, (**G**) *L1CAM*, (**H**) *PTEN*, and (**I**) *EGFR* genes measured by qRT-PCR using *GAPDH* as the reference gene. Expression levels in resistant clones are depicted relative to their respective parental cells. All experiments were performed in biological and technical replicates. The significance of comparisons is denoted by *** $p < 0.001$.

We tested the protein levels of PD-L1 (*CD274*), HIF1α (*HIF1A*), HIF2α (*EPAS1*), and cyclin D1 (*CCND1*) by Western blot analysis (Figure 6; Table 3). These results were largely consistent with the qRT-PCR results. For example, there was a clear increase in PD-L1 expression in the resistant clones of both 786-O and A498 cells compared to the parental cells, and a decrease in levels of HIF2α. For both proteins, however, we observed no expression in Caki-1 cells. Moreover, we observed no expression of HIF1α in Caki-1 cells or 786-O cells, despite repeated replicates. In contrast, in A498 cells, HIF1α was expressed and downregulated in resistant clones. *CCND1* was down-regulated in 786-O-resistant clones but up-regulated in resistant clones of A498 cells. Although expressed in Caki-1 cells, cyclin D1 protein appears to be down-regulated in contrast to the up-regulation of mRNA levels observed by qRT-PCR.

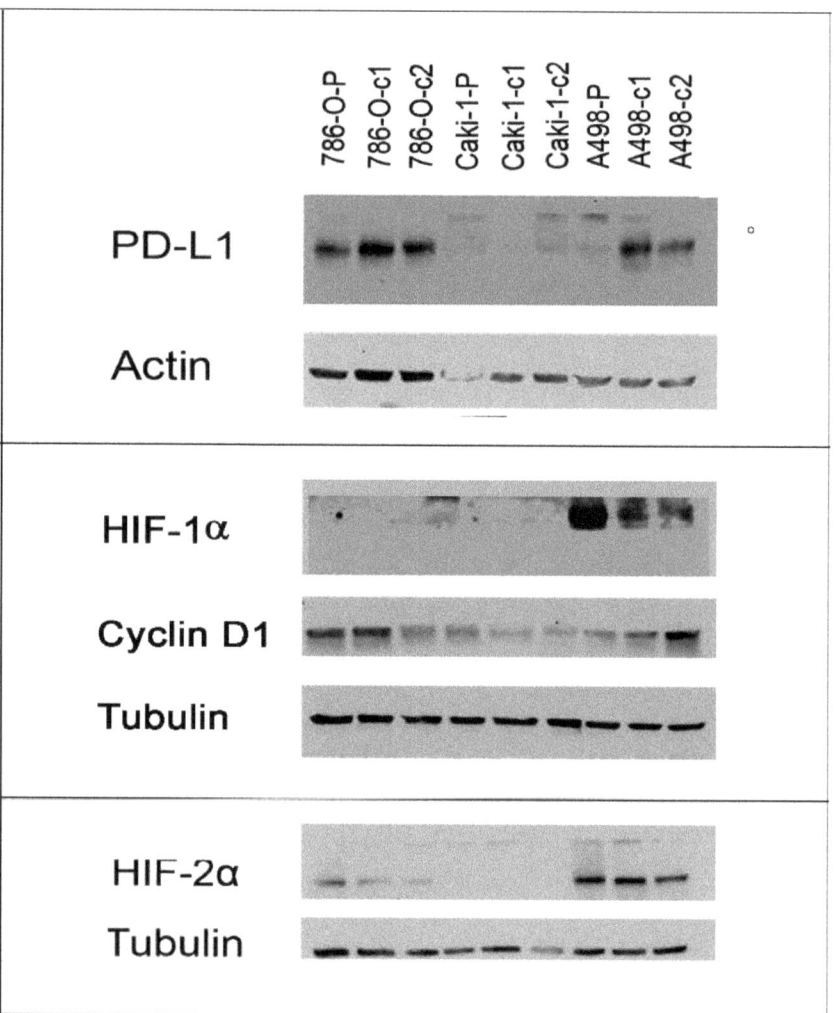

Figure 6. Protein expression in resistant clones and parental control cells of 786-O, Caki-1, and A498 cell lines.

Table 3. Densitometry readings of protein expression showing adjusted densities (%) relative to parental-control cell line.

Cell Line	786-O P	786-O c1	786-O c2	Caki-1 P	Caki-1 c1	Caki-1 c2	A498 P	A498 c1	A498 c2
PD-L1	100	161.3	131.3	100	16.9	35.8	100	1599.3	966.4
HIF1α	ND	ND	ND	ND	ND	ND	100	18.3	14.8
Cyclin D1	100	119.9	77.5	100	56.5	34.9	100	122.0	338.8
HIF2α	100	45.8	24.2	ND	ND	ND	100	128.5	60.8

Quantified using ImageJ software (v.1.8.0) (NIH, Bethesda, MD, USA) and expression adjusted according to respective loading controls using modified ImageJ protocol (http://www.lukemiller.org/ImageJ_gel_analysis.pdf, accessed on 10 August 2021). ND; not detected (i.e., raw value less than 50).

2.4. Gene Ontology and Pathway Analyses

In order to further investigate the potential role of miRNA-regulated genes in sunitinib resistance, we carried out ontology analysis by KEGG pathway enrichment analysis (Tables S7–S9). The number of significantly enriched pathways was highest ($n = 12$) in 786-O cells and lowest in A498 cells ($n = 6$), reflecting the different numbers of genes associated with miRNAs in these cell lines (Figure 3). Reassuringly, the most significant pathway in this analysis for 786-O cells was *miRNAs in cancer* (p-value 4×10^{-9}), which was also significantly enriched in Caki-1 cells despite having non-overlapping genes. The second most highly enriched pathway in this analysis was *proteoglycans in cancer* (p-value 1.6×10^{-5}), which was also significantly enriched in A498 (p-value 8.7×10^{-3}) and Caki-1 cells (p-value 2.2×10^{-5}); again, these pathways had non-overlapping genes in the three cell lines. Other significant pathways commonly shared between different cell lines were the *Human papillomavirus infection* in 786-O and Caki-1 cells (p-values 5.5×10^{-4} and 1.4×10^{-3} respectively) and *fluid shear stress* pathways (p-values 7.7×10^{-3} and 1.4×10^{-3}, respectively). The *PI3K-Akt signalling pathway* was also common between A498 and Caki-1 cells, but not 786-O (p-values 7.7×10^{-3} and 1.4×10^{-3}, respectively).

2.5. Silencing of PD-L1 in 786-O Sunitinib-Resistant Cells Results in an Increased Sensitivity to Sunitinib

As we observed a consistent up-regulation of *CD274* (PD-L1) in all of the resistant clones of all three cell lines and increased protein expression, in 786-O and A498 cells, at least, we hypothesised that this molecule would play an important role in the resistant phenotypes. We therefore silenced this gene in resistant and parental cells to investigate the effect on the resistant phenotype. After confirming the silencing by qRT-PCR (Figure S4) and protein level (Figure 7; Table 4), we carried out sunitinib dose experiments by MTT assay (Table 5). We observed that the silencing of *CD274* led to a significant increase in the sensitivity of 786-O-resistant clones but not in parental cells treated with the same siRNA. This effect was more pronounced in c1 cells, which is consistent with the increased silencing in this clone compared to c2 (84% and 72% reduction in c1 at and 38% and 72% in c2 at 48 h and 72 h, respectively: Figure S5). In contrast, the silencing of *CD274* in A498 or Caki-1 cells did not increase the sensitivity of resistant clones (or parental cells) to sunitinib treatment.

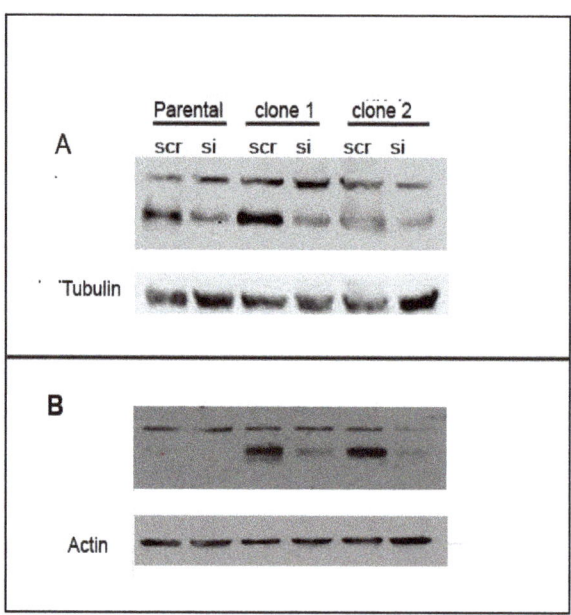

Figure 7. PD-L1 protein expression in 786-O (**A**) and A498 (**B**) parental and resistant cells after treatment with siRNA against CD274 (or scramble control).

Table 4. Densitometry readings of protein expression showing adjusted densities (%) relative to Scramble-control.

Cell Line	P-scr	P-si	c1-scr	c1-P	c2-scr	c2-P
A498	100	0	100	15.8	100	4.5
786-O	100	35.7	100	28.5	100	20.2

Quantified using ImageJ software (v.1.8.0) (NIH, Bethesda, MD, USA) and expression adjusted according to respective loading controls using modified ImageJ protocol (http://www.lukemiller.org/ImageJ_gel_analysis.pdf, accessed on 10 August 2021).

Table 5. IC_{50} values of parental and sunitinib-resistant clones, c1 and c2, of cell lines 786-O, A498, and Caki-1 cell lines after treatment with either anti-CD274 siRNA or a scramble RNA control (SCR).

Cell Line	Replicate	P-SCR	P-siRNA	c1-SCR	c1-siRNA	c2-SCR	c2-siRNA
786-O	A	5.9	4.2	11.0	6.5	10.6	6.6
	B	3.8	4.9	11.7	9.6	8.2	6.5
	C	4.7	6.8	12.3	9.5	9.4	8.0
	Average	4.8	5.3	11.7	8.5 *	9.4	7.0 *
A498	A	5.5	6.31	6.7	7.7	9.6	13.3
	B	9.8	11.8	10.6	12.8	10.2	11.4
	C	14.1	14.8	13	15.4	15.3	20.6
	Average	9.8	11	10.1	12	11.7	15.1
Caki-1	A	9.3	10.8	9	11.4	10	11.5
	B	6.4	6.7	9.5	16.1	11	11.9
	C	9.7	9.2	11	11.4	12	12.4
	Average	8.4	8.9	9.8	13	11	11.9

Values of biological triplicates are indicated by letters A–C. The dose curves used to generate the IC_{50} values can be found in Figures S6–S8. p-values were calculated by comparing siRNA-treated cells with SCR-treated cells by independent t-test and significance denoted by * $p < 0.05$.

3. Discussion

Inactivation of the *VHL* gene and activation of the HIF-VEGF pathway are the major molecular hallmarks of renal carcinoma and form the basis of antiangiogenic therapy such as sunitinib. Sunitinib remains the first-line treatment for mccRCC, and acquired resistance and tumour metastases are the main causes of treatment failure [31]. Consequently, several mechanisms have been proposed, including the up-regulation of *FGF1* [32], the induction of epithelial to mesenchymal transition (EMT) and alternative growth factor signaling [33], and the down-regulation of *PTEN* [18], amongst others. In addition to genes, several studies have established the role of miRNAs and other non-coding RNAs (ncRNAs) in sunitinib resistance [21,23,26,34]. However, very few have used an integrated genomic approach to identify target genes regulated by miRNAs—an approach that lends itself to the possibility of using miRNA-based therapeutics to overcome sunitinib resistance in ccRCC patients.

We, therefore, developed an in vitro model of sunitinib resistance in three different cell lines (786-O, A498, and Caki-1) through prolonged exposure to the drug. All these cell lines were originally sensitive to sunitinib, with an IC_{50} value less than 10 µM (average 8.8 µM), the concentration reached in patient tumour tissue [33]. The generated resistant clones had a significantly higher amount of IC_{50} values greater than 10 µM (average 15.6 µM). Although several studies have investigated miRNA expression in response to sunitinib-treatment, the vast majority have looked at expression after a single dose [22,24,25], rather than prolonged exposure, which could be argued to more accurately reflect acquired resistance [21,23,35].

Unsupervised cluster analysis of miRNA and gene expression data showed that resistant cells not only differed from sunitinib-sensitive cells, but also differed between resistant clones, suggesting differing mechanisms of resistance. This was confirmed by the low levels of overlap (<50%) of differentially expressed genes and miRNAs between the clones. There were 3254, 2313, and 4285 differentially expressed genes identified in 786-O, A498, and Caki-1 cells, respectively. However, gene enrichment analysis using the KEGG pathway database failed to detect any significantly enriched pathways amongst these gene datasets, suggesting that many of these genes were only indirectly linked to the resistant phenotype. In order to resolve this issue, and bearing in mind the association of miRNAs with sunitinib resistance [23,25–27,36–38], we used an integrated genomic approach to identify miRNA-regulated target genes by molecular interaction network analyses. Using this methodology, we identified 76, 6, and 26 miRNA:gene interactions consistently involved in sunitinib resistance for 786-O, A498, and Caki-1 cells, respectively. The much larger number of interactions in 786-O cells most likely reflects the much higher degree of overlap in genes and miRNAs found in this cell line between the clones c1 and c2 (60% cf 32% (A498) and 30% (Caki-1) for miRNAs and 43% vs. 27% vs. 20% of genes).

When we repeated the gene enrichment analysis on the miRNA-regulated genes, we a observed significant enrichment for the *'proteoglycans in cancer'* KEGG pathway in all three cell lines, even though the corresponding gene lists were non-overlapping. Other shared pathways were *'human papillomavirus infection'*, *'fluid shear stress'*, and *'PI3K-Akt signalling'* pathways. Consistent with these findings, Chen et al. also reported that *'proteoglycans in cancer'* and *'PI3K-Akt signalling'* pathways were amongst the most significant pathways identified by meta-analysis of 88 gene expression and next generation sequencing data sets from sunitinib resistance studies containing both in vitro and inpatient-derived xenograft models [29]. Yamagouchi et al. likewise identified the *PI3K-AKT pathway* as significant by KEGG analysis of sunitinib-resistant cells [23]. Moreover, the genes identified in these studies were non-overlapping, with those identified in our study implying a functional relevance of these pathways in sunitinib resistance. Proteoglycans are major components of the extracellular matrix and play important roles in many facets of cancer, including proliferation, adhesion, angiogenesis, and metastasis [39]. Recently, Rausch et al. described the morphometric changes that occur in sunitinib-resistant clones, in which the authors linked the changes of more than 70 genes to cell adhesion, including many proteoglycans [35].

We observed that multiple members of the *miR-17~92* clusters (i.e., *miR-17-5p, miR-17-3p, miR-18a-5p, miR-18a-3p, miR-20a-5p*) and paralogue clusters, including all the members of the *miR-106b~miR-25* (*miR-106b, miR-93-5p,* and *miR-25-5p*) cluster and the *miR-106a-5p,* which is encoded by the *miR-106a~363* cluster, were down-regulated in resistant ccRCC clones. The down-regulation of *miR-18a-5p*, at least, has previously been reported in other sunitinib-resistant ccRCC cell lines (ACHN and RCC23) [23]. Intriguingly, network analyses revealed that the target genes of these miRNAs were non-overlapping in the different cell lines (Table 2). This suggests the involvement of differing gene pathways in resistance mechanisms but implies a convergent regulatory role of these miRNAs in ccRCC, making them potential common targets for modulation that surely warrants further investigation and could potentially be targeted to overcome sunitinib resistance. For example, in 786-O cells, target genes were generally hypoxia and angiogenic-related (i.e., *EPAS1*, *HIF1A*, *MMP2*, and *VLDLR*), whereas, in Caki-1 cells, target genes (i.e., *CCND1*, *BMP2*, *TCEAL1*, and *RND3*) were involved in inflammatory, proliferation, and migration, possibly a reflection of the metastatic phenotype of these cells. Indeed it is tempting to infer that these mechanisms reflect the subclassification of ccRCC into angiogenic and inflammatory tumours that has recently been proposed by Brugarolas et al. [7].

The most regulated gene in 786-O cells was *HIF1A*, which was regulated by down-regulation of multiple members of the *miR-17~92* cluster and *miR-210*, highly suggestive of playing a major role in sunitinib resistance in this cell line. The role of HIF1α in sunitinib treatment and resistance has long been recognised [40]. Yamagouchi et al. similarly found that *HIF1A* was up-regulated in sunitinib-resistant cell lines and that it was targeted by *miR-18a-5p* [23]. Even though there was a clear increase in *HIF1A* expression in the resistant clones of 786-O and Caki-1 cells (Figure 5; Table 3), the HIF1α protein was not detected in these cell lines (Figure 6; Table 4). This is consistent with previous studies, that have shown a lack of protein expression in 786-O cells due to mutations [41,42], and even though Caki-1 cells do encode the intact *HIF1A* gene, the protein is only expressed under hypoxic conditions [43]. The fact that the *HIF1A* transcript, but not the protein, is induced in these cell lines could have functional significance in the resistance mechanism, as several long non-coding RNAs (lncRNAs) are encoded within this gene [44,45], and this is an area we are currently investigating. Although A498 cells also contain a mutated *HIF1A* gene, the HIF1α protein is expressed constitutively under normoxic conditions due to defective *VHL* [43]. We observed that HIF1α expression was down-regulated in A498-resistant clones, a characteristic that was previously described to be the result of sunitinib-associated proteosome degradation [41].

In the Caki-1 miRNA:target gene network, *CCND1* was the most regulated gene which was potentially targeted by five out of thirteen (38%) of down-regulated miRNAs, none of which were found in the 786-O network. Indeed, in contrast to Caki-1 (and A498) resistant clones, 786-O-resistant clones were characterised by *CCND1* mRNA and cyclin D1 protein down-regulation. *CCND1* is not only a marker of proliferation and tumour growth [46], but is also associated with metastatic potential [46,47]. Although the down-regulation of members of the *miR-17~92* cluster is consistent with the up-regulation of *CCND1* observed in Caki-1 and A498-resistant clones [48], the same miRNAs are also down-regulated in 786-O-resistant clones, suggesting a different regulatory mechanism for this cell line, perhaps through the direct targeting by HIF2α [49], which is down-regulated at mRNA and protein levels. Intriguingly, although *CCND1* was strongly up-regulated (8–10-fold) in resistant clones of Caki-1 cells, cyclin D1 protein was down-regulated, as has recently been described [35], suggesting post-transcriptional regulation.

The PD-L1 gene (*CD274*) was also identified in our network analysis as being targeted by *miR-200a*, which we had previously demonstrated was characteristically down-regulated in ccRCC [50], and that was down-regulated in both 786-O and Caki-1-resistant clones (but not A498 cells). *miR-200* has been shown to directly target *CD274*/PD-L1 expression, and, in concert with ZEB1, to play an important role in the initiation of metastasis via the induction of epithelial-to-mesenchymal transition (EMT) and CD8+ TIL immunosuppression [51]. In addition to *miR-200*, *miR-34a* has also been identified as an important regulator of PD-L1 expression [52]. Indeed, a phase 1 clinical trial, using a liposomal mimic of this miRNA (MRX34), included renal carcinoma patients, although the trial was halted due to serious adverse effects [53]. We observed that the levels of *miR-34a* were significantly down-regulated in the resistant clones of all three cell lines. An increase in PD-L1 protein expression in response to transient sunitinib treatment has previously been reported in 786-O and A498 cell lines [17,54]. We extended these observations to the resistant clones of these cell lines, as well as to *CD274* mRNA expression. Indeed, this was the only gene that we found to be consistently up-regulated in all three of the cell lines in this study. It should be noted, however, that we were unable to detect PD-L1 protein expression in the Caki-1 cell line, an observation consistent with previous studies [55,56], presumably due to the lack of HIF1α expression under normoxic conditions in this cell line that also regulates PD-L1 expression [54].

To explore the role of PD-L1 further in the resistant phenotype, we silenced this gene in the three cell lines and observed an increase in the sensitivity to sunitinib of the 786-O-resistant clones but not the parental counterpart cells, nor the Caki-1 or A498 cells. The difference between the response between the cell lines suggests again that there are different resistance mechanisms operating between the cell lines, and that the PD-L1-associated mechanism is most important in 786-O cells. In contrast, in Caki-1 cells, where PD-L1 is not expressed, resistance appears to be regulated through cyclin D1, although this remains to be experimentally confirmed. The lack of effect of PD-L1 silencing on A498 cells, however, is somewhat more surprising, suggesting that the down-regulation of HIF1α that we observed in resistant clones is probably a more dominant mechanism for resistance than PD-L1, as it has been demonstrated that ectopic expression of HIF1α in 786-O cells make them more susceptible to sunitinib [41]. These results suggest that ccRCC patients with *VHL* gene mutations (>50% of patients) [57] that do not express HIF1α (~70% of ccRCC patients [58]) could have an improved response to sunitinib treatment through targeting of PD-L1 by checkpoint inhibitor antibodies such as avelumab that already has FDA-approval for combination treatment in ccRCC [59]. Consistent with this hypothesis, Guo et al. demonstrated that a combination of anti-PD-L1 and sunitinib significantly reduced tumour progression in vivo [17]. Indeed, although immunotherapy targeting the PD-1/PD-L1 axis shows great promise for ccRCC, only 15–25% of patients respond when given it as a monotherapy [60], and there is increasing movement towards combination therapy of antiangiogenic agents and immunotherapy [59,61–64]. We are not aware, however, of any trials to date that have combined sunitinib with anti-PD-L1 immunotherapy. We recognise however, that cell lines may not give a complete reflection of what occurs in ccRCC patients.

In summary, the present study has demonstrated that the use of in vitro models of sunitinib resistance, combined with an integrated genomic approach, can identify divergent mechanisms of sunitinib resistance that could be exploited for the benefit of ccRCC patients.

4. Materials and Methods

4.1. Generation of Sunitinib-Resistant ccRCC Cell Lines

The ccRCC cell lines 786-O (ATCC® CRL1932™), A498 (ATCC® HTB 44™), and Caki-1 (Caki-1ATCC® HTB46™) were obtained from the American Type Culture Collection (ATCC, Manassas, VA, USA). 786-O and A498 cells were grown in RPMI and MEM media respectively, in the presence of 10% fetal calf serum (FCS), 1% *L*-glutamine and 1% penicillin-streptavidin (Fisher Scientific, Waltham, MA, USA). Caki-1 cells were grown in McCoy's 5A (modified) medium with 10% FCS + 1% *L*-glutamine and 1% penicillin-streptavidin (Fisher Scientific, Waltham, MA, USA). Two resistant clones for each cell line were generated by gradually exposing the cells to increasing concentrations of sunitinib (0.5 µM increase per passage) until a final concentration of 10 µM. For each increase in sunitinib concentration, cells were passaged at least twice to remove dead cells. Parental control cells were passaged in parallel without the addition of sunitinib.

4.2. Cell Proliferation Assay

Cells were seeded onto 96-well plates at a density of 2×10^3 cells per well and allowed to attach for 24 h. Afterwards, the cells were treated with differing doses of sunitinib (i.e., 1.25, 2.5, 5, 7.5, 10, 15, 20, 30, and 40 µM) or DMSO as a negative control. Seventy-two hours later, MTT (3-(4,5-Dimethylthiazol-2-yl)-2,5-Diphenyltetrazolium Bromide) was added to the cells before a further incubation at 37 °C for three hours. The reaction was stopped by the addition of DMSO and the resulting absorbance at 570 nm was measured using a Halo LED 96 plate reader (Dynamica Ltd., Livingston, UK). Each sample was measured in triplicate wells and each experiment carried out a minimum of three times.

4.3. RNA Extraction and Microarray Analysis

Total RNA was extracted from cell line material using Trizol in accordance with the manufacturer's instructions (Life Technologies, Paisley, UK). One µg of total RNA was used for Affymetrix Genechip miRNA v.4.0 microarrays, and 200 ng of DNAse treated total RNA were used for Clariom D human microarrays to measure miRNA and gene expression, respectively. The RNA was labelled and hybridised to microarrays in accordance with the manufacturer's instructions (Affymetrix, CA, USA).

Resulting raw intensity data (i.e., cel files) were imported and analysed within Transcriptome Analysis Console (TAC) software version 4.0.2 (Affymetrix, CA, USA). Using this software, we identified differentially expressed miRNAs or genes on the basis of >2-fold up- or down-regulation along with Benjamini–Hochberg multiple corrected p values < 0.05. All microarray data was MIAME compliant, and raw data was deposited in the GEO database (GSE183140). For miRNA microarray analysis, probes were filtered for only human mature miRNAs (i.e., hsa-miR*) (* means wild-card i.e., any miR) and, for gene expression analysis coding, genes were classified as probes and filtered using the group variable 'coding' or 'multiple complex', before removing non-annotated genes that only had a numerical Aceview description.

4.4. Interaction Network Analysis

In order to identify differentially expressed genes that are likely to be regulated by miRNAs, we used the Cytoscape program (v3.8.2) (NIH, Bethesda, MD, USA) [65] to create an (experimentally validated) miRNA-target gene network. In brief, we imported and created a reference network of experimentally validated interactions (n = 10,755) from the miRTarBase dataset consisting of 3502 genes and miRNAs [30]. Differentially expressed miRNAs and genes from microarray analyses were imported into the program and mapped to the reference network. Mapped miRNA:target gene interactions were filtered according to inverse correlations (i.e., up-regulated miRNAs and down-regulated genes and vice versa) for each individual clone, and the intersection between the clonal networks was used to produce common networks, as depicted in Figure 3. These common networks were used for ontology analysis using the STRING app (version 1.6.0) (University of California, San Francisco, CA, USA) to interrogate the KEGG pathway database (release 95.2) implemented in Cytoscape. An overview of the workflow used is depicted in Figure 1.

4.5. Quantitative RT-PCR (qRT-PCR)

To measure levels of individual miRNAs by qRT-PCR, we used 200 ng of total RNA. The RNA was reverse transcribed using the Taqman Megaplex miRNA pool A according to the manufacturer's instructions (Applied Biosystems, Warrington, UK), except in the case where specific miRNAs were not present in this pool, in which individual primers were used. qPCR was carried out with individual Taqman probes in triplicate using a LightCycler® 96 System machine (Roche, Basel, Switzerland). The snoRNA *RNU48* was used as the reference gene for miRNA quantification as previously described [66], and *GAPDH* was used as a control for gene expression. In brief, the mean Ct value of each triplicate was quantified by the ΔC_t method (i.e ΔC_t = mean C_t of *RNU48/GAPDH* minus the mean C_t of miRNA/gene of interest). All qRT-PCR assays were carried out in technical and biological triplicate and expression levels were compared using the Mann–Whitney independent t-test (Graphpad Prism v.5.0, La Jolla, CA, USA).

4.6. PDL-1 Silencing

Cells (4×10^4) were transfected with either 5 nM of ON-TARGET plus human CD274 SMART pool siRNA or a non-targeting scramble control (Dharmacon, Lafayette, CO). Transfection was carried out in 12-well plates using DharmaFECT™ reagent (Dharmacon) according to the manufacturer's protocol. Cells were harvested at 48-, 72-, and 96-h post-transfection, and RNA was extracted using Trizol (Fisher Scientific).

4.7. Western Blotting

Cells were washed with ice-cold PBS twice before lysis in RIPA buffer containing Halt™ protease and phosphatase inhibitor cocktail (Thermo Scientific, Waltham, MA, USA). Protein concentrations were measured by BCA protein assay (Thermo Scientific, Waltham, MA, USA), and equal amounts of protein were run on 10% Mini-PROTEAN TGX Precast Protein Gels (Bio-Rad, Hercules, CA, USA). Proteins were transferred to Amersham Protran 0.45-μm nitrocellulose membranes (Amersham, UK) before blocking for 1 h at room temperature in TBS-Tween 20 (0.05%) (TBS-T) and 5% non-fat milk. Primary antibodies were incubated overnight at 4 °C in TBS-T with 5% non-fat milk, and HRP-conjugated secondary antibodies were incubated for 1 h at room temperature. A list of the antibodies and dilutions can be seen in Table S10.

5. Conclusions

The present study has demonstrated that the use of in vitro models of sunitinib resistance, combined with an integrated genomic approach of miRNA and gene expression, can identify divergent mechanisms of sunitinib resistance that could be exploited for the benefit of ccRCC patients.

Supplementary Materials: The following are available online at https://www.mdpi.com/article/10.3390/cancers13174401/s1, Figure S1: Cell proliferation MTT assays of 786-O resistant clones (c1 and c2) and the parental cell line used to calculate the IC_{50} value in Table 1. Figure S2: Cell proliferation MTT assays of A498 resistant clones (c1 and c2) and the parental cell line used to calculate the IC_{50} value in Table 1. Figure S3: Cell proliferation MTT assays of Caki-1 resistant clones (c1 and c2) and the parental cell line used to calculate the IC_{50} value in Table 1. Figure S4: Unsupervised cluster analysis heatmaps of miRNA expression (**A**–**C**) in 786-O (**A**), A498 (**B**) and Caki-1 (**C**) resistant clones and parental control cell lines. Figure S5: Relative *CD274* mRNA expression measured by qRT-PCR in sunitinib resistant clones, c1 and c2, and parental cells in 786-O (**A**), A498 (**B**) and Caki-1 (**C**) cell lines at 48 and 72 h post-transfection with either siRNA or a scramble control. Figure S6: Cell proliferation MTT assays of 786-O resistant clones (c1 and c2) and the parental cell line transfected with CD274-siRNA or scramble control siRNA. These data were used to calculate the IC_{50} value in Table 3. Figure S7: Cell proliferation MTT assays of A498 resistant clones (c1 and c2) and the parental cell line transfected with CD274-siRNA or scramble control siRNA. Figure S8: Cell proliferation MTT assays of Caki-1 resistant clones (c1 and c2) and the parental cell line transfected with CD274-siRNA or scramble control siRNA. Table S1: List of miRNAs commonly differentially expressed between 786-O parental (P) and resistant clones c1 and c2. Table S2: List of miRNAs commonly differentially expressed between A498 parental (P) and resistant clones c1 and c2. Table S3: List of miRNAs commonly differentially expressed between Caki-1 parental (P) and resistant clones c1 and c2. Table S4: List of top 100 differentially expressed genes between 786-O parental (P) and resistant clones c1 and c2. Arranged according to FDR *F-value*. Table S5: List of top 100 differentially expressed genes between A498 parental (P) and resistant clones c1 and c2. Arranged according to FDR *F-value*. Table S6: List of top 100 differentially expressed genes between Caki-1 parental (P) and resistant clones c1 and c2. Arranged according to FDR *F-value*. Table S7: List of significantly enriched KEGG pathways for 786-O cell line. Table S8: List of significantly enriched KEGG pathways for A498 cell line. Table S9: List of significantly enriched KEGG pathways for Caki-1 cell line. Table S10: List of primary and secondary antibodies used in the Western Blots.

Author Contributions: Conceptualization, M.A. (María Armesto) and C.H.L.; methodology, M.A. (María Armesto); M.M.; M.A. (María Arestin); P.E.; L.M. and A.R.; validation, M.A. (María Armesto); M.A. (María Arestin); J.I.L.; formal analysis, M.A. (María Armesto); J.I.L. and C.H.L.; resources, P.E. and J.I.L. data curation, M.A. (María Armesto); M.A. (María Arestin) and J.I.L.; writing—original draft preparation, M.A. (María Armesto) and C.H.L.; writing—review and editing, all authors. All authors have read and agreed to the published version of the manuscript.

Funding: This research received no external funding.

Institutional Review Board Statement: Not applicable.

Informed Consent Statement: Not applicable.

Data Availability Statement: Data available in a publicly accessible repository. The data presented in this study are openly available in GEO at https://www.ncbi.nlm.nih.gov/geo/, accessed on 26 August 2021, GSE183140.

Acknowledgments: C.H.L. and his research are supported by grants from the IKERBASQUE Foundation for Science, the Starmer–Smith Memorial Fund, Ministerio de Economía y Competitividad (MINECO) of the Spanish Central Government, the ISCIII and FEDER funds (PI12/00663, PIE13/00048, DTS14/00109, PI15/00275, PI18/01710), Departamento de Desarrollo Económico y Competitividad y Departamento de Sanidad of the Basque government, Asociación Española Contra el Cancer (AECC), Diputación Foral de Guipuzcoa (DFG) and Gobierno Vasco, Departamento de Industria (ELKARTEK project code: KK-2018/00038).

Conflicts of Interest: The authors declare no conflict of interest.

References

1. Siegel, R.; Naishadham, D.; Jemal, A. Cancer statistics. *CA Cancer J. Clin.* **2013**, *63*, 11–30. [CrossRef] [PubMed]
2. Nagashima, Y.; Inayama, Y.; Kato, Y.; Sakai, N.; Kanno, H.; Aoki, I.; Yao, M. Pathological and molecular biological aspects of the renal epithelial neoplasms, up-to-date. *Pathol. Int.* **2004**, *54*, 377–386. [CrossRef]
3. Lopez-Beltran, A.; Scarpelli, M.; Montironi, R.; Kirkali, Z. 2004 WHO Classification of the Renal Tumors of the Adults. *Eur. Urol.* **2006**, *49*, 798–805. [CrossRef] [PubMed]
4. Lopez, J.I. Renal tumors with clear cells. A review. *Pathol. Res. Pract.* **2013**, *209*, 137–146. [CrossRef] [PubMed]
5. Tickoo, S.K.; Reuter, V.E. Differential Diagnosis of Renal Tumors With Papillary Architecture. *Adv. Anat. Pathol.* **2011**, *18*, 120–131. [CrossRef]
6. Gupta, K.; Miller, J.D.; Li, J.Z.; Russell, M.W.; Charbonneau, C. Epidemiologic and socioeconomic burden of metastatic renal cell carcinoma (mRCC): A literature review. *Cancer Treat. Rev.* **2008**, *34*, 193–205. [CrossRef]
7. Brugarolas, J.; Rajaram, S.; Christie, A.; Kapur, P. The Evolution of Angiogenic and Inflamed Tumors: The Renal Cancer Paradigm. *Cancer Cell* **2020**, *38*, 771–773. [CrossRef]
8. Motzer, R.J.; Michaelson, M.D.; Redman, B.G.; Hudes, G.R.; Wilding, G.; Figlin, R.A.; Ginsberg, M.S.; Kim, S.T.; Baum, C.M.; DePrimo, S.E.; et al. Activity of SU11248, a Multitargeted Inhibitor of Vascular Endothelial Growth Factor Receptor and Platelet-Derived Growth Factor Receptor, in Patients With Metastatic Renal Cell Carcinoma. *J. Clin. Oncol.* **2006**, *24*, 16–24. [CrossRef]
9. Motzer, R.J.; Hutson, T.; Tomczak, P.; Michaelson, D.; Bukowski, R.M.; Rixe, O.; Oudard, S.; Negrier, S.; Szczylik, C.; Kim, S.T.; et al. Sunitinib versus Interferon Alfa in Metastatic Renal-Cell Carcinoma. *N. Engl. J. Med.* **2007**, *356*, 115–124. [CrossRef]
10. Schueneman, A.J.; Himmelfarb, E.; Geng, L.; Tan, J.; Donnelly, E.; Mendel, D.; McMahon, G.; E Hallahan, D. SU11248 maintenance therapy prevents tumor regrowth after fractionated irradiation of murine tumor models. *Cancer Res.* **2003**, *63*, 4009–4016. [PubMed]
11. Faivre, S.; Demetri, G.; Sargent, W.; Raymond, E. Molecular basis for sunitinib efficacy and future clinical development. *Nat. Rev. Drug Discov.* **2007**, *6*, 734–745. [CrossRef]
12. Calin, G.A.; Cimmino, A.; Fabbri, M.; Ferracin, M.; Wojcik, S.E.; Shimizu, M.; Taccioli, C.; Zanesi, N.; Garzon, R.; Aqeilan, R.I.; et al. MiR-15a and miR-16-1 cluster functions in human leukemia. *Proc. Natl. Acad. Sci. USA* **2008**, *105*, 5166–5171. [CrossRef]
13. Méjean, A.; Ravaud, A.; Thezenas, S.; Colas, S.; Beauval, J.-B.; Bensalah, K.; Geoffrois, L.; Thiery-Vuillemin, A.; Cormier, L.; Lang, H.; et al. Sunitinib Alone or after Nephrectomy in Metastatic Renal-Cell Carcinoma. *N. Engl. J. Med.* **2018**, *379*, 417–427. [CrossRef] [PubMed]
14. Kamli, H.; Gobe, G.C.; Li, L.; Vesey, D.A.; Morais, C. Characterisation of the Morphological, Functional and Molecular Changes in Sunitinib-Resistant Renal Cell Carcinoma Cells. *J. Kidney Cancer VHL* **2018**, *5*, 4009–4016. [CrossRef]
15. Van Der Mijn, J.C.; Broxterman, H.J.; Knol, J.C.; Piersma, S.R.; De Haas, R.R.; Dekker, H.; Pham, T.V.; Van Beusechem, V.W.; Halmos, B.; Mier, J.W.; et al. Sunitinib activates Axl signaling in renal cell cancer. *Int. J. Cancer* **2016**, *138*, 3002–3010. [CrossRef]

16. Han, K.S.; Raven, P.A.; Frees, S.; Gust, K.M.; Fazli, L.; Ettinger, S.; Hong, S.J.; Kollmannsberger, C.; Gleave, M.; So, A.I. Cellular Adaptation to VEGF-Targeted Antiangiogenic Therapy Induces Evasive Resistance by Overproduction of Alternative Endothelial Cell Growth Factors in Renal Cell Carcinoma. *Neoplasia* **2015**, *17*, 805–816. [CrossRef] [PubMed]
17. Guo, X.; Li, R.; Bai, Q.; Jiang, S.; Wang, H. TFE3-PD-L1 axis is pivotal for sunitinib resistance in clear cell renal cell carcinoma. *J. Cell. Mol. Med.* **2020**, *24*, 14441–14452. [CrossRef] [PubMed]
18. Sekino, Y.; Hagura, T.; Han, X.; Babasaki, T.; Goto, K.; Inoue, S.; Hayashi, T.; Teishima, J.; Shigeta, M.; Taniyama, D.; et al. PTEN Is Involved in Sunitinib and Sorafenib Resistance in Renal Cell Carcinoma. *Anticancer Res.* **2020**, *40*, 1943–1951. [CrossRef]
19. Aimudula, A.; Nasier, H.; Yang, Y.; Zhang, R.; Lu, P.; Hao, J.; Bao, Y. PPARα mediates sunitinib resistance via NF-κB activation in clear cell renal cell carcinoma. *Int. J. Clin. Exp. Pathol.* **2018**, *11*, 2389–2400.
20. Khella, H.W.Z.; Butz, H.; Ding, Q.; Rotondo, F.; Evans, K.R.; Kupchak, P.; Dharsee, M.; Latif, A.; Pasic, M.D.; Lianidou, E.; et al. miR-221/222 Are Involved in Response to Sunitinib Treatment in Metastatic Renal Cell Carcinoma. *Mol. Ther.* **2015**, *23*, 1748–1758. [CrossRef]
21. Prior, C.; Perez-Gracia, J.L.; Garcia-Donas, J.; Rodriguez-Antona, C.; Guruceaga, E.; Esteban, E.; Suarez, C.; Castellano, D.; Del Alba, A.G.; Lozano, M.D.; et al. Identification of Tissue microRNAs Predictive of Sunitinib Activity in Patients with Metastatic Renal Cell Carcinoma. *PLoS ONE* **2014**, *9*, e86263. [CrossRef]
22. Osako, Y.; Yoshino, H.; Sakaguchi, T.; Sugita, S.; Yonemori, M.; Nakagawa, M.; Enokida, H. Potential tumor-suppressive role of microRNA-99a-3p in sunitinib-resistant renal cell carcinoma cells through the regulation of RRM2. *Int. J. Oncol.* **2019**, *54*, 1759–1770. [CrossRef]
23. Yamaguchi, N.; Osaki, M.; Onuma, K.; Yumioka, T.; Iwamoto, H.; Sejima, T.; Kugoh, H.; Takenaka, A.; Okada, F. Identification of MicroRNAs Involved in Resistance to Sunitinib in Renal Cell Carcinoma Cells. *Anticancer Res.* **2017**, *37*, 2985–2992. [CrossRef] [PubMed]
24. Lu, L.; Li, Y.; Wen, H.; Feng, C. Overexpression of miR-15b Promotes Resistance to Sunitinib in Renal Cell Carcinoma. *J. Cancer* **2019**, *10*, 3389–3396. [CrossRef]
25. Xiao, W.; Lou, N.; Ruan, H.; Bao, L.; Xiong, Z.; Yuan, C.; Tong, J.; Xu, G.; Zhou, Y.; Qu, Y.; et al. Mir-144-3p Promotes Cell Proliferation, Metastasis, Sunitinib Resistance in Clear Cell Renal Cell Carcinoma by Downregulating ARID1A. *Cell. Physiol. Biochem.* **2017**, *43*, 2420–2433. [CrossRef] [PubMed]
26. Sekino, Y.; Sakamoto, N.; Sentani, K.; Oue, N.; Teishima, J.; Matsubara, A.; Yasui, W. miR-130b Promotes Sunitinib Resistance through Regulation of PTEN in Renal Cell Carcinoma. *Oncology* **2019**, *97*, 164–172. [CrossRef] [PubMed]
27. Yumioka, T.; Osaki, M.; Sasaki, R.; Yamaguchi, N.; Onuma, K.; Iwamoto, H.; Morizane, S.; Honda, M.; Takenaka, A.; Okada, F. Lysosome-associated membrane protein 2 (LAMP-2) expression induced by miR-194-5p downregulation contributes to sunitinib resistance in human renal cell carcinoma cells. *Oncol. Lett.* **2017**, *15*, 893–900. [CrossRef]
28. Butz, H.; Ding, Q.; Nofech-Mozes, R.; Lichner, Z.; Ni, H.; Yousef, G.M. Elucidating mechanisms of sunitinib resistance in renal cancer: An integrated pathological-molecular analysis. *Oncotarget* **2017**, *9*, 4661–4674. [CrossRef]
29. Chen, Y.; Ge, G.; Qi, C.; Wang, H.; Wang, H.; Li, L.; Li, G.; Xia, L. A five-gene signature may predict sunitinib sensitivity and serve as prognostic biomarkers for renal cell carcinoma. *J. Cell. Physiol.* **2018**, *233*, 6649–6660. [CrossRef]
30. Hsu, S.-D.; Lin, F.-M.; Wu, W.-Y.; Liang, C.; Huang, W.-C.; Chan, W.-L.; Tsai, W.-T.; Chen, G.-Z.; Lee, C.-J.; Chiu, C.-M.; et al. miRTarBase: A database curates experimentally validated microRNA–target interactions. *Nucleic Acids Res.* **2010**, *39*, D163–D169. [CrossRef]
31. Rixe, O.; Franco, S.X.; Yardley, D.A.; Johnston, S.R.; Martín, M.; Arun, B.K.; Letrent, S.P.; Rugo, H.S. A randomized, phase II, dose-finding study of the pan-ErbB receptor tyrosine-kinase inhibitor CI-1033 in patients with pretreated metastatic breast cancer. *Cancer Chemother. Pharmacol.* **2009**, *64*, 1139–1148. [CrossRef]
32. Chou, C.-H.; Chang, N.-W.; Shrestha, S.; Hsu, S.-D.; Lin, Y.-L.; Lee, W.-H.; Yang, C.-D.; Hong, H.-C.; Wei, T.-Y.; Tu, S.-J.; et al. miRTarBase 2016: Updates to the experimentally validated miRNA-target interactions database. *Nucleic Acids Res.* **2015**, *44*, D239–D247. [CrossRef]
33. Gotink, K.J.; Broxterman, H.J.; Labots, M.; De Haas, R.R.; Dekker, H.; Honeywell, R.J.; Rudek, M.A.; Beerepoot, L.V.; Musters, R.J.; Jansen, G.; et al. Lysosomal Sequestration of Sunitinib: A Novel Mechanism of Drug Resistance. *Clin. Cancer Res.* **2011**, *17*, 7337–7346. [CrossRef]
34. Li, D.; Li, C.; Chen, Y.; Teng, L.; Cao, Y.; Wang, W.; Pan, H.; Xu, Y.; Yang, D. LncRNA HOTAIR induces sunitinib resistance in renal cancer by acting as a competing endogenous RNA to regulate autophagy of renal cells. *Cancer Cell Int.* **2020**, *20*, 338. [CrossRef]
35. Rausch, M.; Rutz, A.; Allard, P.-M.; Delucinge-Vivier, C.; Docquier, M.; Dormond, O.; Wolfender, J.-L.; Nowak-Sliwinska, P. Molecular and Functional Analysis of Sunitinib-Resistance Induction in Human Renal Cell Carcinoma Cells. *Int. J. Mol. Sci.* **2021**, *22*, 6467. [CrossRef]
36. Gamez-Pozo, A.; Antón-Aparicio, L.M.; Bayona, C.; Borrega, P.; Sancho, M.I.G.; García-Domínguez, R.; de Portugal, T.; Ramos-Vázquez, M.; Pérez-Carrión, R.; Bolós, M.V.; et al. MicroRNA Expression Profiling of Peripheral Blood Samples Predicts Resistance to First-line Sunitinib in Advanced Renal Cell Carcinoma Patients. *Neoplasia* **2012**, *14*, 1144–1152. [CrossRef] [PubMed]
37. Berkers, J.; Govaere, O.; Wolter, P.; Beuselinck, B.; Schöffski, P.; van Kempen, L.; Albersen, M.; Oord, J.V.D.; Roskams, T.; Swinnen, J.; et al. A Possible Role for MicroRNA-141 Down-Regulation in Sunitinib Resistant Metastatic Clear Cell Renal Cell Carcinoma Through Induction of Epithelial-to-Mesenchymal Transition and Hypoxia Resistance. *J. Urol.* **2012**, *189*, 1930–1938. [CrossRef]

38. Gong, L.-G.; Shi, J.-C.; Shang, J.; Hao, J.-G.; Du, X. Effect of miR-34a on resistance to sunitinib in breast cancer by regulating the Wnt/β-catenin signaling pathway. *Eur. Rev. Med. Pharmacol. Sci.* **2019**, *23*, 1151–1157. [PubMed]
39. Ahrens, T.D.; Bang-Christensen, S.R.; Jørgensen, A.M.; Løppke, C.; Spliid, C.B.; Sand, N.T.; Clausen, T.M.; Salanti, A.; Agerbæk, M. The Role of Proteoglycans in Cancer Metastasis and Circulating Tumor Cell Analysis. *Front. Cell Dev. Biol.* **2020**, *8*, 749. [CrossRef] [PubMed]
40. Morais, C. Sunitinib resistance in renal cell carcinoma. *J. Kidney Cancer VHL* **2014**, *1*, 1–11. [CrossRef] [PubMed]
41. Lai, X.-M.; Liu, S.-Y.; Tsai, Y.-T.; Sun, G.-H.; Chang, S.-Y.; Huang, S.-M.; Cha, T.-L. HAF mediates the evasive resistance of anti-angiogenesis TKI through disrupting HIF-1α and HIF-2α balance in renal cell carcinoma. *Oncotarget* **2017**, *8*, 49713–49724. [CrossRef]
42. Hu, C.-J.; Wang, L.-Y.; Chodosh, L.A.; Keith, B.; Simon, M.C. Differential Roles of Hypoxia-Inducible Factor 1α (HIF-1α) and HIF-2α in Hypoxic Gene Regulation. *Mol. Cell. Biol.* **2003**, *23*, 9361–9374. [CrossRef]
43. Swiatek, M.; Jancewicz, I.; Kluebsoongnoen, J.; Zub, R.; Maassen, A.; Kubala, S.; Udomkit, A.; Siedlecki, J.A.; Sarnowski, T.J.; Sarnowska, E. Various forms of HIF -1α protein characterize the clear cell renal cell carcinoma cell lines. *IUBMB Life* **2020**, *72*, 1220–1232. [CrossRef]
44. Wu, Y.; Ding, J.; Sun, Q.; Zhou, K.; Zhang, W.; Du, Q.; Xu, T.; Xu, W. Long noncoding RNA hypoxia-inducible factor 1 alpha-antisense RNA 1 promotes tumor necrosis factor-α-induced apoptosis through caspase 3 in Kupffer cells. *Medicine* **2018**, *97*, e9483. [CrossRef]
45. Zheng, F.; Chen, J.; Zhang, X.; Wang, Z.; Chen, J.; Lin, X.; Huang, H.; Fu, W.; Liang, J.; Wu, W.; et al. The HIF-1α antisense long non-coding RNA drives a positive feedback loop of HIF-1α mediated transactivation and glycolysis. *Nat. Commun.* **2021**, *12*, 1341. [CrossRef] [PubMed]
46. Kim, J.K.; Diehl, J.A. Nuclear cyclin D1: An oncogenic driver in human cancer. *J. Cell. Physiol.* **2009**, *220*, 292–296. [CrossRef]
47. Fusté, N.P.; Fernández-Hernández, R.; Cemeli, T.; Mirantes, C.; Pedraza, N.; Rafel, M.; Torres-Rosell, J.; Colomina, N.; Ferrezuelo, F.; Dolcet, X.; et al. Cytoplasmic cyclin D1 regulates cell invasion and metastasis through the phosphorylation of paxillin. *Nat. Commun.* **2016**, *7*, 11581. [CrossRef] [PubMed]
48. Dankert, J.T.; Wiesehöfer, M.; Czyrnik, E.D.; Singer, B.B.; Von Ostau, N.; Wennemuth, G. The deregulation of miR-17/CCND1 axis during neuroendocrine transdifferentiation of LNCaP prostate cancer cells. *PLoS ONE* **2018**, *13*, e0200472. [CrossRef]
49. Raval, R.R.; Lau, K.W.; Tran, M.G.B.; Sowter, H.M.; Mandriota, S.J.; Li, J.-L.; Pugh, C.; Maxwell, P.; Harris, A.L.; Ratcliffe, P.J. Contrasting Properties of Hypoxia-Inducible Factor 1 (HIF-1) and HIF-2 in von Hippel-Lindau-Associated Renal Cell Carcinoma. *Mol. Cell. Biol.* **2005**, *25*, 5675–5686. [CrossRef]
50. Lawrie, C.H.; Larrea, E.; Larrinaga, G.; Goicoechea, I.; Arestin, M.; Fernandez-Mercado, M.; Hes, O.; Cáceres, F.; Manterola, L.; Lopez, J.I. Targeted next-generation sequencing and non-coding RNA expression analysis of clear cell papillary renal cell carcinoma suggests distinct pathological mechanisms from other renal tumour subtypes. *J. Pathol.* **2013**, *232*, 32–42. [CrossRef] [PubMed]
51. Chen, L.; Gibbons, D.L.; Goswami, S.; Cortez, M.A.; Ahn, Y.-H.; Byers, L.A.; Zhang, X.; Yi, X.; Dwyer, D.; Lin, W.; et al. Metastasis is regulated via microRNA-200/ZEB1 axis control of tumour cell PD-L1 expression and intratumoral immunosuppression. *Nat. Commun.* **2014**, *5*, 5241. [CrossRef] [PubMed]
52. Wang, X.; Li, J.; Dong, K.; Lin, F.; Long, M.; Ouyang, Y.; Wei, J.; Chen, X.; Weng, Y.; He, T.; et al. Tumor suppressor miR-34a targets PD-L1 and functions as a potential immunotherapeutic target in acute myeloid leukemia. *Cell. Signal.* **2015**, *27*, 443–452. [CrossRef] [PubMed]
53. Hong, D.S.; Kang, Y.-K.; Borad, M.; Sachdev, J.; Ejadi, S.; Lim, H.Y.; Brenner, A.J.; Park, K.; Lee, J.-L.; Kim, T.-Y.; et al. Phase 1 study of MRX34, a liposomal miR-34a mimic, in patients with advanced solid tumours. *Br. J. Cancer* **2020**, *122*, 1630–1637. [CrossRef] [PubMed]
54. Liu, X.; Hoang, A.; Zhou, L.; Kalra, S.; Yetil, A.; Sun, M.; Ding, Z.; Zhang, X.; Bai, S.; German, P.; et al. Resistance to Antiangiogenic Therapy Is Associated with an Immunosuppressive Tumor Microenvironment in Metastatic Renal Cell Carcinoma. *Cancer Immunol. Res.* **2015**, *3*, 1017–1029. [CrossRef]
55. Zhu, Q.; Cai, M.-Y.; Weng, D.-S.; Zhao, J.-J.; Pan, Q.-Z.; Wang, Q.-J.; Tang, Y.; He, J.; Li, M.; Xia, J.-C. PD-L1 expression patterns in tumour cells and their association with CD8+ tumour infiltrating lymphocytes in clear cell renal cell carcinoma. *J. Cancer* **2019**, *10*, 1154–1161. [CrossRef] [PubMed]
56. Ruf, M.; Moch, H.; Schraml, P. PD-L1 expression is regulated by hypoxia inducible factor in clear cell renal cell carcinoma. *Int. J. Cancer* **2016**, *139*, 396–403. [CrossRef]
57. Cowey, C.L.; Rathmell, W.K. VHL gene mutations in renal cell carcinoma: Role as a biomarker of disease outcome and drug efficacy. *Curr. Oncol. Rep.* **2009**, *11*, 94–101. [CrossRef]
58. Klatte, T.; Seligson, D.B.; Riggs, S.B.; Leppert, J.T.; Berkman, M.K.; Kleid, M.D.; Yu, H.; Kabbinavar, F.F.; Pantuck, A.J.; Belldegrun, A.S. Hypoxia-Inducible Factor 1 in Clear Cell Renal Cell Carcinoma. *Clin. Cancer Res.* **2007**, *13*, 7388–7393. [CrossRef]
59. Motzer, R.J.; Penkov, K.; Haanen, J.; Rini, B.; Albiges, L.; Campbell, M.T.; Venugopal, B.; Kollmannsberger, C.; Negrier, S.; Uemura, M.; et al. Avelumab plus Axitinib versus Sunitinib for Advanced Renal-Cell Carcinoma. *N. Engl. J. Med.* **2019**, *380*, 1103–1115. [CrossRef]
60. Weinstock, M.; McDermott, D. Targeting PD-1/PD-L1 in the treatment of metastatic renal cell carcinoma. *Ther. Adv. Urol.* **2015**, *7*, 365–377. [CrossRef]

61. Lee, W.S.; Yang, H.; Chon, H.J.; Kim, C. Combination of anti-angiogenic therapy and immune checkpoint blockade normalizes vascular-immune crosstalk to potentiate cancer immunity. *Exp. Mol. Med.* **2020**, *52*, 1475–1485. [CrossRef] [PubMed]
62. Song, Y.; Fu, Y.; Xie, Q.; Zhu, B.; Wang, J.; Zhang, B. Anti-angiogenic Agents in Combination with Immune Checkpoint Inhibitors: A Promising Strategy for Cancer Treatment. *Front. Immunol.* **2020**, *11*, 1956. [CrossRef] [PubMed]
63. Powles, T.; Plimack, E.R.; Soulières, D.; Waddell, T.; Stus, V.; Gafanov, R.; Nosov, D.; Pouliot, F.; Melichar, B.; Vynnychenko, I.; et al. Pembrolizumab plus axitinib versus sunitinib monotherapy as first-line treatment of advanced renal cell carcinoma (KEYNOTE-426): Extended follow-up from a randomised, open-label, phase 3 trial. *Lancet Oncol.* **2020**, *21*, 1563–1573. [CrossRef]
64. Rini, B.I.; Plimack, E.R.; Stus, V.; Gafanov, R.; Hawkins, R.; Nosov, D.; Pouliot, F.; Alekseev, B.; Soulières, D.; Melichar, B.; et al. Pembrolizumab plus Axitinib versus Sunitinib for Advanced Renal-Cell Carcinoma. *N. Engl. J. Med.* **2019**, *380*, 1116–1127. [CrossRef] [PubMed]
65. Smoot, M.E.; Ono, K.; Ruscheinski, J.; Wang, P.-L.; Ideker, T. Cytoscape 2.8: New features for data integration and network visualization. *Bioinformatics* **2010**, *27*, 431–432. [CrossRef]
66. Lawrie, C.H.; Saunders, N.; Soneji, S.; Palazzo, S.; Dunlop, H.M.; Cooper, C.; Brown, P.J.; Troussard, X.; Mossafa, H.; Enver, T.; et al. MicroRNA expression in lymphocyte development and malignancy. *Leukemia* **2008**, *22*, 1440–1446. [CrossRef]

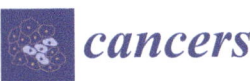

Article

Association between Immune Related Adverse Events and Outcome in Patients with Metastatic Renal Cell Carcinoma Treated with Immune Checkpoint Inhibitors

Agnese Paderi [1], Roberta Giorgione [1], Elisa Giommoni [1], Marinella Micol Mela [1], Virginia Rossi [1], Laura Doni [1], Andrea Minervini [2,3], Marco Carini [2,3], Serena Pillozzi [1] and Lorenzo Antonuzzo [1,3,*]

[1] Clinical Oncology Unit, Careggi University Hospital, Largo Brambilla 3, 50134 Florence, Italy; paderi.agnese@gmail.com (A.P.); roberta.giorgione@unifi.it (R.G.); elisa.giommoni@unifi.it (E.G.); melam@aou-careggi.toscana.it (M.M.M.); virginiarossi89@gmail.com (V.R.); donila@aou-careggi.toscana.it (L.D.); serena.pillozzi@unifi.it (S.P.)
[2] Urology Unit, Careggi University Hospital, Largo Brambilla 3, 50134 Florence, Italy; andrea.minervini@unifi.it (A.M.); marco.carini@unifi.it (M.C.)
[3] Department of Experimental and Clinical Medicine, University of Florence, Largo Brambilla 3, 50134 Florence, Italy
* Correspondence: lorenzo.antonuzzo@unifi.it

Simple Summary: Patients treated with immune-checkpoint inhibitors often experience a wide range of peculiar adverse events, called immune-related adverse events (irAEs). Lately, it has been described that the presence of irAEs may be associated with better clinical response to immunotherapy. The aim of our retrospective study was to observe the onset of the most common side effects and to evaluate their potential prognostic impact in a cohort of metastatic renal cell cancer patients treated with immunotherapy. We confirmed a correlation between irAEs and progression free survival in patients with cutaneous and thyroid adverse reactions as well as in patients that experienced two or more irAEs. Thus, the development of irAEs could act as a clinical marker of efficacy in metastatic renal cell patients treated with immunotherapy.

Abstract: Background: It has been reported that the occurrence of immune-related adverse events (irAEs) in oncological patients treated with immune-checkpoint inhibitors (ICIs) may be associated with favorable clinical outcome. We reported the clinical correlation between irAEs and the efficacy of ICIs in a real-world cohort of metastatic renal cell cancer (mRCC) patients. Methods: We retrospectively evaluated 43 patients with mRCC who were treated with nivolumab or with nivolumab plus ipilimumab. We considered seven specific classes of irAEs including pulmonary, hepatic, gastrointestinal, cutaneous, endocrine, rheumatological, and renal manifestations. We assessed progression-free survival (PFS) of specific irAEs classes compared to the no-irAEs group. Results: Twenty-nine out of 43 patients (67.4%) experienced a total of 49 irAEs registered. The most frequent irAE was thyroid dysfunction ($n = 14$). The median PFS after the beginning of therapy was significantly longer in patients with thyroid dysfunction and cutaneous reactions. In multivariate analysis, thyroid dysfunction was an independent factor for favorable outcome [HR: 0.29 (95% CI 0.11–0.77) $p = 0.013$]. Moreover, experiencing ≥2 irAEs in the same patient correlated in multivariate analysis with better outcome compared with none/one irAE [HR: 0.33 (95% CI 0.13–0.84) $p = 0.020$]. Conclusions: This retrospective study suggests an association between specific irAES (thyroid dysfunction and skin reaction) and efficacy of ICIs in metastatic RCC. Notably, multiple irAEs in a single patient were associated with better tumor response.

Keywords: renal cell carcinoma; immune checkpoint inhibitors; immune related adverse events (irAEs); thyroid; cutaneous; biomarker

Citation: Paderi, A.; Giorgione, R.; Giommoni, E.; Mela, M.M.; Rossi, V.; Doni, L.; Minervini, A.; Carini, M.; Pillozzi, S.; Antonuzzo, L. Association between Immune Related Adverse Events and Outcome in Patients with Metastatic Renal Cell Carcinoma Treated with Immune Checkpoint Inhibitors. *Cancers* **2021**, *13*, 860. https://doi.org/10.3390/cancers13040860

Academic Editors: Claudia Manini and José I. López

Received: 29 December 2020
Accepted: 11 February 2021
Published: 18 February 2021

Publisher's Note: MDPI stays neutral with regard to jurisdictional claims in published maps and institutional affiliations.

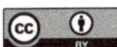

Copyright: © 2021 by the authors. Licensee MDPI, Basel, Switzerland. This article is an open access article distributed under the terms and conditions of the Creative Commons Attribution (CC BY) license (https://creativecommons.org/licenses/by/4.0/).

1. Introduction

The treatment scenario of metastatic renal cell cancer (mRCC) has undergone a complete change in the last few years. Therapeutic options have progressed from non-specific immunotherapy with cytokines to targeted therapy with the development of tyrosine kinase inhibitors (TKI), and more recently to the novel immune checkpoint inhibitors (ICIs) such as anti-programmed death receptor 1 (PD-1), anti-programmed death receptor ligand 1 (PD-L1), and anti-cytotoxic T lymphocytes antigen 4 (CTLA-4) [1]. The CheckMate 025 was the first trial showing the efficacy of nivolumab, a human IgG4 anti-PD-1 antibody, in mRCC patients [2]. Later, the CheckMate 214 trial investigated the combination of nivolumab with another ICI, ipilimumab (anti-CTLA-4), and confirmed the benefit of the association, especially in patients with intermediate and poor-risk disease according to the IMDC (International Metastatic RCC Database Consortium) risk score [3]. More recently, the combined use of an ICI on top of a multitargeted receptor TKI evidenced a survival benefit and is therefore now another therapeutic option for patients with mRCC [4–6]. The opportunities to use ICIs in the future will, most likely, tremendously increase.

With the number of mRCC patients treated with immunotherapy rising year by year, clinicians have found themselves managing a new spectrum of adverse events (AEs) that are specific to this new class of therapeutic agents [7]. As expected, by stimulating the immune system to target malignancies, ICIs have also induced a wide range of immunologic AE (irAEs). The most common reported irAEs involve skin, gastrointestinal tract, endocrine glands, lung, and liver [8]. Little is known about the cellular and molecular mechanisms underlying most irAEs. However, emerging evidence from clinical trials and real-world studies indicate that irAE type and severity depend on the therapeutic target (i.e., CTLA-4 vs. PD-1/PD-L1), tumor type, and patient-intrinsic factors [9,10]. Most irAEs are mild and reversible if detected early and properly managed, but there is a noticeable proportion of patients who have experienced (grade $\geq$ 3) irAEs (31% of patients treated with CTLA-4 vs. 10% treated with PD-1) [11]. It has been reported that the incidence of irAEs is higher in ICI combination therapy than in monotherapy [12]. It must be noted that most clinical trials excluded cancer patients with underlying autoimmune disease or chronic infection. Therefore, irAEs in real-world clinical practice are expected to increase further.

However, despite the improved outcome of cancer treatment by ICIs, efficacy still remains limited. Many studies have searched for biomarkers predictive of response to immunotherapy. Some of these are already used in clinical practice including the PD-L1 tumor prediction score (TPS) and clinical prediction score (CPS) [13,14]. Other markers currently under evaluation include tumor mutational burden (TMB) [15], gene expression scores (GEP) [16], and tumor infiltrating lymphocytes (TILs) [17]. Other studies have suggested that peripheral blood markers could help predict the treatment response, but evidence is still scant [18–20]. In the context of this research irAEs have been proposed as potential clinical markers to predict response to ICI. This relationship, although documented in studies regarding non-small cell lung cancer (NSCLC) and melanoma [21–26] has been less studied in RCC [27–29]. Moreover, current data on the impact of specific types of irAEs on outcomes are not entirely consistent.

Our study represents a real-life observation concerning the onset and management of the most common side effects and the prognostic impact of irAEs in a cohort of mRCC real-world patients treated with nivolumab or nivolumab combined with ipilimumab at our Medical Oncology Unit, AOU Careggi (Firenze, Italy).

2. Materials and Methods

We retrospectively reviewed data from 43 patients treated at the Medical Oncology Unit, Careggi Hospital (Firenze, Italy) from March 2016 to March 2020.

Patient eligibility included age >18, histologically confirmed RCC with metastatic disease, and treatment with an immunotherapy agent. Patients were treated with nivolumab in monotherapy (3 mg/kg every two weeks or flat dose of 240 mg/every two weeks or 480 mg/every four weeks) or with the association of nivolumab 3 mg/kg and ipilimumab

1 mg/kg every three weeks for four cycles, then in monotherapy with nivolumab. PD-L1 status was not requested. Patients received therapy until either disease progression or unacceptable toxicity presented. All patients had measurable disease and the disease progression was evaluated according to the Response Evaluation Criteria in Solid Tumors (RECIST v 1.1).

All patients evaluated had accurate clinical records of the irAEs with a description of their severity and their treatment. Toxicity was assessed according to Common Terminology Criteria for Adverse Events (CTCAE) version 4.0. IrAEs were defined as an adverse event with an immunological basis that required intensive monitoring or treatment with immunosuppressive agents or endocrine therapy. We divided irAEs into seven categories: pulmonary, hepatic, gastrointestinal, cutaneous, endocrine, rheumatological, and renal.

All data were analyzed anonymously; all patients signed an informed consent form for immunotherapy with particular specifications about the occurrence of possible adverse events. This study was conducted in accordance with the World Medical Association Declaration of Helsinki and independently reviewed and approved by the Regional Ethics Committee for Clinical Trials of the Tuscany Region (approval no.: 17332_oss). All patient data were processed anonymously and de-identified prior to analysis.

Statistical analyses. Estimates of PFS in the irAE and non-irAE groups or different irAEs subgroups were calculated using the Kaplan–Meier method, and statistical significance was analyzed using the log-rank test. A significance level of $p < 0.05$ was employed for statistical analyses. First, at the univariate analysis, and then the Cox proportional hazard model was used to calculate the hazard ratios (HRs) and appropriate 95% CIs. Subsequently, the independent effect of each parameter on PFS was investigated by a multivariate Cox regression model. Data were analyzed using the statistical software Jamovi.

3. Results

3.1. Patient Characteristics

Between March 2016 and March 2020, 43 patients with mRCC were treated with ICIs (either nivolumab or nivolumab combined with ipilimumab) at our Medical Oncology Unit, AOU-Careggi (Florence). Table 1 summarizes the patients' clinical features.

Average age of enrolled patients at time of diagnosis was 64 years, ranging from 45 to 79 years; 81.4% ($n = 35$) male, and 18.6% ($n = 8$) female. A total of 53.4% of the patients were current or former smokers. The most frequent histology diagnosis was clear cell (83.7%), followed by papillary and chromophobe renal cancer. Most patients ($n = 39/43$, 91%) had a resected primary tumor. The most frequent site of metastases was lung (65% of patients), followed by lymph nodes (44%), bone (35%), liver (21%), and brain (7%).

Overall, 33 patients (76.7%) received nivolumab in monotherapy while 10 received (23.7%) nivolumab plus ipilimumab. Ten patients (23.2%) received ICI as the first line of therapy and 25 patients (58.1%) as second line. Overall, one patient achieved complete response (2.3%), six partial response (PR) (13.9%), 11 stable disease (SD) (25.6%), and the remaining 25 patients experienced progressive disease (PD) (58.1%).

Among patients treated with nivolumab ($n = 33$), 18 (54.5%) were non responders (defined as patients who experienced a progressive disease as best response), while among patients treated with nivolumab plus ipilimumab ($n = 10$), seven (70%) were non responders.

3.2. Profile of Immune-Related Adverse Event (irAEs)

Twenty-nine out of 43 patients (67.4%) experienced a total of seven different irAE categories (data are reported in Table 2). Baseline clinical features between patients with or without irAEs were not significantly different. In patients who developed irAEs, the median number of days before the onset was 59 days; 14 patients never developed irAEs until the end of the observation phase.

In total, we registered 49 irAEs: 20 (46.5%) developed endocrine-related events, nine (20.9%) developed skin reactions, seven (16.3%) developed hepatitis, five (11.6%)

developed colitis (as diarrhea), four (9.3%) developed arthralgias/myalgias, three patients (9%) developed pneumonia, and one patient (2.3%) developed nephritis.

Table 1. Clinical features of the study population.

Characteristics	No. of Patients (N = 43)	
	Sex	%
Male	35	81.4%
Female	8	18.6%
	Age (years)	
Average	64	
Median	65	
Min–Max	45–79	
	Smoker	
Yes	23	53.5%
No	20	46.5%
	Performance Status at the time of diagnosis	
2	2	4.6%
1	2	4.6%
0	39	90.7%
	Histology	
Clear cells	36	83.7%
Chromophobic cells	2	4.6%
Papillary	5	11.6%
	Therapy line	
1	10	23.3%
2	25	58.1%
3	7	16.3%
4	1	2.3%
	Outcome	
RC	1	2.3%
PR	6	13.9%
SD	11	25.6%
PD	25	58.1%

Table 2. Comparison between irAEs in mRCC patients treated with nivolumab or with nivolumab and ipilimumab.

irAEs	Nivolumab		Nivolumab + Ipilimumab		Total	
	n	%	n	%	n	%
Pneumonitis	3	9.1%	0	0.0%	5	6.9%
Colitis (diarrhea)	5	15.1%	0	0.0%	5	11.6%
Hepatitis	4	12.1%	3	30,0%	7	16.3%
Skin reactions	8	24.2%	1	10.0%	9	20.9%
Nephritis	0	0.0%	1	10.0%	1	2.3%
Arthralgia/myalgia	4	12.1%	0	0,0%	4	9.3%
Endocrine-related events	14	42.4%	6	60.0%	20	46.5%

According to the CTCAE grades, irAEs registered were mainly grades 1 and 2, and were included in a subgroup defined "non-serious AE". Within patients who developed any irAE, 19 experienced a non-serious irAE (65.5%), while 10 patients (34.5%) developed a serious irAE (grade 3 or grade 4). If we consider the total number of irAEs observed ($n = 49$), 12 irAEs were serious (24.5%), while 37 were classified as non-serious (75.5%).

Among the patients only treated in monotherapy with nivolumab ($n = 33$), three (9%) developed pneumonitis, five (15.1%) developed diarrhea, four (12.1%) developed hepatitis, eight (24.4%) developed skin reactions, four (12.1%) developed arthralgia/myalgia, and 14 (42.4%) developed endocrine-related events.

Regarding the cohort of patients treated with nivolumab in combination with ipilimumab ($n = 10$), three (30%) patients developed hepatitis, only one (10%) patient developed a skin reaction, six (60%) patients developed endocrine-related events, and one (10%) patient developed nephritis. No difference in the occurrence of AEs between mono and combination therapy could be found ($p = 0.84$).

Overall, the most frequent AEs were related to endocrine issues (46% of the patients with 19 events), with a percentage up to 40% of the total number of adverse events. The median time to first development of endocrine dysfunction was 80 days. Thyroid dysfunction was by far the most frequently encountered endocrine toxicity ($n = 15/19$), followed by hypophysitis and hyperglycemia. Some patients ($n = 8$) experienced early-stage thyrotoxicosis followed by a permanent stage of hypothyroidism.

3.3. Relationship between irAEs and Patient Outcome

PFS was significantly longer in the group of patients that developed a thyroid dysfunction ($p = 0.028$); the median PFS of the euthyroid group was 121 days (IQR 92–305.) while the median PFS of the thyroid dysfunction group was not reached (Figure 1).

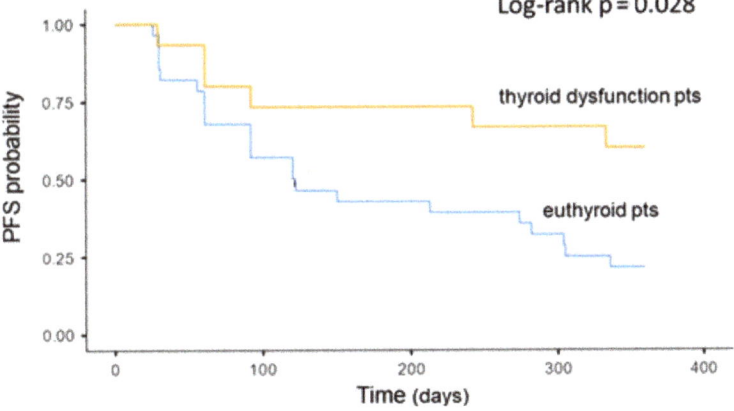

Figure 1. Association between thyroid dysfunction during treatment and oncologic outcomes. Kaplan–Meier plots of progression-free survival. IrAEs = immune-related adverse events; PFS = progression-free survival; pts = patients.

In multivariate analysis, the development of thyroid toxicity was an independent prognostic factor for PFS (HR: 0.34 [95% CI 0.13–0.87] $p = 0.025$) (Table 3). On the other hand, although very rare, hypophysitis was related to significant shorter PFS ($p = 0.048$). Interestingly, endocrine toxicities were significantly higher in patients who had already performed two lines of therapy before immunotherapy ($p = 0.022$).

A significantly longer PFS was also found in patients who experienced skin irAEs ($p = 0.41$). The median PFS of the patients who did not experience skin toxicities was 120 days (IQR 61–336), while the median PFS of the skin irAE group was not reached (Figure 2).

Moreover, in the irAEs group, the PFS was significantly longer in patients who experienced two or more irAEs compared to only one or no irAEs ($p = 0.016$) (Figure 3). In multivariate analysis, the development of two or more irAEs was an independent prognostic factor for PFS (HR: 0.32 [95% CI 0.13–0.79] $p = 0.014$) (Table 3). Age, sex, current or former smoking status, and pathological subtypes were not associated with PFS.

Table 3. Univariate and multivariate analysis of progression-free survival.

Characteristics	Univariate Analysis		Multivariate Analysis	
	HR (95%CI)	p-Value	HR (95%CI)	p-Value
Age, years (≥65)	1.41 (0.66–2.99)	0.373	-	
Gender (female)	0.91 (0.34–2.39)	0.842	-	
Smoking history (current or former)	1.20 (0.57–2.54)	0.625	-	
Histopathology (clear cells)	2.22 (0.88–5.58)	0.089	2.09 (0.72–6.02)	0.173
Skin toxicity (present)	0.33 (0.11–0.95)	0.041	0.36 (0.12–1.06)	0.065
Thyroid disfunction (present)	0.36 (0.15–0.89)	0.028	0.34 (0.13–0.87)	0.025
Number of irAEs (≥2)	0.33 (0.13–0.81)	0.016	0.32 (0.13–0.79)	0.014

HR = hazard ratio; CI = confidence interval; irAEs = immune-related adverse events.

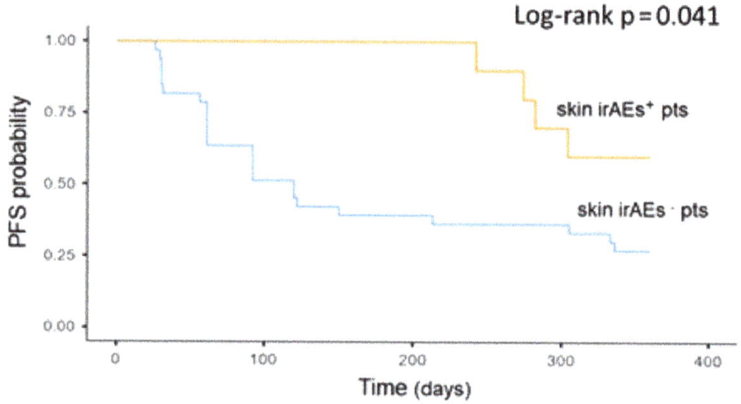

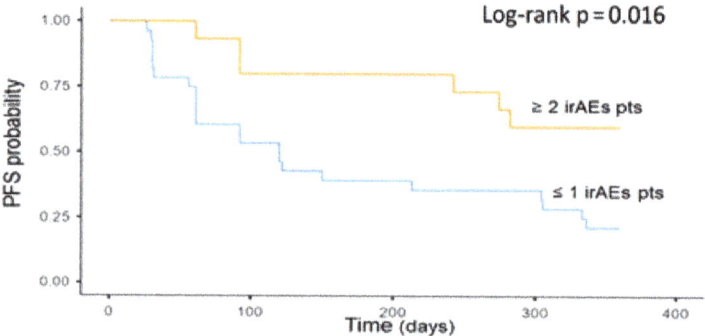

Figure 2. Association between skin toxicity during treatment and oncologic outcomes. Kaplan–Meier plots of progression-free survival. irAEs = immune-related adverse events; PFS = progression-free survival; pts = patients.

Figure 3. Association between multiple irAEs during treatment and oncologic outcomes. Kaplan–Meier plot of progression-free survival. irAEs = immune-related adverse events; PFS = progression-free survival; Pts = patients.

Additionally, we performed a complementary 16-week landmark analysis since patients with longer PFS could have a higher probability of developing AEs, which could lead to analysis bias. The 16-week analysis confirmed that the occurrence of irAEs was significantly associated with prolonged median PFS for patients with skin toxicity and with two or more adverse events (PFS: NR vs. 120 days, $p = 0.005$ and PFS: NR vs. 120 days, $p = 0.029$, respectively) The same analysis for patients with thyroid dysfunction demonstrated similar tendencies, but was not statistically significant ($p = 0.160$).

4. Discussion

Immunotherapy potentiates a patient's immune system to fight cancer, and has become one of the standard treatments for RCC. Immune checkpoint blockade increases antitumor immunity by blocking intrinsic downregulators of immunity such as cytotoxic T-lymphocyte antigen 4 (CTLA-4) and programmed cell death 1 (PD-1) or its ligand, programmed cell death ligand 1 (PD-L1). By enhancing the activity of the immune system, immune checkpoint blockade can induce inflammatory side effects.

Within this study, we aimed to describe toxicities in a real-world cohort of mRCC patients and their potential association with treatment response.

The precise pathophysiology underlying irAEs is yet unknown, but various hypotheses have been made. Some potential mechanisms include increasing T cell activity against antigens that are present both in tumors and healthy tissue and increasing levels of preexisting autoantibodies [30]. Among other theories, the observation that gut microbiota is involved in the functions of intestinal CD4+ and CD8+ T, with anti-tumor immunological activity, is gaining strength and this could impact the efficacy of ICIs [31].

It must be noted that CTLA-4 and PD-1 inhibit the immune response in distinct ways, the first attenuating T-cell activation at a proximal step in the immune response [32] and the latter blocking T cells at later stages of the immune cascade in peripheral tissues [33]. These different functions are reflected in different toxicities. For instance, pneumonitis and thyroiditis appear to be more common with anti-PD-1 therapy, while colitis and hypophysitis seem to be more common with anti-CTLA-4 therapy [11].

Overall, our results confirmed a favorable toxicity profile in patients with mRCC as described in other real-life studies [28,34]. However, colitis was unexpectedly higher in the nivolumab group, however, the total number of cases was very low. We also found a higher frequency of AEs on the endocrine profile compared to previous studies, reaching 46% in our patients compared to 4% as reported by Verzoni [28] or 17.9% reported by Ishihara [29]. The spectrum of endocrinopathies reported in the literature in patients receiving ICIs is quite broad including hypophysitis, thyroiditis, and less frequently, primary adrenal insufficiency, hypogonadism, pancreatitis, hypercalcemia, and diabetes [35,36].The most frequent endocrine toxicities registered in our center in mRCC patients were thyroiditis (either as hypothyroidism or as thyrotoxicosis or both in the same patient), followed by hypophysitis and hyperglycemia. The reasons for such a high rate of endocrine toxicity are unclear. A potential explanation may be a specific search in our practice for signs and symptoms of endocrinopathies that often subtly present themselves with generic symptoms such as fatigue, nausea, and weight changes. Additionally, our patients have often undergone immunotherapy after having already experienced one or more lines of therapy with TKI, drugs that are known to often interfere with the endocrine system, especially the thyroid axis. In fact, endocrine toxicities were significantly higher in patients who had undergone multiple rounds of molecular-targeted therapies before developing endocrine toxicities while on immunotherapy. However, there are currently no studies on this topic. Further explanation could be a longer follow up period, which led to the discovery of a higher number of toxicities.

The correlation between irAEs and patient outcome has been recently described for different cancers [10,37,38]. The occurrence of irAEs has been found to be associated with favorable outcomes in melanoma [21–23], NSCLC [24–26] and, with only a few studies available, also in mRCC [27–29]. These studies corroborate the hypothesis of a direct link between antitumor response and auto-immune reactivity. There are two different hypothesized mechanisms that could lead to irAEs. The first one concerns preexisting self-reactive T-cells being deregulated while the second speculates a cross-reactivity between normal tissues and tumor associated antigens, which share similar targets [39,40].

However, to identify a relationship between AE and treatment response, it is important to consider AE classes individually. Although all patients experiencing irAEs of any class exhibited more favorable outcomes, only patients with thyroid dysfunction and cutaneous toxicity demonstrated significantly higher PFS.

The positive relationship between AEs of the endocrine spectrum and treatment response has been described in a few studies, both analyzed all together or individually as thyroid dysfunction. As above-mentioned, most studies have described a cohort of patients with melanoma [41] or NSCLC [42]. Less is known about endocrine irAEs as a prognostic factor in RCC [28]. Our study confirms this positive relationship with a percentage of responder patients who experienced an endocrine irAE of 64.7%. Interestingly, we noted a specific distribution of the subclasses of endocrine toxicity with respect to the response to treatment: thyroid dysfunction was confirmed to be a positive prognostic indicator while hypopituitarism, although rare, was a negative prognostic factor. However, this result should be carefully interpreted also by taking into account that endocrine toxicities showed two very different profiles between patients treated with combination therapy and monotherapy with nivolumab: thyroiditis were more represented in the group that performed only nivolumab, while all cases of hypophysitis were found in the combination therapy group. The connection that binds endocrine irAEs and efficacy is yet unknown. There are various possible hypotheses described in the literature. One of these assumes that the activation of pre-existing low-grade autoimmunity to thyroid glands could lead to thyroid irAEs and thus select patients with strong baseline immunity [43]. Another hypothesis suggests that thyroid antigens may have a common amino acid sequence with tumor epitopes. Thereby, the cross presentation of those epitopes could be associated with thyroid irAEs and this could facilitate the selection of patients who could benefit from immunotherapy [44].

The relationship between skin irAEs and treatment efficacy has also been previously described, mostly in melanoma and NSCLC [41,45]. A meta-analysis of ICI therapy in melanoma found that vitiligo was significantly associated with both longer PFS and OS [46]. In RCC, the only study that described the relation between skin irAEs and treatment response is the one by Verzoni [28]. Our data confirmed the positive association between skin irAEs and PFS with a significantly longer PFS in patients who experienced skin toxicity. Importantly, this association was confirmed in multivariable analysis, and to our knowledge, this is the first study indicating that this specific irAE represents an independent predictor of ICI efficacy in mRCC patients.

As an additional result, we described a positive correlation between the number of irAEs and patient outcome. Having ≥2 irAEs was associated with longer PFS compared with one or no irAE. This result has already been described in other retrospective real-world studies by Bouhlel [47] and Ricciuti [24], both in NSCLC. To the best of our knowledge, this study is the first to reveal this association in a mRCC cohort of patients. This finding further suggests a mechanistic association between irAEs and immunotherapy efficacy and indicates that the development of multiple immune-mediated toxicities might reflect sustained anti-tumor responses.

It could be argued that patients with longer response to treatment could develop a higher number of irAEs. In an attempt to address this potential confounding factor, we conducted a 16-week landmark analysis. The results confirmed (although the thyroid dysfunction did not reach statistical significance) that the occurrence of irAEs was significantly associated with prolonged median PFS. These findings further underline the association of early onset of irAEs and a durable clinical benefit in mRCC patients treated with immunotherapy.

The limitations in the interpretation of the study results are mainly impacted by the retrospective nature and the small sample size. Further limitations are the selection of patients, which is stricter in clinical trials than in real-life clinical practice. In addition, regarding the determination of outcome and follow up, patients enrolled in clinical trials followed regular and more frequent clinic visits as per pre-determined strict criteria, which are sometimes difficult to follow in a real-life scenario. Moreover, a precise definition and categorization of irAEs is still lacking, and the classification that we performed has not been validated or standardized.

However, despite these limitations, we were able to observe significant results that require further confirmation in prospective studies with larger cohorts.

5. Conclusions

Despite the small sample size, we observed that specific irAEs such as thyroid dysfunction and cutaneous reactions were associated with longer PFS and that patients that experienced more than one AE presented a better response to treatment. These results suggest that irAEs can be a surrogate marker of clinical benefit. Not every toxicity class was significantly associated with better clinical response. However, the two that showed a positive relationship (skin and thyroid), which were also the most frequent, could be very useful in a clinical context. Nevertheless, no definitive conclusions could be derived from these data considering the limited number of patients experiencing any specific class of irAEs.

Given the high percentage of endocrine, and in particular, thyroid AEs, it is essential to implement research and treatment of these particular toxicities during treatment. Since endocrine toxicities often present themselves with vague and unclear clinical pictures, close monitoring by an endocrinologist should be warranted, also given the positive correlation with the patient's outcome and therefore the importance of continuing immunotherapy for these patients. Further prospective studies are necessary to confirm our findings and to investigate the mechanistic association between AEs and clinical response in order to improve therapy with ICIs and the management of their toxicities.

Author Contributions: Conceptualization, S.P. and L.A.; Methodology, V.R. and L.D.; Interpretation of data: E.G., R.G., A.P., and A.M.; Data curation, A.P. and R.G.; Writing—original draft preparation, A.P. and S.P.; Writing—review & editing, L.A. and M.C.; Supervision, M.M.M. and L.A. All authors have read and agreed to the published version of the manuscript.

Funding: This research received no external funding.

Institutional Review Board Statement: This study was conducted in accordance with the World Medical Association Declaration of Helsinki and independently reviewed and approved by the Regional Ethics Committee for Clinical Trials of the Tuscany Region (approval no.: 17332_oss).

Informed Consent Statement: Informed consent was obtained from all subjects involved in the study.

Data Availability Statement: Data available on request to the corresponding author.

Acknowledgments: We thank Susanna Bormioli Weber for the English language editing.

Conflicts of Interest: The authors declare no conflict of interest.

References

1. Longo, D.L.; Choueiri, T.K.; Motzer, R.J. Systemic Therapy for Metastatic Renal-Cell Carcinoma. *N. Engl. J. Med.* **2017**, *376*, 354–366. [CrossRef]
2. Motzer, R.J.; Escudier, B.; McDermott, D.F.; George, S.; Hammers, H.J.; Srinivas, S.; Tykodi, S.S.; Sosman, J.A.; Procopio, G.; Plimack, E.R.; et al. Nivolumab versus Everolimus in Advanced Renal-Cell Carcinoma. *N. Engl. J. Med.* **2015**, *373*, 1803–1813. [CrossRef]
3. Motzer, R.J.; Tannir, N.M.; McDermott, D.F.; Arén Frontera, O.; Melichar, B.; Choueiri, T.K.; Plimack, E.R.; Barthélémy, P.; Porta, C.; George, S.; et al. Nivolumab plus Ipilimumab versus Sunitinib in Advanced Renal-Cell Carcinoma. *N. Engl. J. Med.* **2018**, *378*, 1277–1290. [CrossRef]
4. Motzer, R.J.; Penkov, K.; Haanen, J.; Rini, B.; Albiges, L.; Campbell, M.T.; Venugopal, B.; Kollmannsberger, C.; Negrier, S.; Uemura, M.; et al. Avelumab plus Axitinib versus Sunitinib for Advanced Renal-Cell Carcinoma. *N. Engl. J. Med.* **2019**, *380*, 1103–1115. [CrossRef]

5. Rini, B.I.; Plimack, E.R.; Stus, V.; Gafanov, R.; Hawkins, R.; Nosov, D.; Pouliot, F.; Alekseev, B.; Soulières, D.; Melichar, B.; et al. Pembrolizumab plus Axitinib versus Sunitinib for Advanced Renal-Cell Carcinoma. *N. Engl. J. Med.* **2019**, *380*, 1116–1127. [CrossRef]
6. Choueiri, T.K.; Powles, T.; Burotto, M.; Bourlon, M.T.; Zurawski, B.; Juárez, V.O.; Hsieh, J.J.; Basso, U.; Shah, A.Y.; Suarez, C.; et al. 696O_PR Nivolumab + cabozantinib vs sunitinib in first-line treatment for advanced renal cell carcinoma: First results from the randomized phase 3 CheckMate 9ER trial. *Ann. Oncol.* **2020**, *31* (Suppl. 4), S1159. [CrossRef]
7. De Giorgi, U.; Cartenì, G.; Giannarelli, D.; Basso, U.; Galli, L.; Cortesi, E.; Caserta, C.; Pignata, S.; Sabbatini, R.; Bearz, A.; et al. Safety and efficacy of nivolumab for metastatic renal cell carcinoma: Real-world results from an expanded access programme. *BJU Int.* **2019**, *123*, 98–105. [CrossRef] [PubMed]
8. Ornstein, M.C.; Garcia, J.A. Toxicity of Checkpoint Inhibition in Advanced RCC: A Systematic Review. *Kidney Cancer* **2017**, *1*, 133–141. [CrossRef] [PubMed]
9. Khan, S.; Gerber, D.E. Autoimmunity, checkpoint inhibitor therapy and immune-related adverse events: A review. *Semin. Cancer Biol.* **2020**, *64*, 93–101. [CrossRef] [PubMed]
10. Zhou, X.; Yao, Z.; Yang, H.; Liang, N.; Zhang, X.; Zhang, F. Are immune-related adverse events associated with the efficacy of immune checkpoint inhibitors in patients with cancer? A systematic review and meta-analysis. *BMC Med.* **2020**, *18*, 87. [CrossRef]
11. Khoja, L.; Day, D.; Chen, T.W.W.; Siu, L.L.; Hansen, A.R. Tumour- and class-specific patterns of immune-related adverse events of immune checkpoint inhibitors: A systematic review. *Ann. Oncol.* **2017**, *28*, 2377–2385. [CrossRef] [PubMed]
12. Wolchok, J.D.; Chiarion-Sileni, V.; Gonzalez, R.; Rutkowski, P.; Grob, J.J.; Cowey, C.L.; Lao, C.D.; Wagstaff, J.; Schadendorf, D.; Ferrucci, P.F.; et al. Overall Survival with Combined Nivolumab and Ipilimumab in Advanced Melanoma. *N. Engl. J. Med.* **2017**, *377*, 1345–1356, Erratum in *N. Engl. J. Med.* **2018**, *379*, 2185. [CrossRef] [PubMed]
13. Gong, J.; Chehrazi-Raffle, A.; Reddi, S.; Salgia, R. Development of PD-1 and PD-L1 inhibitors as a form of cancer immunotherapy: A comprehensive review of registration trials and future considerations. *J. Immunother. Cancer* **2018**, *6*, 8. [CrossRef]
14. Lu, S.; Stein, J.E.; Rimm, D.L.; Wang, D.W.; Bell, J.M.; Johnson, D.B.; Sosman, J.A.; Schalper, K.A.; Anders, R.A.; Wang, H.; et al. Comparison of Biomarker Modalities for Predicting Response to PD-1/PD-L1 Checkpoint Blockade: A Systematic Review and Meta-analysis. *JAMA Oncol.* **2019**, *5*, 1195–1204. [CrossRef]
15. Liu, L.; Bai, X.; Wang, J.; Tang, X.R.; Wu, D.H.; Du, S.S.; Du, X.J.; Zhang, Y.W.; Zhu, H.B.; Fang, Y.; et al. Combination of TMB and CNA Stratifies Prognostic and Predictive Responses to Immunotherapy Across Metastatic Cancer. *Clin. Cancer Res.* **2019**, *25*, 7413–7423. [CrossRef]
16. Cristescu, R.; Mogg, R.; Ayers, M.; Albright, A.; Murphy, E.; Yearley, J.; Sher, X.; Liu, X.Q.; Lu, H.; Nebozhyn, M.; et al. Pan-tumor genomic biomarkers for PD-1 checkpoint blockade-based immunotherapy. *Science* **2018**, *362*, eaar3593, Erratum in *Science* **2019**, *363*, eaax1384. [CrossRef]
17. Gettinger, S.N.; Choi, J.; Mani, N.; Sanmamed, M.F.; Datar, I.; Sowell, R.; Du, V.Y.; Kaftan, E.; Goldberg, S.; Dong, W.; et al. A dormant TIL phenotype defines non-small cell lung carcinomas sensitive to immune checkpoint blockers. *Nat. Commun.* **2018**, *9*, 3196. [CrossRef] [PubMed]
18. Tray, N.; Weber, J.S.; Adams, S. Predictive Biomarkers for Checkpoint Immunotherapy: Current Status and Challenges for Clinical Application. *Cancer Immunol. Res.* **2018**, *6*, 1122–1128. [CrossRef]
19. Hopkins, A.M.; Rowland, A.; Kichenadasse, G.; Wiese, M.D.; Gurney, H.; McKinnon, R.A.; Karapetis, C.S.; Sorich, M.J. Predicting response and toxicity to immune checkpoint inhibitors using routinely available blood and clinical markers. *Br. J. Cancer* **2017**, *117*, 913–920. [CrossRef]
20. Darvin, P.; Toor, S.M.; Sasidharan Nair, V.; Elkord, E. Immune checkpoint inhibitors: Recent progress and potential biomarkers. *Exp. Mol. Med.* **2018**, *50*, 1–11. [CrossRef]
21. Freeman-Keller, M.; Kim, Y.; Cronin, H.; Richards, A.; Gibney, G.; Weber, J.S. Nivolumab in Resected and Unresectable Metastatic Melanoma: Characteristics of Immune-Related Adverse Events and Association with Outcomes. *Clin. Cancer Res.* **2016**, *22*, 886–894. [CrossRef] [PubMed]
22. Dupont, R.; Bérard, E.; Puisset, F.; Comont, T.; Delord, J.P.; Guimbaud, R.; Meyer, N.; Mazieres, J.; Alric, L. The prognostic impact of immune-related adverse events during anti-PD1 treatment in melanoma and non-small-cell lung cancer: A real-life retrospective study. *Oncoimmunology* **2019**, *9*, 1682383. [CrossRef] [PubMed]
23. Suo, A.; Chan, Y.; Beaulieu, C.; Kong, S.; Cheung, W.Y.; Monzon, J.G.; Smylie, M.; Walker, J.; Morris, D.; Cheng, T. Anti-PD1-Induced Immune-Related Adverse Events and Survival Outcomes in Advanced Melanoma. *Oncologist* **2020**, *25*, 438–446. [CrossRef] [PubMed]
24. Ricciuti, B.; Genova, C.; De Giglio, A.; Bassanelli, M.; Dal Bello, M.G.; Metro, G.; Brambilla, M.; Baglivo, S.; Grossi, F.; Chiari, R. Impact of immune-related adverse events on survival in patients with advanced non-small cell lung cancer treated with nivolumab: Long-term outcomes from a multi-institutional analysis. *J. Cancer Res. Clin. Oncol.* **2019**, *145*, 479–485. [CrossRef]
25. Sato, Y.; Akamatsu, H.; Murakami, E.; Sasaki, S.; Kanai, K.; Hayata, A.; Tokudome, N.; Akamatsu, K.; Koh, Y.; Ueda, H.; et al. Correlation between immune-related adverse events and efficacy in non-small cell lung cancer treated with nivolumab. *Lung Cancer* **2018**, *115*, 71–74, Erratum in *Lung Cancer* **2018**, *126*, 230–231. [CrossRef] [PubMed]
26. Haratani, K.; Hayashi, H.; Chiba, Y.; Kudo, K.; Yonesaka, K.; Kato, R.; Kaneda, H.; Hasegawa, Y.; Tanaka, K.; Takeda, M.; et al. Association of Immune-Related Adverse Events With Nivolumab Efficacy in Non-Small-Cell Lung Cancer. *JAMA Oncol.* **2018**, *4*, 374–378. [CrossRef]

27. Kobayashi, K.; Iikura, Y.; Hiraide, M.; Yokokawa, T.; Aoyama, T.; Shikibu, S.; Hashimoto, K.; Suzuki, K.; Sato, H.; Sugiyama, E.; et al. Association between Immune-related Adverse Events and Clinical Outcome Following Nivolumab Treatment in Patients With Metastatic Renal Cell Carcinoma. *In Vivo* **2020**, *34*, 2647–2652. [CrossRef] [PubMed]
28. Verzoni, E.; Cartenì, G.; Cortesi, E.; Giannarelli, D.; De Giglio, A.; Sabbatini, R.; Buti, S.; Rossetti, S.; Cognetti, F.; Rastelli, F.; et al. Real-world efficacy and safety of nivolumab in previously-treated metastatic renal cell carcinoma, and association between immune-related adverse events and survival: The Italian expanded access program. *J. Immunother. Cancer* **2019**, *7*, 99. [CrossRef] [PubMed]
29. Ishihara, H.; Takagi, T.; Kondo, T.; Homma, C.; Tachibana, H.; Fukuda, H.; Yoshida, K.; Iizuka, J.; Kobayashi, H.; Okumi, M.; et al. Association between immune-related adverse events and prognosis in patients with metastatic renal cell carcinoma treated with nivolumab. *Urol. Oncol.* **2019**, *37*, 355.e21–355.e29. [CrossRef]
30. Postow, M.A.; Sidlow, R.; Hellmann, M.D. Immune-related adverse events associated with immune checkpoint blockade. *N. Engl. J. Med.* **2018**, *378*, 158–168. [CrossRef]
31. Elkrief, A.; Derosa, L.; Zitvogel, L.; Kroemer, G.; Routy, B. The intimate relationship between gut microbiota and cancer immunotherapy. *Gut Microbes* **2019**, *10*, 424–428. [CrossRef]
32. Krummel, M.F.; Allison, J.P. CTLA-4 engagement inhibits IL-2 accumulation and cell cycle progression upon activation of resting T cells. *J. Exp. Med.* **1996**, *183*, 2533–2540. [CrossRef] [PubMed]
33. Dong, H.; Strome, S.E.; Salomao, D.R.; Tamura, H.; Hirano, F.; Flies, D.B.; Roche, P.C.; Lu, J.; Zhu, G.; Tamada, K.; et al. Tumor-associated B7-H1 promotes T-cell apoptosis: A potential mechanism of immune evasion. *Nat. Med.* **2002**, *8*, 793–800. [CrossRef]
34. Vitale, M.G.; Scagliarini, S.; Galli, L.; Pignata, S.; Lo Re, G.; Berruti, A.; Defferrari, C.; Spada, M.; Masini, C.; Santini, D.; et al. Efficacy and safety data in elderly patients with metastatic renal cell carcinoma included in the nivolumab Expanded Access Program (EAP) in Italy. *PLoS ONE* **2018**, *13*, e0199642. [CrossRef]
35. Scott, E.S.; Long, G.V.; Guminski, A.; Clifton-Bligh, R.J.; Menzies, A.M.; Tsang, V.H. The spectrum, incidence, kinetics and management of endocrinopathies with immune checkpoint inhibitors for metastatic melanoma. *Eur. J. Endocrinol.* **2018**, *178*, 173–180. [CrossRef] [PubMed]
36. Chang, L.S.; Barroso-Sousa, R.; Tolaney, S.M.; Hodi, F.S.; Kaiser, U.B.; Min, L. Endocrine Toxicity of Cancer Immunotherapy Targeting Immune Checkpoints. *Endocr. Rev.* **2019**, *40*, 17–65. [CrossRef]
37. Das, S.; Johnson, D.B. Immune-related adverse events and anti-tumor efficacy of immune checkpoint inhibitors. *J. Immunother. Cancer* **2019**, *7*, 306. [CrossRef] [PubMed]
38. Hussaini, S.; Chehade, R.; Boldt, R.G.; Raphael, J.; Blanchette, P.; Maleki Vareki, S.; Fernandes, R. Association between immune-related side effects and efficacy and benefit of immune checkpoint inhibitors—A systematic review and meta-analysis. *Cancer Treat. Rev.* **2020**, *92*, 102134. [CrossRef]
39. Yoest, J.M. Clinical features, predictive correlates, and pathophysiology of immune-related adverse events in immune checkpoint inhibitor treatments in cancer: A short review. *ImmunoTargets Ther.* **2017**, *6*, 73–82. [CrossRef] [PubMed]
40. Weinmann, S.C.; Pisetsky, D.S. Mechanisms of immune-related adverse events during the treatment of cancer with immune checkpoint inhibitors. *Rheumatology* **2019**, *58* (Suppl. 7), vii59–vii67. [CrossRef]
41. Wu, C.E.; Yang, C.K.; Peng, M.T.; Huang, P.W.; Chang, C.F.; Yeh, K.Y.; Chen, C.B.; Wang, C.L.; Hsu, C.W.; Chen, I.W.; et al. The association between immune-related adverse events and survival outcomes in Asian patients with advanced melanoma receiving anti-PD-1 antibodies. *BMC Cancer* **2020**, *20*, 1018. [CrossRef] [PubMed]
42. Kim, H.I.; Kim, M.; Lee, S.H.; Park, S.Y.; Kim, Y.N.; Kim, H.; Jeon, M.J.; Kim, T.Y.; Kim, S.W.; Kim, W.B.; et al. Development of thyroid dysfunction is associated with clinical response to PD-1 blockade treatment in patients with advanced non-small cell lung cancer. *Oncoimmunology* **2017**, *7*, e1375642. [CrossRef] [PubMed]
43. Ahn, S.; Kim, T.H.; Kim, S.W.; Ki, C.S.; Jang, H.W.; Kim, J.S.; Kim, J.H.; Choe, J.H.; Shin, J.H.; Hahn, S.Y.; et al. Comprehensive screening for PD-L1 expression in thyroid cancer. *Endocr. Relat. Cancer* **2017**, *24*, 97–106. [CrossRef] [PubMed]
44. Vita, R.; Guarneri, F.; Agah, R.; Benvenga, S. Autoimmune thyroid disease elicited by NY-ESO-1 vaccination. *Thyroid* **2014**, *24*, 390–394. [CrossRef]
45. Grangeon, M.; Tomasini, P.; Chaleat, S.; Jeanson, A.; Souquet-Bressand, M.; Khobta, N.; Bermudez, J.; Trigui, Y.; Greillier, L.; Blanchon, M.; et al. Association between Immune-related Adverse Events and Efficacy of Immune Checkpoint Inhibitors in Non-small-cell Lung Cancer. *Clin. Lung Cancer* **2019**, *20*, 201–207. [CrossRef] [PubMed]
46. Teulings, H.E.; Limpens, J.; Jansen, S.N.; Zwinderman, A.H.; Reitsma, J.B.; Spuls, P.I.; Luiten, R.M. Vitiligo-like depigmentation in patients with stage III-IV melanoma receiving immunotherapy and its association with survival: A systematic review and meta-analysis. *J. Clin. Oncol.* **2015**, *33*, 773–781. [CrossRef]
47. Bouhlel, L.; Doyen, J.; Chamorey, E.; Poudenx, M.; Ilie, M.; Gal, J.; Guigay, J.; Benzaquen, J.; Marquette, C.H.; Berthet, J.P.; et al. Occurrence and number of immune-related adverse events are independently associated with survival in advanced non-small-cell lung cancer treated by nivolumab. *Bull. Cancer* **2020**, *107*, 946–958. [CrossRef]

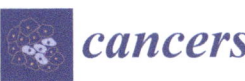

Article

Nivolumab Reduces PD1 Expression and Alters Density and Proliferation of Tumor Infiltrating Immune Cells in a Tissue Slice Culture Model of Renal Cell Carcinoma

Philipp J. Stenzel [1,*], Nina Hörner [1], Sebastian Foersch [1], Daniel-Christoph Wagner [1], Igor Tsaur [2], Anita Thomas [2], Axel Haferkamp [2], Stephan Macher-Goeppinger [1], Wilfried Roth [1], Stefan Porubsky [1,†] and Katrin E. Tagscherer [1,†]

[1] Institute of Pathology, University Medical Center Mainz, 55131 Mainz, Germany; nina.hoerner@unimedizin-mainz.de (N.H.); sebastian.foersch@unimedizin-mainz.de (S.F.); Daniel-Christoph.Wagner@unimedizin-mainz.de (D.-C.W.); sgoeppinger@gmail.com (S.M.-G.); Wilfried.Roth@unimedizin-mainz.de (W.R.); stefan.porubsky@unimedizin-mainz.de (S.P.); katrin.tagscherer@unimedizin-mainz.de (K.E.T.)

[2] Department of Urology, University Medical Center Mainz, 55131 Mainz, Germany; igor.tsaur@unimedizin-mainz.de (I.T.); anita.thomas@unimedizin-mainz.de (A.T.); axel.haferkamp@unimedizin-mainz.de (A.H.)

* Correspondence: philipp.stenzel@unimedizin-mainz.de; Tel.: +49-6131-17-2813; Fax: +49-6131-17-6604

† These authors contributed equally to this project.

Simple Summary: Immune checkpoint inhibitors (ICIs) have become a first-choice therapy option in the treatment of clear cell renal cell carcinoma (ccRCC). A predictive biomarker is urgently needed since not all patients respond and adverse events occur. Therefore, an ex vivo tissue slice culture (TSC) model was tested to investigate the effects of nivolumab on tumor infiltrating immune cells (TIIC). A decrease in programmed death receptor 1 expression, as well as effects on density and proliferation of TIIC, were observed. Thus, the TSC model could serve as a test platform for response prediction to ICIs.

Abstract: Background: In the treatment of clear cell renal cell carcinoma (ccRCC), nivolumab is an established component of the first-line therapy with a favorable impact on progression free survival and overall survival. However, treatment-related adverse effects occur and, to date, there is no approved predictive biomarker for patient stratification. Thus, the aim of this study was to establish an ex vivo tissue slice culture model of ccRCC and to elucidate the impact of nivolumab on tumor infiltrating immune cells. Methods: Fresh tumor tissue of ccRCC was treated with the immune checkpoint inhibitor nivolumab using ex vivo tissue slice culture (TSC). After cultivation, tissue slices were formalin-fixed, immunohistochemically stained and analyzed via digital image analysis. Results: The TSC model was shown to be suitable for ex vivo pharmacological experiments on intratumoral immune cells in ccRCC. PD1 expression on tumor infiltrating immune cells was dose-dependently reduced after nivolumab treatment ($p < 0.01$), whereas density and proliferation of tumor infiltrating T-cells and cytotoxic T-cells were inter-individually altered with a remarkable variability. Tumor cell proliferation was not affected by nivolumab. Conclusions: This study could demonstrate nivolumab-dependent effects on PD1 expression and tumor infiltrating T-cells in TSC of ccRCC. This is in line with results from other scientific studies about changes in immune cell proliferation in peripheral blood in response to nivolumab. Thus, TSC of ccRCC could be a further step to personalized medicine in terms of testing the response of individual patients to nivolumab.

Keywords: nivolumab; clear cell renal cell carcinoma; tissue slice culture; PD1; T-cells

1. Introduction

Renal cell carcinoma (RCC) is among the ten most frequent malignancies worldwide with increasing incidence and decreasing mortality [1]. The decrease in mortality is the consequence of early diagnosis and a broad range of therapy options in advanced and metastasized stages, which applies to 20% of patients at the time of diagnosis and another 20% of patients during the clinical course after initial surgery [2]. For clear cell renal cell carcinoma (ccRCC), the most common histologic subtype of RCC, the combination of either tyrosine kinase inhibitor (TKI) and immune checkpoint inhibitor (ICI) or two ICIs are guideline-recommended first-line treatment options. Four comprehensive clinical trials (Checkmate 214 (ClinicalTrials.gov Identifier: NCT02231749), Keynote 426 (ClinicalTrials.gov Identifier: NCT02853331), Javelin 101 (ClinicalTrials.gov Identifier: NCT02684006), Checkmate9ER (ClinicalTrials.gov Identifier: NCT03141177)) have shown the superiority of either combined ICI therapy (nivolumab + ipilimumab) or combined TKI and ICI therapy (axitinib + pembrolizumab, axitinib + avelumab, cabozantinib + nivolumab) regarding overall survival (OS) or progression free survival (PFS) compared to standard-of-care sunitinib in patients with previously untreated advanced RCC [3–6]. The objective response rate (ORR) for the combination therapies including ICIs ranged from 42% [3] to 59.3% [4] compared to 25.7% to 35.7% for sunitinib alone [3–6]. Complete responses were rare in all studies. Treatment-related adverse events of grade 3 or higher occurred either in the sunitinib group [3] or in the combination therapy group [4,6] or showed no significant difference [5]. With the exception of the Javelin 101 trial, treatment was discontinued due to treatment-related adverse effects, more often in the group with combination therapy. In the Checkmate 214 trial, there were even eight treatment-related deaths in the group treated with the combination of ipilimumab and nivolumab compared to four treatment-related deaths in the sunitinib group [3].

Hence, stratifying patients eligible for therapy including ICIs remains a difficult task and predictive biomarkers are urgently needed. Programmed death receptor ligand 1 (PD-L1) expression of RCC has been examined in the above mentioned clinical trials, but has not been established as a reliable predictive biomarker for ICI [7]. A more dynamic approach is to measure blood parameters before or during ICI treatment. Serum levels of soluble programmed death receptor 1 (sPD1) and sPD-L1 correlated with OS and PFS of patients with RCC [8,9]. In patients with non-small cell lung cancer (NSCLC) an increased proliferation of CD8+ cytotoxic T-cells (CTL) in peripheral blood correlated with response to nivolumab therapy, whereas patients with progressive disease had no change in CTL proliferation or even a decrease [10,11]. In metastasized RCC, a high density of tumor infiltrating PD1+ CTLs correlated with higher ORR and prolonged PFS in a patient cohort treated with nivolumab and is, therefore, a promising candidate predictive biomarker for response to nivolumab [12,13].

In this study, we report our results regarding an ex vivo tissue slice culture (TSC) model with incubation of fresh vital ccRCC tumor tissue with nivolumab for 24 h or 72 h and consecutive quantification of immune cell density, proliferation, and distribution.

2. Materials and Methods

2.1. Patients and Tissue Collection

Twelve patients with ccRCC, surgically treated at the Department of Urology and Pediatric Urology of the University Medical Center Mainz from 2017 to 2020, were included in the study. Tissue collection was approved by ethics approval for the Tissue Biobank, University Medical Center Mainz (ethics approval: 837.031.15 (9799); date of approval: 2 October 2015). After arrival of the surgical specimen in the Institute of Pathology, tumors were macroscopically examined to confirm subtype (golden to yellow cut surface with hemorrhage) and tissue vitality. In cases of doubt, additional microscopic examination by frozen section of the intended area of sampling was performed. Exclusion criteria for tissue collection included a tumor size <1.0 cm to ensure reliable pathologic routine diagnostics, poor tissue quality with a high portion of necrotic tumor tissue, and non-clear cell morphology. Fresh vital tumor tissue (length: 10 mm; diameter: 6 mm) was collected from the tumor periphery by using a defined punching tool (KAI Medical Biopsy Punch, Solingen, Germany), stored in a 4 °C chilled Krebs-Henseleit-Buffer (Sigma-Aldrich/Merck,

Darmstadt, Germany) and referred to the lab for TSC. To match tumor heterogeneity, at least two different tumor localizations were sampled.

2.2. Ex Vivo Tissue Slice Culture

The tissue culture protocol has been described in detail previously [14,15]. Briefly, tumor tissue was cut into slices of 300 µm thickness using a Vibratome VT1200 (Leica Microsystems, Mannheim, Germany). The first and the last slice of each tumor sample was immediately fixated in buffered 4% formalin. The other tissue slices were randomly assigned to control and intervention groups. Tissue slices were incubated at the air-medium-interface in a 12-well plate with appropriate inserts. The used tissue culture medium was DMEM cell culture medium (ATCC, Manassas, CO, USA) with supplements (1% Penicillin/Streptomycin, 10% fetal calf serum (Sigma-Aldrich/Merck, Darmstadt, Germany)) and with or without nivolumab (Opdivo, Bristol-Myers Squibb, Munich, Germany). The medium including nivolumab in the therapy group was changed after 1 h and every additional 24 h. For the time of the experiment, tissue slices were kept in an incubator with a humidified atmosphere, a temperature of 37 °C, and 5% CO_2. After 24 h or 72 h, respectively, tissue slices were harvested, fixated in buffered 4% formalin, and paraffin embedded. Figure 1 provides a detailed overview of the experimental setup.

2.3. Treatment Regimen

Tissue slices were incubated with increasing concentrations of nivolumab (0.1 µg/mL, 1 µg/mL, 10 µg/mL, and 100 µg/mL) or without nivolumab as control. Cultivation was usually performed in triplicates and in cases of limited amount of tumor tissue in duplicates.

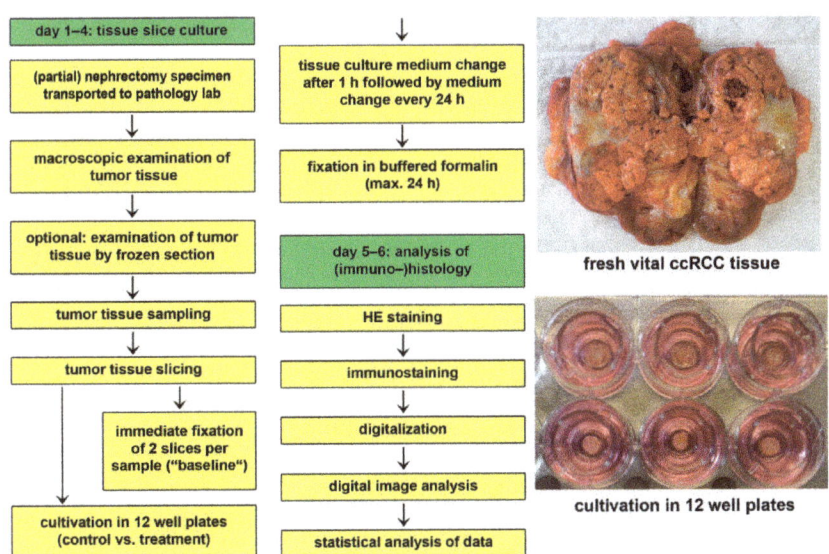

Figure 1. Tissue culture workflow.

2.4. Conventional and Immunohistochemical Staining

Tissue slices were stained with hematoxilyn and eosin (HE) and tumor tissue vitality was confirmed. Slices with necrosis >50% were excluded from further immunohistochemical stainings. Slices were stained with antibodies against Ki67 (MIB-1, Dako, Glostrup, Denmark), PD-L1 (ab213524, Abcam, Cambridge, UK) or double stained using the Envision G/2 Doublestain System or Envision Flex Doublestain System (Dako). The antibody combinations were CD3 (IR503, Dako) + Ki67 (MIB-1, Dako), CD3 (IR503, Dako) + CK AE1/3 (IR053, Dako), CD8 (IR623, Dako) + Ki67 (MIB-1, Dako), PD1 (ab52587, Abcam) + Ki67

(MIB-1, Dako), and PD1 (ab52587, Abcam) + CK AE1/3 (IR053, Dako). All slides were stained with automatized immunostainers (Autostainer Plus, Dako).

2.5. Digital Image Analysis

Digitalization and digital image analysis were performed as previously described using a digital whole slide scanner (Nanozoomer, Hamamatsu Photonics, Hamamatsu, Japan) and the HALO® platform (Indica Labs, Corrales, NM, USA) [16]. Briefly, for the detection and quantification of stain-positive cells, the CytoNuclear module (v1.4–1.6) was used. To differentiate between tumor parenchyma and tumor-associated stroma, a tissue classifier was included. Localization of each detected cell in the tissue and its biomarker profile cells were saved and used for spatial analysis with the proximity tool included in HALO®. Vital and necrotic tumor areas were manually annotated and quantified via digital image analysis. PD-L1 status (tumor proportion score, TPS) was assessed by light microscopy (Olympus BX45, Olympus, Tokio, Japan).

2.6. Spatial Distribution

Tissue slices were immunohistochemically double stained for T-cells (brown) and for tumor cells (red). Digital image analysis was used for detection of T-cells (markup: red), tumor cells (markup: green), and other cells (markup: blue). Tissue was further classified into tumor area (classifier markup: red) and stroma (classifier markup: green) (Figure S1A). T-cells were dichotomized into "T-cells Tumor" and "T-cells Stroma" depending on the T-cells' localization (Figure S1B). The percental distribution of T-cells Tumor and T-cells Stroma within a diameter of 30 µm around tumor cells was quantified using the proximity tool implemented in HALO®.

2.7. Statistical Analysis

Data are given as mean ± standard deviation. In cases of high inter-individual variability of the examined parameters, data were normalized relative to baseline value or to control. For the comparison of two groups, the paired t-test was performed and, for the comparison of three or more groups, the one-way analysis of variance (one-way ANOVA) was performed. The necessary assumptions for the one-way ANOVA were tested with the Shapiro–Wilk test (normal distribution within the individual groups) and the Levene test (homogeneity of variances). In cases, where the assumption of normal distribution within the individual groups was violated, the Kruskal–Wallis test was alternatively performed. Post hoc tests for the one-way ANOVA were the Tukey test and, for the Kruskal–Wallis test, the Dunn test. All calculations were performed using Microsoft Excel (version 2012), R statistical software (version 4.0.3) and Rstudio (version 1.4.1103). Differences with p-values < 0.05 were considered significant.

3. Results

3.1. Characteristics of Patient Collective

Tumor tissues from 12 patients were treated with nivolumab for 24 h (tumors 1–7) or 72 h (tumors 8–12), respectively. Eleven specimens were from primary renal tumors and one from an adrenal gland metastasis. 63.6% ($n = 7$) of primary tumors were organ confined. The median age of patients at the moment of surgery was 65 years (mean 68.3 ± 10.0). Clinical follow-up data was available for nine patients. The median time of follow-up was 10.9 months (min. 1 month, max. 22.9 months, and the mean was 11.4 ± 8.3 months). By the end of follow-up, one patient had died of a disease unrelated to RCC, one was suffering from progressive disease, two showed a stable disease, and five showed no progress. Clinicopathological data including follow up are summarized in Table 1.

Table 1. Clinicopathological information of the patient collective.

Tumor Number	Sex	Age at Surgery	Origin	Tumor Size (cm)	TNM Classification	Grading	Clinical Course after Surgery
1	m	61	Primary tumor	12	pT2b, pNX, cM0, L0, V0, Pn0, R0	G2	Deceased (unrelated to RCC)
2	m	61	Primary tumor	5.5	pT1b, pNX, cM0, L0, V0, Pn0, R0	G1	No information
3	m	82	Primary tumor	3.4	pT3a, pNX, cM0, L0, V0, Pn0, R0	G2	No progress
4	m	64	Primary tumor	3.7	pT1a, pNx, cM0, L0, V0, Pn0, R0	G2	No information
5	m	60	Metastasis	1.2	pT3a, pN0 (0/1), pM1 (ADR), L0, V1, Pn0, R0	G2	Stable disease
6	m	66	Primary tumor	5	pT1b, pNx, cM0, L0, V0, Pn0, R0	G2	No progress
7	m	72	Primary tumor	8	pT3b, pN0(0/1), cM0, L0, V2, Pn0, R1	G2	No progress
8	m	88	Primary tumor	5.8	pT1b, pN0 (0/11), cM0, L0, V0, Pn0, R0	G2	No information
9	m	69	Primary tumor	7.5	pT3a, pN1 (3/11), cM1 (PUL), L0, V0, Pn0, R0	G2	Stable disease
10	m	79	Primary tumor	5.3	pT3a, pNx, cM0, L0, V0, Pn0, R0	G2	No progress
11	w	55	Primary tumor	8	pT2a, pNx, pM1 (OSS), L0, V1, Pn0, R0	G3	Progressive disease
12	m	63	Primary tumor	2.6	pT1a, pNX, cM0, L0, V0, Pn0, R0	G2	No progress

3.2. Tissue Slice Culture Is Possible for up to Three Days but Reduces Tumor Infiltrating Immune Cells

Fresh vital tumor tissue of ccRCC was sampled close to the invasive margin (IM). Post hoc immunostaining of corresponding primary tumors showed that there were tumors with low (Figure S2A) and high (Figure S2B) amounts of tumor infiltrating PD1+ IC which were rather concentrated at the IM. The tumor tissue was cut into 300 µm thick slices and cultivated with increasing concentrations of nivolumab for 24 h or 72 h, respectively. With only one tumor sample which had to be excluded from further analysis due to extensive cultivation related necrosis, the success rate for the establishment of TSC corresponds to 92.3%. All tumors showed clear cell morphology and stayed negative for PD-L1 during TSC (tumor proportion score: 0%). Tumor infiltrating immune cells with PD1 expression (PD1+ IC) could be detected in every tumor (Figure 2). Baseline densities and proliferation rates of tumor infiltrating immune cells showed a high inter-individual variability (Table 2). After 24 h of TSC, the necrotic tumor area was non-significantly compared to baseline, whereas there was a significant increase in necrosis after 72 h (Figure 3A). Overall proliferation, including tumor cells, showed no significant change after 24 h and a non-significant increase after 72 h (Figure 3B). Tumor infiltrating PD1+ IC, proliferating PD1+ IC and proliferating T-cells were not altered significantly after 24 h of cultivation. Tumor infiltrating T-cells, CTL, and proliferating CTL were significantly decreased (Figure 3C). After 72 h of TSC, PD1+ IC, proliferating PD1+ IC, CTL, and proliferating CTL were all significantly decreased compared to baseline. Tumor infiltrating T-cells were not changed after 72 h of TSC and proliferating T-cells non-significantly increased (Figure 3D).

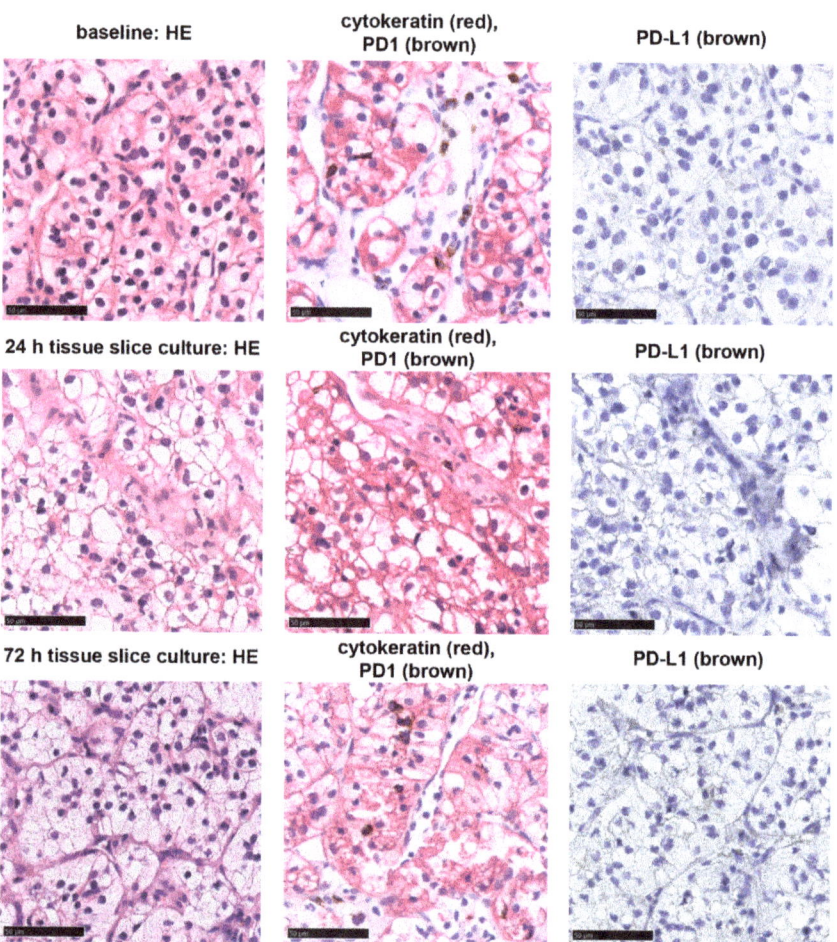

Figure 2. Histological morphology and PD-1/PD-L1 status of tumors. Clear cell morphology of tumors (HE-staining, left), PD1+ immune cells (brown) in the tumor tissue (red) (middle), and PD-L1 expression (brown) at baseline and after tissue slice culture for 24 h or 72 h. Interspersed PD1+ immune cells were present, however the tumor cells showed no PD-L1 expression. Bar indicates 50 µm.

Table 2. PD-L1 status and immune cell densities and proliferation rates at baseline.

Tumor Number	PD-L1 TPS	T-Cells/mm^2	Ki67 + T-Cells/mm^2	CTL/mm^2	Ki67 + CTL/mm^2	PD1+ IC/mm^2	Ki67 + PD1+ IC/mm^2
1	0	1399.0	41.6	187.2	10.3	109.8	2.2
2	0	453.0	22.5	249.4	27.5	252.0	33.1
3	0	741.2	67.8	235.4	59.1	364.2	91.4
4	0	129.8	4.8	96.1	9.7	39.2	2.6
5	0	4696.5	218.3	592.3	122.6	483.0	158.8
6	0	172.9	9.3	113.7	10.3	129.5	10.9
7	0	273.0	9.3	71.5	3.5	85.2	5.2
8	0	66.0	3.4	46.0	1.8	21.3	1.2
9	0	962.1	103.3	472.2	37.5	812.8	64.4
10	0	1994.3	714.1	1785.0	388.9	1580.6	452.6
11	0	543.4	5.7	352.1	20.3	256.4	21.2
12	0	466.7	5.8	300.9	19.4	564.9	65.3
Statistics		T-cells/mm^2	Ki67 + T-cells/mm^2	CTL/mm^2	Ki67 + CTL/mm^2	PD1+ IC/mm^2	Ki67 + PD1+ IC/mm^2
Mean		991.5	100.5	375.2	59.2	391.6	75.7
STD		1297.3	203.2	473.6	109.1	444.3	127.8
Min		66.0	3.4	46.0	1.8	21.3	1.2
Max		4696.5	714.1	1785.0	388.9	1580.6	452.6
Median		505.0	15.9	242.4	19.8	254.2	27.1

Abbreviations: PD-L1: programmed death receptor ligand 1; TPS: tumor proportion score; CTL: CD8+ cytotoxic lymphocytes; PD1+ IC: programmed death receptor 1 expressing immune cells; STD: standard deviation; min: minimum; max: maximum.

3.3. Distinct Reaction Patterns of Tumor Infiltrating Immune Cells in Response to Nivolumab

A decreased density of PD1+ IC after nivolumab treatment was observed across all examined tumors, whereas T-cells and CTL and the corresponding proliferation fractions showed either a nivolumab dependent increase, decrease, or no alteration. Table 3 provides an overview of the reaction patterns of the individual tumors. Tumor 3 showed a significant decrease in PD1+ IC ($p = 0.01$) and a decrease by trend of proliferating PD1+ IC ($p = 0.4$), a consistent non-significant increase in tumor infiltrating T-cells ($p = 0.3$), proliferating T-cells ($p = 0.4$), CTL ($p = 0.5$), and proliferating CTL ($p = 0.6$) after nivolumab treatment (Figure 4A). In contrast, tumor 5 reacted with a significant decrease in PD1+ IC ($p < 0.01$), proliferating PD1+ IC ($p < 0.01$), T-cells ($p = 0.01$) and proliferating T-cells ($p < 0.01$), as well as a non-significant reduction of CTL ($p = 0.4$) and proliferating CTL ($p = 0.3$) (Figure 4B). Tumor 7 showed the third pattern, characterized by minor, non-significant changes in immune cell densities (T-cells: $p = 0.8$; CTL: $p = 0.8$) and proliferation fractions (Ki67+ PD1+ IC: $p = 0.2$; Ki67 + T-cells: $p = 0.5$; Ki67 + CTL: $p = 0.9$); however, the density of PD1+ IC was significantly decreased ($p = 0.001$) (Figure 4C). Overall proliferation (tumor 3: $p = 0.99$; tumor 5: $p = 0.1$; tumor 7: $p = 0.3$) and nivolumab-dependent necrosis (tumor 3: $p = 0.1$; tumor 5: $p = 0.7$; tumor 7: $p = 0.5$) were not significantly changed (Figure 3). The nivolumab-dependent decrease in PD1+ IC was significant after averaging the respective experiments with a duration of 24 h or 72 h (24 h: $p < 0.01$; 72 h: $p < 0.01$); the other parameters showed no significant changes (Figure 4).

Table 3. Nivolumab-dependent reaction patterns of tumor infiltrating immune cell densities and corresponding proliferation rates.

Tumor Number	CD3	CD3-Ki67	CD8	CD8-Ki67	PD1	PD1-Ki67
1	~	~	~	~	-	~
2	-	-	~	~	-	-
3	+	+	+	+	-	-
4	+	+	~	~	-	-
5	-	-	-	-	-	-
6	~	~	~	~	-	-
7	~	~	~	~	-	-
8	~	~	-	+	-	NA
9	~	~	-	-	-	~
10	-	-	~	~	-	~
11	+	-	+	+	-	-
12	-	-	~	-	-	-

Abbreviations: CD3: T-cells; CD3-Ki67: proliferating T-cells; CD8: cytotoxic T-cells; CD8-Ki67: proliferating cytotoxic T-cells; PD1: programmed death receptor expressing immune cells; PD1-Ki67: proliferating programmed death receptor expressing immune cells; + nivolumab-dependent increase; - nivolumab-dependent decrease; ~ no nivolumab-dependent change; NA: data not available.

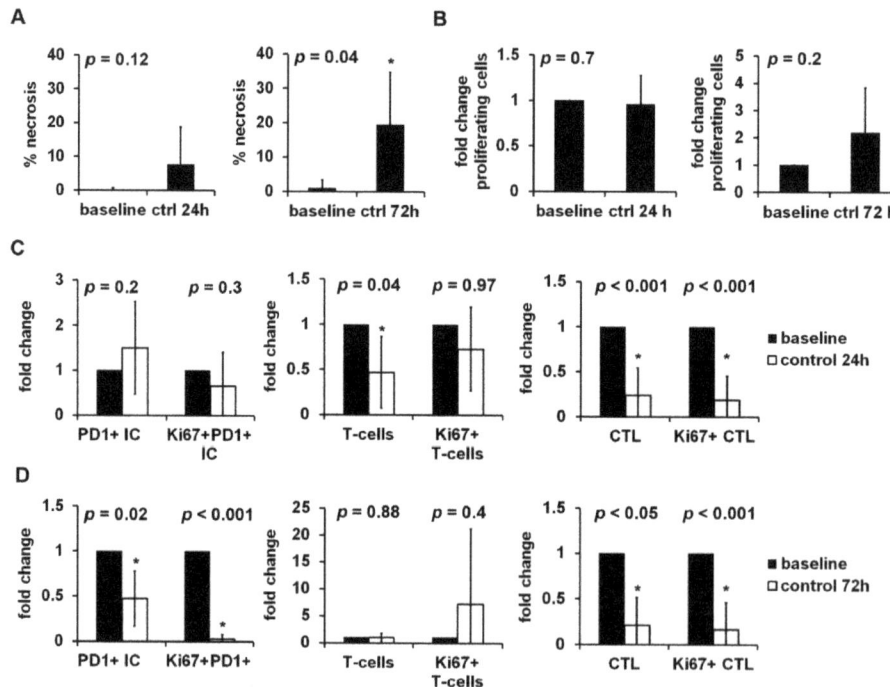

Figure 3. Influence of tissue slice culture (TSC) on tumor vitality, proliferation, and tumor infiltrating immune cells. Tumor tissue of clear cell renal cell carcinoma (ccRCC) was cultivated for 24 h to 72 h. Necrotic tumor area and the immunohistochemical stainings Ki67, Ki67-PD1, Ki67-CD3, and Ki67-CD8 were quantified by digital image analysis. (**A**) The percentage of necrotic tumor after 24 h ($n = 7$) or 72 h ($n = 5$) of TSC compared to baseline. Fold change of (**B**) overall proliferation, (**C**) tumor infiltrating PD1+ immune cells, T-cells, cytotoxic T-cells and their proliferating subsets after 24 h ($n = 7$) or (**D**) 72 h ($n = 5$) of TSC compared to baseline. Data were normalized relative to baseline values, if not stated otherwise, and given as mean ± standard deviation. The paired t-test was used for statistical analysis. *: $p < 0.05$.

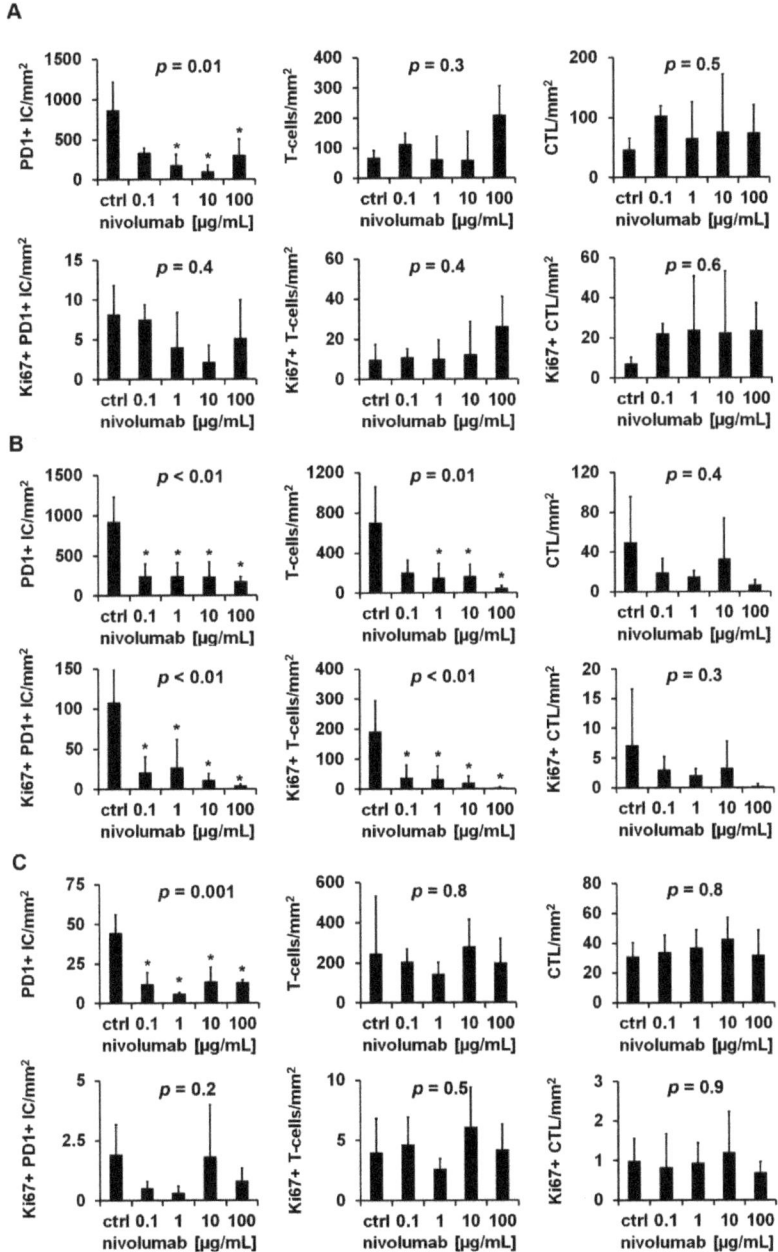

Figure 4. Nivolumab-dependent changes of tumor infiltrating immune cell densities and proliferation rates. Tissue slices of clear cell renal cell carcinoma (ccRCC) were immunohistochemically stained for Ki67-PD1, Ki67-CD3, and Ki67-CD8 after 24 h of cultivation with increasing concentrations of nivolumab. Three representative reaction patterns to nivolumab treatment are shown: (**A**) pattern A (tumor 3) with nivolumab-dependent increased tumor infiltrating T-cells, (**B**) pattern B (tumor 5) with nivolumab-dependent decreased tumor infiltrating T-cells, and (**C**) pattern C (tumor 7) without nivolumab-dependent changes of tumor infiltrating T-cells. Data are given as mean ± standard deviation. For statistical analysis the one-way analysis of variance or the Kruskal–Wallis test with appropriate post hoc tests were used. p-values were corrected with the Bonferroni method. *: $p < 0.05$.

3.4. Spatial Distribution of Tumor Infiltrating Immune Cells under the Influence of Nivolumab

In individual experiments, e.g., tumor 11, a minor shifting of tumor infiltrating T-cells toward tumor cells after treatment with 100 µg/mL nivolumab could be observed (Figure 5A), whereas there was a change in the distribution of stromal T-cells (Figure 5B). After averaging the experiments with a duration of 24 h, the distribution of tumor infiltrating PD1+ IC after nivolumab treatment was unaltered compared to control and the T-cells showed a non-significant shift toward tumor cells (Figure S5A). This effect was even more pronounced, yet still not significant, when looking at the corresponding stromal T-cell fraction (Figure S5A), whereas the stromal PD1+ IC were farther away compared to control. After 72 h, there was no major difference in tumor infiltrating T-cells after nivolumab treatment compared to control (Figure S5B).

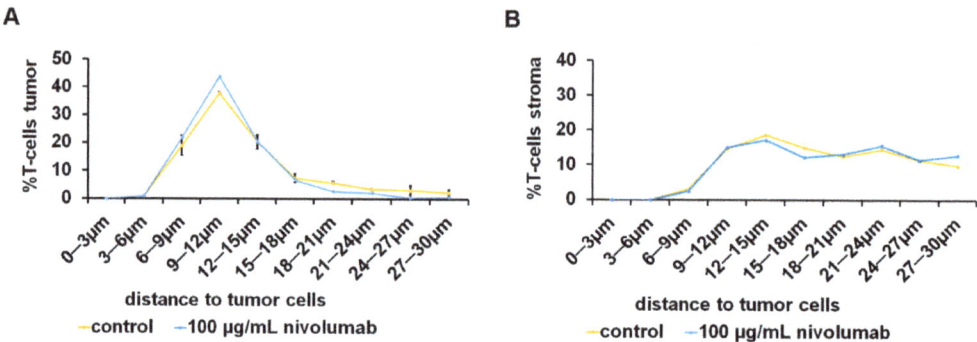

Figure 5. Nivolumab-dependent spatial distribution of tumor infiltrating T-cells. Tumor tissue of clear cell renal cell carcinoma (ccRCC) cultivated 72 h with nivolumab. Tissue slices were immunohistochemically double stained for cytokeratin and CD3. The distance between (**A**) tumor infiltrating T-cells and (**B**) stromal T-cells to tumor cells was calculated by digital image analysis. Data are given as mean ± standard deviation.

4. Discussion

So far, there are no established predictive biomarkers to guide treatment in metastatic RCC. Therefore, a precise test system for response prediction is one option to better stratify patients who will benefit from nivolumab treatment. In this study, an ex vivo TSC model was tested to examine nivolumab-dependent effects on tumor infiltrating immune cells in human ccRCC tumor tissue.

The major finding of this study was the nivolumab-dependent significant reduction of PD1+ IC (Figure 4 and Figure S3). Immunohistochemical PD1 positivity of tumor infiltrating immune cells is widely considered as a biomarker for "exhausted immune cells", but with regard to T-cells and especially CTL, it is rather a biomarker for activated CTL [17,18]. In our previously published study about the prognostic value of tumor infiltrating immune cells in ccRCC, PD1+ IC were associated with a favorable cancer-specific survival [16], indicative that PD1+ CTL comprise tumor-reactive CTL, as was shown in malignant melanoma [19]. Reduced PD1 expression after incubation with PD1-targeting agents, as described in the present study, has been demonstrated before: PD1 expression of peripheral CD8+ T-Cells of patients suffering from PDAC was reduced after incubation with nivolumab and also with pembrolizumab, another therapeutic anti-PD1-antibody [20]. In a xenograft mouse model of colon carcinoma and mammary carcinoma, a reduced frequency of PD1 + CD8+ T-cells and a decrease in PD1 levels below a certain threshold were associated with release from adaptive immune resistance [21]. In principle, this mechanism could also apply to ccRCC TSC. However, methods other than immunohistochemistry (IHC) are required for a more precise PD1 quantification, e.g., flow cytometry. So far, the decreased density in PD1+ IC after nivolumab treatment, assessed by IHC, could serve as a positive control for a successful nivolumab treatment in TSC. For further interpretation of nivolumab-dependent effects, the focus of this study was on the differentially altered densities and proliferation rates of T-Cells and CTL after nivolumab treatment (Figure 4). This is in line with results examining proliferation of peripheral PD1+ CTL in response to nivolumab in NSCLC. Reduced CTL proliferation after nivolumab infusion correlated with progressive disease [10] and an early proliferative response of PD1+ CTL with (partial) response [11,22]. All in all, the number of tumors ($n = 12$) examined in this study was too small for further correlation of the observed reaction patterns and the clinical course of the included patients. Thus, for further validation of the reported results, these experiments need to be conducted in a larger patient cohort.

All of the examined tumors were immunohistochemically negative for PD-L1. However, PD-L1 expression in renal cell carcinoma has been shown to be a strong prognostic factor for poor outcome [23], but it only provides limited value on response prediction to nivolumab. The Checkmate025 [NCT01668784] trial showed the superiority of nivolumab over everolimus as a second-line therapy for patients with advanced RCC independent of PD-L1 expression [24]. Similarly, the consecutive Checkmate214 and Checkmate9ER trials showed the greater benefit of patients with RCC treated with combination therapies including nivolumab compared to the standard of care sunitinib, independent of the PD-L1 status of the primary tumors [3,6]. Thus, a lack of PD-L1 in the tumor tissue seems to have no major impact on response to nivolumab. Therefore, it is reasonable to investigate the effect of nivolumab on tumor infiltrating immune cells in PD-L1 negative ccRCC tumors, too.

The used ex vivo TSC bears several advantages to address this question compared to other established lab-based experimental designs. Firstly, primary and metastatic tumor tissue can be examined with TSC. Cultivation of several samples from different localizations within the tumor tissue allows for modelling tumor heterogeneity, especially with regard to PD-L1 expression [25]. Thus, at least two samples from different tumor localizations were taken. On the other hand, high tumor heterogeneity can result in the high variance of measured data; despite the lack of significant tendencies due to the high variances, these results should also be interpreted as representative for the whole tumor, because they comprise several tumor localizations. Secondly, the tumor microenvironment (TME) which is crucial for interactions between tumor cells and tumor-associated immune cells is transferred into TSC so that associations between therapy effects, e.g., necrosis or proliferation of tumor cells, and the TME can be discovered. One study using the TSC method for pharmacological experiments on RCC highlights the importance of PD-L1 expression and tumor infiltrating CTL [26]. Investigation in the TME can indeed be achieved with air-liquid interface patient-derived organoids or humanized mouse models, too, but establishing these is resource and time intensive [27,28]. Third, differently to common in vitro monolayer cell culture models, the three-dimensional architecture of the tumor is preserved in TSC. This leads to the conception that the tumor tissue reacts similarly in an ex vivo setting compared to the in vivo situation [29–31]. The TSC protocol used in this study has been established for ccRCC tumor tissue and was successfully used in a previous study in our lab (14). Nonetheless, there was increased necrosis of tumor tissue, unrelated to nivolumab treatment (Figure 3A). Tumor necrosis is not uncommon in ccRCC and is a poor prognostic marker for survival [32]. Therefore, a certain amount of tissue necrosis in TSC must be considered inevitable when screened for drug response and can, in principle, be kept low with experiment durations of 24 h (Figure 3A). In terms of the optimization of TSC, protocols studies have so far focused on improving TSC media compositions with regard to tumor cell vitality [33]. Overall proliferation was not significantly changed (Figure 3B) which implies that the used TSC medium composition is suitable to maintain tumor cell proliferation. In contrast, there was a marked drop of immune cell density and proliferation due to TSC alone (Figure 3C,D). CTL were extraordinarily affected which could explain the lack of nivolumab-dependent tumor necrosis in this study (Figure S3). While most TSC studies focus on effects on tumor cells, two have examined tumor infiltrating immune cells in ductal pancreatic adenocarcinoma and gastric carcinoma and found no significant reduction up to day 6 of TSC [34,35]. Thus, in further projects, TSC medium composition should be reevaluated to support both tumor cell and immune cell vitality and proliferation.

In malignant melanoma, responders to ICI had significantly higher CTL densities within 20 μm around tumor cells compared to non-responders [36]. In this study, the spatial distribution of immune cells regarding the distance to tumor cells was investigated, too. The data show only minor nivolumab-dependent effects on the distribution of tumor infiltrating T-cells and PD1+ IC within 30 μm around tumor cells (Figure 5 and Figure S5). This is most likely due to the fact that the ccRCC tumor tissue punches that are used for TSC lack abundant tumor-associated stroma, which means that tumor infiltrating immune cells are close to tumor cells at any time during the experiment. Additionally, intact tissue slices are necessary for the measurement of spatial distribution since tearing of tissue slices is a major confounder. To circumvent these issues, live cell imaging of CTL, as was already established for lung tumor TSC [37], could provide a more detailed insight into the influence of nivolumab on CTL migration through the tumor and number of contacts to tumor cells.

The limitations of the study are: 1. The relatively low number of cases which are sufficient to document the potential and pitfalls of this method but is too low to prove that response to nivolumab can be predicted through TSC and the measurement of tumor infiltrating immune cells; 2. The implementation of clinical studies to correlate the results of this model with clinical therapies and outcomes is needed; 3. The tumor-inherent heterogeneity that—as discussed above—makes sampling at different locations necessary to achieve reliable results. This can turn out to be problematic especially in cases with poor tissue quality or large necrosis.

5. Conclusions

Taken together, the present study provides encouraging data that support the ex vivo TSC approach as a model to predict response to nivolumab in ccRCC. Yet, TSC conditions must be optimized in order to minimize effects on tumor infiltrating immune cells through TSC alone. This together with further research on the correlation of nivolumab-dependent changes in immune cell proliferation as a readout parameter for response of ccRCC patients to nivolumab treatment might be the way to establish TSC as a predictive test system.

Supplementary Materials: The following are available online at https://www.mdpi.com/article/10.3390/cancers13184511/s1. Figure S1: Spatial analysis of tumor infiltrating T-cells; Figure S2: Post hoc immunostaining of clear cell renal cell carcinoma (ccRCC); Figure S3: Nivolumab-dependent changes of overall proliferation and tumor necrosis; Figure S4: Nivolumab-dependent changes of overall proliferation, tumor necrosis and tumor infiltrating immune cell densities and proliferation rates; Figure S5: Nivolumab-dependent spatial distribution of tumor infiltrating PD1+ immune cells and T-cells.

Author Contributions: Conceptualization, P.J.S. and S.M.-G.; Data curation, P.J.S.; Formal analysis, P.J.S.; Investigation, P.J.S.; Methodology, P.J.S. and N.H.; Project administration, P.J.S.; Supervision, W.R., S.P. and K.E.T.; Validation, S.F., D.-C.W., I.T., A.T., A.H., S.M.-G., W.R., S.P. and K.E.T.; Visualization, P.J.S. and K.E.T.; Writing—original draft, P.J.S.; Writing—review & editing, P.J.S., W.R., S.P. and K.E.T. All authors have read and agreed to the published version of the manuscript.

Funding: This research received no external funding.

Institutional Review Board Statement: This study was covered by the ethics approval for the usage of excess tumor tissue within the scope of the terms and regulations of the Tissue Biobank, University Medical Center, Mainz, Germany (837.031.15 (9799); date of approval: 2 October 2015).

Informed Consent Statement: Informed consent was obtained from all subjects involved in the study.

Data Availability Statement: The data presented in this study are available in this article and Supplementary Materials.

Acknowledgments: We thank Ron Unger for the proofreading as well as Silke Mitschke and Bonny Adami for excellent technical assistance. This project was supported by the Tissue Bank of the University Medical Center Mainz.

Conflicts of Interest: The authors declare no conflict of interest.

References

1. Capitanio, U.; Montorsi, F. Renal cancer. *Lancet* **2016**, *387*, 894–906. [CrossRef]
2. Dabestani, S.; Thorstenson, A.; Lindblad, P.; Harmenberg, U.; Ljungberg, B.; Lundstam, S. Renal cell carcinoma recurrences and metastases in primary non-metastatic patients: A population-based study. *World J. Urol.* **2016**, *34*, 1081–1086. [CrossRef]
3. Motzer, R.J.; Tannir, N.M.; McDermott, D.F.; Frontera, O.A.; Melichar, B.; Choueiri, T.K.; Plimack, E.R.; Barthélémy, P.; Porta, C.; George, S.; et al. Nivolumab plus Ipilimumab versus Sunitinib in Advanced Renal-Cell Carcinoma. *N. Engl. J. Med.* **2018**, *378*, 1277–1290. [CrossRef]
4. Rini, B.I.; Plimack, E.R.; Stus, V.; Gafanov, R.; Hawkins, R.; Nosov, D.; Pouliot, F.; Alekseev, B.; Soulières, D.; Melichar, B.; et al. Pembrolizumab plus Axitinib versus Sunitinib for Advanced Renal-Cell Carcinoma. *N. Engl. J. Med.* **2019**, *380*, 1116–1127. [CrossRef]
5. Motzer, R.J.; Penkov, K.; Haanen, J.; Rini, B.; Albiges, L.; Campbell, M.T.; Venugopal, B.; Kollmannsberger, C.; Negrier, S.; Uemura, M.; et al. Avelumab plus Axitinib versus Sunitinib for Advanced Renal-Cell Carcinoma. *N. Engl. J. Med.* **2019**, *380*, 1103–1115. [CrossRef]
6. Choueiri, T.K.; Powles, T.; Burotto, M.; Escudier, B.; Bourlon, M.T.; Zurawski, B.; Juárez, V.M.O.; Hsieh, J.J.; Basso, U.; Shah, A.Y.; et al. Nivolumab plus Cabozantinib versus Sunitinib for Advanced Renal-Cell Carcinoma. *N. Engl. J. Med.* **2021**, *384*, 829–841. [CrossRef]
7. Gibney, G.T.; Weiner, L.M.; Atkins, M.B. Predictive biomarkers for checkpoint inhibitor-based immunotherapy. *Lancet Oncol.* **2016**, *17*, e542–e551. [CrossRef]
8. Incorvaia, L.; Fanale, D.; Badalamenti, G.; Porta, C.; Olive, D.; De Luca, I.; Brando, C.; Rizzo, M.; Messina, C.; Rediti, M.; et al. Baseline plasma levels of soluble PD-1, PD-L1, and BTN3A1 predict response to nivolumab treatment in patients with metastatic renal cell carcinoma: A step toward a biomarker for therapeutic decisions. *Oncoimmunology* **2020**, *9*, 1832348. [CrossRef]
9. Larrinaga, G.; Solano-Iturri, J.D.; Errarte, P.; Unda, M.; Loizaga-Iriarte, A.; Pérez-Fernández, A.; Echevarría, E.; Asumendi, A.; Manini, C.; Angulo, J.C.; et al. Soluble PD-L1 Is an Independent Prognostic Factor in Clear Cell Renal Cell Carcinoma. *Cancers* **2021**, *13*, 667. [CrossRef]
10. Osa, A.; Uenami, T.; Koyama, S.; Fujimoto, K.; Okuzaki, D.; Takimoto, T.; Hirata, H.; Yano, Y.; Yokota, S.; Kinehara, Y.; et al. Clinical implications of monitoring nivolumab immunokinetics in non-small cell lung cancer patients. *JCI Insight* **2018**, *3*, e59125. [CrossRef]
11. Kamphorst, A.O.; Pillai, R.N.; Yang, S.; Nasti, T.H.; Akondy, R.S.; Wieland, A.; Sica, G.L.; Yu, K.; Koenig, L.; Patel, N.T.; et al. Proliferation of PD-1+ CD8 T cells in peripheral blood after PD-1-targeted therapy in lung cancer patients. *Proc. Natl. Acad. Sci. USA* **2017**, *114*, 4993–4998. [CrossRef]
12. Ficial, M.; Jegede, O.A.; Sant'Angelo, M.; Hou, Y.; Flaifel, A.; Pignon, J.-C.; Braun, D.A.; Wind-Rotolo, M.; Sticco-Ivins, M.A.; Catalano, P.J.; et al. Expression of T-Cell Exhaustion Molecules and Human Endogenous Retroviruses as Predictive Biomarkers for Response to Nivolumab in Metastatic Clear Cell Renal Cell Carcinoma. *Clin. Cancer Res.* **2020**, *27*, 1371–1380. [CrossRef]
13. Pignon, J.-C.; Jegede, O.; Shukla, S.A.; Braun, D.A.; Horak, C.E.; Wind-Rotolo, M.; Ishii, Y.; Catalano, P.J.; Grosha, J.; Flaifel, A.; et al. irRECIST for the Evaluation of Candidate Biomarkers of Response to Nivolumab in Metastatic Clear Cell Renal Cell Carcinoma: Analysis of a Phase II Prospective Clinical Trial. *Clin. Cancer Res.* **2019**, *25*, 2174–2184. [CrossRef]
14. Weissinger, D.; Tagscherer, K.E.; Macher-Göppinger, S.; Haferkamp, A.; Wagener, N.; Roth, W. The soluble Decoy Receptor 3 is regulated by a PI3K-dependent mechanism and promotes migration and invasion in renal cell carcinoma. *Mol. Cancer* **2013**, *12*, 120. [CrossRef]
15. Martin, S.Z.; Wagner, D.C.; Hörner, N.; Horst, D.; Lang, H.; Tagscherer, K.E.; Roth, W. Ex vivo tissue slice culture system to measure drug-response rates of hepatic metastatic colorectal cancer. *BMC Cancer* **2019**, *19*, 1030. [CrossRef]
16. Stenzel, P.J.; Schindeldecker, M.; Tagscherer, K.E.; Foersch, S.; Herpel, E.; Hohenfellner, M.; Hatiboglu, G.; Alt, J.; Thomas, C.; Haferkamp, A.; et al. Prognostic and Predictive Value of Tumor-infiltrating Leukocytes and of Immune Checkpoint Molecules PD1 and PDL1 in Clear Cell Renal Cell Carcinoma. *Transl. Oncol.* **2020**, *13*, 336–345. [CrossRef]
17. Simon, S.; Labarriere, N. PD-1 expression on tumor-specific T cells: Friend or foe for immunotherapy? *Oncoimmunology* **2018**, *7*, e1364828. [CrossRef]
18. Okazaki, T.; Honjo, T. The PD-1-PD-L pathway in immunological tolerance. *Trends Immunol.* **2006**, *27*, 195–201. [CrossRef]
19. Gros, A.; Robbins, P.F.; Yao, X.; Li, Y.F.; Turcotte, S.; Tran, E.; Wunderlich, J.R.; Mixon, A.; Farid, S.; Dudley, M.E.; et al. PD-1 identifies the patient-specific CD8$^+$ tumor-reactive repertoire infiltrating human tumors. *J. Clin. Invest.* **2014**, *124*, 2246–2259. [CrossRef]
20. Ding, G.; Shen, T.; Yan, C.; Zhang, M.; Wu, Z.; Cao, L. IFN-γ down-regulates the PD-1 expression and assist nivolumab in PD-1-blockade effect on CD8$^+$ T-lymphocytes in pancreatic cancer. *BMC Cancer* **2019**, *19*, 1053. [CrossRef]
21. Ngiow, S.F.; Young, A.; Jacquelot, N.; Yamazaki, T.; Enot, D.; Zitvogel, L.; Smyth, M.J. A threshold level of intratumor CD8$^+$ T-cell PD1 expression dictates therapeutic response to anti-PD1. *Cancer Res.* **2015**, *75*, 3800–3811. [CrossRef]

22. Kim, K.H.; Cho, J.; Ku, B.M.; Koh, J.; Sun, J.-M.; Lee, S.-H.; Ahn, J.S.; Cheon, J.; Min, Y.J.; Park, S.-H.; et al. The first-week proliferative response of peripheral blood PD-1þCD8þ T cells predicts the response to Anti-PD-1 therapy in solid tumors. *Clin. Cancer Res.* **2019**, *25*, 2144–2154. [CrossRef]
23. Iacovelli, R.; Nolè, F.; Verri, E.; Renne, G.; Paglino, C.; Santoni, M.; Rocca, M.C.; Giglione, P.; Aurilio, G.; Cullurà, D.; et al. Prognostic Role of PD-L1 Expression in Renal Cell Carcinoma. A Systematic Review and Meta-Analysis. *Target Oncol.* **2016**, *11*, 143–148. [CrossRef]
24. Motzer, R.J.; Escudier, B.; McDermott, D.F.; George, S.; Hammers, H.J.; Srinivas, S.; Tykodi, S.S.; Sosman, J.A.; Procopio, G.; Plimack, E.R.; et al. Nivolumab versus Everolimus in Advanced Renal-Cell Carcinoma. *N. Engl. J. Med.* **2015**, *373*, 1803–1813. [CrossRef]
25. Jilaveanu, L.B.; Shuch, B.; Zito, C.R.; Parisi, F.; Barr, M.; Kluger, Y.; Chen, L.; Kluger, H.M. PD-L1 expression in clear cell renal cell carcinoma: An analysis of nephrectomy and sites of metastases. *J. Cancer* **2014**, *5*, 166–172. [CrossRef]
26. Roelants, C.; Pillet, C.; Franquet, Q.; Sarrazin, C.; Peilleron, N.; Giacosa, S.; Guyon, L.; Fontanell, A.; Fiard, G.; Long, J.-A.; et al. Ex-vivo treatment of tumor tissue slices as a predictive preclinical method to evaluate targeted therapies for patients with renal carcinoma. *Cancers* **2020**, *12*, 232. [CrossRef]
27. Neal, J.T.; Li, X.; Zhu, J.; Giangarra, V.; Grzeskowiak, C.L.; Ju, J.; Liu, I.H.; Chiou, S.-H.; Salahudeen, A.A.; Smith, A.R.; et al. Organoid Modeling of the Tumor Immune Microenvironment. *Cell* **2018**, *175*, 1972–1988.e16. [CrossRef]
28. Wang, M.; Yao, L.; Cheng, M.; Cai, D.; Martinek, J.; Pan, C.; Shi, W.; Ma, A.; White, R.W.D.V.; Airhart, S.; et al. Humanized mice in studying efficacy and mechanisms of PD-1-targeted cancer immunotherapy. *FASEB J.* **2018**, *32*, 1537–1549. [CrossRef]
29. Kenerson, H.L.; Sullivan, K.M.; Seo, Y.D.; Stadeli, K.M.; Ussakli, C.; Yan, X.; Lausted, C.; Pillarisetty, V.G.; Park, J.O.; Riehle, K.J.; et al. Tumor slice culture as a biologic surrogate of human cancer. *Ann. Transl. Med.* **2020**, *8*, 114. [CrossRef]
30. Meijer, T.G.; Naipal, K.A.; Jager, A.; Van Gent, D.C. Ex vivo tumor culture systems for functional drug testing and therapy response prediction. *Future Sci. OA* **2017**, *3*, FSO190. [CrossRef]
31. Xu, R.; Zhou, X.; Wang, S.; Trinkle, C. Tumor organoid models in precision medicine and investigating cancer-stromal interactions. *Pharmacol. Ther.* **2021**, *218*, 107668. [CrossRef] [PubMed]
32. Zhang, L.; Zha, Z.; Qu, W.; Zhao, H.; Yuan, J.; Feng, Y.; Wu, B. Tumor necrosis as a prognostic variable for the clinical outcome in patients with renal cell carcinoma: A systematic review and meta-analysis. *BMC Cancer* **2018**, *18*, 870. [CrossRef]
33. Kishan, A.T.N.; Nicole, S.V.; Humberto, S.; van Deurzen Carolien, H.M.; den Bakker Michael, A.; Jan, H.J.H.; Roland, K.; Vreeswijk Maaike, P.G.; Agnes, J.; van Gent, D.C. Tumor slice culture system to assess drug response of primary breast cancer. *BMC Cancer* **2016**, *16*, 78.
34. Jiang, X.; Seo, Y.D.; Chang, J.H.; Coveler, A.; Nigjeh, E.N.; Pan, S.; Jalikis, F.; Yeung, R.S.; Crispe, I.N.; Pillarisetty, V.G. Long-lived pancreatic ductal adenocarcinoma slice cultures enable precise study of the immune microenvironment. *Oncoimmunology* **2017**, *6*, e1333210. [CrossRef]
35. Prill, S.; Rebstock, J.; Tennemann, A.; Körfer, J.; Sönnichsen, R.; Thieme, R.; Gockel, I.; Lyros, O.; Monecke, A.; Wittekind, C.; et al. Tumor-associated macrophages and individual chemo-susceptibility are influenced by iron chelation in human slice cultures of gastric cancer. *Oncotarget* **2019**, *10*, 4731–4742. [CrossRef]
36. Gide, T.; Silva, I.P.; Quek, C.; Ahmed, T.; Menzies, A.M.; Carlino, M.S.; Saw, R.P.; Thompson, J.; Batten, M.; Long, G.V.; et al. Close proximity of immune and tumor cells underlies response to anti-PD-1 based therapies in metastatic melanoma patients. *Oncoimmunology* **2020**, *9*, 1659093. [CrossRef]
37. Peranzoni, E.; Bougherara, H.; Barrin, S.; Mansuet-Lupo, A.; Alifano, M.; Damotte, D.; Donnadieu, E. Ex vivo imaging of resident CD8 T lymphocytes in human lung tumor slices using confocal microscopy. *J. Vis. Exp.* **2017**, *2017*. [CrossRef]

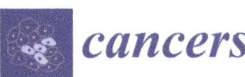

Article

Molecular Subtypes Based on Genomic and Transcriptomic Features Correlate with the Responsiveness to Immune Checkpoint Inhibitors in Metastatic Clear Cell Renal Cell Carcinoma

ByulA Jee [1], Eunjeong Seo [1], Kyunghee Park [2], Yi Rang Kim [3], Sun-ju Byeon [4], Sang Min Lee [1], Jae Hoon Chung [1], Wan Song [1], Hyun Hwan Sung [1], Hwang Gyun Jeon [1], Byong Chang Jeong [1], Seong Il Seo [1], Seong Soo Jeon [1], Hyun Moo Lee [1], Se Hoon Park [5], Woong-Yang Park [2] and Minyong Kang [1,2,6,*]

1 Department of Urology, Samsung Medical Center, Sungkyunkwan University School of Medicine, Seoul 06531, Korea; astherjee@skku.edu (B.J.); ejseo09@skku.edu (E.S.); s2623.lee@samsung.com (S.M.L.); jaehoontasker.chung@samsung.com (J.H.C.); wan.song@samsung.com (W.S.); hyunhwan.sung@samsung.com (H.H.S.); hwanggyun.jeon@samsung.com (H.G.J.); bc2.jung@samsung.com (B.C.J.); seongil.seo@samsung.com (S.I.S.); seongsoo.jeon@samsung.com (S.S.J.); hyunmoo.lee@samsung.com (H.M.L.)
2 Samsung Genome Institute, Samsung Medical Center, Seoul 06531, Korea; kyunghee.park@samsung.com (K.P.); woongyang.park@samsung.com (W.-Y.P.)
3 Oncocross Ltd., Seoul 04168, Korea; 99yirang@oncocross.com
4 Department of Pathology, Hallym University Dongtan Sacred Heart Hospital, Hwaseong 18450, Korea; byeon.sunju@welovedoctor.com
5 Division of Hematology-Oncology, Department of Internal Medicine, Samsung Medical Center, Sungkyunkwan University School of Medicine, Seoul 06531, Korea; sh1767.park@samsung.com
6 Department of Health Sciences and Technology, The Samsung Advanced Institute for Health Sciences & Technology (SAIHST), Sungkyunkwan University, Seoul 06355, Korea
* Correspondence: m79.kang@skku.edu

Simple Summary: Immune checkpoint inhibitors (ICIs), such as programmed cell death protein 1 (PD-1) blockade, have proven to be the most effective agents for the management of many cancer types. Although ICIs are the current standard of care for treating metastatic clear cell renal cell carcinoma (ccRCC), 40–60% of patients still have intrinsic resistance to ICIs across multiple clinical trials. Therefore, identifying optimal biomarkers that can predict either responders or non-responders to ICIs has been of tremendous importance. Here, we generated targeted sequencing and whole transcriptomic sequencing of 60 patients with metastatic ccRCC treated with ICIs. Moreover, transcriptomic analysis was integrated to identify molecular subtypes using a total of 177 tumor samples by merging our data and published data derived from the CheckMate 025 trial. Our results show that these molecular subtypes are associated with specific genomic alterations, distinct molecular pathways, and differential clinical outcomes in patients with metastatic ccRCC treated with ICIs.

Abstract: Clear cell renal cell carcinoma (ccRCC) has been reported to be highly immune to and infiltrated by T cells and has angiogenesis features, but the effect of given features on clinical outcomes followed by immune checkpoint inhibitors (ICIs) in ccRCC has not been fully characterized. Currently, loss of function mutation in *PBRM1*, a PBAF-complex gene frequently mutated in ccRCC, is associated with clinical benefit from ICIs, and is considered as a predictive biomarker for response to anti-PD-1 therapy. However, functional mechanisms of *PBRM1* mutation regarding immunotherapy responsiveness are still poorly understood. Here, we performed targeted sequencing ($n = 60$) and whole transcriptomic sequencing (WTS) ($n = 61$) of patients with metastatic ccRCC treated by ICIs. By integrating WTS data from the CheckMate 025 trial, we obtained WTS data of 177 tumors and finally identified three molecular subtypes that are characterized by distinct molecular phenotypes and frequency of *PBRM1* mutations. Patient clustered subtypes 1 and 3 demonstrated worse responses and survival after ICIs treatment, with a low proportion of *PBRM1* mutation and angiogenesis-poor, but were immune-rich and cell-cycle enriched. Notably, patients clustered in the subtype

2 showed a better response and survival after ICIs treatment, with enrichment of *PBRM1* mutation and metabolic programs and a low exhausted immune phenotype. Further analysis of the subtype 2 population demonstrated that *GATM* (glycine amidinotransferase), as a novel gene associated with *PBRM1* mutation, plays a pivotal role in ccRCC by using a cell culture model, revealing tumor, suppressive-like features in reducing proliferation and migration. In summary, we identified that metastatic ccRCC treated by ICIs have distinct genomic and transcriptomic features that may account for their responsiveness to ICIs. We also revealed that the novel gene *GATM* can be a potential tumor suppressor and/or can be associated with therapeutic efficacy in metastatic ccRCC treated by ICIs.

Keywords: renal cell carcinoma; immune checkpoint inhibitor; responsiveness; molecular features

1. Introduction

Immune checkpoint inhibitors (ICIs), such as programmed cell death protein 1 (PD-1) blockade, have proven to be the most effective agents for the management of many cancer types [1]. Despite the low tumor mutational burden of renal cell carcinoma (RCC), it has unique immunologic features, including high immune infiltration score and increased infiltration by cytotoxic $CD8^+$ T cells, which are known to be associated with the response to PD-1 blockade [2,3]. In this context, recent phase III clinical trials, such as CheckMate 025, CheckMate 214, and KEYNOTE 426, showed that ICIs-based regimens significantly improved the objective response and survival outcomes compared to that of tyrosine kinase inhibitors, particularly in advanced clear cell RCC (ccRCC) [4–7]. Although ICIs are the current standard of care for treating metastatic ccRCC, 40–60% of patients still have intrinsic resistance to ICIs across multiple clinical trials. Therefore, identifying optimal biomarkers that can predict either responders or non-responders to ICIs have been of tremendous importance [8].

While PD-ligand 1 expression is a conventional biomarker for predicting responsiveness to ICIs across various types of malignancies, data on RCC have been heterogeneous, and the predictive value of PD-ligand 1 expression is not clinically practical yet [8]. In contrast to other solid tumors, tumor mutational burden and neoantigen load, which have been the commonly explored predictors for ICIs therapy, were not associated with clinical responses to PD-1 blockade in advanced ccRCC [4]. Additionally, no difference in survival outcomes according to the patterns of $CD8^+$ T cell infiltration in ccRCC patients treated with anti-PD-1 was found [4]. Recently, several studies reported that a loss of function (LOF) mutation in a PBAF-complex gene *PBRM1*, that is commonly mutated in ccRCC, was associated with better clinical benefit (CB) from ICIs [4,9,10]. In this context, a comprehensive understanding of the molecular mechanisms of *PBRM1* mutation in patients with ccRCC treated with ICIs could be critical for the development of a novel biomarker and to help predict which patients are most likely to benefit from ICIs treatment.

Here, targeted sequencing and whole transcriptomic sequencing of 60 patients with metastatic ccRCC treated with ICIs were performed. Moreover, transcriptomic analysis was integrated to identify molecular subtypes using a total of 177 tumor samples and by merging our data and published data derived from the CheckMate 025 trial [4]. Our results show that these molecular subtypes are associated with specific genomic alterations, distinct molecular pathways, and differential clinical outcomes in patients with metastatic ccRCC treated with ICIs.

2. Materials and Methods

2.1. Patients

The data of 60 patients with metastatic ccRCC treated with ICIs, particularly as either first-line (n = 8) (combination of anti-CTLA4 (ipilimumab) or anti-PD-1 (nivolumab)) or second-line (monotherapy of nivolumab) (n = 52) therapy from 2017 to 2020 at Samsung

Medical Center, were retrospectively collected. The Institutional Review Board of our center approved the use of human archival tissues for this study (IRB no. SMC 2020-03-063).

Therapeutic responses of ICIs were determined every 3 to 4 months of treatment using abdomen-pelvis and chest-computed tomography scans. The responses were classified as complete response (CR), partial response (PR), stable disease (SD), or progressive disease (PD), according to the RECIST 1.1 criteria [11]. The clinical benefit (CB), non-clinical benefit (NCB), or intermediate benefit (IB) classification was defined in a previous report [9]. Briefly, CB included patients with CR, PR, or SD with any reduction in tumors lasting at least 6 months. NCB was defined as patients who experienced PD and were discontinued from ICIs therapy within 3 months. All other patients were assigned to the IB group.

2.2. Targeted Sequencing Preprocess

Tumor tissues from 60 patients were used for targeted sequencing of 380 cancer-related genes (CancerSCAN Version 3.1, a targeted-sequencing platform designed at Samsung Medical Center) and extracted from formalin-fixed paraffin-embedded tissues. Most samples had a mean coverage of ~900× with coverage at hotspots well above the mean. The paired-end reads were aligned to the human reference genome (hg19) using BWA (Version 0.7.5). Then, SAMtools (Version 0.1.18), GATK (Version 3.1-1), and Picard (Version 1.93) were used for file handling, local realignment, and removal of duplicate reads, respectively. The base quality scores were recalibrated using the GATK BaseRecalibrator based on known single-nucleotide polymorphisms (SNPs) and indels from dbSNP138.

2.3. RNA-Sequencing Preprocess

To perform RNA sequencing using 60 metastatic ccRCC and 5 adjacent nontumor tissues, total RNA was extracted utilizing the RNA extraction kit (RNeasy Mini Kit, QIAGEN, Maryland, MD, USA), and RNA integrity was verified using a 2100 Bioanalyzer (Agilent, Palo Alto, CA, USA). The libraries for sequencing were generated using the QuantSeq 3′ Library Prep Kit (Lexogen Inc., Vienna, Austria) according to the manufacturer's instructions and sequenced on a HiSeq 2000 system (Illumina, San Diego, CA, USA). The reads were mapped to the hg19 human reference genome using STAR with default parameters. The number of reads mapped to each gene was calculated using RNA-Seq by Expectation-Maximization. Data processing and analysis were performed using the R/Bioconductor libraries. To preprocess the transcriptome data, genes with zero values across samples were filtered out. The data were normalized by subtracting the average expression values of the adjacent nontumor tissues per gene and centering the expression values of each sample and gene. In addition, three ccRCC samples that were outliers with respect to the overall mean and standard deviation and two ccRCC samples without information on the *PBRM1* mutation were filtered.

2.4. Immunohistochemical Analysis

To perform immunohistochemistry using 51 of the 60 available tissues of metastatic ccRCC patients, the Tissue microarray (TMA) method was applied. Briefly, representative tumor tissues (2 mm diameter) were taken from individual paraffin-embedded tumors (donor blocks) and arranged in new recipient paraffin blocks (tissue microarray blocks) using a trephine apparatus. One core tissue was taken from each case. Sections with a thickness of 5 mm were cut from each TMA block, deparaffinized, and dehydrated for immunohistochemical (IHC) staining. Ventana XT Benchmark (Ventana Medical Systems, Oro Valley, AZ, USA) for GATM (1:100 dilution, Catalog #ab32936, Abcam PLC, Cambridge, England, UK) was used IHC staining. Membranous and cytoplasmic staining of GATM was evaluated, and immunoreactivity for GATM was scored as follows: diffuse (more and equal 50% of tumor cells showed immunoreactivity) and moderate to strong expression of GATM was regarded as high expression (2+), diffuse or focal (less than 50% tumor cells showed immunoreactivity) and weak expression of GATM was regarded as low expression (1+), and no expression of GATM was regarded as no (0). Specimens with either weak or high expression of GATM were classified as GATM-positive and specimens with no expression of GATM were considered as GATM-negative. IHC data were reviewed by a well-experienced pathologist (S.-j.B.) who was unaware of other clinical data.

2.5. GSEA (Gene Set Enrichment Analysis) and ssGSEA (Single-Sample GSEA)

To perform the GSEA, the Hallmark gene sets from the Molecular Signatures Database (MSigDB Version 7.0) were used [12]. ssGSEA was computed using the "GSVA" package [13].

2.6. Immune Cell Type and Immune Type

The proportion of immune cell types was calculated using CIBERSORTx [14]. The proportion of 10 immune cell types was calculated by aggregation (for example, the proportion of macrophages was aggregated by macrophages M0, M1, and M2). Immune subtypes, including active and exhausted, were conducted using the nearest template prediction algorithm based on the expression of active and normal stroma signatures [15].

2.7. The Signatures of Differentially Expressed Genes (DEGs)

To identify upregulated or downregulated genes using GSE102806, DEG sets from three conditions were calculated. DEG1 was calculated as shPBRM1 vs. shControl in replicate 1 of the 786-O cell line. DEG2 was calculated as shPBRM1 vs. shControl in replicate 2 of the 786-O cell line. DEG3 was calculated as a *PBRM1* mutation vs. *PBRM1* wild type in the A-704 cell line. DEG4 and DEG5 were calculated from merged data (n = 177). DEG4 was differentially expressed in subtype 2 (Figure S1 and Table S3). DEG5 was calculated as *PBRM1* mutation vs. *PBRM1* wild type. DEGs were subjected to t-test (GSE102806) and permuted t-test (merged data), and the cutoff options were $p < 0.05$, FDR < 0.05, and log2 fold differences > 0.5.

2.8. Statistical Analysis

DEGs were calculated using t-test and permutation t-test. The Kaplan–Meier method was used to estimate PFS and OS. Categorical variables between the two groups were compared using Fisher's exact test. One-way ANOVA was performed for the three groups. Student's t-test was performed for both groups. All statistical analyses were performed using the R software.

2.9. Validation Sets

To merge transcriptomic data for the classification of subtypes, CheckMate 025 data were obtained from Table S4 published in Nature Medicine by Braun et al. [4]. To validate our findings, datasets were obtained from the TCGA-KIRC and GEO websites (accessed date, 17 December 2020; accession numbers: GSE102806 and GSE105288).

2.10. Cell Culture and Treatments

786-O cells transfected with siScramble (siScr) or siPBRM1 (AM16708, Thermo Fisher, Waltham, MA, USA) were seeded before treatment at 60–80% confluent at the time of the experiment. Additionally, 0.5 µM actinomycin D (11805017, Thermo Fisher, Waltham, MA, USA) was used for the indicated time.

2.11. Real-Time qPCR

786-O or Caki cells were transfected with siScr or siPBRM1, and after 48 h, real-time RT-PCR assays were conducted following the manufacturer's instructions. Furthermore, 0.5 µg of total RNA was used as templates for reverse transcription through the ReverTra Ace qPCR RT Master Mix (Toyobo Co., Ltd., Kodakara island, Japan) according to the manufacturer's instructions. Real-time PCR analysis was performed using the QuantStudio system with SYBR Premix Ex Taq (Takara Co., Ltd., Otsu, Japan). GATM F-5′-CAC TAC ATC GGA TCT CGG CTT, GATM R-5′-CTA AGG GGT CCC ATT CGT TGT and USH1C

F-5′-TTC CGG CAT AAG GTG GAT TTT C, USH1C R-5′-GTA CAT TCG CAG CAC ATC ATA GA.

2.12. Cell Migration Assays

A total of 786-O cells were transfected with siRNAs against the control, *PBRM1*, or *GATM*. After 24 h, the 786-O cells seeded on glass-bottomed dishes pre-coated with fibronectin (100 g/mL) were scratched. After the cells reached 90% confluence, the monolayer was scratched with a pipette tip and incubated with a medium containing 300 µM H_2O_2 for 12 h in a humidified CO_2 incubator at 37 °C.

2.13. Colony Formation Assay

Cells were transfected with the indicated siRNAs and seeded at 1000–2000 cells/well in 6-well plates. After 24 h, the medium was replaced with 300 µM H_2O_2 or low-glucose medium (11966025 Thermo Fisher) and incubated. After 7 days, the cells were fixed and stained with crystal violet. Triplicate wells were used for each experiment.

3. Results

3.1. The Characteristics of Genomic Alterations in Patients with ccRCC Treated with ICIs

The baseline demographics of patients with metastatic ccRCC in our cohort are described in Table S1. Additionally, treatment outcomes according to first- and second-line therapies are summarized in Table S2. Next, to evaluate the genomic landscape of patients with metastatic ccRCC (n = 60) treated with ICIs, we focused on targeted sequencing data to identify recurrently mutated genes in our cohort and found 17 recurrently altered genes. The most commonly altered genes in this cohort were *VHL* (n = 34, 56.7%), *PBRM1* (n = 18, 30.0%), *SETD2* (n = 16, 26.7%), and *BAP1* (n = 12, 20.0%), which were generally similar to those previously reported for ccRCC (Figure 1A) [4,9]. Next, when gene-specific alterations were compared between the clinical benefit (CB) group and the non-clinical benefit (NCB) group, only the *PBRM1* mutation among the 17 recurrently altered genes was significantly enriched in the CB group (Fisher's exact test, p = 0.03, odds ratio for CB = 3.67, 95% confidence interval (CI) = 0.98–14.69) (Figure 1B). As expected, patients with the *PBRM1* mutation had significantly prolonged overall survival (OS), not progression-free survival (PFS), compared to those with *PBRM1* wild type (log-rank test, p = 0.018) (Figure 1C). These results indicated that CB following ICIs therapy was more prominent in patients with metastatic ccRCC harboring the *PBRM1* mutation.

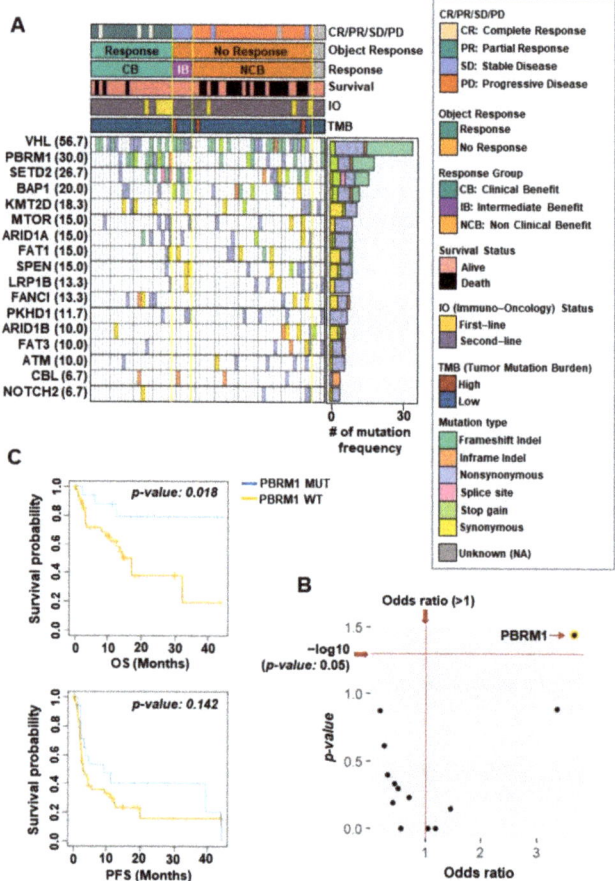

Figure 1. Overall mutational landscape in 60 patients with metastatic clear cell carcinoma treated with immune checkpoint inhibitors. (**A**) Heatmap shows 17 recurrently mutated genes in our cohort ordered by the number of mutation frequencies. (**B**) The plot shows the *p*-value and odds ratio for the 17 genes by performing Fisher's exact test between the clinical benefit versus non-clinical benefit groups. (Red dashed lines denote $p < 0.05$ and odds ratio > 1. Each black dot denotes the 17 recurrently mutated genes). (**C**) Kaplan–Meier plots show the overall survival (top) and progression-free survival (bottom) of patients who did or did not harbor mutations in *PBRM1*. PBRM1 MUT, PBRM1 mutation (blue); PBRM1 WT, PBRM1 wild type (yellow).

3.2. The Characteristics of Molecular Subtypes in Patients with ccRCC Treated with ICIs

To expand our understanding of the molecular phenotypes of metastatic ccRCC treated with ICIs, WTS data were generated using 177 tumor samples by merging our data and CheckMate 025 data. We aimed to identify molecular subtypes by utilizing four signatures associated with *PBRM1*-mutation and *PBRM1* LOF (Loss of Function). Two signatures of *PBRM1*-mutation were previously reported to be differentially expressed genes (DEGs) between patients with and without *PBRM1* mutations [16]. The signatures of *PBRM1* LOF also previously reported that high angiogenesis and less immunomodulation were related to phenotypes of *PBRM1* loss [17]. Unsupervised clustering analysis was performed based on the four signatures associated with *PBRM1* mutation and *PBRM1* LOF and identified three molecular subtypes in 177 patients (Figure 2, top). Patients with subtype 1 (*n* = 64, 36%) were characterized by the moderate expression of upregulated and downregulated genes related to the *PBRM1* mutation with relatively lower expression of angiogenesis and a mixed pattern of immunomodulatory signature. Additionally, 12 patients with subtype 1 showed *PBRM1* mutations (20%). Interestingly, patients with subtype 2 (*n* = 75, 42%) were characterized by consistent expression patterns of upregulated and downregulated genes related to the *PBRM1* mutation, relatively higher expression of angiogenesis, and relatively lower expression of immunomodulatory signature with higher mutation rate of *PBRM1* (*n* = 44, 72%), compared to those with subtypes 1 and 3. The low expressions of immunomodulatory were seen in subtype 2, consistent with previous finding that *PBRM1* loss are associated with a nonimmunogenic tumor phenotype [17]. Patients with subtype 3 (*n* = 38, 22%) were characterized by the inverse expression of both upregulated and downregulated genes related to the *PBRM1* mutation, moderate expression of angiogenesis, and enrichment of higher immunomodulatory signature. Only five patients had the *PBRM1* mutations (8%) in subtype 3 (Figure 2, top).

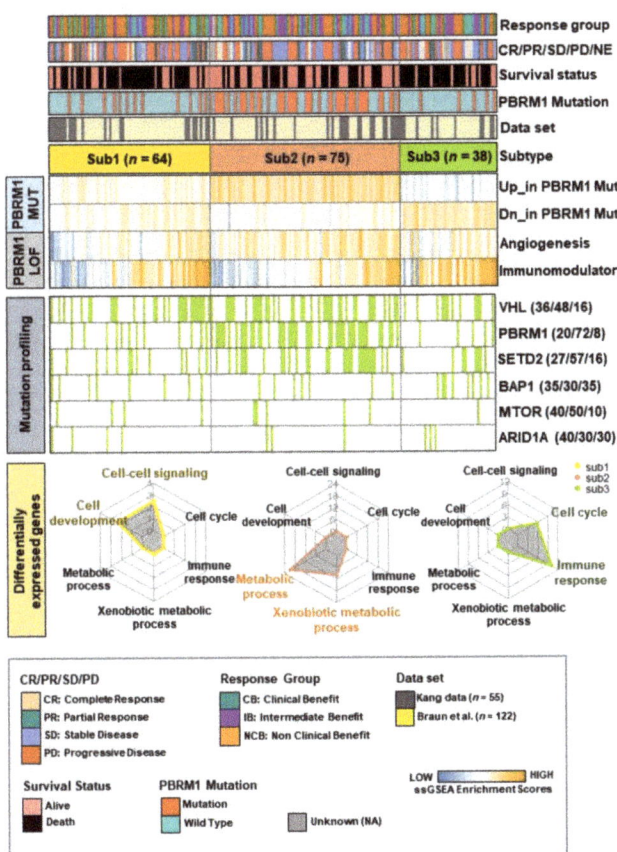

Figure 2. Characteristics of subtypes based on the gene sets associated with *PBRM1* mutation and *PBRM1* loss of function. Heatmap of the single-sample gene set enrichment analysis shows the enrichment scores of the four gene sets in the merged data set (top). Mutation plot shows six commonly mutated genes by overlapping recurrently mutated genes from both our data and the CheckMate 025 data (middle). (Green color denotes harboring mutation). Radar plots show significantly enriched gene ontology terms using upregulated genes in each subtype (bottom).

We further characterized the prevalence of the six commonly mutated genes by overlapping recurrently mutated genes from our data and CheckMate 025 data and found a higher prevalence of alterations such as *VHL* ($n = 36$, 48%), *PBRM1* ($n = 44$, 72%) and *SETD2* ($n = 28$, 57%) in patients in subtype 2 (Figure 2, middle) than that of the other two subtypes. Next, to evaluate the key biological features related to these molecular subtypes, pairwise comparisons of each subtype were performed. Unique upregulated DEGs were identified in each molecular subtype (permuted *t*-test; $p < 0.05$, false discovery rate (FDR) < 0.05, and log2 fold difference > 0.5; Figure S1 and Table S3). First, 397 upregulated genes unique to subtype 1 were enriched in biological process terms for cell–cell signaling (ES = 2.46, $p = 4.39 \times 10^{-4}$) and cell development (ES = 2.34, $p = 2.15 \times 10^{-5}$). Second, 1569 upregulated genes unique to subtype 2 with a high proportion of *PBRM1* mutations were associated with the metabolic process (ES = 25.93, $p = 5.80 \times 10^{-42}$) and xenobiotic metabolism (ES = 12.56, $p = 7.04 \times 10^{-14}$). Finally, 459 upregulated genes unique to subtype 3 showed the activation of genes related to the cell cycle (ES = 12.55, $p = 3.62 \times 10^{-23}$) and immune response (ES = 6.97, $p = 1.19 \times 10^{-10}$) (Figure 2, bottom). Taken together, the molecular stratification of 177 ccRCC tumors, treated with ICIs, was conducted into three subtypes with biologically distinct transcriptomes.

3.3. Subtype 2 Is Associated with Higher Metabolic Processes and Lower Exhausted Immune Types than the Other Two Subtypes

Next, when the treatment responses were examined according to each subtype, significant differences in the clinical responses and benefits were not found (Table S4). To evaluate the prognostic relevance of each subtype, the PFS and OS were compared according to each subtype. Notably, subtype 2, compared to that of subtypes 1 and 3, was significantly associated with OS ($p = 0.0042$) (Figure 3A) but not with PFS ($p = 0.381$) (Figure S2A). To further understand the molecular mechanisms of survival outcomes, transcriptomic pathway programs were explored by performing gene set enrichment analysis (GSEA) and single-sample GSEA (ssGSEA) using Hallmark gene sets ($n = 50$) in each subtype. Overall, 18 gene sets, including inflammatory response, oxidative phosphorylation, and E2F target pathways, were activated in each subtype (one-way analysis of variance (ANOVA) test, $p < 0.0005$, Figure 3B and Figure S2B). Both subtypes 1 and 3 were activated by immune-related pathways (INFLAMMATORY_RESPONSE, COMPLEMENT, and IL6_JAK_STAT3). Subtype 3 differentiated from subtypes 1 and 2 through the enhanced activation of cell cycle progression pathways (G2M_CHECKPOINT, E2F_TARGETS, and MITOTIC_SPINDLE). Particularly, in patients with subtype 2, metabolic-related pathways (OXIDATIVE_PHOSPHORYLATION, FATTY_ACID_METABOLISM, and ADIPOGENESIS), the HYPOXIA and REACTIVE_OXYGEN_SPECIES pathways were activated. Previous reports demonstrated that ccRCC tumors with *PBRM1* mutations were activated with a hypoxic transcriptional signature, which is in agreement with our findings [9,17,18].

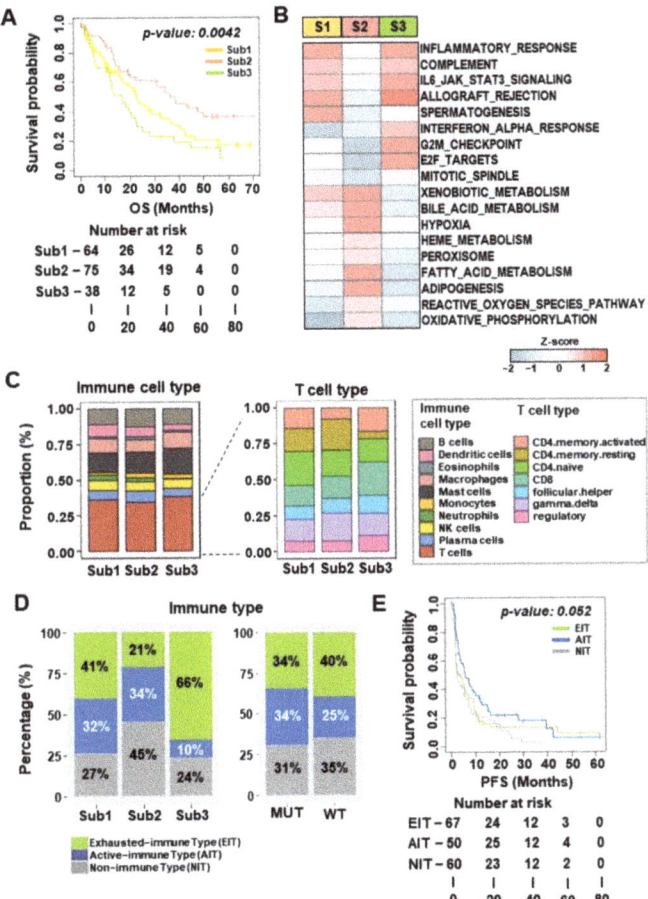

Figure 3. Patients in subtype 2 with enrichment of the *PBRM1* mutation are associated with metabolic pathways and transition of immune types. (**A**) Kaplan–Meier plot analysis of the overall survival for each subtype. (**B**) Heatmap of Hallmark gene sets. The mean Z score of the single-sample gene set enrichment analysis for each gene set was calculated (S1, Sub1; S2, Sub2; S3, Sub3). (**C**) CIBERSORTx findings show the proportion of distinct immune cell subpopulations (left) and the proportion of T cell subpopulations (right). (**D**) Barplots show the percentage of immune types, including active immune, exhausted immune and nonimmune types, in each subtype (left) and in the group with *PBRM1* mutation vs. the group without *PBRM1* mutation (right). (**E**) Kaplan–Meier plot analysis of progression-free survival for each immune type. AIT, active immune type (navy); EIT, exhausted immune type (green); NIT, non-immune type (gray).

3.4. GATM Expression Associated with PBRM1 Mutation as a Novel Biomarker of Therapeutic Response in Patients with ccRCC Treated by ICIs

Next, we aimed to identify key modulating genes associated with subtype 2 harboring a higher proportion of *PBRM1* mutations as well as showing the best survival outcomes. We analyzed cell line data (GSE102806), including 786-O and A-704 cell lines, which were associated with *PBRM1* LOF. First, we generated six gene sets, either upregulated or downregulated DEGs, by comparing treatment samples and control samples (see details in Section 2). To further evaluate the DEGs, including DEG1, DEG2, and DEG3, we applied the merged data of human samples (*n* = 177) using the DEGs and by performing ssGSEA and identified distinct expression patterns in each subtype (Figure 4A). Notably, subtype 2 showed a significantly higher expression of the upregulated DEGs and a lower expression of the downregulated DEGs compared with subtypes 1 and 3. Likewise, tumors harboring the *PBRM1* mutation exhibited a higher expression of the upregulated DEGs, whereas the downregulated DEGs were not related compared with that of the *PBRM1* wild type (Figures 4B and S3A). These results suggested that upregulated DEGs rather than downregulated DEGs derived from cell line data were clearly validated in data derived from human samples showing the distinct characteristics of *PBRM1* LOF.

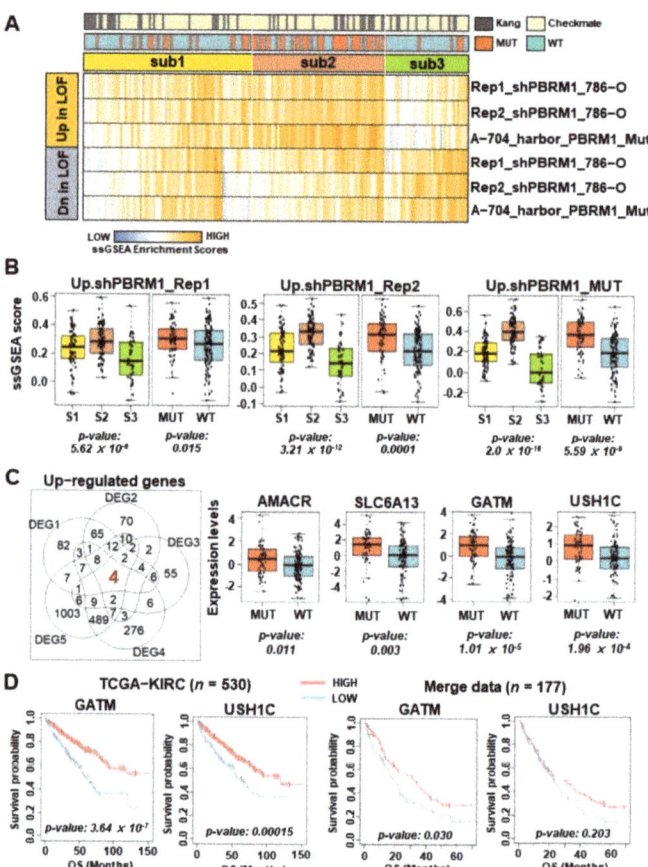

Figure 4. *GATM* expression is related to *PBRM1* mutation and *PBRM1* loss of function. (**A**) Heatmap of enrichment scores for the single-sample gene set enrichment analysis using upregulated and downregulated differentially expressed genes (DEGs) derived from cell line data GSE102806. (**B**) Boxplots summarizing the heatmap in (**A**) for each subtype (left) and in the group with *PBRM1* mutation vs. the group without *PBRM1* mutation (right) (S1, Sub1; S2, Sub2; S3, Sub3). (**C**) Venn diagram shows the overlapping of the five upregulated DEGs (left). Boxplots show the expression levels of *AMACR*, *SLC6A13*, *GATM*, and *USH1C* according to patients with and without *PBRM1* mutation in the merged data (right). (**D**) Kaplan–Meier plots show the overall survival of the patients stratified according the above or below the average *GATM* or *USH1C* in TCGA-KIRC (*n* = 530) and the merged data (*n* = 177). High expression (pink), low expression (sky blue).

Then, five DEGs were used (see details in Section 2), and 4 genes and 0 genes were identified as commonly upregulated or downregulated genes, respectively, by overlapping all five DEGs (Figure 4C, left and Figure S3B). The four identified genes, *AMACR*, *SLC6A3*, *GATM*, and *USH1C*, were upregulated and potentially associated with *PBRM1* mutation (Figure 4C, right). Among them, we focused on *GATM* ($p = 1.01 \times 10^{-5}$) and *USH1C* ($p = 1.94 \times 10^{-4}$), which were significantly differentially expressed in tumors harboring the *PBRM1* mutation. In particular, the *GATM* gene showed a non-tumor-specific expression compared with that of the levels in tumor tissues in The Cancer Genome Atlas Kidney Renal Clear Cell Carcinoma (TCGA-KIRC) data ($n = 607$, $p = 3.07 \times 10^{-7}$; Figure S3C, left) and GSE105288 ($n = 43$, $p = 0.045$; Figure S3D, right). However, the *USH1C* gene showed tumor-specific expression compared with that of the levels of nontumor tissues in TCGA-KIRC data ($p = 6.0 \times 10^{-9}$; Figure S3C, left) and GSE105288 ($p = 0.503$; Figure S3D, right). We then evaluated the clinical relevance of these two genes. When compared according to the expression levels of each gene, there were no differences in DFS (disease-free survival) (Figure S3E) or PFS (Figure S3F). However, a higher expression of *GATM* was consistently correlated with clinical outcomes of OS in TCGA-KIRC data ($p = 3.64 \times 10^{-7}$; Figure 4D, left) and the merged data ($p = 0.030$; Figure 4D, right). A higher expression of *USH1C* was correlated with clinical outcomes of OS in TCGA-KIRC data ($p = 0.00015$; Figure 4D, left), whereas it did not reach statistical significance for OS in the merged data ($p = 0.203$; Figure 4D, right). Accordingly, GATM was prioritized as a potential driver in the following analysis.

3.5. GATM Protein Levels Using Immunohistochemistry Are Related to Favorable Survival

Next, to validate the prognostic role of GATM, we evaluated the GATM protein expression via IHC staining in 51 metastatic ccRCC patients and stratified it into two groups according to the status of GATM expression (GATM-positive and GATM-negative, respectively) (Figure 5A). Then, the association of GATM protein levels with survival outcomes was investigated. Notably, the GATM-positive group had the significantly better PFS ($p = 0.0156$; Figure 5B, top) and OS outcomes ($p = 0.0013$, Figure 5B, bottom) after ICIs therapy compared to GATM-negative group. We further analyzed GATM protein levels based on *PBRM1* mutation status and the molecular subtypes, and found that patients with *PBRM1* mutation exhibited a higher percentage of GATM-positive specimens than patients without the *PBRM1* mutation (Figure 5C, top). Additionally, we observed that subtypes 2 had a highest percentage of GATM-positive cases, whereas subtype 3, with aggressive phenotypes and poor survival, had the lowest percentage of GATM-positive specimens compared to that of subtype 1 and 2 (Figure 5C, bottom). These findings suggested that GATM protein levels are associated with *PBRM1* mutation status and less aggressive phenotypes and exhibit potential clinical utility as a prognostic marker for metastatic ccRCC with ICIs treatment.

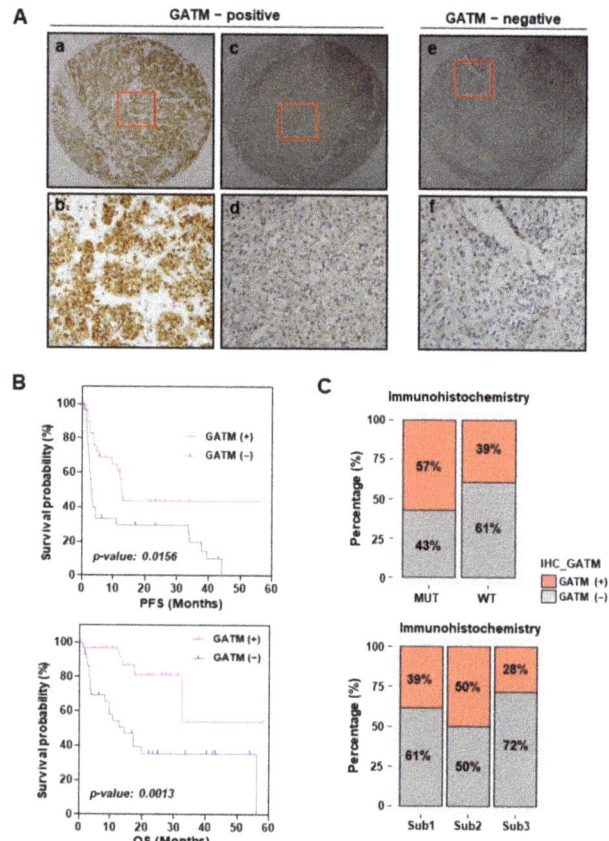

Figure 5. Status of GATM protein expression in immunohistochemistry are related to favorable survival. (**A**) Immunohistochemistry of GATM expression using tissue microarray of 51 patients with metastatic clear cell renal cell carcinoma treated by immune checkpoint blockades. The GATM-positive group includes "high expression" of GATM (a ×4, and b; ×20) and "low expression" of GATM (c; ×4, and d; ×20). The GATM-negative group includes "no expression" of GATM (e; ×4, and f; ×20). (**B**) Kaplan–Meier plot analysis of progression-free survival and overall survival based on the status of GATM protein expression. GATM (+) = GATM-positive group; GATM (−) = GATM-negative group. (**C**) Barplots show the percentage of both GATM-positive (+, crimson), and GATM-negative groups (−, gray), respectively, in the patients with *PBRM1* mutation vs. the patients without *PBRM1* mutation (top), and each subtype (bottom).

3.6. PBRM1 Deficiency and GATM Upregulation in Stress Conditions Reduce Cell Proliferation

We examined whether *GATM* expression is regulated by the loss of *PBRM1* in ccRCC lines. *PBRM1* knockdown in Caki-1 and 786-O cells showed an increase in *GATM* or *USH1C* expression (Figures S4A and 6A). We also tested whether *GATM* expression was regulated by *PBRM1* at the transcriptional level using 0.5 μM actinomycin D (transcriptional inhibitor). As expected, increased levels of *GATM* transcripts were sustained upon *PBRM1* knockdown in 786-O cells treated with actinomycin D compared to that of control cells (Figure 6B). The results indicated that *GATM* expression was increased at the transcriptional level following *PBRM1* knockdown. *PBRM1* has been reported to protect cancer cells under high-stress conditions, and patients with ccRCC harboring *PBRM1* mutations show better responsiveness to PD-1 inhibitors [9,21]. Given the protective roles of *PBRM1* in stress response, we examined whether *GATM* induced by *PBRM1* deletion participated in the anticancer state under stress conditions. An in vitro wound healing assay was performed using 786-O cells. As shown in Figure 6C, 786-O cells transfected with siScr, siPBRM1, or siGATM were scratched and incubated with high concentrations of hydrogen peroxide (H_2O_2) for 12 h. *PBRM1* knockdown in the 786-O cells exposed to H_2O_2 led to little movement compared to that in control cells. Depletion of *GATM* in *PBRM1*-knockdown 786-O cells augmented the migration, and motility by *GATM* knockdown was similar to that in the control cells (Figure 6C). These data indicate that migration ability was lost by *PBRM1* loss-induced *GATM* upregulation.

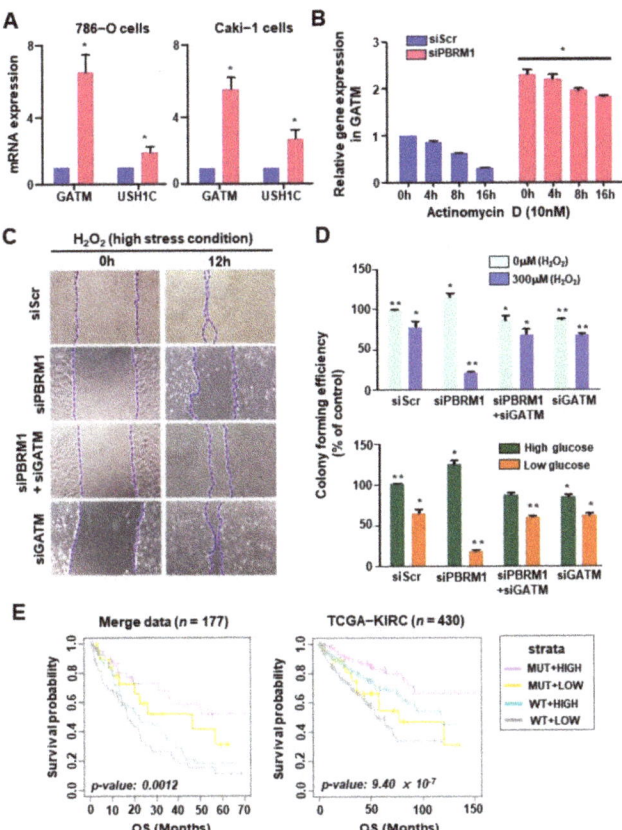

Figure 6. Expression of *GATM* by *PBRM1* knockdown reduces proliferation of clear cell renal cell carcinoma cell lines under stress conditions. (**A**) *GATM* or *USH1C* expression levels in PBRM1 knockdown 786-O or Caki-1 cells. The 786-O or Caki-1 cells were transfected with siScr or siPBRM1 and qRT-PCR analysis was performed. (**B**) *GATM* expression levels in siScr or siPBRM1 were transfected into 786-O cells and treated with 0.5 µM ActD for the indicated time. (**C**) Wound healing assay was performed. The 786-O cells transfected with indicated siRNAs were incubated with medium containing 300 µM H_2O_2 for 12 h. (**D**) Colony formation was performed in *PBRM1* knockdown 786-O cells. The 786-O cells were transfected with the indicated siRNAs and incubated

with a medium containing 300 μM H$_2$O$_2$ or with a low-glucose medium (**E**) Kaplan–Meier plot analysis of overall survival based on *PBRM1* mutation and *GATM* expression using the merge data (*n* = 177, left). PBRM1_MUT+HIGH_GATM (*n* = 42, purple), PBRM1_MUT+LOW_GATM (*n* = 19, yellow), PBRM1_WT+HIGH_GATM (*n* = 55, blue), and PBRM1_WT+LOW_GATM (*n* = 61, gray). Kaplan–Meier plot analysis of overall survival based on *PBRM1* mutation and *GATM* expression using TCGA-KIRC (*n* = 430, right). PBRM1_MUT+HIGH_GATM (*n* = 92, purple), PBRM1_MUT+LOW_GATM (*n* = 46, yellow), PBRM1_WT+HIGH_GATM (*n* = 161, blue), and PBRM1_WT+LOW_GATM (*n* = 131, gray). The *p*-value was calculated using Student's *t*-test: * *p* < 0.05 and ** *p* < 0.01. Data represent means ± SD from a representative experiment of at least two independent repeats (**A**,**B**,**D**).

Next, we examined the effect of *GATM* induced by *PBRM1* knockdown on the proliferation of 786-O cells under stress conditions such as that in H$_2$O$_2$ or low-glucose medium. *PBRM1*-depleted cells incubated with medium containing high concentrations of hydrogen peroxide or low glucose lost the ability to form colonies, which was recovered by silencing *GATM* (Figure 6D). The results suggested that the antiproliferative ability of the *PBRM1* mutation under stress conditions was accompanied by an increase in *GATM* expression.

More importantly, the association of *GATM* expression and *PBRM1* mutations with clinical prognosis was investigated; merged data (*n* = 177) derived from human samples were stratified into four groups according to the status of *PBRM1* mutation and *GATM* expression: (PBRM1_MUT+HIGH_GATM (*n* = 42), PBRM1_MUT+LOW_GATM (*n* = 19), PBRM1_WT+HIGH_GATM (*n* = 55) and PBRM1_WT+LOW_GATM (*n* = 61)). As expected, patients with the *PBRM1* mutation and high expression of *GATM* had the best PFS (*p* = 0.069; Figure S4B, left) and OS outcomes (*p* = 0.0012, Figure 6E, left). The molecular subtypes of the four groups were further analyzed, and it was found that patients in the PBRM1_MUT+HIGH GATM group were enriched in subtype 2 (88%), and patients in the PBRM1_WT+LOW_GATM group were enriched in subtypes 1 (46%) and 3 (48%) (Figure S4C). More importantly, multivariate analysis of the merged data also revealed the prognostic significance of *GATM* expression and *PBRM1* mutation (hazard ratio [HR] = 2.067, 95% confidence interval [CI], 1.147–3.726; *p* = 0.016; Table 1). On further analysis, *PBRM1* mutation and *GATM* expression were associated with significant OS (*p* = 9.40 × 10^{-7}, Figure 6E, right) rather than PFS (*p* = 0.332, Figure S4B, right) in the TCGA-KIRC cohort. Although the TCGA-KIRC cohort was predominately composed of non-ICIs-treated patients, the survival result suggested that patients with the *PBRM1* mutation and high *GATM* expression are consistently associated with superior OS. These retrospective analysis results collectively suggest that the status of the *PBRM1* mutation and *GATM* expression were considered as prognostic key factors of RCC patients.

Table 1. Univariate and multivariate analyses for predicting the overall survival of patients with metastatic clear cell renal cell carcinoma treated with immune checkpoint inhibitors.

Variables		Univariate Analysis		Multivariate Analysis	
		HR (95% CI)	*p*-Value	HR (95% CI)	*p*-Value
Age	<Median	Reference	-	Reference	-
	≥Median	0.855 (0.58–1.26)	0.428	0.895 (0.599–1.339)	0.589
Sex	Female	Reference	-	Reference	-
	Male	2.047 (1.235–3.394)	0.005 **	1.576 (0.939–2.645)	0.085
IMDC	Favor	Reference	-	Reference	-
	Intermediate & Poor	2.134 (1.336–3.409)	0.0015 **	2.012 (1.252–3.233)	0.004 **
PBRM1 & GATM	MUT & HIGH	Reference	-	Reference	-
	MUT & LOW, WT & HIGH, and WT & LOW	2.532 (1.414–4.532)	0.0017 **	2.067 (1.147–3.726)	0.016 *

HR, Hazard Ratio; CI, Confidence Interval; IMDC, International Metastatic RCC Database Consortium; MUT, PBRM1 mutation; WT, PBRM1 wildtype; HIGH, GATM high expression; LOW, GATM low expression (* *p* < 0.05, ** *p* < 0.005).

The *GATM* gene encodes glycine amidinotransferase, catalyzing the rate-limiting step in the synthesis of creatine, which plays a pivotal role in cancer progression and immunotherapy. Previous studies have demonstrated that creatine inhibits the growth of tumor cells both in vitro and in vivo and is associated with the regulation of T cell antitumor immunity [22,23]. In this context, the creatine metabolism level was examined for each subtype ($p = 2.63 \times 10^{-7}$; Figure S4D, left) as well as in patients with the *PBRM1* mutation vs. in patients without the *PBRM1* mutation ($p = 0.048$; Figure S4D, right). Interestingly, patients with subtype 2 and *PBRM1* mutation showed significantly elevated creatine metabolism. Next, the correlation between creatine metabolism and *GATM* expression levels was tested, revealing that the *GATM* expression had a significantly positive correlation with creatine metabolism (correlation coefficient, r = 0.49, $p = 4.61 \times 10^{-12}$, Figure S4E). Collectively, activation of *GATM* may represent an efficient therapeutic approach for ccRCC harboring the *PBRM1* mutation under ICIs by regulating creatine metabolism to enhance antitumor T cell immunity in the tumor microenvironment.

4. Discussion

This study reports a comprehensive molecular analysis of patients with metastatic ccRCC receiving ICIs to investigate the role of tumor genomic and transcriptomic features in determining the response and survival outcomes following ICIs treatment. Our findings are summarized in Figure 7.

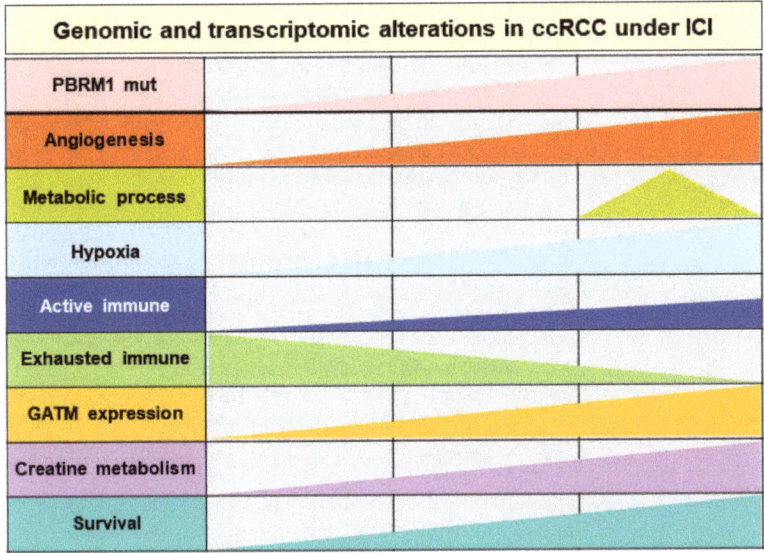

Figure 7. Graphical summary of the dynamics of genomic and transcriptomic aberrations in patients with metastatic clear cell renal cell carcinoma.

The dynamics of genomic and transcriptomic features, including the *PBRM1* mutation, metabolic process, active or exhausted immune types, and *GATM* expression, contributed to the responsiveness and prognosis to immunotherapy in metastatic ccRCC. More importantly, for the first time, we found that *GATM* plays a suppressive role by linking the the *PBRM1* mutation to patients with ccRCC treated with ICIs. Our unsupervised transcriptomic analysis based on signatures related to the the *PBRM1* mutation and *PBRM1* LOF identified three molecular subtypes. This subtyping approach in this study showed concordance with previous reports on gene expression-based subgrouping in large RCC datasets [10,24–26]. Indeed, we found an association between molecular subtypes and differential biological profiles and different prognoses to ICIs in patients with metastatic ccRCC. Patients in subtype 2 demonstrated favorable OS with a higher proportion of them with the *PBRM1* mutation and who are enriched with angiogenesis and metabolic pathways. In contrast, patients in subtypes 1 and 3 showed worse clinical outcomes with a low proportion of them with the *PBRM1* mutation and who are downregulated with angiogenesis signature but upregulated with immune-related and cell-cycle pathways. Overall, the unique features of these subtypes provide their utility in understanding the differential prognosis and responsiveness to ICIs treatment.

One of our key findings is that subtype 2, with a higher proportion of the *PBRM1* mutation, showed enrichment of multiple metabolic pathways, including oxidation and phosphorylation, fatty acid metabolism, adipogenesis, and hypoxia pathways. In fact, hypoxia signaling as a master regulator is associated with the dysregulation of metabolic genes in RCC [27]. Indeed, previous studies have demonstrated that VHL loss and hypoxia-inducible factor stabilization are associated with the reprogramming of metabolic pathways in RCC [28–30]. In summary, our results not only validated previous findings on RCC metabolism but also further explored the metabolic differences among the three subtypes. Interestingly, in-depth transcriptome analysis revealed an unexpected inconsistency between the response to ICIs and immune cell types. Additionally, previous studies demonstrated that *PBRM1* loss shows a nonimmunogenic tumor phenotype associated with ICIs [17], and CD8 T cell infiltration of immunofluorescence in CheckMate025 was not associated with response to PD-1 blockade [4]. Therefore, we investigated whether the association between immune cell types and response to ICIs would be better characterized by considering immune types, including active and exhausted immune subtypes. We found that tumors harboring the the *PBRM1* mutation or molecular subtype 2, which had the best survival outcome, showed a lower percentage of exhausted immune subtype compared to that of tumors with *PBRM1* wild type or subtypes 1 and 3. Previous studies have also shown that high proportion of exhausted immune types in tumor samples results in poor prognosis and an aggressive phenotype [15,31,32]. Taken together, these data suggest that ccRCC tumors can undergo a transition in immune subtypes from active to exhausted types, which may affect the tumor microenvironment to be different response to ICIs.

Moreover, our data indicated that *GATM* is a potential gene-linking *PBRM1* mutation and *PBRM1* LOF. *GATM* encodes glycine amidinotransferase, a mitochondrial enzyme that catalyzes the transfer of guanidinoacetic acid, which is a substrate for creatine synthesis. Interestingly, several studies have demonstrated that creatine inhibits the growth of tumor cells both in vitro and in vivo [22,33,34]. Furthermore, in mouse cancer models, treatment with creatine, either through intraperitoneal injection or through oral administration, effectively suppressed tumor growth, which was associated with a significant reduction in the number of exhausted T cell phenotypes among the tumor-infiltrating $CD8^+$ T cells [22]. The exact mechanism by which creatine or *GATM*-attenuated cancer growth and related to immunotherapy is still unclear; however, a possible tumor-suppressive role of *GATM* was supported by the fact that low expression of *GATM* was associated with poor survival of patients with ccRCC treated with ICIs (as shown in Figure 4D). In addition, the status of GATM protein expression was significantly associated with PFS and OS after ICIs treatment (as shown in Figure 5B). Therefore, the activation of *GATM* has the potential to become an effective approach for enhancing the efficacy of ICIs therapies.

We acknowledged the limitations of the present study. First, the sample size was relatively small, which is the most critical pitfall of our study. To overcome this drawback, data derived from the CheckMate 025 study were merged. Second, a retrospective study was performed and samples were collected; therefore, there was an unavoidable risk of bias, such as selection and misclassification biases. Third, most patients were treated with anti-PD1 monotherapy as a second-line treatment after failure of the first-line targeted therapy. Thus, there was a discrepancy in the time between tumor sampling and anti-PD1 therapy, which means that there was time gap between genomic and/or transcriptomic status and ICIs treatment response status Actually, the population of this study included either first-line therapy (n = 8) or more than second-line treatments that failed withTyrosine Kinase inhibitors (TKIs, n = 52). The selective pressure of multiple lines of TKIs treatment could increase the genomic complexity of tumors and tumor microenvironments, thus influencing responsiveness to ICIs therapy. Fourth, our data were based on WTS analysis, not single-cell sequencing, resulting in a loss of immune cell compartment, which is particularly important for understanding the immune microenvironment and limiting the ability to perform such an immune cell type proportion analysis. Finally, further experiments should be performed to establish causality between the *PBRM1* mutation and *GATM* expression and to determine how *PBRM1-GATM* is involved in the responsiveness to ICIs treatment.

5. Conclusions

This study provides critical insight into genomic and transcriptomic mechanisms such as *PBRM1* mutations, metabolic processes, immune subtypes (active or exhausted), and *GATM* expression that contribute to the response to ICIs therapy in patients with metastatic ccRCC. Moreover, our data underscore the prognostic importance of the *PBRM1* mutation and *GATM* expression in patients with metastatic ccRCC treated with ICIs. Moving forward, it will be important to validate these findings in future clinical trials and to investigate the mechanisms on the interaction between the *PBRM1* mutation and *GATM* expression in the context of ICIs responsiveness.

Supplementary Materials: The following supporting information can be downloaded at: https://www.mdpi.com/article/10.3390/cancers14102354/s1, Figure S1: A heatmap showed up-regulated genes in each subtype; Figure S2: Kaplan-Meier plots for PFS and OS and ssGSEA analysis using HALLMARK gene sets; Figure S3: Kaplan-Meier plots and boxplots based on *GATM* and *USHIC* expressions; Figure S4: Kaplan-Meier plots based on *PBRM1* mutation and *GATM* expression and correlation plot between creatin metabolism and *GATM* expression; Table S1: Baseline clinical characteristics of patients with metastatic renal cell carcinoma (n = 60); Table S2: Baseline outcomes between patients receiving first-line and second-line therapies; Table S3: Upregulated genes in each subtype; Table S4: Clinical features of each subtype.

Author Contributions: Formal analysis, B.J., E.S. and S.-j.B.; resources, S.M.L., J.H.C., W.S., H.H.S., H.G.J., B.C.J., S.I.S., S.S.J., H.M.L. and S.H.P.; data curation, K.P.; writing—original draft preparation, B.J., E.S., S.-j.B. and M.K.; writing—review and editing, B.J. and M.K.; supervision, Y.R.K., W.-Y.P. and M.K.; project administration, M.K.; Funding acquisition, B.J., Y.R.K. and M.K. All authors have read and agreed to the published version of the manuscript.

Funding: This research was supported by the Basic Science Research Program through the National Research Foundation of Korea (NRF) funded by the Ministry of Education (NRF-2018R1A6A3A11046060 and NRF-2021R1I1A1A01040437). This work was also supported by grants from the NRF of Korea funded by the MSIT (NRF-2020R1A2C2007662 and NRF-2020R1C1C1005054). This work was also supported by Hallym University Research Fund (HURF) (no. 2018-30), by research grants from the National R&D Program for Cancer Control, Ministry of Health and Welfare, Republic of Korea (HA17C0039) and the Korea Health Technology R&D Project through the Korea Health Industry Development Institute (KHIDI), funded by the Ministry of Health & Welfare, Republic of Korea (HR20C0025).

Institutional Review Board Statement: The Institutional Review Board of Samsung Medical Center approved the use of human archival tissues for this study (IRB no. SMC 2020-03-063).

Informed Consent Statement: Written informed consent from enrolled patients who were alive during the study period was obtained. Any personal identifiers were removed using an anonymized processing protocol, and all methods used in this study were conducted in accordance with the Declaration of Helsinki guidelines.

Data Availability Statement: Whole transcriptomic sequencing data generated in this study are available from the corresponding author in this study (dr.minyong.kang@gmail.com) upon request.

Acknowledgments: The authors would like to thank the patients and family members who gave their consent on presenting the data in this study, as well as the investigators and research staff involved in this study.

Conflicts of Interest: No potential conflict of interest was reported by the authors.

Abbreviations

ccRCC: clear cell renal cell carcinoma; TCGA: The Cancer Genome Atlas; GSEA: gene set enrichment analysis; ssGSEA: single-sample gene set enrichment analysis; DEG: differentially expressed gene; ES: enrichment score; OS: overall survival; PFS: progression-free survival; ICIs: immune checkpoint inhibitors; PD-1: programmed cell death protein 1; WTS: whole transcriptome sequencing; LOF: loss of function; CB: clinical benefit; NCB: non-clinical benefit.

References

1. Ribas, A.; Wolchok, J.D. Cancer immunotherapy using checkpoint blockade. *Science* **2018**, *359*, 1350–1355. [CrossRef] [PubMed]
2. De Velasco, G.; Miao, D.; Voss, M.H.; Hakimi, A.A.; Hsieh, J.J.; Tannir, N.M.; Tamboli, P.; Appleman, L.J.; Rathmell, W.K.; Van Allen, E.M.; et al. Tumor Mutational Load and Immune Parameters across Metastatic Renal Cell Carcinoma Risk Groups. *Cancer Immunol. Res.* **2016**, *4*, 820–822. [CrossRef] [PubMed]
3. Cristescu, R.; Mogg, R.; Ayers, M.; Albright, A.; Murphy, E.; Yearley, J.; Sher, X.; Liu, X.Q.; Lu, H.; Nebozhyn, M.; et al. Pan-tumor genomic biomarkers for PD-1 checkpoint blockade-based immunotherapy. *Science* **2018**, *362*, eaar3593. [CrossRef] [PubMed]
4. Braun, D.A.; Hou, Y.; Bakouny, Z.; Ficial, M.; Sant' Angelo, M.; Forman, J.; Ross-Macdonald, P.; Berger, A.C.; Jegede, O.A.; Elagina, L.; et al. Interplay of somatic alterations and immune infiltration modulates response to PD-1 blockade in advanced clear cell renal cell carcinoma. *Nat. Med.* **2020**, *26*, 909–918. [CrossRef]
5. Motzer, R.J.; Escudier, B.; McDermott, D.F.; George, S.; Hammers, H.J.; Srinivas, S.; Tykodi, S.S.; Sosman, J.A.; Procopio, G.; Plimack, E.R.; et al. Nivolumab versus Everolimus in Advanced Renal-Cell Carcinoma. *N. Engl. J. Med.* **2015**, *373*, 1803–1813. [CrossRef]
6. Motzer, R.J.; Tannir, N.M.; McDermott, D.F.; Aren Frontera, O.; Melichar, B.; Choueiri, T.K.; Plimack, E.R.; Barthelemy, P.; Porta, C.; George, S.; et al. Nivolumab plus Ipilimumab versus Sunitinib in Advanced Renal-Cell Carcinoma. *N. Engl. J. Med.* **2018**, *378*, 1277–1290. [CrossRef]
7. Rini, B.I.; Plimack, E.R.; Stus, V.; Gafanov, R.; Hawkins, R.; Nosov, D.; Pouliot, F.; Alekseev, B.; Soulieres, D.; Melichar, B.; et al. Pembrolizumab plus Axitinib versus Sunitinib for Advanced Renal-Cell Carcinoma. *N. Engl. J. Med.* **2019**, *380*, 1116–1127. [CrossRef]
8. Xu, W.; Atkins, M.B.; McDermott, D.F. Checkpoint inhibitor immunotherapy in kidney cancer. *Nat. Rev. Urol.* **2020**, *17*, 137–150. [CrossRef]
9. Miao, D.; Margolis, C.A.; Gao, W.; Voss, M.H.; Li, W.; Martini, D.J.; Norton, C.; Bosse, D.; Wankowicz, S.M.; Cullen, D.; et al. Genomic correlates of response to immune checkpoint therapies in clear cell renal cell carcinoma. *Science* **2018**, *359*, 801–806. [CrossRef]
10. Motzer, R.J.; Banchereau, R.; Hamidi, H.; Powles, T.; McDermott, D.; Atkins, M.B.; Escudier, B.; Liu, L.F.; Leng, N.; Abbas, A.R.; et al. Molecular Subsets in Renal Cancer Determine Outcome to Checkpoint and Angiogenesis Blockade. *Cancer Cell* **2020**, *38*, 803–817.e4. [CrossRef]
11. Eisenhauer, E.A.; Therasse, P.; Bogaerts, J.; Schwartz, L.H.; Sargent, D.; Ford, R.; Dancey, J.; Arbuck, S.; Gwyther, S.; Mooney, M.; et al. New response evaluation criteria in solid tumours: Revised RECIST guideline (version 1.1). *Eur. J. Cancer* **2009**, *45*, 228–247. [CrossRef] [PubMed]
12. Liberzon, A.; Birger, C.; Thorvaldsdottir, H.; Ghandi, M.; Mesirov, J.P.; Tamayo, P. The Molecular Signatures Database (MSigDB) hallmark gene set collection. *Cell Syst.* **2015**, *1*, 417–425. [CrossRef]
13. Hanzelmann, S.; Castelo, R.; Guinney, J. GSVA: Gene set variation analysis for microarray and RNA-seq data. *BMC Bioinform.* **2013**, *14*, 7. [CrossRef]
14. Newman, A.M.; Steen, C.B.; Liu, C.L.; Gentles, A.J.; Chaudhuri, A.A.; Scherer, F.; Khodadoust, M.S.; Esfahani, M.S.; Luca, B.A.; Steiner, D.; et al. Determining cell type abundance and expression from bulk tissues with digital cytometry. *Nat. Biotechnol.* **2019**, *37*, 773–782. [CrossRef] [PubMed]
15. Sia, D.; Jiao, Y.; Martinez-Quetglas, I.; Kuchuk, O.; Villacorta-Martin, C.; Castro de Moura, M.; Putra, J.; Camprecios, G.; Bassaganyas, L.; Akers, N.; et al. Identification of an Immune-specific Class of Hepatocellular Carcinoma, Based on Molecular Features. *Gastroenterology* **2017**, *153*, 812–826. [CrossRef] [PubMed]
16. Pena-Llopis, S.; Vega-Rubin-de-Celis, S.; Liao, A.; Leng, N.; Pavia-Jimenez, A.; Wang, S.; Yamasaki, T.; Zhrebker, L.; Sivanand, S.; Spence, P.; et al. BAP1 loss defines a new class of renal cell carcinoma. *Nat. Genet.* **2012**, *44*, 751–759. [CrossRef] [PubMed]
17. Liu, X.D.; Kong, W.; Peterson, C.B.; McGrail, D.J.; Hoang, A.; Zhang, X.; Lam, T.; Pilie, P.G.; Zhu, H.; Beckermann, K.E.; et al. PBRM1 loss defines a nonimmunogenic tumor phenotype associated with checkpoint inhibitor resistance in renal carcinoma. *Nat. Commun.* **2020**, *11*, 2135. [CrossRef]
18. Gao, W.; Li, W.; Xiao, T.; Liu, X.S.; Kaelin, W.G., Jr. Inactivation of the PBRM1 tumor suppressor gene amplifies the HIF-response in VHL-/- clear cell renal carcinoma. *Proc. Natl. Acad. Sci. USA* **2017**, *114*, 1027–1032. [CrossRef]
19. Meng, J.; Lu, X.; Zhou, Y.; Zhang, M.; Ge, Q.; Zhou, J.; Hao, Z.; Gao, S.; Yan, F.; Liang, C. Tumor immune microenvironment-based classifications of bladder cancer for enhancing the response rate of immunotherapy. *Mol. Ther. Oncolytics* **2021**, *20*, 410–421. [CrossRef]

20. Meng, J.; Zhou, Y.; Lu, X.; Bian, Z.; Chen, Y.; Zhou, J.; Zhang, L.; Hao, Z.; Zhang, M.; Liang, C. Immune response drives outcomes in prostate cancer: Implications for immunotherapy. *Mol. Oncol.* **2021**, *15*, 1358–1375. [CrossRef]
21. Piva, F.; Santoni, M.; Matrana, M.R.; Satti, S.; Giulietti, M.; Occhipinti, G.; Massari, F.; Cheng, L.; Lopez-Beltran, A.; Scarpelli, M.; et al. BAP1, PBRM1 and SETD2 in clear-cell renal cell carcinoma: Molecular diagnostics and possible targets for personalized therapies. *Expert Rev. Mol. Diagn.* **2015**, *15*, 1201–1210. [CrossRef] [PubMed]
22. Di Biase, S.; Ma, X.; Wang, X.; Yu, J.; Wang, Y.C.; Smith, D.J.; Zhou, Y.; Li, Z.; Kim, Y.J.; Clarke, N.; et al. Creatine uptake regulates CD8 T cell antitumor immunity. *J. Exp. Med.* **2019**, *216*, 2869–2882. [CrossRef] [PubMed]
23. Miller, E.E.; Evans, A.E.; Cohn, M. Inhibition of rate of tumor growth by creatine and cyclocreatine. *Proc. Natl. Acad. Sci. USA* **1993**, *90*, 3304–3308. [CrossRef] [PubMed]
24. Beuselinck, B.; Job, S.; Becht, E.; Karadimou, A.; Verkarre, V.; Couchy, G.; Giraldo, N.; Rioux-Leclercq, N.; Molinie, V.; Sibony, M.; et al. Molecular subtypes of clear cell renal cell carcinoma are associated with sunitinib response in the metastatic setting. *Clin. Cancer Res.* **2015**, *21*, 1329–1339. [CrossRef] [PubMed]
25. Brannon, A.R.; Reddy, A.; Seiler, M.; Arreola, A.; Moore, D.T.; Pruthi, R.S.; Wallen, E.M.; Nielsen, M.E.; Liu, H.; Nathanson, K.L.; et al. Molecular Stratification of Clear Cell Renal Cell Carcinoma by Consensus Clustering Reveals Distinct Subtypes and Survival Patterns. *Genes Cancer* **2010**, *1*, 152–163. [CrossRef] [PubMed]
26. Hakimi, A.A.; Voss, M.H.; Kuo, F.; Sanchez, A.; Liu, M.; Nixon, B.G.; Vuong, L.; Ostrovnaya, I.; Chen, Y.B.; Reuter, V.; et al. Transcriptomic Profiling of the Tumor Microenvironment Reveals Distinct Subgroups of Clear Cell Renal Cell Cancer: Data from a Randomized Phase III Trial. *Cancer Discov.* **2019**, *9*, 510–525. [CrossRef]
27. Bacigalupa, Z.A.; Rathmell, W.K. Beyond glycolysis: Hypoxia signaling as a master regulator of alternative metabolic pathways and the implications in clear cell renal cell carcinoma. *Cancer Lett.* **2020**, *489*, 19–28. [CrossRef]
28. Hakimi, A.A.; Reznik, E.; Lee, C.H.; Creighton, C.J.; Brannon, A.R.; Luna, A.; Aksoy, B.A.; Liu, E.M.; Shen, R.; Lee, W.; et al. An Integrated Metabolic Atlas of Clear Cell Renal Cell Carcinoma. *Cancer Cell* **2016**, *29*, 104–116. [CrossRef]
29. Linehan, W.M.; Schmidt, L.S.; Crooks, D.R.; Wei, D.; Srinivasan, R.; Lang, M.; Ricketts, C.J. The Metabolic Basis of Kidney Cancer. *Cancer Discov.* **2019**, *9*, 1006–1021. [CrossRef]
30. Pandey, N.; Lanke, V.; Vinod, P.K. Network-based metabolic characterization of renal cell carcinoma. *Sci. Rep.* **2020**, *10*, 5955. [CrossRef]
31. Chen, Y.P.; Wang, Y.Q.; Lv, J.W.; Li, Y.Q.; Chua, M.L.K.; Le, Q.T.; Lee, N.; Colevas, A.D.; Seiwert, T.; Hayes, D.N.; et al. Identification and validation of novel microenvironment-based immune molecular subgroups of head and neck squamous cell carcinoma: Implications for immunotherapy. *Ann. Oncol.* **2019**, *30*, 68–75. [CrossRef] [PubMed]
32. Jee, B.A.; Choi, J.H.; Rhee, H.; Yoon, S.; Kwon, S.M.; Nahm, J.H.; Yoo, J.E.; Jeon, Y.; Choi, G.H.; Woo, H.G.; et al. Dynamics of Genomic, Epigenomic, and Transcriptomic Aberrations during Stepwise Hepatocarcinogenesis. *Cancer Res.* **2019**, *79*, 5500–5512. [CrossRef] [PubMed]
33. Fairman, C.M.; Kendall, K.L.; Hart, N.H.; Taaffe, D.R.; Galvao, D.A.; Newton, R.U. The potential therapeutic effects of creatine supplementation on body composition and muscle function in cancer. *Crit. Rev. Oncol. Hematol.* **2019**, *133*, 46–57. [CrossRef] [PubMed]
34. Li, B.; Yang, L. Creatine in T Cell Antitumor Immunity and Cancer Immunotherapy. *Nutrients* **2021**, *13*, 1633. [CrossRef] [PubMed]

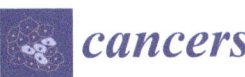

Review

Prognostic Factors for Localized Clear Cell Renal Cell Carcinoma and Their Application in Adjuvant Therapy

Kalle E. Mattila [1],*, Paula Vainio [2] and Panu M. Jaakkola [1]

[1] Department of Oncology and Radiotherapy, FICAN West Cancer Centre, University of Turku, Turku University Hospital, Hämeentie 11, 20521 Turku, Finland; panu.jaakkola@tyks.fi
[2] Department of Pathology, University of Turku, Turku University Hospital, Hämeentie 11, 20521 Turku, Finland; paula.vainio@tyks.fi
* Correspondence: kalle.mattila@tyks.fi; Tel.: +358-2-3130000

Simple Summary: Approximately one fifth of patients with newly diagnosed renal cell carcinoma (RCC) present with metastatic disease and over one third of the remaining patients with localized RCC will eventually have metastases spread to distant sites after complete resection of the primary tumor in the kidney. Usually, disease recurrence is observed within the first five years of follow-up, but late recurrences after five years are seen in up to 10% of patients. Despite novel biomarkers, simple histopathological factors, such as tumor size, tumor grade, and tumor extension into the blood vessels or beyond the kidney, are still valid features in predicting the risk of disease recurrence after surgery. The optimal set of prognostic factors remains unclear. The results from ongoing placebo-controlled adjuvant therapy trials may elucidate prognostic features that help to define high-risk patients for disease recurrence.

Abstract: Approximately 20% of patients with renal cell carcinoma (RCC) present with primarily metastatic disease and over 30% of patients with localized RCC will develop distant metastases later, after complete resection of the primary tumor. Accurate postoperative prognostic models are essential for designing personalized surveillance programs, as well as for designing adjuvant therapy and trials. Several clinical and histopathological prognostic factors have been identified and adopted into prognostic algorithms to assess the individual risk for disease recurrence after radical or partial nephrectomy. However, the prediction accuracy of current prognostic models has been studied in retrospective patient cohorts and the optimal set of prognostic features remains unclear. In addition to traditional histopathological prognostic factors, novel biomarkers, such as gene expression profiles and circulating tumor DNA, are extensively studied to supplement existing prognostic algorithms to improve their prediction accuracy. Here, we aim to give an overview of existing prognostic features and prediction models for localized postoperative clear cell RCC and discuss their role in the adjuvant therapy trials. The results of ongoing placebo-controlled adjuvant therapy trials may elucidate prognostic factors and biomarkers that help to define patients at high risk for disease recurrence.

Keywords: adjuvant therapy; clear cell renal cell carcinoma; biomarker; prediction model; prognostic factor

1. Introduction

Renal cell carcinoma (RCC) is the third most common newly diagnosed urogenital cancer after prostate and bladder cancer. In 2020, the number of new kidney cancer diagnoses was over 400,000 and it caused nearly 180,000 deaths worldwide [1]. The most prevalent histological subtype, clear cell renal cell carcinoma (ccRCC), accounts for 75–80% of all RCCs and has been associated with inferior survival compared to papillary (10–15%) and chromophobe (5%) RCCs [2]. Localized RCC can be treated with curative intent by radical (RN) or partial nephrectomy (PN). PN is preferred for smaller tumors (T1–2N0M0) if technically feasible without compromising the oncological outcome of surgery (negative surgical margins). Small renal tumors might be eligible for radiofrequency ablation. Lymph node dissection (LND) is not routinely performed unless there is a suspicion of metastatic lymph nodes preoperatively or during surgery. If macrovascular invasion is present, tumor thrombus is removed from the renal and caval vein during surgery [3,4].

Unfortunately, approximately 20% of RCC patients present with primarily metastatic disease and over one third of patients will eventually develop distant metastases [5]. Despite recent advances in the medical treatment of advanced RCC (antiangiogenic receptor tyrosine kinase inhibitors (TKI), immune checkpoint inhibitors (ICI) and TKI–ICI combinations), metastatic disease will, in most cases, lead to death. Individualized, risk-based, regular imaging follow-up after surgery for localized RCC for at least five years with thoracic and abdominal CT is recommended to detect disease progression (local recurrence or distant metastases) early. If detected early with few or solitary metastases, the patient may still be curable surgically or with high-dose radiation therapy and may be eligible for oncologic therapies [3,4]. The aim of this review is to provide an overview of the clinical prognostic models for localized ccRCC. Understanding the risk of disease progression after surgery of localized disease is essential for designing postoperative follow-up as well as for designing adjuvant drug trials in localized ccRCC.

2. Histopathological and Clinical Prognostic Factors for Localized ccRCC

The TNM classification of malignant tumors (American Joint Committee on Cancer (AJCC)) has been used since 1977 as a prognostic staging system for multiple solid tumors [6]. The staging of renal cell carcinoma based on pathologic examination and radiological imaging provides crucial prognostic information. Stage I (T1N0M0: tumor $\leq$ 7 cm) and stage II (T2N0M0: tumor > 7 cm) tumors are limited to the kidney, whereas stage III (T3N0, T1–3N1: tumor invades renal vein, perinephric tissues, or presents with regional lymph node metastases) and stage IV (T4N_{any}M0, $T_{any}N_{any}$M1: tumor extends beyond Gerota fascia or presents with distant metastases) tumors extend beyond the kidney [7]. In 1993–2004, 54.7%, 10.6%, 16.1%, and 18.6% of ccRCC tumors in the National Cancer Database were classified as stage I, II, III, and IV, respectively [8]. Stage I and II RCCs had significantly better 5-year survival rates (90.4% and 83.4%) compared to stage III and stage IV RCCs (66.0% and 9.1%) [8]. In a 2004–2015 Surveillance, Epidemiology, and End Results (SEER) database cohort (77% had ccRCC), the pathologic TNM stage was I (64.3%), II (10.9%), III (16.8%), and IV (8%) and the 5-year survival rates after nephrectomy were 97.4%, 89.9%, 77.9%, and 26.7% for stage I, II, III, and IV RCCs, respectively [9]. The proportion of stage I tumors has increased, probably due to the incidental detection of small renal tumors in abdominal imaging studies [8]. The increase in the survival rate of stage III and IV tumors is probably driven by VEGF-targeted TKI therapies introduced in the treatment of advanced RCC in the 2000s.

2.1. Microscopical Histopathological Prognostic Factors

In addition to the TNM stage, several histopathological factors affect the prognosis of localized ccRCC patients. Numerous tumor grading systems have been introduced to assess the histological differentiation of RCC cells. The Fuhrman and the WHO/ISUP grading systems are the most widely used. In 1982, Fuhrman developed a four-tiered grading system that is based on the assessment of nuclear size, nuclear shape, and nucleolar prominence. The estimated 5-year survival rate of RCC patients was 64% (grade I), 34% (grade II), 31% (grade III), and 10% (grade IV) [10]. In 2012, the International Society of Urological Pathology reformed the four-tiered grading system based on the prominence of nucleoli (grades 1–3) and grade 4 tumors showing extreme tumor nuclear pleomorphism, giant cells, or sarcomatoid/rhabdoid dedifferentiation [11].

Approximately 5% of RCCs undergo epithelial to mesenchymal transition and present with sarcomatoid differentiation, and sarcomatoid features have been observed in clear cell, papillary, and chromophobe RCCs [12]. Sarcomatoid morphology is associated with more aggressive cancer behavior: sarcomatoid RCCs (sRCCs) often present with a bulky primary tumor (higher size and stage) and higher tumor grade [12–14]. Metastases are seen in as much as 60–80% of newly diagnosed cases [12] and close to 80% of patients with localized sarcomatoid RCC have been observed to develop disease recurrence within two years after nephrecotomy [15,16]. Sarcomatoid RCCs have unfavorable prognosis compared to ccRCCs regardless of tumor stage: 5-year cancer-specific mortality estimates were 32%, 63%, and 82% for stage I–II, III, and IV sRCCs, compared to 6%, 20%, and 64% for stage I–II, III, and IV ccRCC patients [14].

Tumor necrosis is another established adverse histological feature in RCC. It is associated with a larger tumor size, higher grade, and higher proliferative activity, and it is considered to indicate biologically aggressive tumor behavior [17,18]. The presence of tumor necrosis has been reported in 21–32% of ccRCCs [19,20] and it has also been associated with inferior survival outcomes in multiple studies [20–25]. The combination of WHO/ISUP grading and tumor necrosis outperformed WHO/ISUP grading after adjusting for TNM stage. Researchers observed that the presence of tumor necrosis affected the prognosis, especially in WHO/ISUP grade 3 tumors. The 10-year cancer-specific survival was 62% in grade 3 tumors without necrosis but only 30% in grade 3 tumors with necrosis [26].

RCCs are highly vascularized, and microscopic vascular invasion is observed in 5.6–45% of tumors [19]. Tumor cells can spread via blood and lymph vessels to distant sites (lungs, bones, liver, etc.) and lymph nodes. Microvascular invasion is defined as tumor cells within small vessels in the tumor pseudocapsule, tumor, or renal parenchyma adjacent to the tumor [27]. Microvascular invasion (MVI) was more commonly present in ccRCC (29%) than in non-ccRCC (12%) and it was associated with metastatic spread and inferior survival in ccRCC patients [28]. MVI was found to be associated with a larger tumor size, higher Fuhrman grade, more advanced T stage, the presence of lymph node and distant metastases, as well as a shorter survival time in univariate but not in multivariate analysis [29]. In another cohort of RCC patients (93% had ccRCC), MVI was observed to correlate with metastases and shorter disease-free survival as well as cancer-specific survival [30].

Partial nephrectomy (PN) is the standard of treatment for small renal tumors if technically feasible. Positive surgical margins (PSM) have been observed in up to 18% of patients after surgery for localized RCC [31–34]. However, the effect of PSM on oncologic outcomes (recurrence-free and cancer-specific survival) is controversial. Local tumor recurrence in the surgical bed is uncommon. In a retrospective study, local tumor bed recurrence was found in only 1.9% of patients who underwent PN, and PSM were found in 15.9% of patients with local tumor bed recurrence, compared to 3% in the control group [35]. However, PSM is more common in patients with other adverse features (higher tumor stage, grade, multiple tumors, solitary kidney) and local recurrences are also observed in patients with negative surgical margins [32,33,35]. Therefore, imaging surveillance is preferred over radical nephrectomy in patients with PSM after PN.

2.2. Macroscopical Histopathological Prognostic Factors

Tumor extension into perirenal tissues, renal vein, and regional lymph nodes might be discovered in preoperative radiological imaging or during surgery but sometimes only after microscopical evaluation of resected tumor and regional lymph nodes. Tumor invasion into perirenal tissues (perirenal fat, renal sinus fat) or macrovascular invasion into the renal vein and inferior vena cava (IVC) or local lymph nodes (T3N0, T1–3N1, stage III) lead to inferior oncologic outcomes compared to stage I and II tumors [8,9]. Perinephric fat, renal sinus fat, and renal vein invasion were present in 26%, 9%, and 29% of T3a tumors and patients with multiple extrarenal extensions had inferior progression-free and overall survival [36]. The association of concomitant fat invasion and renal vein invasion with poorer cancer-specific survival has also been observed in other studies [37–39]. Upper pole RCCs may invade directly into the adrenal gland. These tumors are classified as T4 as well as tumors extending beyond Gerota's fascia, leading to worse oncologic outcomes compared to T1–3N0/Nx tumors [8,9].

Tumor extension into the renal vein and inferior vena cava has been observed in 23% and 7–13% of patients, respectively [40,41]. Patients with venous invasion had significantly shorter survival compared to tumors limited to the kidney [41]. The Mayo Clinic's thrombus classification is commonly used to classify the level of tumor extension into the IVC [42]. The prognostic significance of the tumor thrombus level is controversial. In a retrospective multicenter evaluation of tumor thrombus level, 78%, 16%, and 5% of the patients had tumor extension into the renal vein, IVC below diaphragm, and above diaphragm, respectively [43]. The level of tumor thrombus in the IVC (below or above diaphragm) was not statistically significantly associated with the survival time, but patients with tumor thrombus in the IVC had shorter survival (18–26 months) compared to patients with tumor thrombus in the renal vein (52 months) [41,43]. In another multicenter study (89.9% had ccRCC), a higher tumor thrombus level was independently associated with shorter cancer-specific survival [44]. Notably, the patients in these studies were treated before modern TKI and ICI therapies. In a contemporary analysis of 6340 patients who underwent surgery for localized RCC (93.4% had ccRCC), only 3.6% of the patients had venous tumor thrombus and the level of thrombus was not associated with the risk of recurrence or death [45].

Lymph node dissection (LND) is not routinely performed during nephrectomy unless there is a suspicion of metastatic lymph nodes preoperatively or during surgery, and local lymph node status usually remains unknown (Nx). LND has not proven therapeutic but is a prognostic procedure to assess metastatic spread to regional (hilar, abdominal, para-aortic, and para caval) lymph nodes. In the SEER database analysis, 24.8% of patients (59.4% had ccRCC) underwent lymph node dissection (LND) and metastatic lymph nodes were observed in 17.1% (9.3% of T2 and 21.6% of T3) of the patients who underwent LND [46]. In another study, local lymph node metastases were present in 11% of non-metastatic RCC patients (90.7% had ccRCC) who underwent nephrectomy [47]. The patients with regional lymph node metastases (T1–3N1) have as poor survival as stage IV patients [47,48]. The 5-year survival rates were 61.9%, 22.7%, and 15.6% for stage III lymph node negative, stage III lymph node positive, and stage IV patients, respectively (78.1% had ccRCC) [48].

3. Prognostic Models for Localized RCC

There are several postoperative prognostic models to assess the risk of RCC recurrence or death after surgery of localized RCC based on histopathological features, such as TNM stage, tumor size, tumor grade, coagulative necrosis, and microvascular invasion, and clinical manifestations, such as symptoms of the disease. Kattan et al. introduced the first nomogram in 2001 to assess the risk of disease recurrence for localized RCC [49], followed by the UISS, the SSIGN, the Cindolo, the Leibovich, the Sorbellini, and the Karakiewicz algorithms [50–55]. There are differences in the required prediction features and the prediction outcomes between these models. The majority (88–100%) of the patients included in these models have had clear cell RCC, although the Kattan, the UISS, the Cindolo, and the Karakiewicz models also included patients with papillary and chromophobe RCC. Because of marked differences in the histopathology and prognosis of clear cell, papillary, and chromophobe RCC subtypes, similar prediction models may not be optimal for different histological subtypes. Grading of chromophobe carcinoma is not recommended [19,27], which limits eligible prediction models for this subtype. Leibovich et al. introduced different algorithms for each histological subtype, aiming to improve the prediction accuracy. The study cohort included 75% clear cell, 17% papillary, and 6% chromophobe RCC patients [56]. Recently, Mattila et al. developed a prediction model for localized ccRCC that comprised only three features and included an easy-to-use nomogram for clinicians [57]. The properties of different prognostic models for localized RCC are described in Table 1.

Table 1. Postoperative prognostic models for localized RCC.

Reference	RCC Subtype	Prediction Outcome	Number of Risk Groups	Prediction Features	Number of Patients
Kattan (2001) [49]	Clear Cell, Papillary, and Chromophobe RCC	Recurrence-Free Survival	Not Defined	Symptoms (Incidental, Local, Systemic), Histology, Tumor Size, 1997 T Stage	612
UISS (2001) [50]	Clear Cell, Papillary, and Chromophobe RCC	Overall Survival	5	1997 TNM Stage, Fuhrman Grade, ECOG Performance Status	661
SSIGN (2002) [51]	Clear Cell RCC	Cancer-Specific Survival	10	1997 TNM Stage, Tumor Size (<5 cm, ≥5 cm), Tumor Grade, Necrosis	1801
Cindolo (2003) [52]	Clear Cell, Papillary, and Chromophobe RCC	Recurrence-Free Survival	Not Defined	Symptoms (Asymptomatic, Symptomatic), Tumor Size	660
Leibovich (2003) [53]	Clear Cell RCC	Metastasis-Free Survival	8 (0–2 low, 3–5 Intermediate, ≥6 High)	2002 TNM Stage, Regional Lymph Node Involvement	479
Sorbellini MSKCC (2005) [54]	Clear Cell RCC	Recurrence-Free Survival	Not Defined	Tumor Size, 2002 TNM Stage, Fuhrman Grade, Necrosis, Microvascular Invasion, Presentation (Incidental, Local Symptoms, Systemic Symptoms)	701 + Validation Cohort 200
Karakiewicz (2007) [55]	Clear Cell, Papillary, and Chromophobe RCC	Cancer-Specific Survival	Not Defined	2002 TNM Stage, Tumor Size, Fuhrman Grade, Symptoms (Non, Local, Systemic)	2530 + Validation Cohort 1377
Leibovich (2018) [56]	Clear Cell, Papillary, and Chromophobe RCC	Progression-Free and Cancer-Specific Survival	19	Constitutional Symptoms (Yes, No), Tumor Grade, Coagulative Necrosis, Sarcomatoid Differentiation, Tumor Size, Perinephric or Renal Sinus Fat Invasion, Tumor Thrombus Level, Extension Beyond Kidney, and Nodal Involvement	3633
Mattila (2021) [57]	Clear Cell RCC	Metastasis-Free Survival	3 (Low, Intermediate, High)	Tumor Size, Fuhrman Grade, Microvascular Invasion	196 + Validation Cohort 714

The prediction accuracy (concordance index, C-index) of these prognostic models had exceeded 0.8: SSIGN 0.82–0.84 [51], Leibovich 2003 0.82, Sorbellini 0.82, Leibovich 2018 0.83–0.86, Mattila 0.76–0.84. However, these prediction models are based on the analysis of retrospective patient cohorts. A prospective validation of prediction models in a cohort of 1647 nonmetastatic (≥T1b grade 3–4 or $T_{any}N1M0$) ccRCC patients enrolled in a sorafenib adjuvant therapy trial (ASSURE) resulted in considerably lower C-indices (0.57–0.69) for the UISS, SSIGN, Leibovich 2003, Kattan, MSKCC, Yayciogly, Karakiewicz, Cindolo, and 2002 TNM staging systems. All models demonstrated the best prediction accuracy during the first two years of follow-up after surgery [58]. Higher prediction accuracy for the first two years of follow-up was also found when comparing the Mattila and the Leibovich 2003 models: C-indices were 0.81–0.88 (Mattila) and 0.76–0.88 (Leibovich 2003) during 0–24 months and 0.78–0.84 (Mattila) and 0.71–0.82 (Leibovich 2003) during 24–90 months [57]. Late disease recurrence after 5 years of follow-up has been observed in 5–11% of patients with localized RCC [59], and the prediction of these late events remains imprecise with present prognostic models [58].

4. Current Applications of Biomarkers in Localized RCC

While current clinical prognostic models do not use any genetic or other biomarkers, several genetic alterations have been described for RCC. In ccRCC, the inactivation of the von Hippel–Lindau (VHL) gene is the best-described and most widely occurring genetic change seen in most sporadic ccRCCs. The inactivation of the VHL tumor suppressor can occur by numerous point mutations (over 150 described) or by suppressing transcription by methylation of the promoter areas. The inactivation of VHL function results in the activation of hypoxia-inducible transcription factors (HIF-1a and -2a) of the cellular oxygen sensing pathway, leading to the up- or downregulation of over 300 genes. These include the upregulation of proangiogenic genes, such as vascular endothelial growth factor (VEGF) [60]. In particular, HIF-2a has been shown to drive a more aggressive phenotype in ccRCC [61,62]. Since VHL inactivation has been detected from 80% to nearly all ccRCCs and is the first and universal genetic alteration in ccRCC [63,64], it does not function as a prognostic factor.

Further analyses of tumor mutations and gene expression profiles have revealed genetic features associated with prognosis in localized ccRCC. In addition to loss of VHL function, mutations in tumor suppressor genes PBRM1, BAP1, and SETD2, which function as chromatin and histone modifiers, and the PI3K/AKT pathway have been identified in nephrectomy specimens included in the Cancer Genome Atlas [65,66]. PBRM1 and BAP1 mutations have been associated with unfavorable prognosis in ccRCC [67,68]. Patients with PBMR1 or BAP1 loss had increased risk of death from RCC but it was not statistically significant after adjusting for the SSIGN score [67]. The association of gene expression profiles and RCC survival has been studied widely. A scoring system based on 16 genes discovered in gene expression analysis was observed to predict disease recurrence in localized clear cell RCCs that were stratified by stage and adjusted for tumor size, tumor grade, and the Leibovich score [69], and its prognostic ability has been validated among stage III ccRCC patients in the sunitinib adjuvant therapy trial [70]. Another gene expression signature biomarker (ClearCode34) was developed to classify good- and poor-risk clear cell RCCs and was significantly associated with RFS, OS, and CSS [71]. The cell cycle proliferation (CCP) score assay, which measures the activation of 31 genes involved in cellular proliferation, was observed to be an independent predictor of disease recurrence after nephrectomy in 565 localized RCC patients (81% ccRCC) and it outperformed the prediction accuracy of the Karakiewicz nomogram (C-index 0.87 vs. 0.84) [72].

Cell-free circulating tumor DNA (ctDNA) is a potential prognostic biomarker in multiple cancer types. Fragments of tumor DNA are released into circulation after tumor cell death and by active secretion. ctDNA can be detected from body fluids (plasma, pleural effusion, ascites, cerebrospinal fluid, and urine) with multiple methods, including polymerase chain reaction-based assays, such as droplet digital PCR (ddPCR), or next-generation DNA sequencing (NGS) [73]. Plasma or urine samples containing ctDNA fragments are easy to collect and liquid biopsy is particularly valuable when invasive tumor biopsy is not feasible or there is only a limited amount of tumor tissue available. Moreover, ctDNA may reflect heterogeneous tumor mutations better than single-site tumor biopsy and reveal therapeutically actionable mutations. Elevated ctDNA levels may reveal disease recurrence/progression before radiologically detected disease progression and thus molecular residual disease is a compelling biomarker to monitor disease recurrence after radical surgery for the primary tumor. Detectable ctDNA (molecular residual disease) has been shown to predict disease recurrence after radical surgery for localized cancer in multiple tumor types, including melanoma [74,75], colorectal cancer [76,77], and NSCLC [78,79].

Interestingly, detectable plasma ctDNA was found to be a predictive biomarker for adjuvant atezolizumab therapy after surgery of urothelial carcinoma [80]. However, a sufficient amount of ctDNA has to be present to cross the detection limit.

CtDNA has also been analyzed from plasma and urine samples of RCC patients, although studies are still scarce compared to NSCLC, colorectal cancer, melanoma, and urothelial cancer, and have mostly been done in metastatic RCC patients. Patients with metastatic ccRCC had higher plasma levels of cell-free DNA compared to localized ccRCC and healthy control patients, and higher plasma cell-free DNA levels predicted disease recurrence after nephrectomy [81]. Untargeted sequencing methods revealed detectable ctDNA in plasma or urine samples of 30–40% of RCC patients with localized and metastatic disease, and detectable ctDNA in plasma, but not in urine, was more common in patients with larger tumors and with venous tumor thrombus [82]. The rate of detectable ctDNA in RCC patients has varied markedly based on the method used (NGS panel) and patient cohort (localized or metastatic). Targeted analysis of ctDNA using an RCC-targeted NGS panel (including BAP1, KDM5C, MET, MTOR, PBRM1, PIK3CA, PTEN, SETD2, TP53, and VHL genes) revealed detectable plasma ctDNA in only 18.6% of the patients (mostly metastatic ccRCC) [82]. CtDNA analysis of plasma samples from 220 patients with metastatic RCC with a 74-gene panel revealed genomic alterations in 79% of the patients. The most frequently observed mutations included TP53 (35%), VHL (23%), EGFR (17%), NF1 (16%), and ARID1A (12%) [83]. In a smaller series of metastatic RCC patients (76% ccRCC), 18/34 (53%) of the patients had detectable plasma ctDNA and it was associated with tumor burden (the sum of longest diameter of all measurable lesions) but not with IMDC risk groups or tumor histology [84].

Upregulated programmed death ligand-1 (PD-L1 or B7-H1) expression on the surface of tumor cells is an important mechanism of tumor immune evasion. The interaction of PD-L1 and PD-1 receptors in tumor-infiltrating lymphocytes (especially cytotoxic T cells) hampers the immune response against cancer cells [85]. Although different studies have used variable methods to define PD-L1 positivity in RCC (different antibodies in immunohistochemistry, tumor cell or immune cell positivity, positivity cut-off %), PD-L1 expression has unequivocally been an adverse prognostic feature. PD-L1 expression can be found in tumor cells and in tumor-infiltrating lymphocytes (TILs) and both features have been associated with inferior survival in RCC [86]. PD-L1-positive tumor cells have been observed in 20–24% of ccRCCs and the 5-year cancer-specific survival rate of these patients was 42–47%, compared to 66–83% in PD-L1-negative patients [87,88].

In addition to a higher stage and higher tumor grade, sRCCs are found to have increased PD-L1 expression compared to ccRCCs. Genomic amplifications at 9p24.1 are more frequently found in sRCC tumors (6%) compared to ccRCC tumors (0.6%). These amplifications included JAK2, PD-L1, and PD-L2 genes, leading to upregulated PD-L1 expression [89]. In the IMmotion151 trial evaluating bevacizumab and atezolizumab vs. sunitinb in first-line metastatic RCC patients, sarcomatoid features were found in 16% (142/915) of patients. In addition, 61% of sarcomatoid RCCs (86/142) were PD-L1-positive ($\geq$1% tumor-infiltrating immune cells positive), compared to 40% of PD-L1-positive cases among all study patients (362/915) [90,91]. In the CheckMate 214 trial evaluating ipilimumab and nivolumab vs. sunitinib in treatment-naive metastatic ccRCC patients, 13% of all patients (145/1096) had sarcomatoid features and only 4% (6/145) had an IMDC favorable risk score. Of 139 sRCC patients with IMDC intermediate or poor risk scores, 50% were PD-L1-positive ($\geq$1% tumor cells positive), compared to 26% of all IMDC intermediate- or poor-risk patients [92]. This feature renders sRCCs more susceptible to ICI than to antiangiogenic TKI therapies, and the introduction of ICI has significantly improved treatment outcomes in patients with advanced sRCC [90,92].

In addition to gene expression profiles, ctDNA, and PD-L1 expression levels, the prognostic ability of epigenetic biomarkers, such as DNA methylation, expression of microRNAs, and long noncoding RNA, is being studied. Cell-free DNA methylation analysis from plasma and urine samples has been introduced as a potential method detect early-stage RCC patients from among healthy control patients [93]. However, none of these biomarkers are yet recommended in the international RCC guidelines [4,94], nor have they been adopted into widespread clinical use. The aim of future studies is to supplement current prognostic algorithms with novel biomarkers to improve their prediction accuracy and validate these findings in independent patient cohorts.

5. Prognostic Markers and Adjuvant Therapies for Localized ccRCC

The efficacy of antiangiogenic TKI therapies and immune checkpoint inhibitors (ICI) in the treatment of advanced ccRCC has led to adjuvant therapy trials aiming to reduce the risk of disease recurrence and improve the overall survival (OS) of patients with localized RCC after radical or partial nephrectomy. Before TKI and ICI therapies, cytokines (interferon-alpha and high-dose interleukin-2) showed modest clinical activity (response rates of 15–31%) in stage IV RCC [95] and were also studied in the adjuvant setting. However, cytokine and tumor vaccine adjuvant therapy trials failed to improve recurrence-free and overall survival [94–98].

The next attempt to improve RFS and OS was made with VEGF-targeted TKI adjuvant therapies. Five large, prospective, multicenter trials with sunitinib (S-TRAC), sunitinib and sorafenib (ASSURE), pazopanib (PROTECT), axitinib (ATLAS), and sorafenib (SORCE) were conducted [99–103]. The design of adjuvant therapy trials and results are described in Table 2. There were various inclusion criteria for intermediate- and high-risk patients and the proportion of higher-risk ($\geq$T3 or N1) patients was different across these adjuvant trials. The inclusion criteria for the S-TRAC trial were modified from the UISS criteria (T3N0M0 Fuhrman grade $\geq$ 2 and ECOG performance status $\geq$ 1, T4N0M0 any Fuhrman grade, any ECOG PS, or T_{any}N1-2M0). The ASSURE and the PROTECT trials required Fuhrman grade $\geq$ 3 for lower-risk (T1b-T2) tumors, whereas the ATLAS trial included >T2 tumors regardless of Fuhrman grade. The SORCE trial was the only trial that directly adopted the existing prognostic algorithm (the Leibovich score (2003)) for classifying patients into intermediate- (3–5 points) or high-risk (6–11 points) groups for disease recurrence. The proportion of lower-risk patients (T1-2, stage I and II) ranged from 11% to 35% in the ATLAS, PROTECT, ASSURE, and SORCE trials [100–103].

Table 2. The results from phase III randomized adjuvant TKI and ICI trials in RCC.

Trial	Treatment	Inclusion Criteria	Median DFS/HR of Disease Recurrence or Death	Discontinuation Rate Due to AE/(AE + Patient Withdrawal) [#]
S-TRAC [99]	Sunitinib vs. Placebo 12 Months	$\geq$T3N0 (gr $\geq$ 2, ECOG $\geq$ 1) or T_{any}N1	6.8 Years, HR 0.76 (0.59–0.98) vs. 5.6 Years	28% vs. 6%
ASSURE [100]	Sunitinib vs. Sorafenib vs. Placebo 12 Months	$\geq$T1b (gr 3–4) N0 or T_{any}N1	5.8 Years, HR 1.17 (0.90–1.52) vs. 6.1 Years, HR 0.97 (0.75–1.28) vs. 6.6. Years	44% [#] vs. 45% [#] vs. 11% [#]
PROTECT [101]	Pazopanib vs. Placebo 12 Months	T2 (gr 3–4) N0, T3–4N0, or T_{any}N1	HR 0.86 (0.70–1.06)	35% vs. 5%
ATLAS [102]	Axitinib vs. Placebo 12–36 Months	$\geq$T2N0 or T_{any}N1	HR 0.87 (0.660–1.147)	23% vs. 11%
SORCE [103]	Sorafenib 12 Months vs. Sorafenib 36 Months vs. Placebo	Intermediate Risk (Score 3–5) or High Risk (Score $\geq$ 6) According to Leibovich (2003)	HR 0.94 (0.77–1.14) Sorafenib 12 Months vs. Placebo HR 1.01 (0.82–1.23) Sorafenib 36 Months vs. Placebo	44% [#] vs. 49% [#] vs. 12%
KEYNOTE-564 [104]	Pembrolizumab vs. Placebo 12 Months	T2 (gr 3–4 or Sarcomatoid) N0, T3–4N0, T_{any}N1, or Resected M1	HR 0.68 (0.53–0.87)	21% vs. 2%

[#] indicates AE + patient withdrawal.

All adjuvant TKI trials were placebo-controlled and aimed to show the DFS benefit, but only S-TRAC yielded a positive result, with a 1.2-year improvement in the DFS of the sunitinib arm. Tumor cell PD-L1 expression was not statistically significantly associated with DFS, whereas high tumor CD8+ T-cell density was predictive for longer DFS in the sunitinib arm of the S-TRAC trial [105]. The S-TRAC, PROTECT, and ATLAS trials included only ccRCC patients, and the majority (79% and 84%) of patients enrolled in the ASSURE and SORCE trials had ccRCC. Usually, the protocol-specified duration of adjuvant TKI therapy was 12 months. The ATLAS and the SORCE trials included cohorts with adjuvant TKI therapy up to 36 months, but the longer duration of TKI therapy did not lead to improved DFS. Adjuvant TKI therapy caused substantial toxicity (grade 3–4 adverse events 49–72%) and a significant proportion of the patients (23–49%) discontinued adjuvant TKI therapy because of intolerable toxicity or refused to continue study therapy (96–100). Currently, adjuvant TKI therapy is not recommended after complete resection of the primary tumor in the international RCC guidelines due to the substantial toxicity and the lack of OS benefit [4,94].

Immune checkpoint inhibitors (ICI) have replaced cytokines in the immune therapy of advanced RCC and are also being studied in randomized placebo-controlled prospective clinical trials in the adjuvant and neoadjuvant setting. IMmotion010 is evaluating 12-month adjuvant therapy with PD-L1 inhibitor atezolizumab, PROSPER neoadjuvant therapy (nivolumab two doses), followed by 9-month adjuvant therapy with PD-1 inhibitor nivolumab and CheckMate 914 6-month adjuvant therapy with the combination of CTLA-4 inhibitor ipilimumab and PD-1 inhibitor nivolumab in resected localized ccRCC patients, and RAMPART 12-month durvalumab adjuvant therapy and 12-month adjuvant CTLA-4 and PD-L1 inhibitor (tremelimumab and durvalumab) combination therapy. The first results of these trials are expected to be published in 2022–2024. The results from the KEYNOTE-564 trial evaluating 12-month adjuvant therapy with pembrolizumab in resected intermediate- or high-risk ccRCC patients showed a statistically significantly longer recurrence-free survival rate in the pembrolizumab arm compared to the placebo arm at 24 months (77.3% vs. 68.1%, HR for recurrence or death 0.68 (0.53–0.87)) (Table 2) [105]. As this was the first analysis, a longer follow-up will be needed to confirm the survival outcomes of the pembrolizumab adjuvant therapy. However, ICI may finally become a practice-changing adjuvant treatment option for RCC patients after complete resection of the primary tumor and lymph node or distant metastases.

6. Discussion

Numerous traditional histopathological factors and an increasing number of biomarkers have been identified to affect the postoperative prognosis of patients with localized ccRCC. The individual assessment of the risk for disease recurrence after radical or partial nephrectomy is important to tailor the intensity of postoperative follow-up imaging. Moreover, accurate risk assessment for disease recurrence is essential to select optimal patients for adjuvant therapy trials. However, there is no consensus regarding which is the best model or biomarker to choose to guide the clinical decision making. Limitations in the availability of biomarker analyses, time required to obtain the results, costs from the analyses, and, in particular, the lack of sufficient clinical validation still limit the use of prognostic biomarkers in clinical practice. Useful risk assessment tools for clinicians should be easy-to-use and include only a moderate amount of readily available risk factors (e.g., 3–5 traditional histopathological factors). Different clinicopathological features may be available in different centers. In the future, biomarkers, including those from plasma and urine (liquid biopsies), may supplement these prognostic algorithms.

Prognostic models with traditional histopathological and clinical factors should be easy-to-use and readily available. However, only the SORCE trial had incorporated a prognostic algorithm into the inclusion criteria of the trial. Adjuvant TKI trials underscored the fact that careful patient selection is required to avoid substantial toxicity and enrich higher-risk patients for adjuvant therapy. A meta-analysis of adjuvant TKI trials showed a DFS benefit in the high-risk (T3, Fuhrman grade 3–4; T4, or N1) population but not in the low-risk population (pooled HR for DFS 0.85 (0.75–0.97) and 0.98 (0.82–1.17), respectively) [106]. The optimal selection criteria for the high-risk localized ccRCC population remain to be defined. The results from the biomarker analyses of current neoadjuvant and adjuvant trials with ICI may shed more light on the issue.

7. Conclusions

Prognostic factors and validated prediction models help to evaluate the risk for disease recurrence after complete surgical resection of localized ccRCC. Better models to reduce follow-up imaging in low-risk patients and optimize the selection of patients for adjuvant trials are required. The combination of clinical and histopathological features with novel biomarkers may improve the prediction accuracy of prognostic models. The optimal set of prognostic factors and biomarkers to define high-risk patients for disease recurrence may be discovered in ongoing placebo-controlled randomized prospective clinical trials.

Author Contributions: Conceptualization, K.E.M., P.V. and P.M.J.; writing—original draft preparation, K.E.M., P.V. and P.M.J.; writing—review and editing, K.E.M., P.V. and P.M.J.; supervision, P.M.J. All authors have read and agreed to the published version of the manuscript.

Funding: This research work was supported by the Finnish Cancer Unions and Turku University Hospital (project 13031).

Conflicts of Interest: The authors declare no conflict of interest.

References

1. Sung, H.; Ferlay, J.; Siegel, R.L.; Laversanne, M.; Soerjomataram, I.; Jemal, A.; Bray, F. Global Cancer Statistics 2020: GLOBOCAN Estimates of Incidence and Mortality Worldwide for 36 Cancers in 185 Countries. *CA Cancer J. Clin.* **2021**, *3*, 209–249. [CrossRef]
2. Leibovich, B.C.; Lohse, C.M.; Crispen, P.L.; Boorjian, S.A.; Thompson, R.H.; Blute, M.L.; Cheville, J.C. Histological subtype is an independent predictor of outcome for patients with renal cell carcinoma. *J. Urol.* **2010**, *183*, 1309–1315. [CrossRef]
3. Ljungberg, B.; Bensalah, K.; Canfield, S.; Dabestani, S.; Hofmann, F.; Hora, M.; Kuczyk, M.A.; Lam, T.; Marconi, L.; Merseburger, A.S.; et al. EAU guidelines on renal cell carcinoma: 2014 update. *Eur. Urol.* **2015**, *67*, 913–924. [CrossRef]
4. Motzer, R.J.; Jonasch, E.; Boyle, S.; Carlo, M.I.; Manley, B.; Agarwal, N.; Alva, A.; Beckermann, K.; Choueiri, T.K.; Costello, B.A.; et al. NCCN guidelines insights: Kidney cancer, version 1.2021. *J. Natl. Compr. Cancer Netw.* **2020**, *18*, 1160–1170. [CrossRef]
5. Capitanio, U.; Montorsi, F. Renal cancer. *Lancet* **2016**, *387*, 894–906. [PubMed]
6. Swami, U.; Nussenzveig, R.H.; Haaland, B.; Agarwal, N. Revisiting AJCC TNM staging for renal cell carcinoma: Quest for improvement. *Ann. Transl. Med.* **2019**, *7*, S18. [CrossRef] [PubMed]
7. Bierley, J.D.; Gospodarowicz, M.K.; Wittekind, C. *TNM Classification of Malignant Tumours*, 8th ed.; John Wiley & Sons, Inc.: Hoboken, NJ, USA, 2017.
8. Kane, C.J.; Mallin, K.; Ritchey, J.; Cooperberg, M.R.; Carroll, P.R. Renal cell cancer stage migration: Analysis of the national cancer data base. *Cancer* **2008**, *113*, 78–83. [CrossRef]
9. Cheaib, J.G.; Patel, H.D.; Johnson, M.H.; Gorin, M.A.; Haut, E.R.; Canner, J.K.; Allaf, M.E.; Pierorazio, P.M. Stage-specific Conditional survival in renal cell carcinoma after nephrectomy. *Urol. Oncol.* **2020**, *38*, e1–e6. [CrossRef] [PubMed]
10. Fuhrman, S.A.; Lasky, L.C.; Limas, C. Prognostic significance of morphologic parameters in renal cell carcinoma. *Am. J. Surg. Pathol.* **1982**, *6*, 655–663.
11. Delahunt, B.; Srigley, J.R.; Egevad, L.; Montironi, R.; International Society for Urological Pathology. International society of urological pathology grading and other prognostic factors for renal neoplasia. *Eur. Urol.* **2014**, *66*, 795–798. [CrossRef]
12. Blum, K.A.; Gupta, S.; Tickoo, S.K.; Chan, T.A.; Russo, P.; Motzer, R.J.; Karam, J.A.; Hakimi, A.A. Sarcomatoid renal cell carcinoma: Biology, natural history and management. *Nat. Rev. Urol.* **2020**, *17*, 659–678. [CrossRef]
13. Cheville, J.C.; Lohse, C.M.; Zincke, H.; Weaver, A.L.; Leibovich, B.C.; Frank, I.; Blute, M.L. Sarcomatoid renal cell carcinoma: An examination of underlying histologic subtype and an analysis of associations with patient outcome. *Am. J. Surg. Pathol.* **2004**, *28*, 435–441. [CrossRef]
14. Trudeau, V.; Larcher, A.; Sun, M.; Boehm, K.; Dell'Oglio, P.; Sosa, J.; Tian, Z.; Fossati, N.; Briganti, A.; Shariat, S.F.; et al. Comparison of oncologic outcomes between sarcomatoid and clear cell renal cell carcinoma. *World J. Urol.* **2016**, *34*, 1429–1436. [CrossRef]
15. Mian, B.M.; Bhadkamkar, N.; Slaton, J.W.; Pisters, P.W.; Daliani, D.; Swanson, D.A.; Pisters, L.L. Prognostic factors and survival of patients with sarcomatoid renal cell carcinoma. *J. Urol.* **2002**, *167*, 65–70. [CrossRef]
16. Merrill, M.M.; Wood, C.G.; Tannir, N.M.; Slack, R.S.; Babaian, K.N.; Jonasch, E.; Pagliaro, L.C.; Compton, Z.; Tamboli, P.; Sircar, K.; et al. Clinically nonmetastatic renal cell carcinoma with sarcomatoid dedifferentiation: Natural history and outcomes after surgical resection with curative intent. *Urol. Oncol.* **2015**, *33*, e21–e166. [CrossRef]

17. Pichler, M.; Hutterer, G.C.; Chromecki, T.F.; Jesche, J.; Kampel-Kettner, K.; Rehak, P.; Pummer, K.; Zigeuner, R. Histologic tumor necrosis is an independent prognostic indicator for clear cell and papillary renal cell carcinoma. *Am. J. Clin. Pathol.* **2012**, *137*, 283–289. [CrossRef]
18. Lam, J.S.; Shvarts, O.; Said, J.W.; Pantuck, A.J.; Seligson, D.B.; Aldridge, M.E.; Bui, M.H.; Liu, X.; Horvath, S.; Figlin, R.A.; et al. Clinicopathologic and molecular correlations of necrosis in the primary tumor of patients with renal cell carcinoma. *Cancer* **2005**, *103*, 2517–2525. [CrossRef]
19. Delahunt, B.; Cheville, J.C.; Martignoni, G.; Humphrey, P.A.; Magi-Galluzzi, C.; McKenney, J.; Egevad, L.; Algaba, F.; Moch, H.; Grignon, D.J.; et al. The international society of urological pathology (ISUP) grading system for renal cell carcinoma and other prognostic parameters. *Am. J. Surg. Pathol.* **2013**, *37*, 1490–1504. [CrossRef]
20. Khor, L.Y.; Dhakal, H.P.; Jia, X.; Reynolds, J.P.; McKenney, J.K.; Rini, B.I.; Magi-Galluzzi, C.; Przybycin, C.G. Tumor necrosis adds prognostically significant information to grade in clear cell renal cell carcinoma: A study of 842 consecutive cases from a single institution. *Am. J. Surg. Pathol.* **2016**, *40*, 1224–1231. [CrossRef]
21. Sengupta, S.; Lohse, C.M.; Leibovich, B.C.; Frank, I.; Thompson, R.H.; Webster, W.S.; Zincke, H.; Blute, M.L.; Cheville, J.C.; Kwon, E.D. Histologic coagulative tumor necrosis as a prognostic indicator of renal cell carcinoma aggressiveness. *Cancer* **2005**, *104*, 511–520. [CrossRef]
22. Katz, M.D.; Serrano, M.F.; Grubb, R.L.; Skolarus, T.A.; Gao, F.; Humphrey, P.A.; Kibel, A.S. Percent microscopic tumor necrosis and survival after curative surgery for renal cell carcinoma. *J. Urol.* **2010**, *183*, 909–914. [CrossRef]
23. Foria, V.; Surendra, T.; Poller, D.N. Prognostic relevance of extensive necrosis in renal cell carcinoma. *J. Clin. Pathol.* **2005**, *58*, 39–43. [CrossRef]
24. Lee, S.E.; Byun, S.S.; Oh, J.K.; Lee, S.C.; Chang, I.H.; Choe, G.; Hong, S.K. Significance of macroscopic tumor necrosis as a prognostic indicator for renal cell carcinoma. *J. Urol.* **2006**, *176*, 1332–1338. [CrossRef]
25. Renshaw, A.A.; Cheville, J.C. Quantitative tumour necrosis is an independent predictor of overall survival in clear cell renal cell carcinoma. *Pathology* **2015**, *47*, 34–37. [CrossRef]
26. Delahunt, B.; McKenney, J.K.; Lohse, C.M.; Leibovich, B.C.; Thompson, R.H.; Boorjian, S.A.; Cheville, J.C. A novel grading system for clear cell renal cell carcinoma incorporating tumor necrosis. *Am. J. Surg. Pathol.* **2013**, *37*, 311–322. [CrossRef]
27. Moch, H.; Humphrey, P.A.; Ulbright, T.M.; Reuter, V.E. *WHO Classification of Tumours of the Urinary System and Male Genital Organs. WHO Classification of Tumours*, 4th ed.; International Agency for Research on Cancer: Lyon, France, 2016; Volume 8.
28. Bedke, J.; Heide, J.; Ribback, S.; Rausch, S.; de Martino, M.; Scharpf, M.; Haitel, A.; Zimmermann, U.; Pechoel, M.; Alkhayyat, H.; et al. Microvascular and lymphovascular tumour invasion are associated with poor prognosis and metastatic spread in renal cell carcinoma: A validation study in clinical practice. *BJU Int.* **2018**, *121*, 84–92. [CrossRef]
29. Lang, H.; Lindner, V.; Letourneux, H.; Martin, M.; Saussine, C.; Jacqmin, D. Prognostic value of microscopic venous invasion in renal cell carcinoma: Long-term follow-up. *Eur. Urol.* **2004**, *46*, 331–335. [CrossRef]
30. Kroeger, N.; Rampersaud, E.N.; Patard, J.J.; Klatte, T.; Birkhauser, F.D.; Shariat, S.F.; Lang, H.; Rioux-Leclerq, N.; Remzi, M.; Zomorodian, N.; et al. Prognostic value of microvascular invasion in predicting the cancer specific survival and risk of metastatic disease in renal cell carcinoma: A multicenter investigation. *J. Urol.* **2012**, *187*, 418–423. [CrossRef]
31. Van Poppel, H. Efficacy and safety of nephron-sparing surgery. *Int. J. Urol.* **2010**, *17*, 314–326. [CrossRef]
32. Antic, T.; Taxy, J.B. Partial nephrectomy for renal tumors: Lack of correlation between margin status and local recurrence. *Am. J. Clin. Pathol.* **2015**, *143*, 645–651. [CrossRef]
33. Bansal, R.K.; Tanguay, S.; Finelli, A.; Rendon, R.; Moore, R.B.; Breau, R.H.; Lacombe, L.; Black, P.C.; Kawakami, J.; Drachenberg, D.; et al. Positive surgical margins during partial nephrectomy for renal cell carcinoma: Results from canadian kidney cancer information system (CKCis) collaborative. *Can. Urol. Assoc. J.* **2017**, *11*, 182–187. [CrossRef]
34. Schiavina, R.; Mari, A.; Bianchi, L.; Amparore, D.; Antonelli, A.; Artibani, W.; Brunocilla, E.; Capitanio, U.; Fiori, C.; Di Maida, F.; et al. Predicting positive surgical margins in partial nephrectomy: A prospective multicentre observational study (the RECORd 2 project). *Eur. J. Surg. Oncol.* **2020**, *46*, 1353–1359. [CrossRef]
35. Wood, E.L.; Adibi, M.; Qiao, W.; Brandt, J.; Zhang, M.; Tamboli, P.; Matin, S.F.; Wood, C.G.; Karam, J.A. Local tumor bed recurrence following partial nephrectomy in patients with small renal masses. *J. Urol.* **2018**, *199*, 393–400. [CrossRef]
36. Shah, P.H.; Lyon, T.D.; Lohse, C.M.; Cheville, J.C.; Leibovich, B.C.; Boorjian, S.A.; Thompson, R.H. Prognostic evaluation of perinephric fat, renal sinus fat, and renal vein invasion for patients with pathological stage T3a clear-cell renal cell carcinoma. *BJU Int.* **2019**, *123*, 270–276. [CrossRef]
37. Stuhler, V.; Rausch, S.; Kroll, K.; Scharpf, M.; Stenzl, A.; Bedke, J. The prognostic value of fat invasion and tumor expansion in the hilar veins in pT3a renal cell carcinoma. *World J. Urol.* **2021**, *39*, 3367–3376. [CrossRef]
38. da Costa, W.H.; Moniz, R.R.; da Cunha, I.W.; Fonseca, F.P.; Guimaraes, G.C.; de Cassio Zequi, S. Impact of renal vein invasion and fat invasion in pT3a renal cell carcinoma. *BJU Int.* **2012**, *109*, 544–548. [CrossRef]
39. Baccos, A.; Brunocilla, E.; Schiavina, R.; Borghesi, M.; Rocca, G.C.; Chessa, F.; Saraceni, G.; Fiorentino, M.; Martorana, G. Differing risk of cancer death among patients with pathologic T3a renal cell carcinoma: Identification of risk categories according to fat infiltration and renal vein thrombosis. *Clin. Genitourin. Cancer* **2013**, *11*, 451–457. [CrossRef]
40. Campbell, S.; Novick, A.; Bukowski, R. Treatment of locally advanced renal cell carcinoma. In *Urology*; Campbell, S., Walsh, P., Eds.; W. B. Saunders Co.: Philadelphia, PA, USA, 2007; pp. 1619–1622.

41. Ljungberg, B.; Stenling, R.; Osterdahl, B.; Farrelly, E.; Aberg, T.; Roos, G. Vein invasion in renal cell carcinoma: Impact on Metastatic behavior and survival. *J. Urol.* **1995**, *154*, 1681–1684. [CrossRef]
42. Neves, R.J.; Zincke, H. Surgical treatment of renal cancer with vena cava extension. *Br. J. Urol.* **1987**, *59*, 390–395. [CrossRef]
43. Wagner, B.; Patard, J.J.; Mejean, A.; Bensalah, K.; Verhoest, G.; Zigeuner, R.; Ficarra, V.; Tostain, J.; Mulders, P.; Chautard, D.; et al. Prognostic value of renal vein and inferior vena cava involvement in renal cell carcinoma. *Eur. Urol.* **2009**, *55*, 452–459. [CrossRef]
44. Tilki, D.; Nguyen, H.G.; Dall'Era, M.A.; Bertini, R.; Carballido, J.A.; Chromecki, T.; Ciancio, G.; Daneshmand, S.; Gontero, P.; Gonzalez, J.; et al. Impact of histologic subtype on cancer-specific survival in patients with renal cell carcinoma and tumor thrombus. *Eur. Urol.* **2014**, *66*, 577–583. [CrossRef]
45. Shiff, B.; Breau, R.H.; Mallick, R.; Pouliot, F.; So, A.; Tanguay, S.; Kapoor, A.; Lattouf, J.B.; Lavallee, L.; Fairey, A.; et al. Prognostic significance of extent of venous tumor thrombus in patients with non-metastatic renal cell carcinoma: Results from a Canadian multi-institutional collaborative. *Urol. Oncol.* **2021**, *39*, 836.e19–836.e27. [CrossRef]
46. Marchioni, M.; Bandini, M.; Pompe, R.S.; Martel, T.; Tian, Z.; Shariat, S.F.; Kapoor, A.; Cindolo, L.; Briganti, A.; Schips, L.; et al. The impact of lymph node dissection and positive lymph nodes on cancer-specific mortality in contemporary pT2-3 non-metastatic renal cell carcinoma treated with radical nephrectomy. *BJU Int.* **2018**, *121*, 383–392. [CrossRef]
47. Sun, M.; Bianchi, M.; Hansen, J.; Abdollah, F.; Trinh, Q.D.; Lughezzani, G.; Shariat, S.F.; Montorsi, F.; Perrotte, P.; Karakiewicz, P.I. Nodal involvement at nephrectomy is associated with worse survival: A stage-for-stage and grade-for-grade analysis. *Int. J. Urol.* **2013**, *20*, 372–380. [CrossRef]
48. Srivastava, A.; Rivera-Nunez, Z.; Kim, S.; Sterling, J.; Farber, N.J.; Radadia, K.D.; Patel, H.V.; Modi, P.K.; Goyal, S.; Parikh, R.; et al. Impact of pathologic lymph node-positive renal cell carcinoma on survival in patients without metastasis: Evidence in support of expanding the definition of stage IV kidney cancer. *Cancer* **2020**, *126*, 2991–3001. [CrossRef]
49. Kattan, M.W.; Reuter, V.; Motzer, R.J.; Katz, J.; Russo, P. A postoperative prognostic nomogram for renal cell carcinoma. *J. Urol.* **2001**, *166*, 63–67. [CrossRef]
50. Zisman, A.; Pantuck, A.J.; Dorey, F.; Said, J.W.; Shvarts, O.; Quintana, D.; Gitlitz, B.J.; deKernion, J.B.; Figlin, R.A.; Belldegrun, A.S. Improved prognostication of renal cell carcinoma using an integrated staging system. *J. Clin. Oncol.* **2001**, *19*, 1649–1657. [CrossRef]
51. Parker, W.P.; Cheville, J.C.; Frank, I.; Zaid, H.B.; Lohse, C.M.; Boorjian, S.A.; Leibovich, B.C.; Thompson, R.H. Application of the stage, size, grade, and necrosis (SSIGN) score for clear cell renal cell carcinoma in contemporary patients. *Eur. Urol.* **2017**, *71*, 665–673. [CrossRef]
52. Cindolo, L.; de la Taille, A.; Messina, G.; Romis, L.; Abbou, C.C.; Altieri, V.; Rodriguez, A.; Patard, J.J. A preoperative clinical prognostic model for non-metastatic renal cell carcinoma. *BJU Int.* **2003**, *92*, 901–905. [CrossRef]
53. Leibovich, B.C.; Blute, M.L.; Cheville, J.C.; Lohse, C.M.; Frank, I.; Kwon, E.D.; Weaver, A.L.; Parker, A.S.; Zincke, H. Prediction of progression after radical nephrectomy for patients with clear cell renal cell carcinoma: A stratification tool for prospective clinical trials. *Cancer* **2003**, *97*, 1663–1671. [CrossRef]
54. Sorbellini, M.; Kattan, M.W.; Snyder, M.E.; Reuter, V.; Motzer, R.; Goetzl, M.; McKiernan, J.; Russo, P. A postoperative prognostic nomogram predicting recurrence for patients with conventional clear cell renal cell carcinoma. *J. Urol.* **2005**, *173*, 48–51. [CrossRef]
55. Karakiewicz, P.I.; Suardi, N.; Capitanio, U.; Jeldres, C.; Ficarra, V.; Cindolo, L.; de la Taille, A.; Tostain, J.; Mulders, P.F.A.; Bensalah, K.; et al. A preoperative prognostic model for patients treated with nephrectomy for renal cell carcinoma. *Eur. Urol.* **2009**, *55*, 287–295. [CrossRef]
56. Leibovich, B.C.; Lohse, C.M.; Cheville, J.C.; Zaid, H.B.; Boorjian, S.A.; Frank, I.; Thompson, R.H.; Parker, W.P. Predicting oncologic outcomes in renal cell carcinoma after surgery. *Eur. Urol.* **2018**, *73*, 772–780. [CrossRef]
57. Mattila, K.E.; Laajala, T.D.; Tornberg, S.V.; Kilpelainen, T.P.; Vainio, P.; Ettala, O.; Bostrom, P.J.; Nisen, H.; Elo, L.L.; Jaakkola, P.M. A three-feature prediction model for metastasis-free survival after surgery of localized clear cell renal cell carcinoma. *Sci. Rep.* **2021**, *11*, 8650–8659. [CrossRef]
58. Correa, A.F.; Jegede, O.A.; Haas, N.B.; Flaherty, K.T.; Pins, M.R.; Adeniran, A.; Messing, E.M.; Manola, J.; Wood, C.G.; Kane, C.J.; et al. Predicting disease recurrence, early progression, and overall survival following surgical resection for high-risk localized and locally advanced renal cell carcinoma. *Eur. Urol.* **2021**, *80*, 20–31. [CrossRef]
59. Park, Y.H.; Baik, K.D.; Lee, Y.J.; Ku, J.H.; Kim, H.H.; Kwak, C. Late recurrence of renal cell carcinoma >5 years after surgery: Clinicopathological characteristics and prognosis. *BJU Int.* **2012**, *110*, 553. [CrossRef]
60. Pugh, C.W.; Ratcliffe, P.J. The von hippel-lindau tumor suppressor, hypoxia-inducible factor-1 (HIF-1) degradation, and cancer pathogenesis. *Semin. Cancer Biol.* **2003**, *13*, 83–89. [CrossRef]
61. Gordan, J.D.; Bertout, J.A.; Hu, C.J.; Diehl, J.A.; Simon, M.C. HIF-2alpha promotes hypoxic cell proliferation by enhancing C-Myc transcriptional activity. *Cancer Cell* **2007**, *11*, 335–347. [CrossRef]
62. Miikkulainen, P.; Hogel, H.; Seyednasrollah, F.; Rantanen, K.; Elo, L.L.; Jaakkola, P.M. Hypoxia-inducible factor (HIF)-prolyl hydroxylase 3 (PHD3) maintains high HIF2A mRNA levels in clear cell renal cell carcinoma. *J. Biol. Chem.* **2019**, *294*, 3760–3771. [CrossRef]
63. Kaelin, W.G. The von hippel-lindau tumor suppressor protein and clear cell renal carcinoma. *Clin. Cancer Res.* **2007**, *13*, 680s–684s. [CrossRef]

64. Gerlinger, M.; Rowan, A.J.; Horswell, S.; Math, M.; Larkin, J.; Endesfelder, D.; Gronroos, E.; Martinez, P.; Matthews, N.; Stewart, A.; et al. Intratumor heterogeneity and branched evolution revealed by multiregion sequencing. *N. Engl. J. Med.* **2012**, *366*, 883–892. [CrossRef]
65. Cancer Genome Atlas Research Network. Comprehensive molecular characterization of clear cell renal cell carcinoma. *Nature* **2013**, *499*, 43–49. [CrossRef]
66. Hakimi, A.A.; Pham, C.G.; Hsieh, J.J. A clear picture of renal cell carcinoma. *Nat. Genet.* **2013**, *45*, 849–850. [CrossRef]
67. Joseph, R.W.; Kapur, P.; Serie, D.J.; Parasramka, M.; Ho, T.H.; Cheville, J.C.; Frenkel, E.; Parker, A.S.; Brugarolas, J. Clear cell renal cell carcinoma subtypes identified by BAP1 and PBRM1 expression. *J. Urol.* **2016**, *195*, 180–187. [CrossRef]
68. Carril-Ajuria, L.; Santos, M.; Roldan-Romero, J.M.; Rodriguez-Antona, C.; de Velasco, G. Prognostic and predictive value of PBRM1 in clear cell renal cell carcinoma. *Cancers* **2019**, *12*, 16. [CrossRef]
69. Rini, B.; Goddard, A.; Knezevic, D.; Maddala, T.; Zhou, M.; Aydin, H.; Campbell, S.; Elson, P.; Koscielny, S.; Lopatin, M.; et al. A 16-gene assay to predict recurrence after surgery in localised renal cell carcinoma: Development and validation studies. *Lancet Oncol.* **2015**, *16*, 676–685. [CrossRef]
70. Rini, B.I.; Escudier, B.; Martini, J.F.; Magheli, A.; Svedman, C.; Lopatin, M.; Knezevic, D.; Goddard, A.D.; Febbo, P.G.; Li, R.; et al. Validation of the 16-gene recurrence score in patients with locoregional, high-risk renal cell carcinoma from a phase III trial of adjuvant sunitinib. *Clin. Cancer Res.* **2018**, *24*, 4407–4415. [CrossRef]
71. Ghatalia, P.; Rathmell, W.K. Systematic review: ClearCode 34—A validated prognostic signature in clear cell renal cell carcinoma (ccRCC). *Kidney Cancer* **2018**, *2*, 23–29. [CrossRef]
72. Morgan, T.M.; Mehra, R.; Tiemeny, P.; Wolf, J.S.; Wu, S.; Sangale, Z.; Brawer, M.; Stone, S.; Wu, C.L.; Feldman, A.S. A multigene signature based on cell cycle proliferation improves prediction of mortality within 5 yr of radical nephrectomy for renal cell carcinoma. *Eur. Urol.* **2018**, *73*, 763–769. [CrossRef]
73. Busser, B.; Lupo, J.; Sancey, L.; Mouret, S.; Faure, P.; Plumas, J.; Chaperot, L.; Leccia, M.T.; Coll, J.L.; Hurbin, A.; et al. Plasma circulating tumor DNA levels for the monitoring of melanoma patients: Landscape of available technologies and clinical applications. *Biomed. Res. Int.* **2017**, *2017*, 5986129. [CrossRef]
74. Lee, R.J.; Gremel, G.; Marshall, A.; Myers, K.A.; Fisher, N.; Dunn, J.A.; Dhomen, N.; Corrie, P.G.; Middleton, M.R.; Lorigan, P.; et al. Circulating tumor DNA predicts survival in patients with resected high-risk stage II/III melanoma. *Ann. Oncol.* **2018**, *29*, 490–496. [CrossRef]
75. Tan, L.; Sandhu, S.; Lee, R.J.; Li, J.; Callahan, J.; Ftouni, S.; Dhomen, N.; Middlehurst, P.; Wallace, A.; Raleigh, J.; et al. Prediction and monitoring of relapse in stage III melanoma using circulating tumor DNA. *Ann. Oncol.* **2019**, *30*, 804–814. [CrossRef]
76. Lee, C.S.; Kim, H.S.; Schageman, J.; Lee, I.K.; Kim, M.; Kim, Y. Postoperative circulating tumor DNA can predict high risk patients with colorectal cancer based on next-generation sequencing. *Cancers* **2021**, *13*, 4190. [CrossRef]
77. Tarazona, N.; Gimeno-Valiente, F.; Gambardella, V.; Zuniga, S.; Rentero-Garrido, P.; Huerta, M.; Rosello, S.; Martinez-Ciarpaglini, C.; Carbonell-Asins, J.A.; Carrasco, F.; et al. Targeted next-generation sequencing of circulating-tumor DNA for tracking minimal residual disease in localized colon cancer. *Ann. Oncol.* **2019**, *30*, 1804–1812. [CrossRef]
78. Peng, M.; Huang, Q.; Yin, W.; Tan, S.; Chen, C.; Liu, W.; Tang, J.; Wang, X.; Zhang, B.; Zou, M.; et al. Circulating tumor DNA as a prognostic biomarker in localized non-small cell lung cancer. *Front. Oncol.* **2020**, *10*, 561598. [CrossRef]
79. Chaudhuri, A.A.; Chabon, J.J.; Lovejoy, A.F.; Newman, A.M.; Stehr, H.; Azad, T.D.; Khodadoust, M.S.; Esfahani, M.S.; Liu, C.L.; Zhou, L.; et al. Early detection of molecular residual disease in localized lung cancer by circulating tumor DNA profiling. *Cancer Discov.* **2017**, *7*, 1394–1403. [CrossRef]
80. Powles, T.; Assaf, Z.J.; Davarpanah, N.; Banchereau, R.; Szabados, B.E.; Yuen, K.C.; Grivas, P.; Hussain, M.; Oudard, S.; Gschwend, J.E.; et al. ctDNA guiding adjuvant immunotherapy in urothelial carcinoma. *Nature* **2021**, *595*, 432–437. [CrossRef]
81. Wan, J.; Zhu, L.; Jiang, Z.; Cheng, K. Monitoring of plasma cell-free DNA in predicting postoperative recurrence of clear cell renal cell carcinoma. *Urol. Int.* **2013**, *91*, 273–278. [CrossRef]
82. Smith, C.G.; Moser, T.; Mouliere, F.; Field-Rayner, J.; Eldridge, M.; Riediger, A.L.; Chandrananda, D.; Heider, K.; Wan, J.C.M.; Warren, A.Y.; et al. Comprehensive characterization of cell-free tumor DNA in plasma and urine of patients with renal tumors. *Genome Med.* **2020**, *12*, 23–28. [CrossRef]
83. Pal, S.K.; Sonpavde, G.; Agarwal, N.; Vogelzang, N.J.; Srinivas, S.; Haas, N.B.; Signoretti, S.; McGregor, B.A.; Jones, J.; Lanman, R.B.; et al. Evolution of circulating tumor DNA profile from first-line to subsequent therapy in metastatic renal cell carcinoma. *Eur. Urol.* **2017**, *72*, 557–564. [CrossRef]
84. Maia, M.C.; Bergerot, P.G.; Dizman, N.; Hsu, J.; Jones, J.; Lanman, R.B.; Banks, K.C.; Pal, S.K. Association of circulating tumor DNA (ctDNA) detection in metastatic renal cell carcinoma (mRCC) with tumor burden. *Kidney Cancer* **2017**, *1*, 65–70. [CrossRef]
85. Blank, C.; Gajewski, T.F.; Mackensen, A. Interaction of PD-L1 on tumor cells with PD-1 on tumor-specific T cells as a mechanism of immune evasion: Implications for tumor immunotherapy. *Cancer Immunol. Immunother.* **2005**, *54*, 307–314. [CrossRef]
86. Carlsson, J.; Sundqvist, P.; Kosuta, V.; Falt, A.; Giunchi, F.; Fiorentino, M.; Davidsson, S. PD-L1 Expression is associated with poor prognosis in renal cell carcinoma. *Appl. Immunohistochem. Mol. Morphol.* **2020**, *28*, 213–220. [CrossRef]
87. Thompson, R.H.; Kuntz, S.M.; Leibovich, B.C.; Dong, H.; Lohse, C.M.; Webster, W.S.; Sengupta, S.; Frank, I.; Parker, A.S.; Zincke, H.; et al. Tumor B7-H1 is associated with poor prognosis in renal cell carcinoma patients with long-term follow-up. *Cancer Res.* **2006**, *66*, 3381–3385. [CrossRef]

88. Abbas, M.; Steffens, S.; Bellut, M.; Eggers, H.; Grosshennig, A.; Becker, J.U.; Wegener, G.; Schrader, A.J.; Grunwald, V.; Ivanyi, P. Intratumoral expression of programmed death ligand 1 (PD-L1) in patients with clear cell renal cell carcinoma (ccRCC). *Med. Oncol.* **2016**, *33*, 80. [CrossRef]
89. Gupta, S.; Cheville, J.C.; Jungbluth, A.A.; Zhang, Y.; Zhang, L.; Chen, Y.B.; Tickoo, S.K.; Fine, S.W.; Gopalan, A.; Al-Ahmadie, H.A.; et al. JAK2/PD-L1/PD-L2 (9p24.1) amplifications in renal cell carcinomas with sarcomatoid transformation: Implications for clinical management. *Mod. Pathol.* **2019**, *32*, 1344–1358. [CrossRef]
90. Rini, B.I.; Motzer, R.J.; Powles, T.; McDermott, D.F.; Escudier, B.; Donskov, F.; Hawkins, R.; Bracarda, S.; Bedke, J.; De Giorgi, U.; et al. Atezolizumab plus bevacizumab versus sunitinib for patients with untreated metastatic renal cell carcinoma and sarcomatoid features: A prespecified subgroup analysis of the IMmotion151 clinical trial. *Eur. Urol.* **2021**, *79*, 659–662. [CrossRef]
91. Rini, B.I.; Powles, T.; Atkins, M.B.; Escudier, B.; McDermott, D.F.; Suarez, C.; Bracarda, S.; Stadler, W.M.; Donskov, F.; Lee, J.L.; et al. Atezolizumab plus bevacizumab versus sunitinib in patients with previously untreated metastatic renal cell carcinoma (IMmotion151): A multicentre, open-label, phase 3, randomised controlled trial. *Lancet* **2019**, *393*, 2404–2415. [CrossRef]
92. Motzer, R.J.; Tannir, N.M.; McDermott, D.F.; Aren Frontera, O.; Melichar, B.; Choueiri, T.K.; Plimack, E.R.; Barthelemy, P.; Porta, C.; George, S.; et al. Nivolumab plus ipilimumab versus sunitinib in advanced renal-cell carcinoma. *N. Engl. J. Med.* **2018**, *378*, 1277–1290. [CrossRef]
93. Nuzzo, P.V.; Berchuck, J.E.; Korthauer, K.; Spisak, S.; Nassar, A.H.; Abou Alaiwi, S.; Chakravarthy, A.; Shen, S.Y.; Bakouny, Z.; Boccardo, F.; et al. Detection of renal cell carcinoma using plasma and urine cell-free DNA methylomes. *Nat. Med.* **2020**, *26*, 1041–1043. [CrossRef]
94. Escudier, B.; Porta, C.; Schmidinger, M.; Rioux-Leclercq, N.; Bex, A.; Khoo, V.; Grunwald, V.; Gillessen, S.; Horwich, A.; ESMO Guidelines Committee. Renal cell carcinoma: ESMO clinical practice guidelines for diagnosis, treatment and follow-updagger. *Ann. Oncol.* **2019**, *30*, 706–720. [CrossRef]
95. Janowitz, T.; Welsh, S.J.; Zaki, K.; Mulders, P.; Eisen, T. Adjuvant therapy in renal cell carcinoma-past, present, and future. *Semin. Oncol.* **2013**, *40*, 482–491. [CrossRef]
96. Pizzocaro, G.; Piva, L.; Colavita, M.; Ferri, S.; Artusi, R.; Boracchi, P.; Parmiani, G.; Marubini, E. Interferon adjuvant to radical nephrectomy in robson stages II and III renal cell carcinoma: A multicentric randomized study. *J. Clin. Oncol.* **2001**, *19*, 425–431. [CrossRef]
97. Messing, E.M.; Manola, J.; Wilding, G.; Propert, K.; Fleischmann, J.; Crawford, E.D.; Pontes, J.E.; Hahn, R.; Trump, D.; Eastern Cooperative Oncology Group/Intergroup Trial. Phase III study of interferon Alfa-NL as adjuvant treatment for resectable renal cell carcinoma: An eastern cooperative oncology group/intergroup trial. *J. Clin. Oncol.* **2003**, *21*, 1214–1222. [CrossRef]
98. Clark, J.I.; Atkins, M.B.; Urba, W.J.; Creech, S.; Figlin, R.A.; Dutcher, J.P.; Flaherty, L.; Sosman, J.A.; Logan, T.F.; White, R.; et al. Adjuvant high-dose bolus interleukin-2 for patients with high-risk renal cell carcinoma: A cytokine working group randomized trial. *J. Clin. Oncol.* **2003**, *21*, 3133–3140. [CrossRef]
99. Ravaud, A.; Motzer, R.J.; Pandha, H.S.; George, D.J.; Pantuck, A.J.; Patel, A.; Chang, Y.H.; Escudier, B.; Donskov, F.; Magheli, A.; et al. Adjuvant sunitinib in high-risk renal-cell carcinoma after nephrectomy. *N. Engl. J. Med.* **2016**, *375*, 2246–2254. [CrossRef]
100. Haas, N.B.; Manola, J.; Uzzo, R.G.; Flaherty, K.T.; Wood, C.G.; Kane, C.; Jewett, M.; Dutcher, J.P.; Atkins, M.B.; Pins, M.; et al. Adjuvant sunitinib or sorafenib for high-risk, non-metastatic renal-cell carcinoma (ECOG-ACRIN E2805): A double-blind, placebo-controlled, randomised, phase 3 trial. *Lancet* **2016**, *387*, 2008–2016. [CrossRef]
101. Motzer, R.J.; Haas, N.B.; Donskov, F.; Gross-Goupil, M.; Varlamov, S.; Kopyltsov, E.; Lee, J.L.; Melichar, B.; Rini, B.I.; Choueiri, T.K.; et al. Randomized phase III trial of adjuvant pazopanib versus placebo after nephrectomy in patients with localized or locally advanced renal cell carcinoma. *J. Clin. Oncol.* **2017**, *35*, 3916–3923. [CrossRef]
102. Gross-Goupil, M.; Kwon, T.G.; Eto, M.; Ye, D.; Miyake, H.; Seo, S.I.; Byun, S.S.; Lee, J.L.; Master, V.; Jin, J.; et al. Axitinib versus placebo as an adjuvant treatment of renal cell carcinoma: Results from the phase III, randomized ATLAS trial. *Ann. Oncol.* **2018**, *29*, 2371–2378. [CrossRef]
103. Eisen, T.; Frangou, E.; Oza, B.; Ritchie, A.W.S.; Smith, B.; Kaplan, R.; Davis, I.D.; Stockler, M.R.; Albiges, L.; Escudier, B.; et al. Adjuvant sorafenib for renal cell carcinoma at intermediate or high risk of relapse: Results from the SORCE randomized phase III intergroup trial. *J. Clin. Oncol.* **2020**, *38*, 4064–4075. [CrossRef]
104. Choueiri, T.K.; Tomczak, P.; Park, S.H.; Venugopal, B.; Ferguson, T.; Chang, Y.H.; Hajek, J.; Symeonides, S.N.; Lee, J.L.; Sarwar, N.; et al. Adjuvant pembrolizumab after nephrectomy in renal-cell carcinoma. *N. Engl. J. Med.* **2021**, *385*, 683–694. [CrossRef]
105. George, D.J.; Martini, J.F.; Staehler, M.; Motzer, R.J.; Magheli, A.; Escudier, B.; Gerletti, P.; Li, S.; Casey, M.; Laguerre, B.; et al. Immune biomarkers predictive for disease-free survival with adjuvant sunitinib in high-risk locoregional renal cell carcinoma: From randomized phase III S-TRAC study. *Clin. Cancer Res.* **2018**, *24*, 1554–1561. [CrossRef]
106. Massari, F.; Di Nunno, V.; Mollica, V.; Graham, J.; Gatto, L.; Heng, D. Adjuvant tyrosine kinase inhibitors in treatment of renal cell carcinoma: A meta-analysis of available clinical trials. *Clin. Genitourin. Cancer* **2019**, *17*, e339–e344. [CrossRef]

Article

The Hypoxic Microenvironment Induces Stearoyl-CoA Desaturase-1 Overexpression and Lipidomic Profile Changes in Clear Cell Renal Cell Carcinoma

Juan Pablo Melana [1], Francesco Mignolli [2], Tania Stoyanoff [1], María V. Aguirre [1], María A. Balboa [3,4], Jesús Balsinde [3,4,*,†] and Juan Pablo Rodríguez [1,*,†]

[1] Laboratorio de Investigaciones Bioquímicas de la Facultad de Medicina (LIBIM), Instituto de Química Básica y Aplicada del Nordeste Argentino (IQUIBA-NEA), Universidad Nacional del Nordeste, Consejo Nacional de Investigaciones Científicas y Técnicas (UNNE-CONICET), Corrientes 3400, Argentina; jpmelana@med.unne.edu.ar (J.P.M.); taniastoyanoff@gmail.com (T.S.); vikyaguirre@yahoo.com (M.V.A.)

[2] Instituto de Botánica del Nordeste, Facultad de Ciencias Agrarias (UNNE-CONICET), Universidad Nacional del Nordeste, Corrientes 3400, Argentina; fmignolli80@gmail.com

[3] Instituto de Biología y Genética Molecular, Consejo Superior de Investigaciones Científicas (CSIC), 47003 Valladolid, Spain; mbalboa@ibgm.uva.es

[4] Centro de Investigación Biomédica en Red de Diabetes y Enfermedades Metabólicas Asociadas (CIBERDEM), 28029 Madrid, Spain

* Correspondence: jbalsinde@ibgm.uva.es (J.B.); rodriguezcasco@med.unne.edu.ar (J.P.R.); Tel.: +34-983-423-062 (J.B.); Tel.: +54-937-9469-4464 (J.P.R.)

† These authors contributed equally to this work.

Simple Summary: Clear cell renal cell carcinoma (ccRCC) is characterized by a high rate of cell proliferation and an extensive accumulation of lipids. Uncontrolled cell growth usually generates areas of intratumoral hypoxia that define the tumor phenotype. In this work, we show that, under these microenvironmental conditions, stearoyl-CoA desaturase-1 is overexpressed. This enzyme induces changes in the cellular lipidomic profile, increasing the oleic acid levels, a metabolite that is essential for cell proliferation. This work supports the idea of considering stearoyl-CoA desaturase-1 as an exploitable therapeutic target in ccRCC.

Abstract: Clear cell renal cell carcinoma (ccRCC) is the most common histological subtype of renal cell carcinoma (RCC). It is characterized by a high cell proliferation and the ability to store lipids. Previous studies have demonstrated the overexpression of enzymes associated with lipid metabolism, including stearoyl-CoA desaturase-1 (SCD-1), which increases the concentration of unsaturated fatty acids in tumor cells. In this work, we studied the expression of SCD-1 in primary ccRCC tumors, as well as in cell lines, to determine its influence on the tumor lipid composition and its role in cell proliferation. The lipidomic analyses of patient tumors showed that oleic acid (18:1n-9) is one of the major fatty acids, and it is particularly abundant in the neutral lipid fraction of the tumor core. Using a ccRCC cell line model and in vitro-generated chemical hypoxia, we show that SCD-1 is highly upregulated (up to 200-fold), and this causes an increase in the cellular level of 18:1n-9, which, in turn, accumulates in the neutral lipid fraction. The pharmacological inhibition of SCD-1 blocks 18:1n-9 synthesis and compromises the proliferation. The addition of exogenous 18:1n-9 to the cells reverses the effects of SCD-1 inhibition on cell proliferation. These data reinforce the role of SCD-1 as a possible therapeutic target.

Keywords: kidney; hypoxia; tumor microenvironment; SCD-1; oleic acid

1. Introduction

Renal cell carcinoma (RCC) is the most common malignancy of the urinary system. Although the incidence of RCC has remained stable, the mortality rates have decreased by only 0.9% each year from 2007 to 2016 [1,2].

Clear cell renal cell carcinoma (ccRCC) represents the most common subtype (>80%) of RCC. The most striking phenotypic feature of ccRCC is its clear cell morphology, which has been linked to a high lipid and glycogen accumulation [3]. Neutral lipids such as triacylglycerol (TAG) and cholesterol esters (CE) are stored in prominent cytoplasmic lipid droplets (LD), which are critical for cell growth and maintenance of the cell membrane [4]. Although the presence of these droplets in ccRCC is critical for sustained tumorigenesis, their contribution to lipid homeostasis and tumor cell viability is not completely understood [5].

A ubiquitous metabolic event in cancer is the constitutive activation of the pathway for fatty acid biosynthesis. Saturated fatty acids (SFAs), monounsaturated fatty acids (MUFAs) and polyunsaturated fatty acids (PUFAs) are synthetized to sustain the growing demand for phospholipids (PLs) that are used for the assembly of new membranes, energy storage and cell signaling [6–8]. The activation of enzymes such as ATP-citrate lyase (ACL), acetyl-CoA carboxylase (ACC) and fatty acid synthase (FAS) leading to an increased synthesis of SFAs has been extensively studied [9–12]. SFAs later become MUFAs by the action of stearoyl-CoA desaturase-1 (SCD-1) [13]. SCD-1 is a $\Delta 9$-fatty acyl-CoA desaturase that catalyzes the insertion of a double bond in the cis-$\Delta 9$ position of several saturated fatty acyl-CoAs—mainly, palmitoyl-CoA and stearoyl-CoA—to produce palmitoleoyl- and oleoyl-CoA, respectively [14]. It has been reported that these unsaturated fatty acids affect several crucial biological functions of tumor cells, such as proliferation, signaling, invasiveness and apoptosis. It was shown that oleic acid (18:1n-9), one of the most prevalent free fatty acids (FFAs) in human plasma, increases the proliferation of human prostate, breast and renal cancer cells [15,16]. As noted above, it was suggested that SCD-1 could be a therapeutic target in oncology, since its pharmacological inhibition induces tumor cell apoptosis [14,17–21]. Controversially, it is known that certain fatty acids such as 18:1n-9 exert anticancer effects on many tumors, inhibiting cell proliferation and favoring apoptosis [22,23].

Solid tumors such as ccRCC often show hypoxic areas as a result of uncontrolled tumor growth, without a proper development of its associated vascular network [13]. Hypoxia inducible factors (HIF-1α and HIF-2α) are commonly stabilized key players connected to cell growth and metabolic reprogramming in ccRCC. Both factors modulate tumoral hypoxic responses through altering the cell energy metabolism, including the modification of glucose consumption [24] and the expression of a lipid metabolism-associated gene [13,25,26].

We have previously shown that SCD-1 expression correlates with other cellular markers of the tumor hypoxic microenvironment, such as EPO, EPO-R, VEGF and VEGF-R in ccRCC [27]. However, up to now, tumor hypoxia in ccRCC has not been associated with the induction of SCD-1 and its consequent modification of the tumor lipidomic profile.

In this work, we demonstrate that cellular hypoxia favors the induction of SCD-1, and this influences the cellular lipid phenotype. Furthermore, we observed that SCD-1 inhibition deprives cells of essential lipid metabolites for cell proliferation. These data provide evidence to consider SCD-1 as an exploitable therapeutic target in ccRCC.

2. Materials and Methods

2.1. Patients and Sampling Procedures

Samples of ccRCC (n = 12) were obtained from patients treated for radical nephrectomy in the Urology Unit of the Hospital Dr. José Ramón Vidal (Corrientes, Argentina) between 2015 and 2018. The normal distal tissues and ccRCC of the same affected kidney were surgically removed. Samples were aseptically transported to the laboratory and quickly processed. They were then fixed for histopathology and immunohistochemistry procedures.

The design and methods of this research were approved by the Bioethics Committee of the Medical Research Department at Dr. José Ramón Vidal Hospital in Corrientes,

Argentina. Written informed consent was obtained from each donor. The researchers received the samples in an anonymous manner.

2.2. Cell lines, Proliferation and Viability Assays

Caki-1 and Caki-2 cell lines (derived from ccRCC), originally from the American Type Cell Culture Collection, were generously provided by Dr. Alfredo Martínez Ramírez (Centro de Investigaciones Biomédicas de La Rioja, Logroño, Spain) and Dr. Ricardo Sánchez Prieto (Universidad de Castilla-La Mancha, Albacete, Spain), respectively. The cells were cultured in McCoy's 5a medium modified (Thermo Fisher, Madrid, Spain) with 10% fetal bovine serum and 50 µg/mL of gentamicin (Invitrogen, Carlsbad, CA, USA) at 37 °C under humidified conditions with 5% CO_2. Cell proliferation and viability were measured with a Neubauer chamber and also using the CellTiter 96® AQueous One Solution Cell Proliferation Assay Kit (Promega, Madison, WI, USA).

For in vitro experiments, cells were subcultured every 3 to 4 days after reaching 80–90% confluence. The cells were trypsinized, centrifuged and resuspended in the medium at a suitable density. Experiments utilizing exogenous 18:1n-9 were performed under serum-restrictive conditions (1%) [28].

2.3. Hypoxic Microenvironment

To achieve a hypoxic microenvironment similar to the tumor and the effects of HIF stabilization, Caki-2 cells were exposed to different nontoxic concentrations of $CoCl_2$ in McCoy's 5a medium modified with 1% fetal bovine serum [29–35]. It has been previously shown that $CoCl_2$ inhibits the hydroxylation of HIF-1α, thus stabilizing HIF-1α and achieving the desired hypoxic effect [36–39].

2.4. Real-Time Quantitative PCR (RT-qPCR)

SCD-1, HIF-1A and HIF-2A mRNA were determined by RT-qPCR. Total RNA was extracted using the TRIzol reagent method (Invitrogen) according to the manufacturer's protocols. The obtained total RNA was purified using Ambion® TURBO DNA-free™. First-strand cDNA was obtained by using the Moloney murine leukemia virus reverse transcriptase (Promega) from 1 µg of RNA. qPCRs were then performed using specific primers for SCD-1 as follows: 5′-TTCCTACCTGCAAGTTCTACACC-3′ (forward) and 5′-CCGAGCTTTGTAAGAGCGGT-3′ (reverse) with a product of 116 bp. HIF-1A: 5′-TGCTGGGGCAATCAATGGAT-3′ (forward) and 5′-CTACCACGTACTGCTGGCAA-3′ (reverse) with a product of 590 bp. HIF-2A: 5′-TATAGTGACCCCGTCCACGT-3′ (forward) and 5′-AGGGCAACACACACAGGAAA-3′ (reverse) with a product of 572 bp. B-ACTIN: 5′-CATGTACGTTGCTATCCAGGC-3′ (forward) and 5′-CTCCTTAATGTCACGCACGAT-3′ (reverse) with a product of 250 bp was used as the housekeeping gene.

All primers were tested for specificity using the primer BLAST program available at the National Center for Biotechnology Information website (www.ncbi.nlm.nih.gov; accessed on 1 February 2020). Cycling conditions were: 1 cycle at 95 °C for 12 min, 40 cycles at 95 °C for 15 s, 60 °C for 20 s, 72 °C for 20 s and a final extension at 72 °C for 10 min.

2.5. SCD-1 Inhibition Assays

CAY 10566, a potent selective SCD-1 inhibitor, was purchased from Cayman Chemical (Ann Arbor, MI, USA), dissolved in DMSO and used (3 µM) according to the manufacturer's recommendations (noncytotoxic concentrations). Caki-2 cells were cultured in McCoy's 5a medium modified with 1% fetal bovine serum.

2.6. Analyses of Fatty Acids by Gas Chromatography Coupled to Mass Spectrometry (GC/MS)

Cellular lipids were extracted using the method of Bligh and Dyer [40]. After the addition of the appropriate standards, lipids were separated by thin-layer chromatography (TLC) using as the stationary phase silica gel 60 and a mobile phase consisting of

n-hexane/ethyl ether/acetic acid (70:30:1 $v/v/v$) [41]. Glycerolipids and glycerophospholipids were transmethylated with 500 µL of 0.5-M KOH in methanol for 30 min at 37 °C, and 500 µL of 0.5-M HCl was added to neutralize. For the transmethylation of cholesterol esters, the samples were resuspended in 400-µL methyl propionate and 600 µL of 0.84-M KOH in methanol for 1 h at 37 °C. Afterward, 50 mL and 1 mL of acetic acid and water, respectively, were added to neutralize. Analysis of the fatty acid methyl esters was carried out using an Agilent 7890A gas chromatograph coupled to an Agilent 5975C mass-selective detector operated in the electron impact mode (EI, 70 eV) equipped with an Agilent 7693 autosampler and an Agilent DB23 column (60-m length × 250-µm internal diameter × 0.15-µm film thickness) under the conditions described previously [42–45]. Data analysis was carried out with Agilent G1701EA MSD Productivity Chemstation software, revision E.02.00.

2.7. Confocal Microscopy

Caki-2 cells attached to coverslips were incubated for 24 h in McCoy 5a medium modified with different concentrations of $CoCl_2$ and a positive control with 30-µM oleic acid. Cells were then washed with phosphate-buffered saline and incubated with BODIPY 493/503 staining solution (2 µg/mL) for 15 min at 37 °C. Cells were subsequently washed, fixed with 4% paraformaldehyde and washed again. The coverslips were mounted on slides with a DAPI reagent (1 µg/mL). Untreated cells were used as negative controls. Fluorescence was monitored by microscopy using a Bio-Rad confocal system Radiance 2100 laser scanner (Bio-Rad, Richmond, VA, USA). The images were analyzed with ImageJ software.

2.8. Apoptosis Detection by Flow Cytometry

The effect of SCD-1 inhibition on apoptosis was evaluated by flow cytometry. Based on the preliminary time–course data, the exposure time was set to 18 h, and apoptosis was analyzed by labeling with the annexin V-fluorescein isothiocyanate (FITC) apoptosis detection kit (BD Bioscience, San Jose, CA, USA), which recognizes phosphatidylserine exposure on the outer leaflet of the plasma membrane. After washing the cells, cell fluorescence was quantified by flow cytometry in FL1 (Gallios; Beckman Coulter, Barcelona, Spain). Data were analyzed with FlowJo software version 8.7. The propidium iodide (PI; Sigma-Aldrich, Madrid, Spain) uptake was analyzed by incubating cells with 50-µg/mL PI in PBS in the dark for 5 min. Fluorescence was quantified by flow cytometry in FL3. Data were analyzed with FlowJo version 8.7.

2.9. Statistics

Statistics were performed using GraphPad Prism 8.0 via an unpaired t-test or one-way analysis of variance (ANOVA), followed by Bonferroni's or Tukey's comparison tests. Differences were considered to be significant at $p < 0.05$.

3. Results

3.1. The Lipidomic Profile of ccRCC Is Dependent on the Tumor Area Analyzed

ccRCC tumors frequently show visible macroscopic differences with defined boundaries between the center and external areas. Therefore, we first performed a lipidomic analysis of fatty acids by GC/MS of two arbitrarily separated tumor sections: the core and periphery. Figure 1 shows that the fatty acid profile of cellular PLs did not show marked differences when the control was compared with the different tumor sections: core or periphery. Both had similar amounts and types of fatty acids, with the exception of oleic acid (18:1n-9) and arachidonic acid (20:4n-6), which were increased in the core. In contrast, the distribution of fatty acids in the TAG and CE fractions showed a higher amount of lipids in the core (Figure 1B,C). Palmitic acid (16:0), stearic acid (18:0) and, particularly, 18:1n-9 were greatly increased in the core compared to normal tissue or periphery.

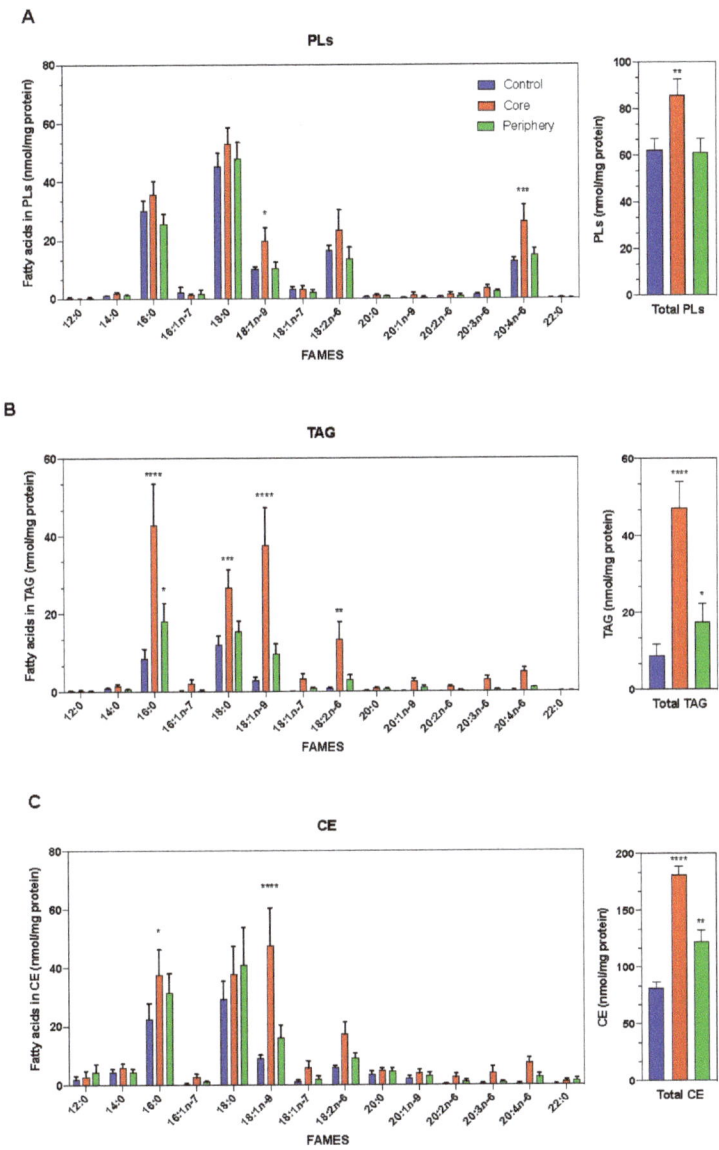

Figure 1. Lipidomic profile of ccRCC. (**A**) The profile of major phospholipid fatty acids in healthy distal normal tissue (blue bars) or tumors (core and periphery: red and green, respectively) were determined by GC/MS after converting the fatty acid glyceryl esters into fatty acid methyl esters. (**B,C**) Profile of fatty acids present in neutral lipids (TAG and CE). Data are expressed as the means ± SEM ($n = 12$). * $p < 0.05$, ** $p < 0.01$, *** $p < 0.001$ and **** $p < 0.0001$, significantly different from the control.

Since interindividual genotypic variations create great variability in primary cell culture models derived from tumors [46], in the following series of experiments, we used the Caki-1 and Caki-2 cell lines as an in vitro model of ccRCC. To compare the lipidomic profile of the Caki-1/-2 cell lines, we first analyzed the total cellular fatty acid content.

Similar to that observed in tumors, Figure 2 shows that the most abundant fatty acids in these cell lines were also 16:0, 18:0, 18:1*n*-9 and 20:4*n*-6. Although the two cell lines showed a similar fatty acid distribution, Caki-2 had a slightly higher amount of 18:1*n*-9. While both cell lines are ccRCC models, Caki-2 was established from a primary clear cell carcinoma of the kidney, and Caki-1 was derived from a skin metastasis. Consequently, we decided to use the Caki-2 cell line for the in vitro experiments.

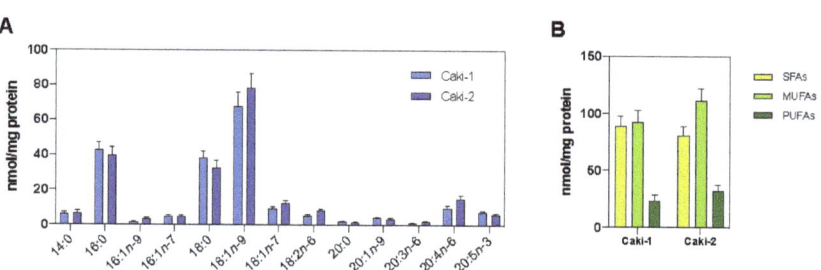

Figure 2. Lipidomic fatty acids profile of the Caki-1 and Caki-2 cell lines. (**A**) Total cellular fatty acid content. (**B**) Distribution of SFAs, MUFAs and PUFAs. Data are expressed as the means ± SEM and are representative of three independent experiments.

3.2. The Hypoxic Microenvironment Promotes SCD-1 Overexpression, Lipid Droplet Formation and Changes in the Cellular Fatty Acids Profile

Differences in the lipid composition, depending on the area of the tumor analyzed, should be in line with the expression pattern of the enzymes involved in their cellular metabolic pathways. Likewise, enzyme induction is strictly linked to the tumor microenvironment. Analyzing renal tumors, we previously showed that there is a statistical association of some hypoxia markers (e.g., *HIF-1A*) with the expression of *SCD-1* [27]. Thus, to investigate whether this physiological condition is actually responsible, at least in part, for SCD-1 induction, the Caki-2 cells were treated with different $CoCl_2$ concentrations for 24 h to generate chemical hypoxia in vitro [30,39].

We first determined the cytotoxicity after the treatment with $CoCl_2$ for 24 h and cell proliferation rates (growth constants (k) and cell doubling times; Supplementary Materials Figure S1). We observed that concentrations below 300 µM did not affect the cellular viability [47], but higher concentrations, up to 400 µM, induced cell death (5–10%). To verify that this salt did indeed generate cellular hypoxia, we evaluated by RT-qPCR the expression of hypoxia markers such as *HIF-1A* and *HIF-2A* (Figure 3A). Under the same conditions, the expression of *SCD-1* mRNA significantly increased (up to 200-fold) with 300-µM $CoCl_2$ (Figure 3B). We hypothesized that this increase in SCD-1 would be expected to lead to elevated amounts of intracellular 18:1*n*-9, which, in turn, would induce modifications in the lipid profile and/or cytoplasmic morphological changes. Hence we next evaluated the Caki-2 cells treated with 30-µM 18:1*n*-9 as a positive control for LD formation [48] with the cells treated with $CoCl_2$ (0–300 µM) by confocal microscopy. Using BODIPY® staining, we detected increased LD biogenesis that was dependent on the hypoxic conditions (Figure 3C).

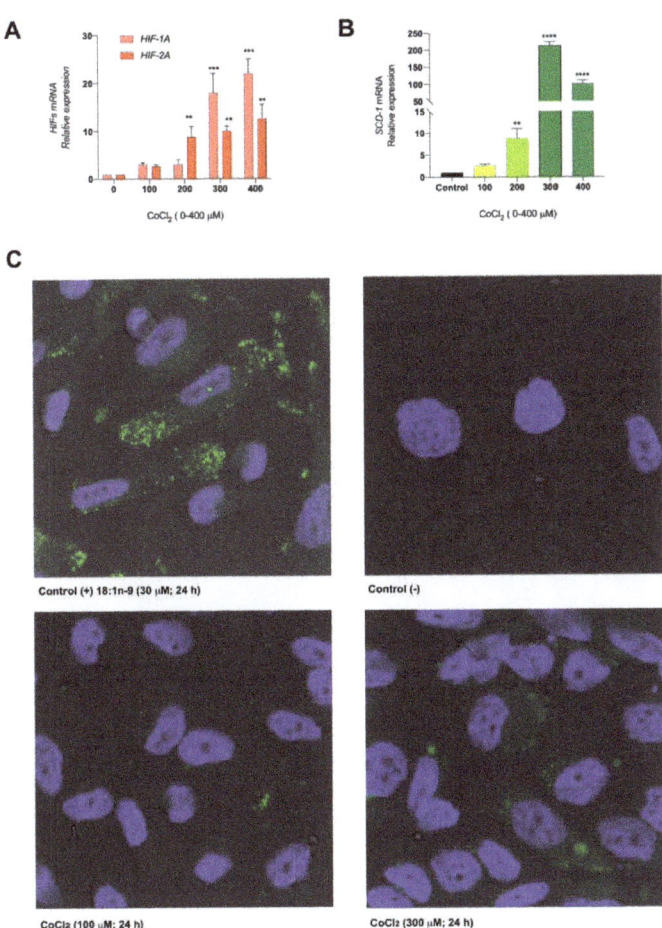

Figure 3. Chemical hypoxia promotes SCD-1 expression in vitro. (**A**) Caki-2 cells were exposed to different concentrations of CoCl$_2$ (0–400 μM) for 24 h, and the development of the hypoxic microenvironment was tested with the expression of *HIF-1A* and *HIF-2A* by RT-qPCR. (**B**) Then, *SCD-1* overexpression was detected under the same experimental conditions by RT-qPCR. (**C**) The evaluation of LD formation was determined by confocal microscopy. Caki-2 cells were exposed to 18:1n-9 (30 μM) for 24 h as a positive control for LD formation. Magnification 400×. Data are expressed as the means ± SEM and are representative of three independent experiments. ** $p < 0.01$, *** $p < 0.001$ and **** $p < 0.0001$, significantly different from the control.

In line with these phenotypic modifications, we evaluated the hypoxia-induced lipidomic changes in Caki-2 cells using GC/MS. Notably, the saturated fatty acids (16:0 and 18:0) experienced a significant reduction ($p < 0.001$) in all treatments in the PL fraction (Figure 4A). Consistent with the induction of *SCD-1* and the appearance of cytoplasmic LD, we observed a significant increase in 18:1n-9 but only in the TAG and CE fractions under hypoxic conditions ($p < 0.01$) (Figure 4B,C).

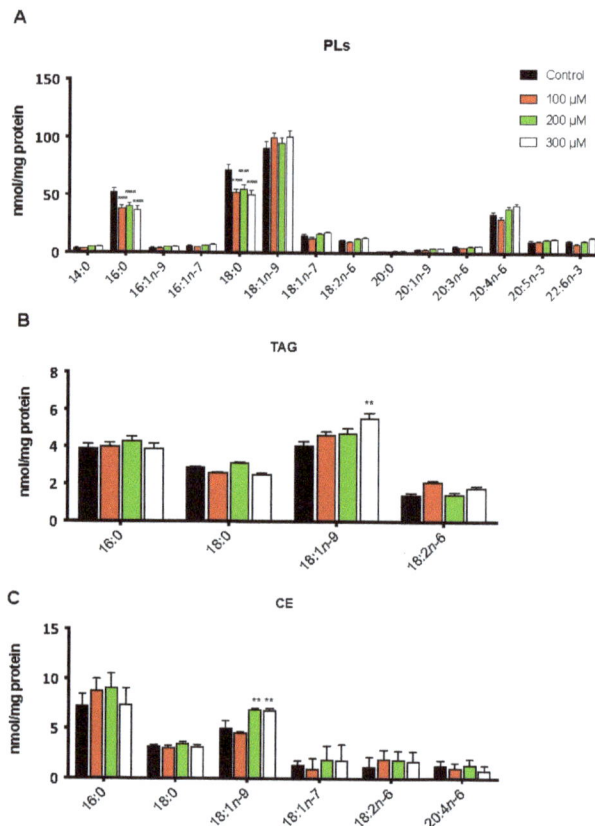

Figure 4. Lipidomic profile of the Caki-2 cells under hypoxic conditions. The cells were treated with the indicated concentrations of $CoCl_2$, and (**A**) the fatty acid contents in the phospholipids (PL), (**B**) triacylglycerol (TAG) and (**C**) cholesterol esters (CE) were determined by GC/MS. Data are expressed as the means ± SEM and are representative of three independent experiments. ** $p < 0.01$ and **** $p < 0.0001$, significantly different from the control.

3.3. Oleic Acid Is Essential for ccRCC Cell Proliferation

As additional evidence for the role of SCD-1 in the biosynthesis of MUFAs, the pharmacological inhibition of the enzyme was performed in Caki-2 cells using the selective inhibitor CAY 10566 at a nontoxic concentration (3 μM) for 24 h [49]. As shown in Figure 5A, marked lipid changes in the 18:0 and 18:1n-9 levels were detected. The total cellular fatty acid profile, considering all the lipid fractions simultaneously, showed a significant increase of 18:0, with a consequent decrease of 18:1n-9 ($p < 0.01$).

In line with that demonstrated by other authors with different methodologies [50], we noted that prolonged exposure times (longer than 24 h) to the enzyme inhibitor (3 μM) induced drastic decreases in the cell viability (34.65% ± 2.97; $p < 0.001$).

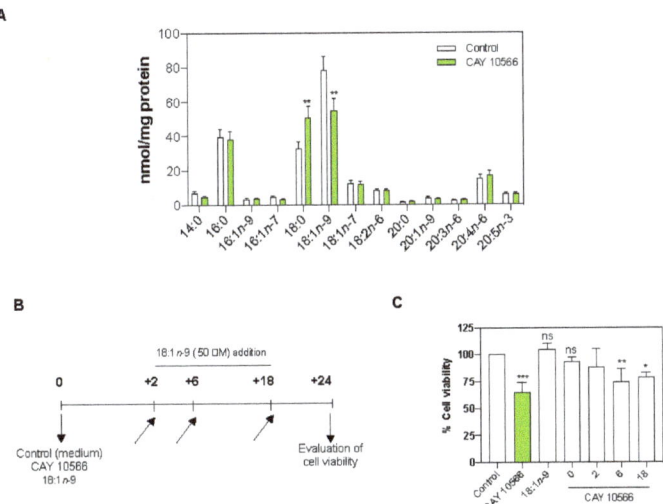

Figure 5. SCD-1 pharmacological inhibition. (**A**) Caki-2 cells were treated with the enzyme inhibitor CAY 10566 (3 µM) for 24 h. (**B**) Experimental design used in SCD-1 inhibition (slanted arrows indicate the addition of 18:1n-9 at different times). (**C**) Cell viability was measured with the CellTiter 96® kit. In all cases, the cells were cultured with 1% fetal bovine serum. Data are expressed as the means ± SEM and are representative of three independent experiments. * $p < 0.05$, ** $p < 0.01$ and *** $p < 0.001$, significantly different from the control.

If the reduced cellular levels of 18:1n-9 play a role in arresting the cell growth or triggering apoptosis, its addition to the cell culture would restore, at least in part, the cell proliferation. In order to check this hypothesis, 18:1n-9 (50 µM) was added at different times (Figure 5B,C) to Caki-2 cells with and without a treatment with CAY 10566 (3 µM). We observed that the addition of 18:1n-9, along with CAY 10566 or two hours after, preserved the cell viability; this effect was not observed if the fatty acid was added at later time points (Figure 5C).

In addition to evaluating the cell viability with CellTiter, we determined whether the inhibition of SCD-1 with CAY 10566 induced apoptosis in ccRCC. The Caki-2 cells were stained with annexin V-FITC and propidium iodide (50 µg/mL), as detailed in the Materials and Methods. Figure 6 shows that the cells treated with CAY 10566 manifested a small increase in apoptotic cell death, which was fully preventable if 18:1n-9 was present in the incubation media. Collectively, these data suggest that the decrease in cell viability that the cells experienced when SCD-1 was inhibited by CAY 10566 (Figure 5) was due to a reduced proliferation rate rather than drug-induced apoptotic cell death.

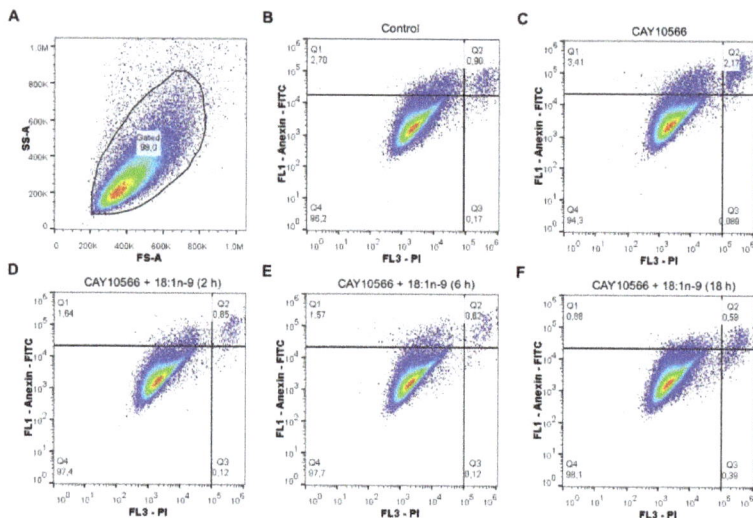

Figure 6. Analysis of the apoptotic markers in Caki-2 cells treated with a SCD-1 inhibitor and 18:1*n*-9. Apoptotic changes in the plasma membrane were detected by simultaneous staining with annexin V-fluorescein isothiocyanate (FITC) (FL1) and propidium iodide (PI; FL3) (**A**) Gating strategy in the control and treated cells. (**B**,**C**) Cells were untreated (control) or treated with 3-µM CAY 10566, respectively. (**D**–**F**) Afterward, 18:1*n*-9 (50 µM) was added to the cells at 2, 6 and 18 h, respectively.

4. Discussion

ccRCC tumors characteristically show a bright yellow color in the center as a result of its abundant lipid content and a variegated appearance in the boundary with hemorrhage, necrosis and/or fibrosis with a frequently well-circumscribed capsule or pseudo-capsule that separates the tumor from the adjacent tissues [51]. In order to address these differences in tumor heterogeneity, we developed a separate core and periphery analysis compared to the normal distal tissues, similarly to other ccRCC-focused studies [52,53]. In all the samples individually analyzed, the highest lipid content in the core was a constant pattern, despite the interindividual differences usually determined in the oncological analysis [54–56]. Consistent with these results, Saito et al., developing a broader study of untargeted lipidomics, determined that these tumors have large accumulations of CE and TAG among the other lipids [53].

These imbalances are obviously associated with the particular conditions that tumor cells show to adapt their metabolism to an uncontrolled and continuous growth [57]. Several enzymes within the fatty acid biosynthesis pathway have been found to be essential for cancer cell growth or survival and are currently tracked as possible targets for therapeutic development [13,58]. Among them, SCD-1 was demonstrated to be a key regulator of the MUFA/SFA balance in several cancer cells, and its blockade triggers apoptosis [8,59,60]. In particular, SCD-1 was shown to be overexpressed in ccRCC [1] and, therefore, proposed as a possible therapeutic target for future pharmacological actions [61]. However, in none of these previous studies was enzyme inhibition associated with the lipidomic cell profile and its hypoxic context.

We previously associated the expression of cellular hypoxia markers with SCD-1 overexpression in a large number of tumor samples (n = 24) [27]. In this study using Caki-2 cells exposed to in vitro chemical hypoxia [47], we effectively determined that the enzyme was highly overexpressed, mimicking the microenvironmental conditions of the tumor core. In this sense, although there is evidence that SCD-1 can be modulated by post-transcriptional mechanisms involving ubiquitin proteasome-dependent and -independent pathways [62], the levels of mammalian SCD-1 appear to be principally determined by its rate of transcription [6].

Adapting to hypoxic stress is pivotal in tumor progression and determining tumor malignancy [25,63,64]. Since cellular hypoxia increases 18:1n-9 production, the Caki-2 cells showed increased LD biogenesis, and this was in line with the dose of $CoCl_2$ used. Additionally, we used an 18:1n-9 overload of the same cells to simultaneously demonstrate that the 18:1n-9 increase is responsible for the increased LD production. The accumulation of these droplets is a sign of adaptation to stress and/or increased cell confluence [65]. The lipotoxicity that the increased synthesis of lipids brings about is neutralized, at least in part, with the production of these organelles [66,67]. LD biogenesis and degradation need to be discussed in the context of the synthesis and turnover of their major components: neutral lipids. Their synthesis is driven by the availability of precursors like TAG and CE [68,69]. Thus, we next performed a lipidomic analysis, under hypoxic conditions, using GC/MS to measure the levels of fatty acids in PLs and neutral lipids. In the PL fraction, large decreases were observed only in the SFAs (16:0 and 18:0), consequent with the increased expression of SCD-1. However, we did not observe changes at the 18:1n-9 level in this fraction. Conversely, the increases in 18:1n-9 were observed in neutral lipids, mainly in CE. Since these decreases in the SFAs are not quantitatively related to the newly formed 18:1n-9 by SCD-1 catalysis, most of 18:1n-9 must be redirected to mitochondrial β-oxidation [70] or, more likely (given the hypoxic context), released to the extracellular space. Thus, all types of cancer overexpressing this enzyme show high rates of cell proliferation, and this can only be done in cell contexts with high metabolic energy production [6,8,18,19,60,71]. On the other hand, Kamphorst et al. [72] found in other tumor lines (breast, lung and cervix) that hypoxia inhibits the catalytic activity of SCD-1 (since it uses oxygen as an electron acceptor) and shows that 18:1n-9 could be imported from the extracellular space.

The essential role of SCD-1 in cancer cell mitogenesis was unambiguously demonstrated by several works in which the suppression of SCD-1 by genetic and pharmacological means led to a slower rate of cell proliferation and decreased survival [61]. In this study, we observed that the viability of CAY 10566-treated Caki-2 cells was strongly correlated with the degree of inactivation of SCD-1, firmly establishing a positive relationship between the rate of MUFA synthesis and cell replication. Thus, at different times, we restored 18:1n-9 in the cell culture and observed that the cell viability improved, compared with CAY 10566-treated Caki-2 cells. Taken together, the lipidomic profile and cell viability experiments allowed us to assume that changes in the 18:1n-9 levels are critical for these tumor cells. Simultaneously, it has been observed that the excess content of long-chain fatty acids, especially SFAs, triggers programmed cell death in a process known as lipid-mediated toxicity or lipoapoptosis [73]. Thus, these two effects (SFA increase and 18:1n-9 decrease, caused by SCD-1 inhibition) evidently synergize and explain the cytotoxicity observed by long-term pharmacological inhibition.

Finally, the findings described here support the concept that SCD-1 may be a potentially useful target for ccRCC treatments [61,74]. The specific design of small-molecule inhibitors of SCD-1 activity could be of great potential for possible therapeutic agents [75]. Likewise, the association of SCD-1 inhibitors with therapeutic agents that target signaling pathways and their receptors (i.e., tyrosine kinase-mediated cascades, such as pazopanib, sunitinib, axitinib and cabozantinib, or temsirolimus, which targets mTOR, among others) already in use in medical oncology could also be an attractive option for future implementation [2]. Despite these hypothetical considerations, establishing the value of SCD-1 inhibitors as a protective agent for the treatment of ccRCC will require more extensive experimental testing and careful preclinical validation.

5. Conclusions

In this work, we provided evidence supporting the hypothesis that the lipid composition of ccRCC depends on the hypoxic microenvironment prevailing in certain areas, such as the center of the tumor. Our results added to this concept by demonstrating that there is a tumor microheterogeneity in terms of the fatty acid distribution in different lipid species such as PLs, TAG and CE. In line with the above, we showed that SCD-1 is particularly influenced by hypoxia, since it is overexpressed under these conditions and catalyzes the conversion of 18:0 into 18:1n-9, favoring tumor cell proliferation. In addition, we provided evidence to reinforce the idea that SCD-1 is a meaningful pharmacological target pondering the global hypoxic context of the tumor microenvironment.

Supplementary Materials: The following are available online at https://www.mdpi.com/article/10.3390/cancers13122962/s1: Figure S1: Cell proliferation rates (growth constants (k) and cell-doubling times) in all the conditions tested. Data are expressed as the means ± SEM and are representative of three independent experiments.

Author Contributions: Conceptualization: J.P.M., J.B. and J.P.R. Methodology: J.P.M., F.M. and T.S. Software: J.P.R. and F.M. Validation: J.B. and M.A.B. Formal analysis: J.P.R. and F.M. Investigation: J.P.M. Resources: J.B., M.V.A., J.P.R. and F.M. Data curation: M.V.A. and M.A.B. Writing—original draft preparation: J.P.M., J.B. and J.P.R. Writing—review and editing: J.P.M., J.P.R., M.A.B. and J.B. Visualization: J.P.M. and J.P.R. Supervision: J.P.R., M.V.A., M.A.B. and J.B. Project administration: J.P.R., M.V.A. and J.B. Funding acquisition: J.P.R., M.A.B. and J.B. All authors have read and agreed to the published version of the manuscript.

Funding: This research was funded by the Spanish Ministry of Science and Innovation, grant number PID2019-105989RB-I00, and Universidad Nacional del Nordeste de Argentina, grant number PI 18-I009. CIBERDEM is an initiative of Instituto de Salud Carlos III.

Institutional Review Board Statement: This study was conducted according to the guidelines of the Declaration of Helsinki and was approved by the Department of Medical Research and Bioethics Committee of the José Ramón Vidal Hospital in Corrientes, Argentina (date of approval, June 30 2015).

Informed Consent Statement: Informed consent was obtained from all the subjects involved in the study.

Data Availability Statement: The datasets used during the current study are available from the corresponding author upon reasonable request.

Acknowledgments: The authors thank Juan Todaro for the excellent technical advice.

Conflicts of Interest: The authors declare no conflict of interest. The funders had no role in the design of the study; in the collection, analyses or interpretation of the data; in the writing of the manuscript or in the decision to publish the results.

References

1. Wang, H.; Zhang, Y.; Lu, Y.; Song, J.; Huang, M.; Zhang, J.; Huang, Y. The role of stearoyl-coenzyme A desaturase 1 in clear cell renal cell carcinoma. *Tumour Biol.* **2015**, *37*, 479–489. [CrossRef]
2. Motzer, R.J.; Jonasch, E.; Michaelson, M.D.; Nandagopal, L.; Gore, J.L.; George, S.; Alva, A.; Haas, N.; Harrison, M.R.; Plimack, E.R.; et al. NCCN guidelines insights: Kidney cancer, version 2.2020. *J. Natl. Compr. Cancer Netw.* **2019**, *17*, 1278–1285. [CrossRef] [PubMed]
3. Tun, H.W.; Marlow, L.A.; von Roemeling, C.A.; Cooper, S.J.; Kreinest, P.; Wu, K.; Luxon, B.A.; Sinha, M.; Anastasiadis, P.Z.; Copland, J.A. Pathway signature and cellular differentiation in clear cell renal cell carcinoma. *PLoS ONE* **2010**, *5*, e10696. [CrossRef]
4. Abramczyk, H.; Surmacki, J.; Kopeć, M.; Olejnik, A.K.; Lubecka-Pietruszewska, K.; Fabianowska-Majewska, K. The role of lipid droplets and adipocytes in cancer. Raman imaging of cell cultures: MCF10A, MCF7, and MDA-MB-231 compared to adipocytes in cancerous human breast tissue. *Analyst* **2015**, *140*, 2224–2235. [CrossRef]
5. Ackerman, D.; Tumanov, S.; Qiu, B.; Michalopoulou, E.; Spata, M.; Azzam, A.; Xie, H.; Simon, M.C.; Kamphorst, J.J. Triglycerides promote lipid homeostasis during hypoxic stress by balancing fatty acid saturation. *Cell Rep.* **2018**, *24*, 2596–2605.e5. [CrossRef] [PubMed]
6. Igal, R.A. Stearoyl-Coa desaturase-1: A novel key player in the mechanisms of cell proliferation, programmed cell death and transformation to cancer. *Carcinogenesis* **2010**, *31*, 1509–1515. [CrossRef]
7. Beloribi-Djefaflia, S.; Vasseur, S.; Guillaumond, F. Lipid metabolic reprogramming in cancer cells. *Oncogenesis* **2016**, *5*, e189. [CrossRef]

8. Roongta, U.V.; Pabalan, J.G.; Wang, X.; Ryseck, R.P.; Fargnoli, J.; Henley, B.J.; Yang, W.P.; Zhu, J.; Madireddi, M.T.; Lawrence, R.M.; et al. Cancer cell dependence on unsaturated fatty acids implicates stearoyl-CoA desaturase as a target for cancer therapy. *Mol. Cancer Res.* **2011**, *9*, 1551–1561. [CrossRef] [PubMed]
9. Zhou, Y.; Bollu, L.R.; Tozzi, F.; Ye, X.; Bhattacharya, R.; Gao, G.; Dupre, E.; Xia, L.; Lu, J.; Fan, F.; et al. ATP citrate lyase mediates resistance of colorectal cancer cells to SN38. *Mol. Cancer Ther.* **2013**, *12*, 2782–2791. [CrossRef]
10. Wang, C.; Ma, J.; Zhang, N.; Yang, Q.; Jin, Y.; Wang, Y. The acetyl-CoA carboxylase enzyme: A target for cancer therapy? *Expert Rev. Anticancer Ther.* **2015**, *15*, 667–676. [CrossRef]
11. Ueda, K.; Nakatsu, Y.; Yamamotoya, T.; Ono, H.; Inoue, Y.; Inoue, M.K.; Mizuno, Y.; Matsunaga, Y.; Kushiyama, A.; Sakoda, H.; et al. Prolyl isomerase Pin1 binds to and stabilizes acetyl CoA carboxylase 1 protein, thereby supporting cancer cell proliferation. *Oncotarget* **2019**, *10*, 1637–1648. [CrossRef]
12. Svensson, R.U.; Parker, S.J.; Eichner, L.J.; Kolar, M.J.; Wallace, M.; Brun, S.N.; Lombardo, P.S.; Van Nostrand, J.L.; Hutchins, A.; Vera, L.; et al. Inhibition of acetyl-CoA carboxylase suppresses fatty acid synthesis and tumor growth of non-small-cell lung cancer in preclinical models. *Nat. Med.* **2016**, *22*, 1108–1119. [CrossRef]
13. Santos, C.R.; Schulze, A. Lipid metabolism in cancer. *FEBS J.* **2012**, *279*, 2610–2623. [CrossRef]
14. Igal, R.A. Roles of stearoylCoA desaturase-1 in the regulation of cancer cell growth, survival and tumorigenesis. *Cancers* **2011**, *3*, 2462–2477. [CrossRef]
15. Liotti, A.; Cosimato, V.; Mirra, P.; Calì, G.; Conza, D.; Secondo, A.; Luongo, G.; Terracciano, D.; Formisano, P.; Beguinot, F.; et al. Oleic acid promotes prostate cancer malignant phenotype via the G protein-coupled receptor FFA1/GPR40. *J. Cell. Physiol.* **2018**, *233*, 7367–7378. [CrossRef]
16. Liu, Z.; Xiao, Y.; Yuan, Y.; Zhang, X.; Qin, C.; Xie, J.; Hao, Y.; Xu, T.; Wang, X. Effects of oleic acid on cell proliferation through an integrin-linked kinase signaling pathway in 786-O renal cell carcinoma cells. *Oncol. Lett.* **2013**, *5*, 1395–1399. [CrossRef]
17. Chen, L.; Ren, J.; Yang, L.; Li, Y.; Fu, J.; Li, Y.; Tian, Y.; Qiu, F.; Liu, Z.; Qiu, Y. Stearoyl-CoA desaturase-1 mediated cell apoptosis in colorectal cancer by promoting ceramide synthesis. *Sci. Rep.* **2016**, *6*, 19665. [CrossRef]
18. Hess, D.; Chisholm, J.W.; Igal, R.A. Inhibition of stearoyl-CoA desaturase activity blocks cell cycle progression and induces programmed cell death in lung cancer cells. *PLoS ONE* **2010**, *5*, e11394. [CrossRef] [PubMed]
19. Scaglia, N.; Chisholm, J.W.; Igal, R.A. Inhibition of stearoylCoA desaturase-1 inactivates acetyl-CoA carboxylase and impairs proliferation in cancer cells: Role of AMPK. *PLoS ONE* **2009**, *4*, e6812. [CrossRef] [PubMed]
20. Mukherjee, A.; Kenny, H.A.; Lengyel, E. Unsaturated fatty acids maintain cancer cell stemness. *Cell Stem Cell* **2017**, *20*, 291–292. [CrossRef] [PubMed]
21. Suburu, J.; Chen, Y.Q. Lipids and prostate cancer. *Prostaglandins Other Lipid Mediat.* **2012**, *98*, 1–10. [CrossRef]
22. Jiang, L.; Wang, W.; He, Q.; Wu, Y.; Lu, Z.; Sun, J.; Liu, Z.; Shao, Y.; Wang, A. Oleic acid induces apoptosis and autophagy in the treatment of tongue squamous cell carcinomas. *Sci. Rep.* **2017**, *7*, 1–11. [CrossRef]
23. Carrillo, C.; Cavia, M.D.M.; Alonso-Torre, S.R. Efecto antitumoral del ácido oleico; mecanismos de acción; revisión científica. *Nutr. Hosp.* **2012**, *27*, 1860–1865. [PubMed]
24. Massari, F.; Ciccarese, C.; Santoni, M.; Brunelli, M.; Piva, F.; Modena, A.; Bimbatti, D.; Fantinel, E.; Santini, D.; Cheng, L.; et al. Metabolic alterations in renal cell carcinoma. *Cancer Treat. Rev.* **2015**, *41*, 767–776. [CrossRef]
25. Zhang, Y.; Wang, H.; Zhang, J.; Lv, J.; Huang, Y. Positive feedback loop and synergistic effects between hypoxia-inducible factor-2α and stearoyl-CoA desaturase-1 promote tumorigenesis in clear cell renal cell carcinoma. *Cancer Sci.* **2013**, *104*, 416–422. [CrossRef] [PubMed]
26. Arreola, A.; Cowey, C.L.; Coloff, J.L.; Rathmell, J.C.; Rathmell, W.K. HIF1α and HIF2α exert distinct nutrient preferences in renal cells. *PLoS ONE* **2014**, *9*, e98705. [CrossRef]
27. Stoyanoff, T.R.; Rodríguez, J.P.; Todaro, J.S.; Espada, J.D.; Melana Colavita, J.P.; Brandan, N.C.; Torres, A.M.; Aguirre, M.V. Tumor biology of non-metastatic stages of clear cell renal cell carcinoma; overexpression of stearoyl desaturase-1, EPO/EPO-R system and hypoxia-related proteins. *Tumor Biol.* **2016**, *37*, 13581–13593. [CrossRef] [PubMed]
28. Peck, B.; Schulze, A. Lipid Desaturation—The next step in targeting lipogenesis in cancer? *FEBS J.* **2016**, *15*, 2767–2778. [CrossRef]
29. Micucci, C.; Matacchione, G.; Valli, D.; Orciari, S.; Catalano, A. HIF2α is involved in the expansion of CXCR4-positive cancer stem-like cells in renal cell carcinoma. *Br. J. Cancer* **2015**, *113*, 1178–1185. [CrossRef]
30. Jin, G.; Liu, B.; You, Z.; Bambakidis, T.; Dekker, E.; Maxwell, J.; Halaweish, I.; Linzel, D.; Alam, H.B.; Arbor, A. Development of a novel neuroprotective strategy: Combined treatment with hypothermia and valproic acid improves survival in hypoxic hippocampal cells. *Surgery* **2015**, *156*, 221–228. [CrossRef]
31. Lazarowski, A.; Caltana, L.; Merelli, A.; Rubio, M.D.; Ramos, A.J.; Brusco, A. Neuronal mdr-1 gene expression after experimental focal hypoxia—A new obstacle for neuroprotection? *J. Neurol. Sci.* **2007**, *258*, 84–92. [CrossRef] [PubMed]
32. Du, J.; Sun, B.; Zhao, X.; Gu, Q.; Dong, X.; Mo, J.; Sun, T.; Wang, J.; Sun, R.; Liu, Y. Hypoxia promotes vasculogenic mimicry formation by inducing epithelial-mesenchymal transition in ovarian carcinoma. *Gynecol. Oncol.* **2014**, *133*, 575–583. [CrossRef]
33. Nishii, K.; Nakaseko, C.; Jiang, M.; Shimizu, N.; Takeuchi, M.; Schneider, W.J.; Bujo, H. The soluble form of LR11 protein is a regulator of hypoxia-induced, urokinase-type plasminogen activator receptor (uPAR)-mediated adhesion of immature hematological cells. *J. Biol. Chem.* **2013**, *288*, 11877–11886. [CrossRef] [PubMed]
34. Borsi, E.; Perrone, G.; Terragna, C.; Martello, M.; Dico, A.F.; Solaini, G.; Baracca, A.; Sgarbi, G.; Pasquinelli, G.; Valente, S.; et al. Hypoxia inducible factor-1 alpha as a therapeutic target in multiple myeloma. *Oncotarget* **2014**, *5*, 1779–1792. [CrossRef]

35. Chiang, C.K.; Nangaku, M.; Tanaka, T.; Iwawaki, T.; Inagi, R. Endoplasmic reticulum stress signal impairs erythropoietin production: A role for ATF4. *Am. J. Physiol. Cell Physiol.* **2013**, *304*, 342–353. [CrossRef]
36. Gao, Y.H.; Wu, Z.X.; Xie, L.Q.; Li, C.X.; Mao, Y.Q.; Duan, Y.T.; Han, B.; Han, S.F.; Yu, Y.; Lu, H.J.; et al. VHL deficiency augments anthracycline sensitivity of clear cell renal cell carcinomas by down-regulating ALDH2. *Nat. Commun.* **2017**, *8*, 15337. [CrossRef] [PubMed]
37. Chen, L.; Xia, G.; Qiu, F.; Wu, C.; Denmon, A.P.; Zi, X. Physapubescin selectively induces apoptosis in VHL-null renal cell carcinoma cells through down-regulation of HIF-2α and inhibits tumor growth. *Sci. Rep.* **2016**, *6*, 32582. [CrossRef] [PubMed]
38. Shinojima, T.; Oya, M.; Takayanagi, A.; Mizuno, R.; Shimizu, N.; Murai, M. Renal cancer cells lacking hypoxia inducible factor (HIF)-1α expression maintain vascular endothelial growth factor expression through HIF-2α. *Carcinogenesis* **2007**, *28*, 529–536. [CrossRef] [PubMed]
39. Wu, D.; Yotnda, P. Induction and testing of hypoxia in cell culture. *J. Vis. Exp.* **2011**, *54*, e2899. [CrossRef] [PubMed]
40. Bligh, E.G.; Dyer, W.J. A Rapid method of total lipid extraction and purification. *Can. J. Biochem. Physiol.* **1959**, *37*, 911–917. [CrossRef] [PubMed]
41. Diez, E.; Balsinde, J.; Aracil, M.; Schüller, A. Ethanol induces release of arachidonic acid but not synthesis of eicosanoids in mouse peritoneal macrophages. *Biochim. Biophys. Acta* **1987**, *921*, 82–89. [CrossRef]
42. Rodríguez, J.P.; Guijas, C.; Astudillo, A.M.; Rubio, J.M.; Balboa, M.A.; Balsinde, J. Sequestration of 9-hydroxystearic acid in fahfa (fatty acid esters of hydroxy fatty acids) as a protective mechanism for colon carcinoma cells to avoid apoptotic cell death. *Cancers* **2019**, *11*, 524. [CrossRef]
43. Astudillo, A.M.; Pérez-Chacón, G.; Balgoma, D.; Gil-De-Gómez, L.; Ruipérez, V.; Guijas, C.; Balboa, M.A.; Balsinde, J. Influence of cellular arachidonic acid levels on phospholipid remodeling and CoA-independent transacylase activity in human monocytes and U937 cells. *Biochim. Biophys. Acta* **2011**, *1811*, 97–103. [CrossRef] [PubMed]
44. Guijas, C.; Meana, C.; Astudillo, A.M.; Balboa, M.A.; Balsinde, J. Foamy monocytes are enriched in cis-7-hexadecenoic fatty acid, 16:1n-9, a possible biomarker for early detection of cardiovascular disease. *Cell Chem. Biol.* **2016**, *23*, 689–699. [CrossRef] [PubMed]
45. Astudillo, A.M.; Meana, C.; Guijas, C.; Pereira, L.; Lebrero, P.; Balboa, M.A.; Balsinde, J. Occurrence and biological activity of palmitoleic acid isomers in phagocytic cells. *J. Lipid Res.* **2018**, *59*, 237–249. [CrossRef] [PubMed]
46. Liu, S.; Yang, Z.; Li, G.; Li, C.; Luo, Y.; Gong, Q.; Wu, X.; Li, T.; Zhang, Z.; Xing, B.; et al. Multi-omics analysis of primary cell culture models reveals genetic and epigenetic basis of intratumoral phenotypic diversity. *Genom. Proteom. Bioinform.* **2019**, *17*, 576–589. [CrossRef] [PubMed]
47. Colavita, J.P.M.; Todaro, J.S.; de Sousa, M.; May, M.; Gomez, N.; Yaneff, A.; Di Siervi, N.; Aguirre, M.V.; Guijas, C.; Ferrini, L.; et al. Multidrug resistance protein 4 (MRP4/ABCC4) is overexpressed in clear cell renal cell carcinoma (ccRCC) and is essential to regulate cell proliferation. *Int. J. Biol. Macromol.* **2020**, *161*, 836–847. [CrossRef]
48. Valdearcos, M.; Esquinas, E.; Meana, C.; Gil-de-Gómez, L.; Guijas, C.; Balsinde, J.; Balboa, M.A. Subcellular localization and role of lipin-1 in human macrophages. *J. Immunol.* **2011**, *186*, 6004–6013. [CrossRef] [PubMed]
49. Koeberle, A.; Shindou, H.; Harayama, T.; Shimizu, T. Palmitoleate is a mitogen, formed upon stimulation with growth factors, and converted to palmitoleoyl-phosphatidylinositol. *J. Biol. Chem.* **2012**, *287*, 27244–27254. [CrossRef] [PubMed]
50. Qin, X.Y.; Su, T.; Yu, W.; Kojima, S. Lipid desaturation-associated endoplasmic reticulum stress regulates MYCN gene expression in hepatocellular carcinoma cells. *Cell Death Dis.* **2020**, *11*, 66. [CrossRef]
51. Grignon, D.J.; Che, M. Clear cell renal cell carcinoma. *Clin. Lab. Med.* **2005**, *25*, 305–316. [CrossRef]
52. Ricketts, C.J.; Linehan, W.M. Intratumoral heterogeneity in kidney cancer. *Nat. Genet.* **2014**, *46*, 214–215. [CrossRef] [PubMed]
53. Saito, K.; Arai, E.; Maekawa, K.; Ishikawa, M.; Fujimoto, H.; Taguchi, R.; Matsumoto, K.; Kanai, Y.; Saito, Y. Lipidomic signatures and associated transcriptomic profiles of clear cell renal cell carcinoma. *Sci. Rep.* **2016**, *6*, 28932. [CrossRef]
54. Sankin, A.; Hakimi, A.A.; Mikkilineni, N.; Ostrovnaya, I.; Silk, M.T.; Liang, Y.; Mano, R.; Chevinsky, M.; Motzer, R.J.; Solomon, S.B.; et al. The impact of genetic heterogeneity on biomarker development in kidney cancer assessed by multiregional sampling. *Cancer Med.* **2014**, *3*, 1485–1492. [CrossRef] [PubMed]
55. Okegawa, T.; Morimoto, M.; Nishizawa, S.; Kitazawa, S.; Honda, K. Intratumor heterogeneity in primary kidney cancer revealed by metabolic profiling of multiple spatially separated samples within tumors. *EBioMedicine* **2017**, *19*, 31–38. [CrossRef]
56. Casuscelli, J.; Vano, Y.; Herve, W.; Hsieh, J.J. Molecular classification of renal cell carcinoma and its implication in future clinical practice. *Kidney Cancer* **2017**, *1*, 3–13. [CrossRef] [PubMed]
57. Zhang, F. Dysregulated lipid metabolism in cancer. *World J. Biol. Chem.* **2012**, *3*, 167–174. [CrossRef]
58. Currie, E.; Schulze, A.; Zechner, R.; Walther, T.C.; Farese, R.V. Cellular fatty acid metabolism and cancer. *Cell Metab.* **2013**, *18*, 153–161. [CrossRef]
59. Minville-Walz, M.; Pierre, A.S.; Pichon, L.; Bellenger, S.; Fèvre, C.; Bellenger, J.; Tessier, C.; Narce, M.; Rialland, M. Inhibition of stearoyl-CoA desaturase 1 expression induces CHOP-dependent cell death in human cancer cells. *PLoS ONE* **2010**, *5*, e14363. [CrossRef]
60. Mason, P.; Liang, B.; Li, L.; Fremgen, T.; Murphy, E.; Quinn, A.; Madden, S.L.; Biemann, H.P.; Wang, B.; Cohen, A.; et al. SCD1 inhibition causes cancer cell death by depleting mono-unsaturated fatty acids. *PLoS ONE* **2012**, *7*, e33823. [CrossRef] [PubMed]

61. Von Roemeling, C.A.; Marlow, L.A.; Wei, J.J.; Cooper, S.J.; Caulfield, T.R.; Wu, K.; Tan, W.W.; Tun, H.W.; Copland, J.A. Stearoyl-CoA desaturase 1 is a novel molecular therapeutic target for clear cell renal cell carcinoma. *Clin. Cancer Res.* **2013**, *19*, 2368–2380. [CrossRef]
62. Kato, H.; Sakaki, K.; Mihara, K. Ubiquitin-proteasome-dependent degradation of mammalian ER stearoyl-CoA desaturase. *J. Cell Sci.* **2006**, *119*, 2342–2353. [CrossRef]
63. Koumenis, C. ER Stress, Hypoxia Tolerance and Tumor Progression. *Curr. Mol. Med.* **2006**, *6*, 55–69. [CrossRef]
64. Abou Khouzam, R.; Goutham, H.V.; Zaarour, R.F.; Chamseddine, A.N.; Francis, A.; Buart, S.; Terry, S.; Chouaib, S. Integrating tumor hypoxic stress in novel and more adaptable strategies for cancer immunotherapy. *Semin. Cancer Biol.* **2020**, *65*, 140–154. [CrossRef]
65. Guštin, E.; Jarc, E.; Kump, A.; Petan, T. Lipid droplet formation in hela cervical cancer cells depends on cell density and the concentration of exogenous unsaturated fatty acids. *Acta Chim. Slov.* **2017**, *64*, 549–554. [CrossRef]
66. Herms, A.; Bosch, M.; Ariotti, N.; Reddy, B.J.N.; Fajardo, A.; Fernández-Vidal, A.; Alvarez-Guaita, A.; Fernández-Rojo, M.A.; Rentero, C.; Tebar, F.; et al. Cell to cell heterogeneity in lipid droplets suggests a mechanism to reduce lipotoxicity. *Curr. Biol.* **2013**, *23*, 1489–1496. [CrossRef] [PubMed]
67. Kohlwein, S.D.; Veenhuis, M.; van der Klei, I.J. Lipid droplets and peroxisomes: Key players in cellular lipid homeostasis or a matter of fat-store'em up or burn'em down. *Genetics* **2013**, *193*, 1–50. [CrossRef] [PubMed]
68. Fujimoto, T.; Ohsaki, Y.; Cheng, J.; Suzuki, M.; Shinohara, Y. Lipid droplets: A classic organelle with new outfits. *Histochem. Cell Biol.* **2008**, *130*, 263–279. [CrossRef]
69. Guijas, C.; Rodríguez, J.P.; Rubio, J.M.; Balboa, M.A.; Balsinde, J. Phospholipase A_2 regulation of lipid droplet formation. *Biochim. Biophys. Acta* **2014**, *1841*, 1661–1671. [CrossRef] [PubMed]
70. Tamura, K.; Horikawa, M.; Sato, S.; Miyake, H.; Setou, M. Discovery of lipid biomarkers correlated with disease progression in clear cell renal cell carcinoma using desorption electrospray ionization imaging mass spectrometry. *Oncotarget* **2019**, *10*, 1688–1703. [CrossRef]
71. Noto, A.; Raffa, S.; De Vitis, C.; Roscilli, G.; Malpicci, D.; Coluccia, P.; Di Napoli, A.; Ricci, A.; Giovagnoli, M.R.; Aurisicchio, L.; et al. Stearoyl-CoA desaturase-1 is a key factor for lung cancer-initiating cells. *Cell Death Dis.* **2013**, *4*, e947. [CrossRef]
72. Kamphorst, J.J.; Cross, J.R.; Fan, J.; De Stanchina, E.; Mathew, R.; White, E.P.; Thompson, C.B.; Rabinowitz, J.D. Hypoxic and Ras-transformed cells support growth by scavenging unsaturated fatty acids from lysophospholipids. *Proc. Natl. Acad. Sci. USA* **2013**, *110*, 8882–8887. [CrossRef]
73. Schaffer, J.E. Lipotoxicity: When tissues overeat. *Curr. Opin. Lipidol.* **2003**, *14*, 281–287. [CrossRef] [PubMed]
74. Peck, B.; Schug, Z.T.; Zhang, Q.; Dankworth, B.; Jones, D.T.; Smethurst, E.; Patel, R.; Mason, S.; Jiang, M.; Saunders, R.; et al. Inhibition of fatty acid desaturation is detrimental to cancer cell survival in metabolically compromised environments. *Cancer Metab.* **2016**, *4*, 6. [CrossRef] [PubMed]
75. Imamura, K.; Tomita, N.; Kawakita, Y.; Ito, Y.; Ono, K.; Nii, N. Discovery of novel and potent stearoyl coenzyme A desaturase 1 (SCD1) inhibitors as anticancer agents. *Bioorg. Med. Chem.* **2017**, *25*, 3768–3779. [CrossRef] [PubMed]

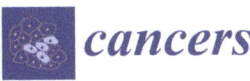

Article

PBRM1 Immunohistochemical Expression Profile Correlates with Histomorphological Features and Endothelial Expression of Tumor Vasculature for Clear Cell Renal Cell Carcinoma

Kazuho Saiga [1,†], Chisato Ohe [1,*,†], Takashi Yoshida [2], Haruyuki Ohsugi [2], Junichi Ikeda [1,2], Naho Atsumi [1], Yuri Noda [1], Yoshiki Yasukochi [3], Koichiro Higasa [3], Hisanori Taniguchi [2], Hidefumi Kinoshita [2] and Koji Tsuta [1]

[1] Department of Pathology, Kansai Medical University, 2-3-1 Shin-machi, Hirakata 573-1191, Japan; saigakaz@hirakata.kmu.ac.jp (K.S.); ikedaj@hirakata.kmu.ac.jp (J.I.); naatsumi@hirakata.kmu.ac.jp (N.A.); nodayur@hirakata.kmu.ac.jp (Y.N.); tsutakoj@hirakata.kmu.ac.jp (K.T.)

[2] Department of Urology and Andrology, Kansai Medical University, 2-3-1 Shin-machi, Hirakata 573-1191, Japan; yoshidtk@takii.kmu.ac.jp (T.Y.); ohsugih@hirakata.kmu.ac.jp (H.O.); taniguhi@hirakata.kmu.ac.jp (H.T.); kinoshih@hirakata.kmu.ac.jp (H.K.)

[3] Department of Genome Analysis, Institute of Biomedical Science, Kansai Medical University, 2-5-1 Shin-machi, Hirakata 573-1010, Japan; yasukocy@hirakata.kmu.ac.jp (Y.Y.); higasako@hirakata.kmu.ac.jp (K.H.)

* Correspondence: ohec@hirakata.kmu.ac.jp
† These authors contributed equally to this study.

Simple Summary: The PBRM1 protein, whose gene is the most frequently mutated one in clear cell renal cell carcinoma (ccRCC) following *von Hippel-Lindau*, has been proposed as a potential biomarker for ccRCC. However, the association of the PBRM1 immunohistochemical expression with histomorphological features of ccRCC and the endothelial expression of tumor vasculature, which is an important role of the tumor microenvironment related to treatment response, is little known. Recently, our research team has established a vascularity-based architectural classification of ccRCC correlated with angiogenesis and immune gene expression signatures, which could provide prognostic information and function as a surrogate for treatment selection. In the present study, we found the PBRM1 expression was correlated with the architectural patterns. Furthermore, we demonstrated that endothelial expression tended to be lost in cases with low PBRM1 expression. This correlation implied the orchestrated expression of PBRM1, raising the possibility that the cancer cells and their microenvironment interact in ccRCC.

Abstract: Loss of the polybromo-1 (PBRM1) protein has been expected as a possible biomarker for clear cell renal cell carcinoma (ccRCC). There is little knowledge about how PBRM1 immunohistochemical expression correlates with the histomorphological features of ccRCC and the endothelial expression of tumor vasculature. The present study evaluates the association of architectural patterns with the PBRM1 expression of cancer cells using a cohort of 425 patients with nonmetastatic ccRCC. Furthermore, we separately assessed the PBRM1 expression of the endothelial cells and evaluated the correlation between the expression of cancer cells and endothelial cells. PBRM1 loss in cancer cells was observed in 148 (34.8%) patients. In the correlation analysis between architectural patterns and PBRM1 expression, macrocyst/microcystic, tubular/acinar, and compact/small nested were positively correlated with PBRM1 expression, whereas alveolar/large nested, thick trabecular/insular, papillary/pseudopapillary, solid sheets, and sarcomatoid/rhabdoid were negatively correlated with PBRM1 expression. PBRM1 expression in vascular endothelial cells correlated with the expression of cancer cells (correlation coefficient = 0.834, $p < 0.001$). PBRM1 loss in both cancer and endothelial cells was associated with a lower recurrence-free survival rate ($p < 0.001$). Our PBRM1 expression profile indicated that PBRM1 expression in both cancer and endothelial cells may be regulated in an orchestrated manner.

Keywords: clear cell renal cell carcinoma; histomorphological features; PBRM1; immunohistochemistry; architectural patterns; endothelial cells

Citation: Saiga, K.; Ohe, C.; Yoshida, T.; Ohsugi, H.; Ikeda, J.; Atsumi, N.; Noda, Y.; Yasukochi, Y.; Higasa, K.; Taniguchi, H.; et al. PBRM1 Immunohistochemical Expression Profile Correlates with Histomorphological Features and Endothelial Expression of Tumor Vasculature for Clear Cell Renal Cell Carcinoma. *Cancers* 2022, 14, 1062. https://doi.org/10.3390/cancers14041062

Academic Editors: Claudia Manini and José I. López

Received: 17 January 2022
Accepted: 16 February 2022
Published: 20 February 2022

Publisher's Note: MDPI stays neutral with regard to jurisdictional claims in published maps and institutional affiliations.

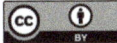

Copyright: © 2022 by the authors. Licensee MDPI, Basel, Switzerland. This article is an open access article distributed under the terms and conditions of the Creative Commons Attribution (CC BY) license (https://creativecommons.org/licenses/by/4.0/).

1. Introduction

Clear cell renal cell carcinoma (ccRCC), the most frequently diagnosed histologic subtype of adult RCC [1], is associated with a hyperangiogenic state due to the overproduction of vascular endothelial growth factor (VEGF) by loss of *von Hippel-Lindau (VHL)* gene function [2]. In addition to targeted therapy for these angiogenesis pathways such as VEGF receptor—tyrosine kinase inhibitors (TKIs) [3], novel systemic immunotherapy agents have improved patient survival in metastatic RCC [4,5]. However, predictive biomarkers for both the prognostic and therapeutic implications of RCC remain lacking in a clinical setting [6].

Recent genomic advances using exome sequencing revealed that the *PBRM1* gene encoding the protein polybromo-1, which is a subunit of the SWI/SNF chromatin remodeling complex, is a second major ccRCC cancer gene, following the *VHL* gene [7,8]. Several studies have shown that the loss of PBRM1 protein has been confirmed as a possible biomarker for ccRCC, which is associated with adverse pathological factors and poor patient outcomes [9,10]. Subsequently, our research team presented a novel scoring system to predict recurrence after radical surgery using standard pathologic factors incorporating immunohistochemical (IHC) expression of PBRM1 [11]. Furthermore, because *PBRM1* is considered not only a key driver gene of ccRCC but also a key regulator of tumor cell-autonomous immune response in ccRCC, the influence of PBRM1 loss on the response to immune checkpoint inhibitors (ICIs) has been investigated [7,12,13].

Recently, we first demonstrated that histological phenotypes, such as clear or eosinophilic types, were significantly correlated with survival outcomes and response to TKIs and ICIs in patients with ccRCC, which could be applied as a predictive marker for treatment selection [14]. Additionally, we established the vascularity-based architectural classification of ccRCC in accordance with nine architectural patterns, which corresponded to both angiogenesis and immune gene expression signatures [15]. Although the prognostic and therapeutic significance for architectural patterns of ccRCC has been shown [16,17], there is little knowledge on how genomics and subsequent protein expressions are reflected in histomorphological features [18].

To evaluate the association of the PBRM1 expression with histomorphological features, we semiquantitatively re-evaluated the expression by using the PBRM1-stained slides used in our previous study [11]. In addition, we noticed that the expression in vascular endothelial cells, which has been used as one of the internal positive controls in some studies [10,11], tended to decrease or disappear in the PBRM1 loss cases. However, there is little evidence regarding PBRM1 expression of the tumor vasculature, which plays an important role in the tumor microenvironment [19]. In the present study, we aimed to evaluate whether the histomorphological features of ccRCC correlate with the PBRM1 expression of cancer cells. Furthermore, we separately evaluated the PBRM1 expression of the vascular endothelial cells and examined the PBRM1 expression profiles of cancer cells and endothelial cells.

2. Materials and Methods

2.1. Case Selection

This study was performed under the institutional review board's approval at Kansai Medical University Hospital (No. 2018109 and No. 2020222). As in our previous report [15], data for 436 patients who underwent extirpative surgery for nonmetastatic ccRCC were identified from the institutional database between 2006 and 2017. Of these, 11 patients were excluded from this study due to an insufficient supply of pathological materials for immunohistochemistry. Thus, 425 cases with nonmetastatic ccRCC (cT1-4N0-1M0) were retrospectively analyzed. Our institutional database of RCC contains pathological findings, which were re-evaluated by a genitourinary pathologist (C.O.) based on the 2016 World Health Organization (WHO) classification [20] and the 2017 TNM staging system [21] as previously described [11,14,15]. All ccRCCs were histologically diagnosed when the carcinoma contained typical ccRCC histology and/or showed diffuse membranous positivity of carbonic anhydrase IX by immunohistochemistry [20]. Pathological prognostic factors, including pathological TNM stage, WHO/International Society of Urological Pathology (WHO/ISUP) grade, and necrosis, were collected [22].

2.2. Evaluation of Histomorphological Features

All histomorphological features were evaluated by C.O., blinded to clinical outcomes, using whole-tissue sections of H&E-stained slides. Histological phenotype, based on cytoplasmic features, such as clear, mixed, or eosinophilic, and vascularity-based architectural classification, based on nine architectural patterns, such as compact/small nested, macrocyst/microcystic, tubular/acinar, alveolar/large nested, thick trabecular/insular, papillary/pseudopapillary, solid sheets, and sarcomatoid and rhabdoid, were determined at the highest-grade area as previously described [15].

2.3. Tissue Microarray (TMA) Construction and Immunohistochemistry of PBRM1

As previously described [11,23,24], TMA was constructed from duplicate 2 mm cores of representative tumor locations (including the highest-grade area) in each case. The morphological patterns of each core were also assessed based on the nine architectural patterns included in the vascularity-based architectural classification [15]. A primary antibody against PBRM1 (rabbit polyclonal, dilution 1:200; Atlas Antibodies AB, Bromma, Sweden) was used according to the manufacturer's protocols of the Ventana Discovery Ultra Autostainer (Roche Diagnostics, Indianapolis, IN, USA). PBRM1 was visualized with OptiView and an amplification kit (Ventana Medical System, Tucson, AZ, USA). The same PBRM1-stained slides from our previous study [11] were used in the present study. The nuclear expression of cancer cells was semiquantitatively assessed, referring to the internal positive controls (inflammatory cells or stromal fibroblasts), using the H-score. The score was determined by multiplying the staining intensity (0, none; 1, weak; 2, moderate; and 3, strong) and the percentage of positive cells (range: 0–300). The final scores (average H-score for the two cores) were determined as previously described [23]: H-score ≤ 20 was considered for PBRM1 loss, and H-score > 20 was considered for PBRM1 retention in cancer cells. An IHC evaluation was performed by two pathologists (K.S. and C.O.), and discordant cases were resolved by consensus. Next, we separately evaluated the nuclear expression of endothelial cells within the tumor area and scored them as follows: 0, none; 1, focal weak; 2, diffuse weak; or 3, diffuse strong. The scores of endothelial cells were finally stratified as PBRM1 loss (score: 0–1) and PBRM1 retention (score: 2–3). The representative PBRM1 expressions of cancer cells and endothelial cells are presented in Figure 1.

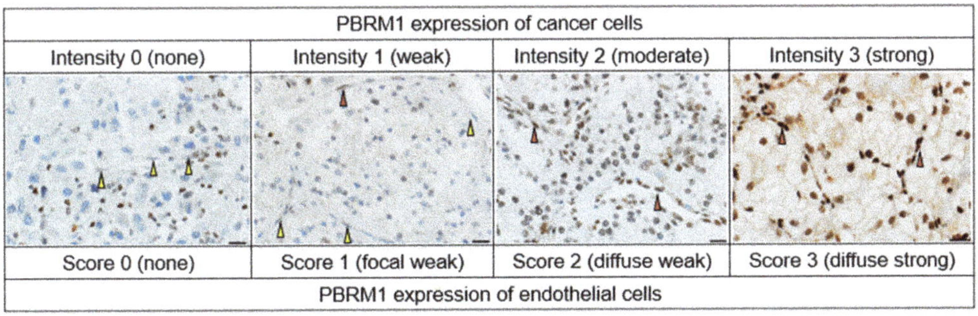

Figure 1. Representative PBRM1 expressions of cancer cells and endothelial cells. The staining intensity of cancer cells is assessed as follows: 0, none (internal control shows positive staining); 1, weak; 2, moderate; 3, strong. The score of endothelial cells is separately assessed as follows: 0, none; 1, focal weak; 2, diffuse weak; or 3, diffuse strong. The negative and positive expressions of endothelial cells are indicated by yellow and red arrows, respectively. Scale bar: 20 µm.

2.4. Statistical Analysis

Statistical analyses were performed using EZR version 1.54 (Saitama Medical Center, Jichi, Japan) [25]. A two-sided $p < 0.05$ was considered statistically significant. A Chi-squared test for categorical variables was used to evaluate the statistical significance among two or more groups. The t-statistic in linear regression analysis and one-way ANOVA analysis were used to evaluate the statistical significance among the architectural patterns. Interobserver agreement was statistically assessed using kappa statistics. Correlations between the two variables were evaluated using Spearman's rank correlation test. Recurrence-free survival (RFS; recurrence was calculated on imaging from the date of surgery to the date of recurrence) was assessed using the Kaplan–Meier method with the log-rank test.

3. Results

3.1. Patients' Characteristics and PBRM1 Expression in Cancer Cells

The median age of the patients was 65 years (IQR, 56–73 years). The male to female ratio was 2.8:1 (312 males and 113 females). The rate of TNM stage III or IV, WHO/ISUP grade 3 or 4, and the presence of necrosis was 24.0% (102/425), 32.3% (137/425), and 15.3% (65/425), respectively. Of the 425 patients, 57 (13.4%) experienced a recurrence of ccRCC during a median follow-up of 62.6 months (IQR, 33.8–94.0 months).

Cases with PBRM1 loss and PBRM1 retention were observed in 148 (34.8%) and 277 (65.2%) patients, respectively. The interobserver variability showed good agreement between the two pathologists (kappa = 0.84). The PBRM1 expression of clinicopathological factors is shown in Table 1.

Table 1. PBRM1 expression in cancer cells with clinicopathological factors in 425 cases with non-metastatic ccRCC.

Variables	PBRM1 Retention	PBRM1 Loss
Gender, n (%)		
Female	81 (71.7)	32 (28.3)
Male	196 (62.8)	116 (37.2)
TNM stage, n (%)		
I	242 (78.1)	68 (21.9)
II	3 (23.1)	10 (76.9)
III	32 (32.0)	68 (68.0)
IV	0 (0.0)	2 (100.0)
WHO/ISUP grade, n (%)		
1	58 (96.7)	2 (3.3)
2	155 (68.0)	73 (32.0)
3	58 (52.7)	52 (47.3)
4	6 (22.2)	21 (77.8)
Necrosis, n (%)		
Absent	256 (71.1)	104 (28.9)
Present	21 (32.3)	44 (67.7)
Histological phenotype, n (%)		
Clear	201 (77.3)	59 (22.7)
Mixed	71 (49.0)	74 (51.0)
Eosinophilic	5 (25.0)	15 (75.0)
Vascularity-based architectural classification, n (%)		
Category 1	218 (79.0)	58 (21.0)
Category 2	55 (45.1)	67 (54.9)
Category 3	4 (14.8)	23 (85.2)
Recurrence, n (%)	11 (19.3)	46 (80.7)
Cancer-specific mortality, n (%)	2 (13.3)	13 (86.7)

3.2. Association of PBRM1 Expression in Cancer Cells with Clinicopathological Factors

Loss of PBRM1 expression was significantly associated with worsened pathological prognostic factors, such as TNM stage, WHO/ISUP grade, and the presence of necrosis (all $p < 0.001$; Figure 2A). Regarding the association of PBRM1 expression with histomorphological features, cases with PBRM1 loss were significantly observed in the eosinophilic type, which is related to high gene expression signature scores of effector T-cells, immune checkpoint molecules, and epithelial and mesenchymal transitions [14], among other histologic phenotypes. Similarly, cases with PBRM1 loss were significantly observed in category 3, which is associated with a low gene signature of angiogenesis and high gene signatures of effector T-cell and immune checkpoint [15], among vascularity-based architectural categories (both $p < 0.001$; Figure 2B).

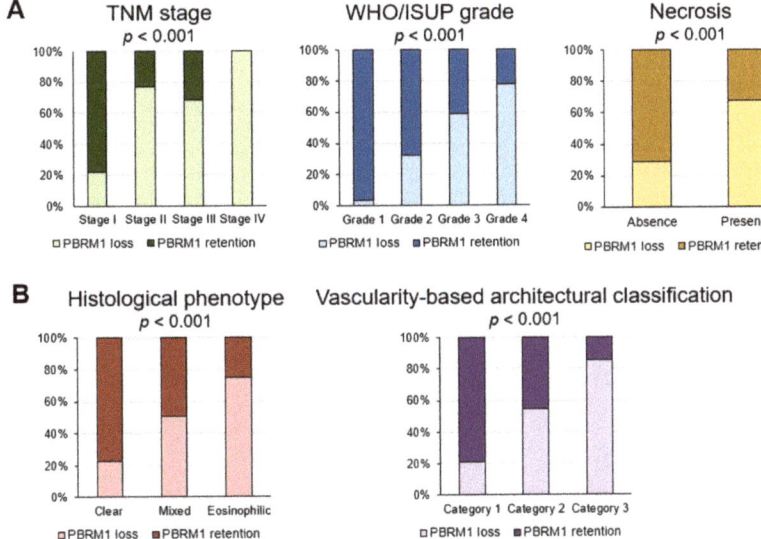

Figure 2. Association of PBRM1 expression in cancer cells with pathological factors. (**A**) Percentage of cases of PBRM1 expression and conventional pathological prognostic factors; (**B**) Percentage of cases of PBRM1 expression and histological phenotype and vascularity-based architectural classification.

3.3. Association of PBRM1 Expression in Cancer Cells with Architectural Patterns

Regarding the association of PBRM1 expression with architectural patterns in the highest-grade area, tumors with PBRM1 loss were observed in 50/177 (28.2%) of compact/small nested, 1/36 (2.8%) in macrocyst/microcystic, 7/63 (11.1%) in tubular/acinar, 20/47 (42.6%) in alveolar/large nested, 37/55 (67.3%) in thick trabecular/insular, 10/20 (50%) in papillary/pseudopapillary, 8/9 (88.9%) in solid sheet, and 15/18 (83.3%) in sarcomatoid/rhabdoid patterns (Table 2). Representative images of PBRM1 expression in each architectural pattern are shown in Figure 3.

Table 2. PBRM1 expression in cancer cells with histomorphological features in 425 cases with nonmetastatic ccRCC.

Architectural Patterns, n (%)	PBRM1 Retention	PBRM1 Loss
Compact/Small nested	127 (71.8)	50 (28.2)
Macrocyst/Microcystic	35 (97.2)	1 (2.8)
Tubular/Acinar	56 (88.9)	7 (11.1)
Alveolar/Large nested	27 (57.4)	20 (42.6)
Thick trabecular/Insular	18 (32.7)	37 (67.3)
Papillary/Pseudopapillary	10 (50.0)	10 (50.0)
Solid sheets	1 (11.1)	8 (88.9)
Sarcomatoid/Rhabdoid	3 (16.7)	15 (83.3)

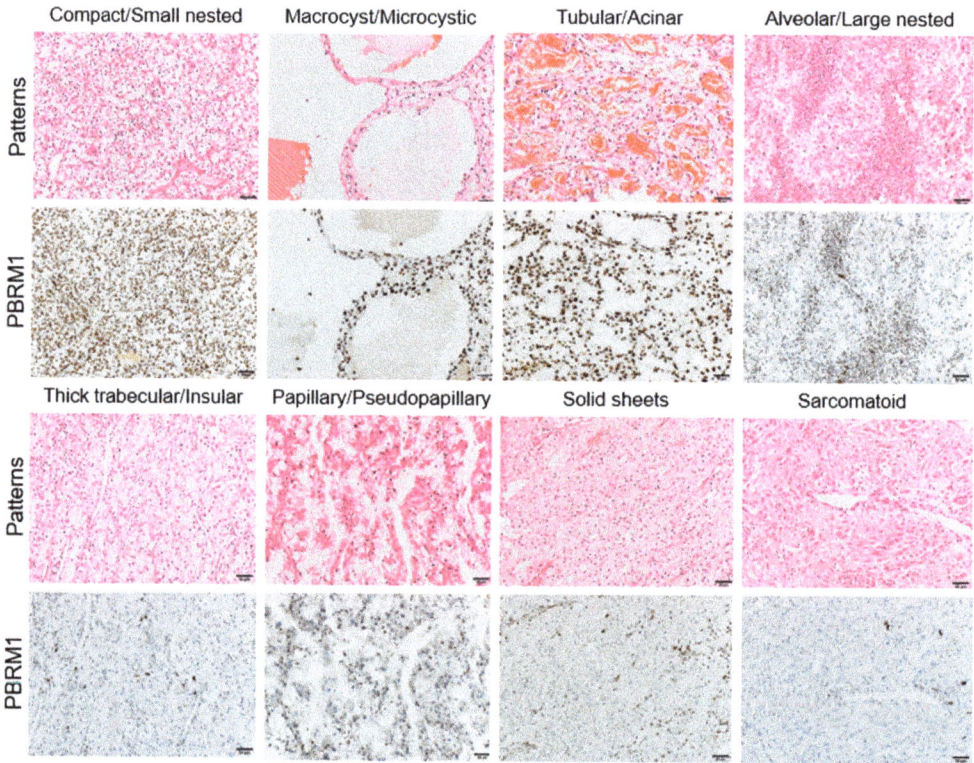

Figure 3. Representative images of each architectural pattern and PBRM1 immunohistochemical expression. Compact/small nested, macrocyst/microcystic, and tubular/acinar patterns are highly associated with PBRM1 retention, whereas the other patterns are highly associated with PBRM1 loss. Scale bar: 20 μm.

To evaluate the correlation between architectural patterns and PBRM1 expression (H-score), multiple linear regression analysis was performed (Figure 4). Macrocyst/microcystic (t statistic = 7.734, $p < 0.001$), tubular/acinar (t statistic = 4.228, $p < 0.001$), and compact/small nested (t statistic = 1.95, $p = 0.0519$) were positively correlated with the PBRM1 expression although compact/small nested was not statistically significant. On the other hand, thick trabecular/insular (t statistic = -5.98, $p < 0.001$), sarcomatoid/rhabdoid (t statistic = -3.829, $p < 0.001$), solid sheets (t statistic = -2.965, $p = 0.0032$), alveolar/large nested (t statistic = -2.935, $p = 0.0035$), and papillary/pseudopapillary (t statistic = -2.016, $p = 0.0444$) were negatively correlated with the PBRM1 expression.

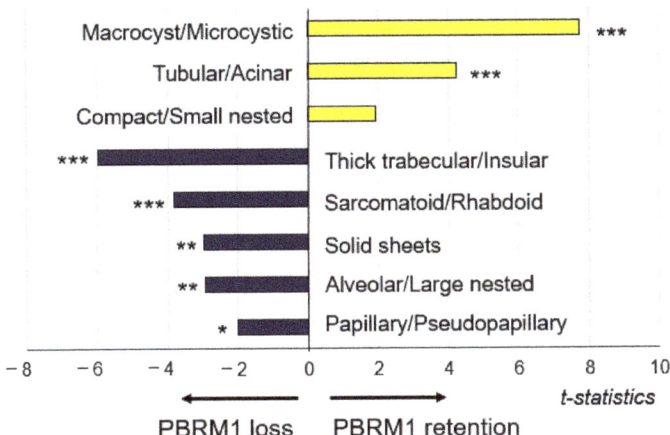

Figure 4. Association of architectural patterns with PBRM1 expression in cancer cells; correlation analysis between architectural patterns in the highest-grade area and PBRM1 expression ($n = 425$). * $p < 0.05$, ** $p < 0.01$, *** $p < 0.001$ using multiple linear regression analysis.

Of 403 cases where two cores were assessed for PBRM1 expression (22 out of 425 cases were missing one core), 77 (19.1%) showed heterogeneity of PBRM1 expression (H-score ≤ 20 vs. >20) between cores. Therefore, we examined whether PBRM1 expression was correlated with the architectural patterns of the corresponding area by assessing a total of 828 cores. It was revealed that PBRM1 expression was correlated with the architectural patterns among all of the evaluated cores. Notably, this association between PBRM1 expression and the architectural patterns assessed in the highest-grade area, namely, macrocyst/microcystic, tubular/acinar, and compact/small nest, had significantly higher PBRM1 expressions (H-score) compared to the other patterns ($p < 0.001$, $p < 0.001$, and $p < 0.05$, respectively) (Figure 5).

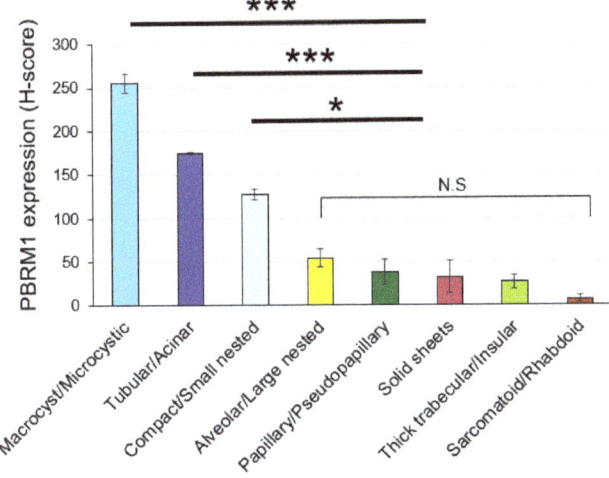

Figure 5. Association of architectural patterns with PBRM1 expression in cancer cells based on H-score in each TMA core ($n = 828$). The histogram shows the mean ± standard error of the mean H-score of PBRM1 expression in cancer cells. One-way analysis of variance with the Tukey test was used for statistical analysis (N.S. means not statistically significant: * $p < 0.05$, *** $p < 0.001$).

3.4. Association between Cancer Cells and Endothelial Cells

3.4.1. Correlation between PBRM1 Expression in Cancer Cells and Endothelial Cells

A positive correlation between PBRM1 expression in cancer cells and endothelial cells was confirmed (correlation coefficient = 0.834, $p < 0.001$; Figure 6A).

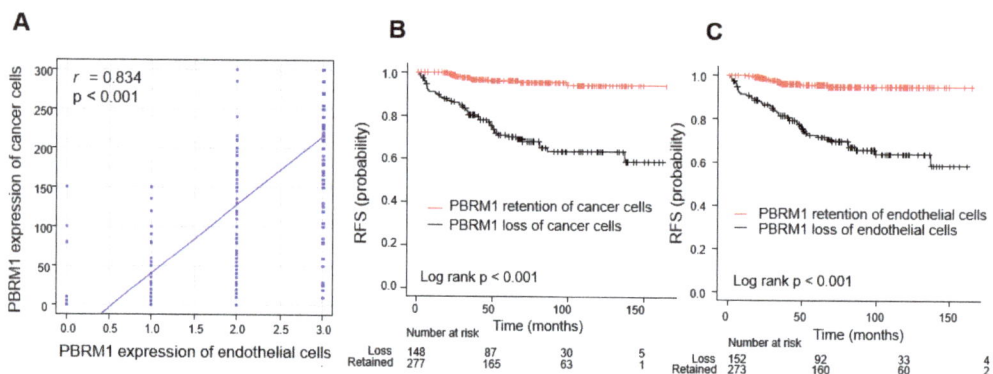

Figure 6. Association between cancer cells and endothelial cells. (**A**) Correlation between PBRM1 expression in cancer cells and endothelial cells. Correlations between the two variables were evaluated using Spearman's rank correlation test. (**B,C**) Kaplan–Meier curve of recurrence-free survival (RFS) stratified by PBRM1 expression. (**B**) PBRM1 expression of cancer cells. (**C**) PBRM1 expression of endothelial cells.

3.4.2. Prognostic Significance of PBRM1 Expression in Cancer Cells and Endothelial Cells

Survival curve analysis showed that the 5-year RFS rate was significantly lower in patients with PBRM1 loss than in those with PBRM1 retained in cancer cells (71.1% versus 96.1%, $p < 0.001$; Figure 6B). Similarly, the 5-year RFS rate was significantly lower in patients with PBRM1 loss than in those with PBRM1 retained in endothelial cells (72.5 versus 95.6%, $p < 0.001$; Figure 6C).

4. Discussion

Typical histological features of ccRCC consist of neoplastic cells with clear cytoplasm and a vascular network of small and thin-walled blood vessels, activated by hypoxia-inducible factors following *VHL* inactivation [20]. Although the most common architectural pattern of ccRCC is compact/small nested with an extensive vascular network, the morphologic intratumoral heterogeneity of ccRCC has been recognized [15–17]. Recent findings have shown that *VHL* mono-driver tumors are characterized by low-grade and indolent behavior with minimum intratumoral heterogeneity [26]. In contrast, tumors characterized by high-grade and aggressive behavior include multiple clonal drivers that exhibit truncal aberrations of ccRCC epigenetic-related genes: the SWI/SNF chromatin remodeling complex gene *PBRM1*, histone deubiquitinate gene *BAP1*, and histone methyltransferase gene *SETD2* [8,26]. Högner et al. also showed that the combined loss of PBRM1 and VHL may contribute to tumor aggressiveness [27]. However, little is known about the ways these genetic abnormalities impact the histomorphological features of ccRCC.

In the current study, we provided several insights into the PBRM1 IHC expression profile of ccRCC. First, we revealed the association of PBRM1 expression with histological phenotype based on cytoplasmic features [14] and vascularity-based architectural classification [15] (Figure 2B), both of which stratify patient prognosis. For histological phenotype, the eosinophilic type was significantly correlated with PBRM1 loss, followed by mixed type, whereas for vascularity-based architectural classification, category 3 was significantly enriched in the PBRM1 loss group, followed by category 2. These results indicated that PBRM1 loss was correlated with novel poor prognostic factors based on histomorphological features. Consistent with the previous reports [28–31], we showed the adverse prognostic factors of ccRCC, such as high TNM stage and WHO/ISUP grade or presence of necrosis, were significantly associated with PBRM1 loss (Figure 2A). While a study of localized RCC using TMA failed to show the prognostic role of PBRM1 loss after adjusting for the significant prognostic clinicopathological parameters [32], multivariable models of our prior study showed that PBRM1-negativity is an independent prognostic factor for RFS [11]. Thus, our findings suggest that the additional epigenetic change increases the aggressiveness of ccRCC and results in a poor prognosis.

Second, we showed architectural patterns based on a vascularity-based architectural classification [15], assessed in the highest-grade area in 425 nonmetastatic ccRCC, correlated with the PBRM1 expression profile. Macrocyst/microcystic, tubular/acinar, and compact/small nested patterns characterized by enrichment of the vascular network (corresponded to category 1) were positively correlated with PBRM1 expression, whereas alveolar/large nested, thick trabecular/insular, and papillary/pseudopapillary patterns characterized by the widely spaced-out vascular network (corresponded to category 2), or solid sheets and sarcomatoid/rhabdoid patterns characterized by scattered vascularity without a vascular network (corresponded to category 3) were negatively correlated with the PBRM1 expression (Figure 4). These results indicate that PBRM1 expression patterns differ among the architectural patterns of ccRCC with or without an extensive vascular network.

Third, in the evaluation of 828 cores considering intratumor heterogeneity, we also demonstrated architectural patterns in macrocyst/microcystic, tubular/acinar, and compact/small nested associated with significantly higher PBRM1 expression (H-score) compared to the other patterns (Figure 5), which suggested that PBRM1 expression profile correlated well with the ccRCC architectural patterns, even with intratumoral heterogeneity. Although intratumoral heterogeneity of ccRCC has been reported based on DNA sequencing and chromosome aberration analysis [33], we showed that loss of PBRM1 protein reflects morphologic heterogeneity and aggressive architectural patterns of ccRCC.

The role of PBRM1 protein expression for clinical decisions is not only being a biomarker of prognostic prediction but also providing information on molecular mechanisms and potential therapeutic targets. In the present study, we showed the prognostic predictive ability of PBRM1 loss in nonmetastatic ccRCC, while Cai et al. also showed that PBRM1 could improve the predictive accuracy for survival outcomes of metastatic RCC patients treated with tyrosine kinase inhibitors (TKIs) [34]. Recently, the effectiveness of systemic therapies (TKIs vs. ICIs) in patients with the *PBRM1* mutation status of ccRCC has also been investigated [12,13,35–37]. Although some studies have shown that patients with PBRM1 loss in ccRCC experience increased clinical benefit from ICIs [12,35], data on the effect of PBRM1 loss regarding immune responsiveness are inconsistent [13,36,37]. According to our previous study, category 3 of the vascularity-based architectural classification, which is related to loss of PBRM1 expression, was significantly associated with an inflamed and excluded immunophenotype in the localized ccRCC cohort and significantly enriched in effector-T cell and immune checkpoint gene signatures in the TCGA-KIRC cohort [15]. We have also shown that in ccRCC, including eosinophilic features related to loss of PBRM1 expression, significant clinical benefit was observed in the ICI therapy group compared to the TKI therapy group ($p = 0.035$) [14].

Contrary to our findings, however, some studies showed that *PBRM1* mutations were associated with increased angiogenesis, decreased immune infiltrates, and poor response to ICIs [13,37]. While these controversial findings have yet to be resolved, the *PBRM1* mutation does not directly determine the loss of the corresponding protein or function [38]. Because some discrepancies between *PBRM1* mutation and PBRM1 IHC expression have been reported, a comprehensive investigation, including *PBRM1* mutation, PBRM1 expression, and histomorphological features, should be conducted. Recently, Lin et al. evaluated the influence of PBRM1 loss for treatment response, focusing on the "immunogenic" tumor microenvironment [13]. However, the "non-immunogenic" tumor microenvironment, including endothelial cells, is also an important factor for appropriate treatment strategies because combined therapies of TKIs and ICIs have been applied for metastatic ccRCC [19,39]. Nevertheless, there are a few studies focusing on the expression of PBRM1 in endothelial cells of ccRCC.

To the best of our knowledge, we are the first to have demonstrated that the PBRM1 IHC expression of endothelial cells is correlated with the expression of cancer cells, which suggests that the vascular endothelial cells may also be genetically or immunohistochemically abnormal (Figure 6). Although we should consider the possibility of a marked reduction in the protein expression due to insufficient or unequal fixation [40], positive expression of internal control such as inflammatory cells or stromal fibroblasts was confirmed in the present study (Figure 1). Angiogenesis also plays a central role in ccRCC tumorigenesis and progression, regulating the immune landscape through abnormal tumor vessel formation [39]. Our observation showed that the tumor vasculature among the vascularity-based architectural pattern of category 1 vs. categories 2 and 3 was different. The specific mechanism underlying the association of decreased PBRM1 expression with the architectural patterns without a vascular network is still unclear, but the interaction of cancer cells and endothelial cells may be suggested. In the current treatment strategies, including angiogenic therapy, the understanding of the epigenetic abnormality between cancer cells and endothelial cells should be considered. Further investigation by single-cell analysis is required to determine the mechanism of the interaction between cancer cells and endothelial cells in the tumor microenvironment.

Our current work has some limitations. The PBRM1 expression was evaluated using only TMA, including the highest-grade area. Even considering intratumoral heterogeneity, however, we showed that the PBRM1 expression was correlated with the architectural patterns. Next, we semiquantitatively assessed PBRM1 IHC expression in cancer cells using an H-score. Furthermore, we could not validate the association of architectural patterns with *PBRM1* mutation status. Despite these limitations, we comprehensively showed the association of the PBRM1 expression profile with clinicopathological factors, including detailed histomorphological features.

5. Conclusions

We demonstrated that PBRM1 expression of cancer cells correlated with histomorphological features of ccRCC and correlated with the expression of vascular endothelial cells. Our PBRM1 expression profile indicated that PBRM1 expression in both cancer and endothelial cells may be regulated in an orchestrated manner.

Author Contributions: Conceptualization, K.S., C.O., T.Y. and K.T.; Data curation, T.Y., J.I. and H.O.; Formal analysis, C.O., T.Y. and J.I.; Investigation, K.S. and C.O.; Methodology, C.O., T.Y., N.A. and Y.N.; Resources, H.O., Y.Y. and H.T.; Supervision, K.H., H.K. and K.T.; Visualization, C.O.; Writing—original draft, K.S. and C.O. All authors have read and agreed to the published version of the manuscript.

Funding: This research was funded by the Japan Society for the Promotion of Science KAKENHI fund (Grants No. 19K16875 to C.O. and Grants No. 20K16457 to H.O.).

Institutional Review Board Statement: The study was conducted according to the guidelines of the Declaration of Helsinki and approved by the Institutional Review Board of Kansai Medical University Hospital (No. 2018109 and No. 2020222).

Informed Consent Statement: Informed consent was obtained in the form of opt-out on the website of Kansai Medical University Hospital. No one expressed a refusal.

Data Availability Statement: The data are available upon reasonable request by contacting the corresponding author.

Acknowledgments: We are grateful to Ryosuke Yamaka for his technical assistance in the construction of tissue microarray.

Conflicts of Interest: C.O. received research funding from Chugai Pharmaceutical Co. Ltd. outside the submitted work. The funders had no role in the design of the study; in the collection, analyses, or interpretation of data; in the writing of the manuscript, or in the decision to publish the results. The remaining authors declare no conflicts of interest.

References

1. Shuch, B.; Amin, A.; Armstrong, A.J.; Eble, J.N.; Ficarra, V.; Lopez-Beltran, A.; Martignoni, G.; Rini, B.I.; Kutikov, A. Understanding pathologic variants of renal cell carcinoma: Distilling therapeutic opportunities from biologic complexity. *Eur. Urol.* **2015**, *67*, 85–97. [CrossRef] [PubMed]
2. George, D.J.; Kaelin, W.G., Jr. The von Hippel-Lindau protein, vascular endothelial growth factor, and kidney cancer. *N. Engl. J. Med.* **2003**, *349*, 419–421. [CrossRef] [PubMed]
3. Rini, B.I. Vascular endothelial growth factor-targeted therapy in metastatic renal cell carcinoma. *Cancer* **2009**, *115*, 2306–2312. [CrossRef] [PubMed]
4. Motzer, R.J.; Escudier, B.; McDermott, D.F.; George, S.; Hammers, H.J.; Srinivas, S.; Tykodi, S.S.; Sosman, J.A.; Procopio, G.; Plimack, E.R.; et al. Nivolumab versus Everolimus in Advanced Renal-Cell Carcinoma. *N. Engl. J. Med.* **2015**, *373*, 1803–1813. [CrossRef] [PubMed]
5. Motzer, R.J.; Tannir, N.M.; McDermott, D.F.; Arén Frontera, O.; Melichar, B.; Choueiri, T.K.; Plimack, E.R.; Barthélémy, P.; Porta, C.; George, S.; et al. Nivolumab plus Ipilimumab versus Sunitinib in Advanced Renal-Cell Carcinoma. *N. Engl. J. Med.* **2018**, *378*, 1277–1290. [CrossRef] [PubMed]
6. Schmidt, A.L.; Siefker-Radtke, A.; McConkey, D.; McGregor, B. Renal Cell and Urothelial Carcinoma: Biomarkers for New Treatments. *Am. Soc. Clin. Oncol. Educ. Book* **2020**, *40*, 1–11. [CrossRef]
7. Varela, I.; Tarpey, P.; Raine, K.; Huang, D.; Ong, C.K.; Stephens, P.; Davies, H.; Jones, D.; Lin, M.L.; Teague, J.; et al. Exome sequencing identifies frequent mutation of the SWI/SNF complex gene PBRM1 in renal carcinoma. *Nature* **2011**, *469*, 539–542. [CrossRef]
8. The Cancer Genome Atlas Research Network. Comprehensive molecular characterization of clear cell renal cell carcinoma. *Nature* **2013**, *499*, 43–49. [CrossRef] [PubMed]
9. Da Costa, W.H.; Rezende, M.; Carneiro, F.C.; Rocha, R.M.; da Cunha, I.W.; Carraro, D.M.; Guimaraes, G.C.; de Cassio Zequi, S. Polybromo-1 (PBRM1), a SWI/SNF complex subunit is a prognostic marker in clear cell renal cell carcinoma. *BJU Int.* **2014**, *113*, E157–E163. [CrossRef]
10. Joseph, R.W.; Kapur, P.; Serie, D.J.; Parasramka, M.; Ho, T.H.; Cheville, J.C.; Frenkel, E.; Parker, A.S.; Brugarolas, J. Clear Cell Renal Cell Carcinoma Subtypes Identified by BAP1 and PBRM1 Expression. *J. Urol.* **2016**, *195*, 180–187. [CrossRef]
11. Ohsugi, H.; Yoshida, T.; Ohe, C.; Ikeda, J.; Sugi, M.; Kinoshita, H.; Tsuta, K.; Matsuda, T. The SSPN Score, a Novel Scoring System Incorporating PBRM1 Expression, Predicts Postoperative Recurrence for Patients with Non-metastatic Clear Cell Renal Cell Carcinoma. *Ann. Surg. Oncol.* **2021**, *28*, 2359–2366. [CrossRef] [PubMed]
12. Miao, D.; Margolis, C.A.; Gao, W.; Voss, M.H.; Li, W.; Martini, D.J.; Norton, C.; Bossé, D.; Wankowicz, S.M.; Cullen, D.; et al. Genomic correlates of response to immune checkpoint therapies in clear cell renal cell carcinoma. *Science* **2018**, *359*, 801–806. [CrossRef] [PubMed]
13. Liu, X.D.; Kong, W.; Peterson, C.B.; McGrail, D.J.; Hoang, A.; Zhang, X.; Lam, T.; Pilie, P.G.; Zhu, H.; Beckermann, K.E.; et al. PBRM1 loss defines a nonimmunogenic tumor phenotype associated with checkpoint inhibitor resistance in renal carcinoma. *Nat. Commun.* **2020**, *11*, 2135. [CrossRef] [PubMed]
14. Yoshida, T.; Ohe, C.; Ikeda, J.; Atsumi, N.; Ohsugi, H.; Sugi, M.; Higasa, K.; Saito, R.; Tsuta, K.; Matsuda, T.; et al. Eosinophilic features in clear cell renal cell carcinoma correlate with outcomes of immune checkpoint and angiogenesis blockade. *J. Immunother. Cancer* **2021**, e002922. [CrossRef] [PubMed]
15. Ohe, C.; Yoshida, T.; Amin, M.B.; Atsumi, N.; Ikeda, J.; Saiga, K.; Noda, Y.; Yasukochi, Y.; Ohashi, R.; Ohsugi, H.; et al. Development and validation of a vascularity-based architectural classification for clear cell renal cell carcinoma: Correlation with conventional pathological prognostic factors, gene expression patterns, and clinical outcomes. *Mod. Pathol.* **2021**, 1–9. [CrossRef]
16. Verine, J.; Colin, D.; Nheb, M.; Prapotnich, D.; Ploussard, G.; Cathelineau, X.; Desgrandchamps, F.; Mongiat-Artus, P.; Feugeas, J.P. Architectural Patterns are a Relevant Morphologic Grading System for Clear Cell Renal Cell Carcinoma Prognosis Assessment: Comparisons with WHO/ISUP Grade and Integrated Staging Systems. *Am. J. Surg. Pathol.* **2018**, *42*, 423–441. [CrossRef]
17. Cai, Q.; Christie, A.; Rajaram, S.; Zhou, Q.; Araj, E.; Chintalapati, S.; Cadeddu, J.; Margulis, V.; Pedrosa, I.; Rakheja, D.; et al. Ontological analyses reveal clinically-significant clear cell renal cell carcinoma subtypes with convergent evolutionary trajectories into an aggressive type. *EBioMedicine* **2020**, *51*, 102526. [CrossRef]
18. Peña-Llopis, S.; Vega-Rubín-de-Celis, S.; Liao, A.; Leng, N.; Pavía-Jiménez, A.; Wang, S.; Yamasaki, T.; Zhrebker, L.; Sivanand, S.; Spence, P.; et al. BAP1 loss defines a new class of renal cell carcinoma. *Nat. Genet.* **2012**, *44*, 751–759. [CrossRef]
19. Heidegger, I.; Pircher, A.; Pichler, R. Targeting the Tumor Microenvironment in Renal Cell Cancer Biology and Therapy. *Front. Oncol.* **2019**, *9*, 490. [CrossRef]
20. Moch, H.; Humphrey, P.A.; Ulbright, T.M.; Reuter, V.E. *WHO Classification of Tumours of the Urinary System and Male Genital Organs*, 4th ed.; IARC: Lyon, France, 2016.

21. Brierley, J.D.; Gospodarowics, M.K.; Wittekind, C. Union for International Cancer Control. In *TNM Classification of Malignant Tumours*, 8th ed.; Wiley: New York, NY, USA, 2017.
22. Delahunt, B.; Srigley, J.R.; Judge, M.J.; Amin, M.B.; Billis, A.; Camparo, P.; Evans, A.J.; Fleming, S.; Griffiths, D.F.; Lopez-Beltran, A.; et al. Data set for the reporting of carcinoma of renal tubular origin: Recommendations from the International Collaboration on Cancer Reporting (ICCR). *Histopathology* **2019**, *74*, 377–390. [CrossRef]
23. Ikeda, J.; Ohe, C.; Yoshida, T.; Ohsugi, H.; Sugi, M.; Tsuta, K.; Kinoshita, H. PD-L1 Expression and Clinicopathological Factors in Renal Cell Carcinoma: A Comparison of Antibody Clone 73-10 with Clone 28-8. *Anticancer Res.* **2021**, *41*, 4577–4586. [CrossRef] [PubMed]
24. Yoshida, T.; Ohe, C.; Ikeda, J.; Atsumi, N.; Saito, R.; Taniguchi, H.; Ohsugi, H.; Sugi, M.; Tsuta, K.; Matsuda, T.; et al. Integration of NRP1, RGS5, and FOXM1 expression, and tumour necrosis, as a postoperative prognostic classifier based on molecular subtypes of clear cell renal cell carcinoma. *J. Pathol. Clin. Res.* **2021**, *7*, 590–603. [CrossRef] [PubMed]
25. Kanda, Y. Investigation of the freely available easy-to-use software 'EZR' for medical statistics. *Bone Marrow Transplant.* **2013**, *48*, 452–458. [CrossRef] [PubMed]
26. Kapur, P.; Christie, A.; Rajaram, S.; Brugarolas, J. What morphology can teach us about renal cell carcinoma clonal evolution. *Kidney Cancer J.* **2020**, *18*, 68–76. [CrossRef]
27. Högner, A.; Krause, H.; Jandrig, B.; Kasim, M.; Fuller, T.F.; Schostak, M.; Erbersdobler, A.; Patzak, A.; Kilic, E. PBRM1 and VHL expression correlate in human clear cell renal cell carcinoma with differential association with patient's overall survival. *Urol. Oncol.* **2018**, *36*, 94-e1. [CrossRef]
28. Pawłowski, R.; Mühl, S.M.; Sulser, T.; Krek, W.; Moch, H.; Schraml, P. Loss of PBRM1 expression is associated with renal cell carcinoma progression. *Int. J. Cancer* **2013**, *132*, E11–E17. [CrossRef] [PubMed]
29. Nam, S.J.; Lee, C.; Park, J.H.; Moon, K.C. Decreased PBRM1 expression predicts unfavorable prognosis in patients with clear cell renal cell carcinoma. *Urol. Oncol.* **2015**, *33*, e9–e16. [CrossRef]
30. Wang, Z.; Peng, S.; Guo, L.; Xie, H.; Wang, A.; Shang, Z.; Niu, Y. Prognostic and clinicopathological value of PBRM1 expression in renal cell carcinoma. *Clin. Chim. Acta* **2018**, *486*, 9–17. [CrossRef]
31. Bihr, S.; Ohashi, R.; Moore, A.L.; Rüschoff, J.H.; Beisel, C.; Hermanns, T.; Mischo, A.; Corrò, C.; Beyer, J.; Beerenwinkel, N.; et al. Expression and Mutation Patterns of PBRM1, BAP1 and SETD2 Mirror Specific Evolutionary Subtypes in Clear Cell Renal Cell Carcinoma. *Neoplasia* **2019**, *21*, 247–256. [CrossRef]
32. Kim, S.H.; Park, W.S.; Park, E.Y.; Park, B.; Joo, J.; Joung, J.Y.; Seo, H.K.; Lee, K.H.; Chung, J. The prognostic value of BAP1, PBRM1, pS6, PTEN, TGase2, PD-L1, CA9, PSMA, and Ki-67 tissue markers in localized renal cell carcinoma: A retrospective study of tissue microarrays using immunohistochemistry. *PLoS ONE* **2017**, *12*, e0179610. [CrossRef]
33. Gerlinger, M.; Rowan, A.J.; Horswell, S.; Math, M.; Larkin, J.; Endesfelder, D.; Gronroos, E.; Martinez, P.; Matthews, N.; Stewart, A.; et al. Intratumor heterogeneity and branched evolution revealed by multiregion sequencing. *N. Engl. J. Med.* **2012**, *366*, 883–892. [CrossRef] [PubMed]
34. Cai, W.; Wang, Z.; Cai, B.; Yuan, Y.; Kong, W.; Zhang, J.; Chen, Y.; Liu, Q.; Huang, Y.; Huang, J.; et al. Expression of PBRM1 as a prognostic predictor in metastatic renal cell carcinoma patients treated with tyrosine kinase inhibitor. *Int. J. Clin. Oncol.* **2020**, *25*, 338–346. [CrossRef] [PubMed]
35. Braun, D.A.; Ishii, Y.; Walsh, A.M.; Van Allen, E.M.; Wu, C.J.; Shukla, S.A.; Choueiri, T.K. Clinical Validation of PBRM1 Alterations as a Marker of Immune Checkpoint Inhibitor Response in Renal Cell Carcinoma. *JAMA Oncol.* **2019**, *5*, 1631–1633. [CrossRef] [PubMed]
36. Dizman, N.; Lyou, Y.; Salgia, N.; Bergerot, P.G.; Hsu, J.; Enriquez, D.; Izatt, T.; Trent, J.M.; Byron, S.; Pal, S. Correlates of clinical benefit from immunotherapy and targeted therapy in metastatic renal cell carcinoma: Comprehensive genomic and transcriptomic analysis. *J. Immunother. Cancer* **2020**, e000953. [CrossRef] [PubMed]
37. McDermott, D.F.; Huseni, M.A.; Atkins, M.B.; Motzer, R.J.; Rini, B.I.; Escudier, B.; Fong, L.; Joseph, R.W.; Pal, S.K.; Reeves, J.A.; et al. Clinical activity and molecular correlates of response to atezolizumab alone or in combination with bevacizumab versus sunitinib in renal cell carcinoma. *Nat. Med.* **2018**, *24*, 749–757. [CrossRef] [PubMed]
38. Piva, F.; Giulietti, M.; Occhipinti, G.; Santoni, M.; Massari, F.; Sotte, V.; Iacovelli, R.; Burattini, L.; Santini, D.; Montironi, R.; et al. Computational analysis of the mutations in BAP1, PBRM1 and SETD2 genes reveals the impaired molecular processes in renal cell carcinoma. *Oncotarget* **2015**, *6*, 32161–32168. [CrossRef]
39. D'Aniello, C.; Berretta, M.; Cavaliere, C.; Rossetti, S.; Facchini, B.A.; Iovane, G.; Mollo, G.; Capasso, M.; Pepa, C.D.; Pesce, L.; et al. Biomarkers of Prognosis and Efficacy of Anti-angiogenic Therapy in Metastatic Clear Renal Cancer. *Front. Oncol.* **2019**, *9*, 1400. [CrossRef]
40. Sato, M.; Kojima, M.; Nagatsuma, A.K.; Nakamura, Y.; Saito, N.; Ochiai, A. Optimal fixation for total preanalytic phase evaluation in pathology laboratories. A comprehensive study including immunohistochemistry, DNA, and RNA assays. *Pathol. Int.* **2014**, *64*, 209–216. [CrossRef]

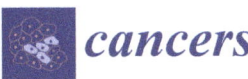

Review

Radiogenomics in Clear Cell Renal Cell Carcinoma: A Review of the Current Status and Future Directions

Sari Khaleel [1], Andrew Katims [2], Shivaram Cumarasamy [2], Shoshana Rosenzweig [2], Kyrollis Attalla [2], A Ari Hakimi [1] and Reza Mehrazin [2,*]

[1] Memorial Sloan Kettering Cancer Center, Department of Urology, New York, NY 10065, USA; khaleels@mskcc.org (S.K.); hakimia@mskcc.org (A.A.H.)
[2] Department of Urology, Icahn School of Medicine at Mount Sinai, New York, NY 10029, USA; andrew.katims@mountsinai.org (A.K.); shivaram.cumarasamy@mountsinai.org (S.C.); shoshana.rosenzweig@icahn.mssm.edu (S.R.); kyrollis.attalla@mountsinai.org (K.A.)
* Correspondence: reza.mehrazin@mountsinai.org

Simple Summary: Clear renal cell carcinoma (ccRCC) is the most common type of renal cancer. As with other malignancies, knowledge of the genetic makeup of ccRCC tumors may provide insights for tumor management and outcomes. However, this normally requires obtaining tissue specimens from the tumor by invasive interventions—surgery or biopsy. Radiogenomics is a field that aims to non-invasively predict the genetic makeup of the tumor based on the tumor's appearance on conventional imaging, such as CT scans. To achieve this, radiogenomics uses complex machine learning (artificial intelligence) algorithms to process imaging data and build predictive models that can infer a tumor's genetic makeup and clinical outcomes from its features on conventional imaging. In this article, we searched scientific literature databases for radiogenomic studies in ccRCC, offering a review and critical analysis of these studies. More research and validation are needed before applying radiogenomics in clinical practice.

Abstract: Radiogenomics is a field of translational radiology that aims to associate a disease's radiologic phenotype with its underlying genotype, thus offering a novel class of non-invasive biomarkers with diagnostic, prognostic, and therapeutic potential. We herein review current radiogenomics literature in clear cell renal cell carcinoma (ccRCC), the most common renal malignancy. A literature review was performed by querying PubMed, Medline, Cochrane Library, Google Scholar, and Web of Science databases, identifying all relevant articles using the following search terms: "radiogenomics", "renal cell carcinoma", and "clear cell renal cell carcinoma". Articles included were limited to the English language and published between 2009–2021. Of 141 retrieved articles, 16 fit our inclusion criteria. Most studies used computed tomography (CT) images from open-source and institutional databases to extract radiomic features that were then modeled against common genomic mutations in ccRCC using a variety of machine learning algorithms. In more recent studies, we noted a shift towards the prediction of transcriptomic and/or epigenetic disease profiles, as well as downstream clinical outcomes. Radiogenomics offers a platform for the development of non-invasive biomarkers for ccRCC, with promising results in small-scale retrospective studies. However, more research is needed to identify and validate robust radiogenomic biomarkers before integration into clinical practice.

Keywords: radiogenomics; translational; clear cell renal cell carcinoma

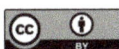

1. Introduction

Renal cell carcinoma (RCC) is the most common malignant kidney tumor, accounting for approximately 85% of cases [1]. Clear cell carcinoma (ccRCC) is the most common histologic RCC subtype, particularly in advanced RCC (approximately 60–70%, and 90%, respectively) [2]. With increased use of computed tomography (CT) and magnetic resonance-guided imaging (MRI), the incidence of RCC is rising in developed countries, usually at the clinically localized stage [3]. Despite the advancements in cross-sectional imaging technology, their ability to differentiate RCC subtypes and their underlying molecular profiles remain limited [4,5].

One approach to improve the diagnostic ability of conventional imaging has been the adoption of advanced computational and statistical methods to process high throughput radiologic features extracted from conventional imaging, giving rise to the field of radiomics [6]. In parallel, our understanding of the genomic profiles of cancers and their potential as diagnostic, prognostic, and therapeutic biomarkers has been advanced by the application of complex computational and statistical methods to analyze high-throughput next-generation sequencing data, allowing for complex genomic, transcriptomic, and epigenomic analyses of tumor specimens. Such analyses in the field of RCC have revealed that in addition to histologic variance, RCC is a genetically diverse disease, with distinct molecular genomic and transcriptomic profiles that correlate with clinical outcomes such as recurrence, progression, and response to systemic therapies [7–10].

Despite the above advances in molecular and radiologic profiling of RCC in general and ccRCC in particular, the current prognostic models remain based on clinical, pathologic, and laboratory characteristics, with the pathologic stage heavily influencing cancer-specific survival [11–14]. The reliance of these models on pathologic staging makes them inherently invasive, requiring tissue diagnosis based on surgical extirpation or tissue biopsy, with no standardized non-invasive or pre-treatment biomarkers that can be used to classify RCC or predict tumor behavior. This limitation applies to genomic profiling tools, as well, as they also require tissue extraction for their analyses, along with complex and cost-prohibitive translational infrastructures that currently limit their applicability in clinical practice.

Radiogenomics is a novel field that circumvents the above challenges by utilizing computational machine learning algorithms to correlate radiomic features of disease (radiologic phenotype) with its underlying molecular profile (genotype), thereby offering a platform for the development of non-invasive biomarkers to aid in treatment decisions and disease [15,16]. Of note, while the term "radiogenomics" has been used interchangeably with "radiomics" in literature to describe the study of radiologic features of predictive treatment outcomes, "radiogenomics" is more commonly used to describe the study of the molecular changes underlying the radiologic phenotype of a disease process, including genetic mutations, gene expression, and methylation (epigenetic) changes [15–19].

Here, we present an in-depth review of the current state of radiogenomics in ccRCC, and examine the variety of innovative computational models that have been developed in this field to infer the molecular profile of ccRCC from its radiologic phenotype, concluding with a discussion of the field's current limitations and future directions.

2. Methods

A literature review was performed by querying the PubMed, Medline, Cochrane Library, Google Scholar, and Web of Science databases. We attempted to identify all articles pertaining to radiogenomics and ccRCC. The search terms included "radiogenomics and . . . " one of the following MeSH search terms: "renal cell carcinoma", "clear cell renal cell carcinoma", "kidney cancer", or "renal cancer". Titles and abstracts of the articles retrieved from the above search were then screened for relevance. Inclusion criteria were (1) publication in the English language, (2) publication between 1/2009 and 9/2021, (3) and article topic pertaining to radiogenomics of ccRCC. Exclusion criteria included (1) publication before 1/2009, (2) not published in the English language, (3) study topics not pertaining to ccRCC or radiogenomics, (4) duplicate articles, and (5) non-primary literature, e.g., abstracts, review articles, and letters to the editor, which were excluded after being reviewed to identify any missed primary studies.

3. Results

Overall, 141 articles were identified in our initial search, of which 16 fit our inclusion criteria described above. Radiogenomic features related to mutational status were the most commonly described and targeted features for modeling (eight articles), followed by gene expression (five articles) and epigenetic features (one article). Only two articles developed clinical prognostic models utilizing radiogenomic data. Most articles focused on multiphasic, contrast-enhanced CT scan as the modality of choice, with two paper(s) discussing MRI features. A PRISMA flow chart of our search with inclusion and exclusion criteria can be seen in Figure 1. A list of the included articles along with a summary of their methodology and targeted predictive outcomes can be found in Table 1.

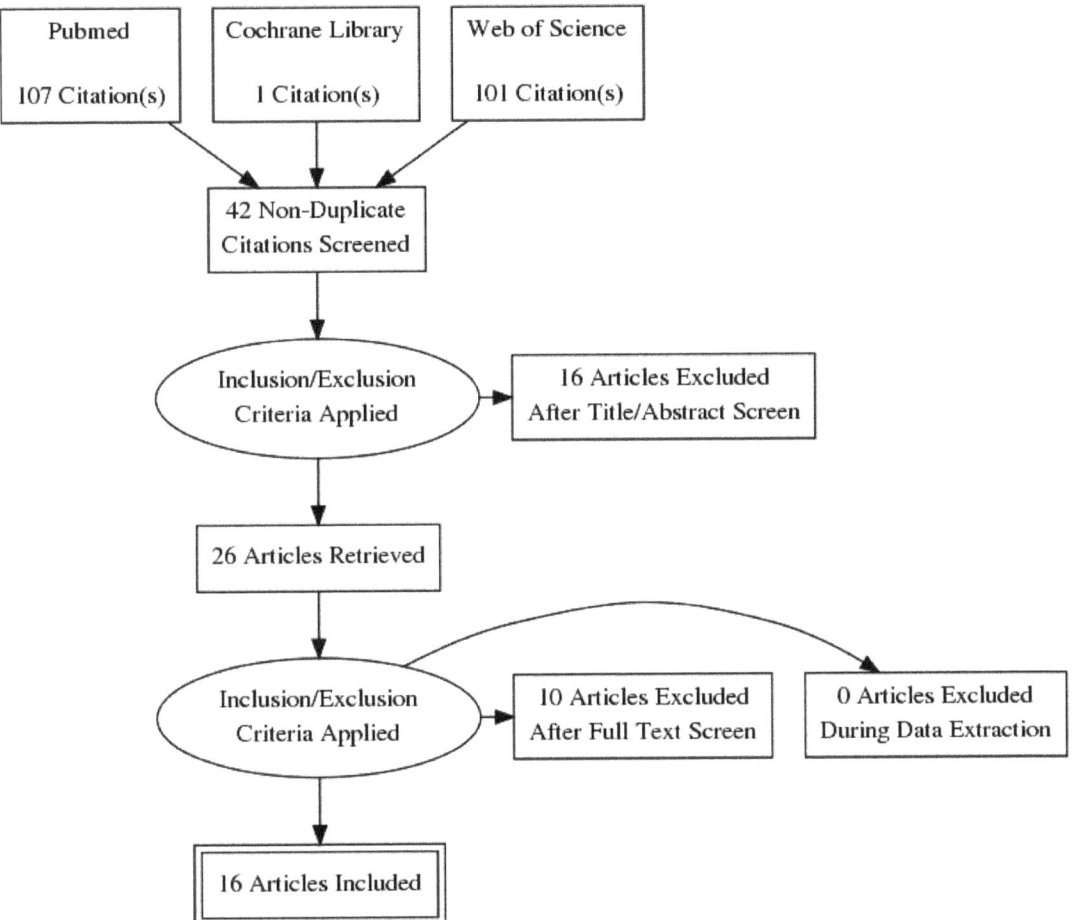

Figure 1. PRISMA flow diagram of article selection criteria.

Table 1. Summary of included radiogenomic studies in this review. Studies were selected based on the literature search strategy summarized in the methods section and Figure 1. Most studies utilized studies from the publicly available TCGA-KIRC cohort, specifically focusing on patients in that database with corresponding imaging studies in the TCIA portal.

Author and Year	Imaging Modality	Primary Outcome of Interest	Machine Learning Algorithm	Summary of Results	Notes
Karlo et al. (2014) [20]	Multiphase CT	Investigate association between CT features of ccRCC and mutations in VHL, PBRM1, SETD2, KDM5C, or BAP1	N/A—Development of a predictive model was not intended	Mutations of VHL were significantly associated with well-defined tumor margins, nodular tumor enhancement, and gross appearance of intratumoral vascularity. Mutations of KDM5C and BAP1 were significantly associated with evidence of renal vein invasion. Mutations of SETD2, KDM5C, and BAP1 were absent in multicystic clear cell RCC; mutations of VHL and PBRM1 were significantly more common among solid clear cell RCC	Retrospective review of institutional cohort of 233 patients with ccRCC and known mutation status for genes of interest.
Shinagare et al. (2015) [21]	Multiphase CT and MRI	Investigate association between CT/MRI features of ccRCC and mutations in VHL, BAP1, PBRM1, SETD2, KDM5C, and MUC4	N/A—Development of a predictive model was not intended		Retrospective review of 103 patients with CT and/or MRI images; majority (81) were CT-only.
Chen et al. (2018) [22]	Multiphase CT	Create a ML model to differentiate ccRCC tumors by radiomic features reflective of genetic mutation profile (VHL, PBRM1, BAP1)	Multi-classifier multi-objective (MO) and MO optimization algorithm	Model AUC $\geq$ 0.86, sensitivity $\geq$ 0.75, and specificity $\geq$ 0.80	Used a relatively small (57 patients) institutional cohort for training and validation. The model was designed to predict multiple rather than single outcome (mutation).
Li et al. (2019) [23]	Multiphase CT	Create a ML model to differentiate ccRCC from non-ccRCC tumors by radiomic features	Random forest (RF) and minimum redundancy maximum relevance (mRMR)	Model AUC of 0.949 and an accuracy of 92.9% vs. an AUC of 0.851 and an accuracy of 81.2% for the RF and mRMR models, respectively	Used a large (255 patients) institutional cohort for training and validation. Secondary outcome was correlation of predictive features with VHL mutational status, with false discovery rate p-value < 0.05.
Kocack et al. (2019) [24]	Multiphase CT	Create a ML model to differentiate ccRCC tumors by radiomic features reflective of PBRM1 mutation status	Artificial neural network (ANN) and RF algorithms	Model accuracy of 88.2% (AUC = 0.925) vs. 95.0% (AUC = 0.987) for the ANN vs. RF models	Used only 45 patient studies from the TCGA-KIRC cohort for training the model (29 PBRM1-unmutated, 16 PBRM1-mutated).

Table 1. *Cont.*

Author and Year	Imaging Modality	Primary Outcome of Interest	Machine Learning Algorithm	Summary of Results	Notes
Kocack et al. (2020) [25]	Multiphase CT	Create a ML model to differentiate ccRCC tumors by radiomic features reflective of *BAP1* mutation status	RF algorithm	Model specificity of 78.8% and precision of 81% for presence and absence of *BAP1* mutations, respectively	Used 65 patients from TCGA-KIRC for training the model (13 with and 52 without *BAP1* mutation).
Feng et al. (2020) [26]	Multiphase CT	Create a ML model to differentiate ccRCC tumors by radiomic features reflective of *BAP1* mutation status	RF algorithm	Model AUC = 0.77, sensitivity of 0.72, specificity of 0.87, and precision of 0.65	Used 56 patients (9 *BAP1*-mutated, 45 *BAP1*-unmutated) TCGA-KIRC for training the model.
Ghosh et al. (2015) [27]	Multiphase CT	Create a ML model to differentiate ccRCC tumors by radiomic features reflective of *BAP1* mutation status	RF algorithm	AUCs of 0.66, 0.62, 0.71, and 0.52 for the non-contrast, cortico-medullary, nephrographic, and excretory phases, respectively	Used TCGA-KIRC for training and validation cohorts (78 patients). Developed separate classifiers for *BAP1* in the non-contrast, cortico-medullary, nephrographic, and excretory phases. Utilized 3D feature extraction to evaluate intra-tumoral heterogeneity.
Bowen et al. (2019) [7]	Multiphase CT	Describe radiomic features associated of molecular TCGA subtypes (m1-m4)	N/A—Development of a predictive model was not intended	The m1 subgroup had well-defined tumor margins (vs. ill-defined, OR = 2.104; CI 1.024-4.322). The m3 subgroup was less frequently associated with well-defined tumor margins (OR = 0.421; CI 0.212-0.834); more collecting system invasion (OR = 2.164; CI 1.090-4.294) and renal vein invasion (OR 2.120; CI 1.078-4.168). There were no significant CT findings with the m2 or m4 subgroups	TCGA cohort was used for this assessment.
Marigliano et al. (2019) [28]	Multiphase CT	Describe radiomic features associated with miRNA expression	N/A—Development of a predictive model was not intended	There were no significantly associated texture-specific features with expression of any of the evaluated miRNAs	Pilot study using small institutional cohort of 20 patients.

Table 1. *Cont.*

Author and Year	Imaging Modality	Primary Outcome of Interest	Machine Learning Algorithm	Summary of Results	Notes
Yin et al. (2018) [29]	PET and MRI	Develop a combined PET/MRI model + other features to predict ccRCC molecular subtype (ccA vs. ccB)	ML was not used to build the predictive model	Correct classification rate was 87% vs. 95.6% using the radiomic signature alone vs. the combined signature (radiomic signature + several clinical features)	Very small training/test subset (23 specimens from 8 primary ccRCC patients). Sparse partial least squares discriminant analysis (SPLS-DA) was used to build their predictive models.
Cen et al. (2019) [30]	Multiphase CT	Identify CT imaging features predictive of high *RUNX3* methylation levels	N/A—Development of a predictive model was not intended	Well vs. poorly defined margin status (OR 2.685; CI 1.057–6.820), and present/absent intratumoral vascularity (OR 3.286; CI 1.367–7.898) were all significant independent predictors of high *RUNX3* methylation on multivariate regression	
Huang et al. (2021) [31]	Multiphase CT	Development of a radiogenomic model to predict overall survival in ccRCC using gene expression data	LASSO-COX regression to identify a prognostic radiomic signature, then RF to combine the radiomic and prognostic gene signatures	The radiogenomic model outperformed the radiomic features-only model at predicting overall survival at 1, 3 and 5 years (average AUCs for 1-, 3-, and 5-year survival of 0.814 vs. 0.837, 0.74 vs. 0.806, and 0.689 vs. 0.751, respectively)	Trained model using TCGA-KIRC dataset (205 patients).
Jamshidi et al. (2015) [32]	Multiphase CT	Development of a radiogenomic risk score (RSS) to predict gene expression results from a microarray assay	None—Multivariate regression was used to identify features most predictive of variation in supervised principal component (SPC) gene expression analysis	Significant correlation of RSS with the microarray gene signature (R = 0.57, $p < 0.001$; classification accuracy 70.1%, $p < 0.001$) Significant correlation of RSS with disease-specific survival: log-rank $p < 0.001$	RSS was developed from data in a 70-patient cohort, with validation in a separate cohort (70 for validation of the signature's correlation with micro-array results, 77 for correlation of signature with disease-free survival).
Jamshidi et al. (2016) [33]	Multiphase CT	Correlation of RSS developed in above study with radiologic progression free survival (rPFS) in a cohort of 41 mRCC patients undergoing CRN and pre-surgical bevacizumab	None—Purpose of study was to compare rPFS in the low- vs. high-RSS cohorts	Patients with a low RSS vs. high RSS had longer rPFS (25 months vs. 6 months; $p = 0.005$) and OS (37 months vs. 25 months; $p = 0.03$)	

Table 1. *Cont.*

Author and Year	Imaging Modality	Primary Outcome of Interest	Machine Learning Algorithm	Summary of Results	Notes
Udayakumar et al. (2021) [34]	Dynamic contrast-enhanced MRI	Correlation of enhancement scores for tumors with their TME expression signature	None	Enhancement-high tumors exhibited upregulated angiogenesis-related TME gene signatures, while enhancement-low areas exhibited higher levels of T-cell infiltration signatures. Better PFS with TKI in the enhancement-high compared to enhancement-low tumor groups (adjusted $p < 0.0001$), but no significant difference in PFS with IO between the two groups	Cutoff for determining tumors to have high or low enhancement/angiogenesis/infiltration was relative to the median value of the distribution of these values in the training cohort. Authors did not utilize any previously published TME signatures for angiogenesis or immune infiltration.

3.1. Key Genetic Mutations in ccRCC

Key gene mutations identified in ccRCC include *VHL*, *PBRM1*, *BAP1*, *SETD2*, and *KDM5C*; most of which are located on the short arm of chromosome 3 [35]. Key genetic mutations and their radiogenomic characteristics as well as prognostic value are discussed below, and are summarized in Table 2.

Table 2. Summary of the top 5 most common gene mutations in ccRCC.

Gene Mutation	Frequency in ccRCC (%)	Protein Function	Clinical and Prognostic Implications	Associated Features on CT Imaging
VHL	>90%	Tumor Suppressor	None	Defined tumor margins, nodular tumor enhancement, intratumor vascularity
PRBM1	40–50%	Tumor Suppressor	Inconsistent clinical significance in localized ccRCC; may be predictive of better prognosis and response to immune checkpoint inhibitors in metastatic ccRCC	Solid ccRCC
BAP1	10–15%	Tumor Suppressor	Poor prognosis	Renal vein invasion, ill-defined tumor margins, and intratumor calcificationsAbsent in multicystic ccRCC
SET2D	10–15%	Tumor Suppressor	Poor prognosis	Inconsistent Absent in multicystic ccRCC
KDM5C	6–7%	Tumor Suppressor	Good prognosis	Renal vein invasion Absent in multicystic ccRCC

3.1.1. VHL

VHL gene alteration is the most common mutation in solid ccRCC, with very high frequency (>90%) of biallelic inactivation due to deletion, mutation, or loss of heterozygosity [36,37]. As normal *VHL* protein complexes with other proteins to degrade hypoxia-inducible factor (HIF), *VHL* loss or mutation results in constitutive activation of HIF, promoting cell growth and neo-angiogenesis through the VEGF pathway [38]. Despite its prevalence in ccRCC, the presence of a *VHL* mutation in patients with ccRCC has no prognostic value [10,36,39,40].

3.1.2. PBRM1

PBRM1 is the second most commonly mutated tumor suppressor gene in ccRCC (40–50%), and is often co-deleted with *VHL*. This gene encodes for a nucleosome remodeling complex which limits DNA accessibility to RNA polymerase and transcription factors [35,41]. The prognostic value of *PBRM1* mutation is unclear, with a recent meta-analysis suggesting that mutation and/or loss of in *PBRM1* is a poor prognostic factor in localized disease and a good prognostic factor in advanced disease [42,43]. Other analyses suggest that *PBRM1* mutation status may be predictive of response to immune checkpoint inhibitors [44,45]. *PBRM1* mutations are most associated with solid ccRCC on imaging [20,21].

3.1.3. BAP1

BAP1 gene, present on the short arm of chromosome 3, is mutated in 10–15% of ccRCC, and is typically mutually exclusive of *PBRM1* mutation [35,46]. This tumor suppressor gene encodes a ubiquitin carboxyl-terminal hydrolase that regulates with downstream targets involved in cell breakdown and replication, with *BAP1* inactivation resulting in uncontrolled cell proliferation [41,47]. *BAP1* mutation has been associated with more aggressive disease and lower overall survival in ccRCC, with coagulative necrosis and high Furman grade on tumor pathology [48,49].

Typical radiologic features associated with *BAP1* mutation include renal vein invasion, ill-defined tumor margins, and intratumor calcifications. Of note, *BAP1* mutations were absent in multicystic ccRCC [20,21].

3.1.4. SETD2

As with *BAP1*, *SETD2* is a tumor suppressor gene located on the short arm of chromosome 3, and is mutated in approximately 10–15% of ccRCC [35]. *SETD2* loss has been associated with poor prognosis in nonmetastatic ccRCC [48]. Radiomic analyses note *SETD2* mutation to be absent in multicystic ccRCC, with no consistent CT imaging findings predictive of *SETD2* mutation in solid ccRCC [20,21].

3.1.5. KDM5C

KDM5C is mutated in approximately 6–7% of ccRCC [35]. The prognostic value of *KDM5C* remains debated, with one series noting an association with prolonged survival in metastatic ccRCC [50]. Tumors with *KDM5C* mutation were consistently associated with renal vein invasion on CT and absent in multicystic ccRCC [20,21].

3.2. Overview of Radiogenomics Workflow

As mentioned earlier, radiomics refers to the extraction and analysis of quantitative imaging features from cross-sectional imaging modalities, while radiogenomics refers to the study of the translational phenotype underlying these imaging features [51]. A typical radiogenomic workflow is shown in Figure 2. First, the region of interest (ROI), being the tumor and/or specific tumor sub-region(s), is "segmented", i.e., outlined in all slices of the imaging study using manual or semi-automated segmentation software, generating a 3D rendering of the ROI. Next, specialized software is used to extract hundreds to thousands of radiomic features from the ROI "agnostically", with no knowledge of its clinical context or molecular profile, such as malignant/benign status, RCC subtype, or mutational profile. Extracted features may include first-order statistics of voxel intensity and distribution, as well as higher level metrics of tumor shape, texture, and 2D/3D features, extracted from one or more phases of the imaging study. Next, machine learning (ML) algorithms are used to process these raw features to identify the subset of features that are predictive of an outcome of interest, which in radiogenomics would include specific gene mutation, gene expression profile, or clinical outcome [52]. The radiogenomic model constructed from this subset of features is usually "trained" using one dataset, followed by external cross-validation in an independent dataset.

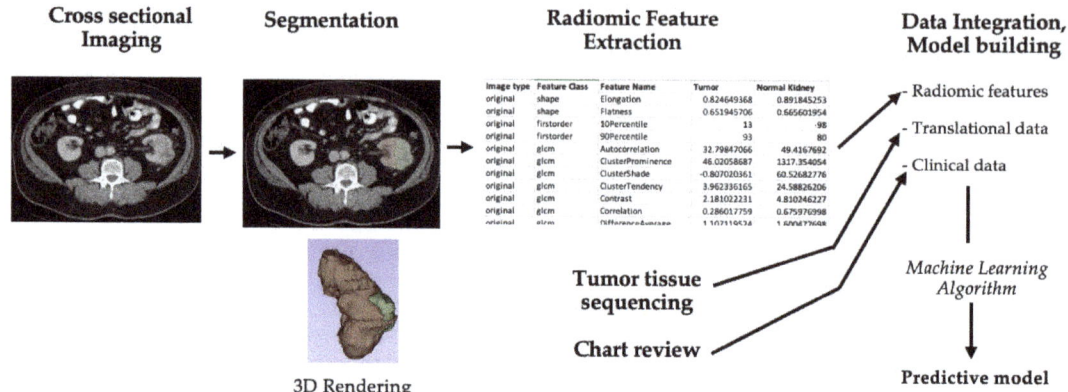

Figure 2. Flowchart showing typical radiogenomic workflow. Using cross-sectional images, a region of interest (ROI) that contains either the whole tumor or subregions within the tumor can be identified and outlined using manual in process called segmentation, using semi-automated, or automated segmentation software. Some segmentation software, such as 3D Slicer (shown above) allow for further ROI rendering in 3D dimensions. Quantitative radiomic features are extracted from ROI using separate or built-in radiomic feature extraction modules. Finally, this data is integrated with corresponding tumor molecular profile, as well as patient clinical data. These data are then processed using machine learning algorithms to develop diagnostic, predictive, or prognostic models for outcomes of interest.

3.3. Mutational Radiogenomic Biomarkers

In this section, we review articles that develop radiogenomic models to predict tumor gene mutational profile in ccRCC, which mostly focused on the previously discussed *PBRM1* and *BAP1* mutations.

Chen et al. (2018) presented a radiogenomic predictive model to predict multiple ccRCC gene mutations (*VHL*, *PBRM1*, and *BAP1*) using quantitative CT features. To achieve this, they developed a new multi-classifier multi-objective (MCMO) model to train their model against multiple objectives (ccRCC mutations of interest) rather than a single objective. After training their model using an institutional cohort of 57 patients, it was validated using The Cancer Genome Atlas's Kidney-Renal Cell Carcinoma (TCGA-KIRC) cohort. Their model achieved prediction accuracy of 0.81, 0.78, and 0.90 for *VHL*, *PBRM1*, and *BAP1* genes, respectively, with AUC $\geq$ 0.86, sensitivity $\geq$ 0.75, and specificity $\geq$ 0.80 [22].

Focusing on *PBRM1* mutation, which is a likely good prognostic factor in advanced ccRCC [42,53], Kocack et al. (2019) developed two predictive radiogenomic models using artificial neural network algorithm (ANN) and RF algorithms to differentiate ccRCC tumors by *PBRM1* mutations status in the TCGA-KIRC cohort (45 patients; 29 without and 16 with *PBRM1* mutation). Their ANN model demonstrated an accuracy of 88.2% (AUC = 0.925) compared to 95.0% (AUC = 0.987) with the RF algorithm. However, they did not directly evaluate their model's correlation with clinical outcomes [24].

The same group (Kocak et al., 2020) then developed an RF-based radiogenomic model for the prediction of *BAP1* mutation status, which carries poor prognostic implications in ccRCC [20,21,25], in a subset of 65 patients from TCGA-KIRC (13 with and 52 without *BAP1* mutation). This model correctly classified *BAP1* mutation status in 84.6% of cases (AUC = 0.897) [20,21,25]. The same algorithm (RF) and dataset (TCGA-KIRC) were used by Feng et al. (2020) to also predict *BAP1* mutation status, but using different segmentation and radiomic feature extraction platforms; the model accurately classified 83% (AUC = 0.77) of *BAP1* mutation status with a sensitivity of 0.72, specificity of 0.87, and precision of 0.65 [26]. Finally, targeting *BAP1* status as well, Ghosh et al. (2015) developed four imaging phase-specific *BAP1* classifiers for the non-contrast, cortico-medullary, nephrographic, and excretory phases of CT studies from the TCGA-KIRC cohort (78 patients). Interestingly, their model utilized 3D feature extraction to evaluate intra-tumoral heterogeneity (ITH), which they hypothesized reflected *BAP1* mutational status [27]. In contrast, none of the previously discussed studies considered ITH in their model design, despite its known prevalence and influence on clinicopathological and molecular assessment of ccRCC, as one tumor area's molecular profile may be different from another's, with downstream implications for the extracted radiomic features in these models [54,55].

3.4. Beyond Gene Mutations: Transcriptomic and Epigenetic Radiogenomic Biomarkers

As discussed earlier, the clinical relevance of some of the most common mutations in ccRCC remains unclear, particularly given the low prevalence of some of these mutations, limiting their potential as clinical biomarkers [20,21,35–39,41–50,56]. In contrast, transcriptional (gene-expression based) signatures have been shown to be better tools for classifying ccRCC into clinically-relevant molecular subtypes [57,58]. Such subgrouping classifications include clear cell type A (ccA) and clear cell type B (ccB) described by Brannon et al. using microarray data. Using these tumor classifications, they noted a prognostic difference between the two groups; ccA was significantly associated with better survival compared to ccB [8]. As transcriptomic research shifted from microarray to next-generation RNA-sequencing (RNA-Seq) technology, Brooks et al. developed a 34-gene expression signature, ClearCode34, for the classification of localized ccRCC tumors to ccA and ccB categories using RNA-Seq data [57]. Another attempt at transcriptomic profiling of ccRCC performed by the TCGA group using unsupervised clustering of RNA-Seq data identified four subgroups, m1–m4. Supervised clustering of these subgroups against ccA/ccB subgrouping noted cluster m1 to correspond to ccA, m2–m3 to correspond to cluster ccB, and m4 to correspond to the 15% of tumors that did not align with either ccA or ccB. As with ccA, the m1 subgroup had a survival advantage over m2–m4, sharing some of its genes with the *PBRM1* mutation group and functions within the chromatin remodeling process. In contrast, the m3 subgroup harbored mutations of *PTEN* and *CDKN2A*, while patients within the m4 subgroup exhibited a higher frequency of *BAP1* mutations [35]. Furthermore, these subtypes were associated with distinct radiomic features; the m1 subgroup had well-defined tumor margins (vs. ill-defined, OR = 2.104; CI 1.024–4.322), while the m3 subtype was less frequently associated with well-defined tumor margins (OR = 0.421; CI 0.212–0.834) and had more collecting system invasion (OR = 2.164; CI 1.090–4.294) and renal vein invasion (OR 2.120; CI 1.078–4.168). There were no significant CT findings with the m2 or m4 subgroups [7].

In this section, we explore radiogenomic models that correlate radiologic tumor "phenotype" to its underlying transcriptomic and epigenetic molecular profile, rather than genetic mutational profile. In addition to their ability to reflect variations in individual tumor gene expression and hypermethylation patterns, these models are potentially more applicable to clinical practice than radiogenomic models that predict only genomic mutational profile, given the ability of their targeted molecular expression profiles to better reflect survival and therapeutic outcomes [29,30].

3.4.1. Transcriptomic Radiogenomic Biomarkers

Using the aforementioned transcriptomic ccA/ccB ccRCC subtype, Yin et al. developed a model utilizing radiomic features extracted from MRI/PET data to classify ccRCC into ccA or ccB subtypes, using sparse partial least squares discriminant analysis (SPLS-DA) to build two predictive models—one with the radiomic features alone, and one incorporating clinical characteristics, mRNA, microvascular density, and molecular subtype information. The correct classification rate was 87% vs. 95.6% using the radiomic signature alone vs. the combined signature, respectively [29]. However, the study utilized a small cohort (23 specimens from eight primary ccRCC patients), and PET imaging is not usually used for evaluation nor surveillance of localized ccRCC.

3.4.2. Epigenetic Radiogenomic Biomarkers

At the epigenetic level, DNA methylation, particularly the runt-related transcription factor 3 (RUNX3) gene, has been correlated with overall survival [30]. Cen et al. (2019) evaluated the correlation between RUNX3 methylation levels and certain imaging features on CT in ccRCC. Among somatic CT findings, margin status (ill vs. well-defined; OR 2.685; CI 1.057–6.820) and intratumoral vascularity (present or absent; OR 3.286; CI 1.367–7.898) were significant independent predictors of high RUNX3 methylation levels on multivariate logistic regression [30].

3.5. Beyond Predicting Molecular Profile: Radiogenomic Models as Clinical Biomarkers

While the above reviewed studies present impressive analyses and methods for inferring tumor biology using radiomic features, the clinical relevance of their proposed features and models remains unproven without direct assessment of their ability to predict clinical outcomes. In this section, we review a few notable radiogenomic studies that go beyond correlating only radiomic and molecular features to also demonstrating a direct correlation between their radiogenomic biomarkers with clinical outcomes for ccRCC.

Focusing on radiologic features predictive of survival outcomes, Huang et al. performed radiogenomic analysis of CT imaging for ccRCC cases with corresponding RNA expression data in the TCGA-KIRC cohort. LASSO-COX regression was used to identify prognostic radiomic features and prognostic gene signatures. An RF algorithm was then used to combine prognostic and radiomic features into a radiogenomic prognostic model. The radiogenomic model outperformed the radiomic features-only model at predicting overall survival at 1, 3, and 5 years (average AUCs for 1-, 3-, and 5-year survival of 0.814 vs. 0.837, 0.74 vs. 0.806, and 0.689 vs. 0.751, respectively) [31].

In another study, Jamshidi et al. constructed a radiogenomic risk score (RSS) using a cohort of patients who underwent nephrectomy with corresponding micro-array-derived gene expression data. Following CT imaging feature extraction, multivariate regression was used to identify features most predictive of variation in supervised principal component (SPC) gene expression analysis. These features were used to constitute their RSS, which was validated in a separate patient cohort (70 for validation of the signature's correlation with micro-array results, 77 for correlation of signature with disease-free survival). The RRS exhibited a statistically significant correlation with micro-array SPC variation (R = 0.57, $p < 0.001$, classification accuracy 70.1%, $p < 0.001$) and disease-specific survival (log-rank $p < 0.001$), accounting for stage, grade, and performance status (multivariate Cox model $p < 0.05$, log-rank $p < 0.001$) [32]. In a separate study, the RRS was validated in a cohort of 41 mRCC patients undergoing cytoreductive nephrectomy (CRN) and pre-surgical bevacizumab, noting that it was able to stratify radiological progression-free survival (rPFS) in this cohort; patients with a low RSS vs. high RSS had longer rPFS (25 months vs. 6 months; $p = 0.005$) and OS (37 months vs. 25 months; $p = 0.03$) [33].

Focusing on micro-RNA (miRNA) expression in RCC, Marigliano et al. (2019) evaluated the correlation between a variety of radiomic features extracted from a cohort of 20 ccRCC patients, and their expression levels of selected microRNAs. Specifically, they examined the correlation of these features with miR-21-5p, miR-210-3p, miR-185-5p, miR-221-3p, and miR-145-5p, which had been shown to correlate with clinical outcomes in ccRCC [59]. They found no significant correlation between their extracted features and expression of any of their evaluated miRNAs [28].

While the molecular profiling of tumors using transcriptomic and epigenetic signatures offers more clinically meaningful biomarkers than genomic mutational signatures, it overlooks the critical role of the tumor's stromal and immune background, collectively referred to as the tumor microenvironment (TME), in the prognosis and therapeutic response of ccRCC. This role has been increasingly recognized with the rise of immunotherapy (IO) regimens, which target the immune component of the TME as monotherapy or in combination with TKI agents, which target the angiogenic component of the TME, as well [60–63].

In this regard, Udayakumar et al. (2021) utilized dynamic contrast-enhanced MRI (DCE-MRI) imaging to identify areas of high and low colocalized enhancement within tumor regions of 49 ccRCC patients undergoing DCE-MRI prior to nephrectomy, followed by targeted sampling and RNA-sequencing of nephrectomy specimen regions corresponding to these areas. They found enhancement-high tumors to exhibit upregulated angiogenesis-related TME gene expression signatures, while enhancement-low areas exhibited higher levels of immune (T-cell infiltration) TME signatures, confirmed by immunohistochemical analysis. They then validated their model's ability to predict response to TKI or immunotherapy (IO) treatments in a cohort of 19 patients with metastatic ccRCC, noting better PFS with TKI in the enhancement-high compared to enhancement-low tumor groups (adjusted $p < 0.0001$), but no significant difference in PFS with IO between the two groups [34].

4. Discussion

In this review, we provided an overview of radiogenomic studies in ccRCC, the most common subtype of RCC, and renal malignancies in general. While the majority of studies focused on developing models for the prediction of tumor gene mutational profiles, we noted a shift towards the prediction of gene expression patterns and epigenetic changes within the tumor as well as the tumor microenvironment, which provide better insights into tumor biology and potential therapeutic response than isolated gene mutation profiles. A minority of the reviewed models were also shown to be predictive of relevant clinical outcomes, such as cancer-specific survival and response to systemic therapy in advanced ccRCC. Such models may complement the management of localized renal tumors to confirm whether the tumor exhibits high- or low-risk features that may warrant more aggressive management vs. surveillance, and in advanced ccRCC to determine the optimal systemic treatment regimens based on radiogenomic assessment of the tumor and its microenvironment.

However, the clinical applicability of these models remains limited by several factors. First, all the predictive models presented by the reviewed studies were developed using relatively small cohorts, mostly utilizing the same publicly available cohort (TCGA-KIRC), potentially overfitting their models to this cohort, with only a few performing external validation in independent cohorts. Second, the quality of CT studies is dependent on a variety of technical factors, such as the CT scanner, acquisition mode, and voxel reconstruction algorithms, thereby affecting the quality of extracted radiomic data. Third, the extracted radiomic features come from segmented tumor images, which are usually manually or semi-automatically delineated by a human user—a process that is inherently subjective and liable to inter-observer variability. Fourth, there are no standardized protocols or software tools for radiomic feature extraction, with the concern that the hundreds to thousands of radiomic features extracted by one software package are often redundant and difficult to replicate by other software packages [64], thus limiting the external validity of the models developed from these features. The Image Biomarker Standardization Initiative is a recent attempt at addressing this issue, establishing a standardized set of unique radiomics features [65], although compliance with this initiative has yet to be seen in radiogenomics publications. This lack of a unified radiomic feature extraction protocol or terminology limits our ability to compare the subsets of predictive radiomic features across different models, which consequently limits the ability to identify any consistent radiomic features across different models. Furthermore, it hinders attempts to identify the biologic processes that may underlie changes in these radiomic features. Fifth, most of the models did not consider intra-tumoral heterogeneity, despite its known influence on clinicopathological and molecular assessment of ccRCC, with different tumor regions expressing different pathologic phenotypes and molecular profiles, with implications for therapeutic response. Therefore, a radiogenomic model that was trained to treat the entire tumor region as a single homogenous entity may not accurately predict a tumor's molecular profile or its correlated clinical outcomes. Finally, while the ultimate measure of any biomarker is to show reliable and independent correlation with clinical outcomes, complementing standard-of-care biomarkers and predictive tools, most of these studies focused on developing models to predict molecular profiles without directly demonstrating clinical relevance as an independent biomarker of key prognostic and therapeutic outcomes, or in combination with established predictive models and nomograms. These are critical limitations that must be addressed for radiogenomics to be reliably used as a tool in clinical practice.

Despite these limitations, the above studies demonstrate the potential of radiogenomics as a non-invasive biomarker of tumor biology, utilizing complex computational tools to identify radiologic tumor features that correlate with genomic, transcriptomic, and/or epigenetic features of the tumor, and their downstream clinical implications.

5. Conclusions

The field of radiogenomics is a potentially promising tool in constructing personalized cancer care, offering a novel non-invasive translational biomarker that can be used for molecular profiling of clear cell renal carcinoma. However, this field remains relatively immature, and all the reviewed studies in the field rely on retrospective analyses, with no large-scale prospective trials, a critical requirement for the implementation of this technology in clinical practice.

Author Contributions: Conceptualization, A.K. and R.M; methodology, A.K., S.C. and S.K.; writing—original draft preparation, S.K. and A.K.; writing—review and editing, S.K., A.K., K.A., A.A.H. and R.M.; visualization, S.K. and S.R.; supervision, A.A.H. and R.M. All authors have read and agreed to the published version of the manuscript.

Funding: This research received no external funding.

Conflicts of Interest: The authors declare no conflict of interest.

References

1. Motzer, R.J.; Jonasch, E.; Michaelson, M.D.; Nandagopal, L.; Gore, J.L.; George, S.; Alva, A.; Haas, N.; Harrison, M.R.; Plimack, E.R.; et al. NCCN Guidelines Insights: Kidney Cancer, Version 2.2020. *J. Natl. Compr. Canc. Netw.* **2019**, *17*, 1278–1285. [CrossRef] [PubMed]
2. Linehan, W.M. Genetic basis of kidney cancer: Role of genomics for the development of disease-based therapeutics. *Genome Res.* **2012**, *22*, 2089–2100. [CrossRef] [PubMed]
3. Patel, H.D.; Gupta, M.; Joice, G.A.; Srivastava, A.; Alam, R.; Allaf, M.E.; Pierorazio, P.M. Clinical Stage Migration and Survival for Renal Cell Carcinoma in the United States. *Eur. Urol. Oncol.* **2019**, *2*, 343–348. [CrossRef] [PubMed]
4. Johnson, D.C.; Vukina, J.; Smith, A.B.; Meyer, A.M.; Wheeler, S.B.; Kuo, T.M.; Tan, H.J.; Woods, M.E.; Raynor, M.C.; Wallen, E.M.; et al. Preoperatively misclassified, surgically removed benign renal masses: A systematic review of surgical series and United States population level burden estimate. *J. Urol.* **2015**, *193*, 30–35. [CrossRef]
5. Sasaguri, K.; Takahashi, N. CT and MR imaging for solid renal mass characterization. *Eur. J. Radiol.* **2018**, *99*, 40–54. [CrossRef]
6. Avanzo, M.; Stancanello, J.; El Naqa, I. Beyond imaging: The promise of radiomics. *Phys. Med.* **2017**, *38*, 122–139. [CrossRef]
7. Bowen, L.; Xiaojing, L. Radiogenomics of Clear Cell Renal Cell Carcinoma: Associations Between mRNA-Based Subtyping and CT Imaging Features. *Acad. Radiol.* **2019**, *26*, e32–e37. [CrossRef]
8. Brannon, A.R.; Reddy, A.; Seiler, M.; Arreola, A.; Moore, D.T.; Pruthi, R.S.; Wallen, E.M.; Nielsen, M.E.; Liu, H.; Nathanson, K.L.; et al. Molecular Stratification of Clear Cell Renal Cell Carcinoma by Consensus Clustering Reveals Distinct Subtypes and Survival Patterns. *Genes Cancer* **2010**, *1*, 152–163. [CrossRef]
9. Vuong, L.; Kotecha, R.R.; Voss, M.H.; Hakimi, A.A. Tumor Microenvironment Dynamics in Clear-Cell Renal Cell Carcinoma. *Cancer Discov.* **2019**, *9*, 1349–1357. [CrossRef]
10. Hakimi, A.A.; Voss, M.H.; Kuo, F.; Sanchez, A.; Liu, M.; Nixon, B.G.; Vuong, L.; Ostrovnaya, I.; Chen, Y.B.; Reuter, V.; et al. Transcriptomic Profiling of the Tumor Microenvironment Reveals Distinct Subgroups of Clear Cell Renal Cell Cancer: Data from a Randomized Phase III Trial. *Cancer Discov.* **2019**, *9*, 510–525. [CrossRef]
11. Sun, M.; Shariat, S.F.; Cheng, C.; Ficarra, V.; Murai, M.; Oudard, S.; Pantuck, A.J.; Zigeuner, R.; Karakiewicz, P.I. Prognostic factors and predictive models in renal cell carcinoma: A contemporary review. *Eur. Urol.* **2011**, *60*, 644–661. [CrossRef] [PubMed]
12. Heng, D.Y.; Xie, W.; Regan, M.M.; Warren, M.A.; Golshayan, A.R.; Sahi, C.; Eigl, B.J.; Ruether, J.D.; Cheng, T.; North, S.; et al. Prognostic factors for overall survival in patients with metastatic renal cell carcinoma treated with vascular endothelial growth factor-targeted agents: Results from a large, multicenter study. *J. Clin. Oncol.* **2009**, *27*, 5794–5799. [CrossRef] [PubMed]

13. Frank, I.; Blute, M.L.; Cheville, J.C.; Lohse, C.M.; Weaver, A.L.; Zincke, H. An outcome prediction model for patients with clear cell renal cell carcinoma treated with radical nephrectomy based on tumor stage, size, grade and necrosis: The SSIGN score. *J. Urol.* **2002**, *168*, 2395–2400. [CrossRef]
14. Zisman, A.; Pantuck, A.J.; Dorey, F.; Said, J.W.; Shvarts, O.; Quintana, D.; Gitlitz, B.J.; DeKernion, J.B.; Figlin, R.A.; Belldegrun, A.S. Improved prognostication of renal cell carcinoma using an integrated staging system. *J. Clin. Oncol.* **2001**, *19*, 1649–1657. [CrossRef] [PubMed]
15. Rutman, A.M.; Kuo, M.D. Radiogenomics: Creating a link between molecular diagnostics and diagnostic imaging. *Eur. J. Radiol.* **2009**, *70*, 232–241. [CrossRef]
16. Lo Gullo, R.; Daimiel, I.; Morris, E.A.; Pinker, K. Combining molecular and imaging metrics in cancer: Radiogenomics. *Insights Imaging* **2020**, *11*, 1. [CrossRef]
17. Mazurowski, M.A. Radiogenomics: What it is and why it is important. *J. Am. Coll. Radiol.* **2015**, *12*, 862–866. [CrossRef]
18. Story, M.D.; Durante, M. Radiogenomics. *Med. Phys.* **2018**, *45*, e1111–e1122. [CrossRef]
19. Bodalal, Z.; Trebeschi, S.; Nguyen-Kim, T.D.L.; Schats, W.; Beets-Tan, R. Radiogenomics: Bridging imaging and genomics. *Abdom. Radiol.* **2019**, *44*, 1960–1984. [CrossRef]
20. Karlo, C.A.; Di Paolo, P.L.; Chaim, J.; Hakimi, A.A.; Ostrovnaya, I.; Russo, P.; Hricak, H.; Motzer, R.; Hsieh, J.J.; Akin, O. Radiogenomics of clear cell renal cell carcinoma: Associations between CT imaging features and mutations. *Radiology* **2014**, *270*, 464–471. [CrossRef]
21. Shinagare, A.B.; Vikram, R.; Jaffe, C.; Akin, O.; Kirby, J.; Huang, E.; Freymann, J.; Sainani, N.I.; Sadow, C.A.; Bathala, T.K.; et al. Radiogenomics of clear cell renal cell carcinoma: Preliminary findings of The Cancer Genome Atlas-Renal Cell Carcinoma (TCGA-RCC) Imaging Research Group. *Abdom. Imaging* **2015**, *40*, 1684–1692. [CrossRef] [PubMed]
22. Chen, X.; Zhou, Z.; Hannan, R.; Thomas, K.; Pedrosa, I.; Kapur, P.; Brugarolas, J.; Mou, X.; Wang, J. Reliable gene mutation prediction in clear cell renal cell carcinoma through multi-classifier multi-objective radiogenomics model. *Phys. Med. Biol.* **2018**, *63*, 215008. [CrossRef] [PubMed]
23. Li, Z.C.; Zhai, G.; Zhang, J.; Wang, Z.; Liu, G.; Wu, G.Y.; Liang, D.; Zheng, H. Differentiation of clear cell and non-clear cell renal cell carcinomas by all-relevant radiomics features from multiphase CT: A VHL mutation perspective. *Eur. Radiol.* **2019**, *29*, 3996–4007. [CrossRef] [PubMed]
24. Kocak, B.; Durmaz, E.S.; Ates, E.; Ulusan, M.B. Radiogenomics in Clear Cell Renal Cell Carcinoma: Machine Learning-Based High-Dimensional Quantitative CT Texture Analysis in Predicting PBRM1 Mutation Status. *AJR Am. J. Roentgenol.* **2019**, *212*, W55–W63. [CrossRef] [PubMed]
25. Kocak, B.; Durmaz, E.S.; Kaya, O.K.; Kilickesmez, O. Machine learning-based unenhanced CT texture analysis for predicting BAP1 mutation status of clear cell renal cell carcinomas. *Acta Radiol.* **2020**, *61*, 856–864. [CrossRef]
26. Feng, Z.; Zhang, L.; Qi, Z.; Shen, Q.; Hu, Z.; Chen, F. Identifying BAP1 Mutations in Clear-Cell Renal Cell Carcinoma by CT Radiomics: Preliminary Findings. *Front Oncol.* **2020**, *10*, 279. [CrossRef]
27. Ghosh, P.; Tamboli, P.; Vikram, R.; Rao, A. Imaging-genomic pipeline for identifying gene mutations using three-dimensional intra-tumor heterogeneity features. *J. Med. Imaging* **2015**, *2*, 041009. [CrossRef]
28. Marigliano, C.; Badia, S.; Bellini, D.; Rengo, M.; Caruso, D.; Tito, C.; Miglietta, S.; Palleschi, G.; Pastore, A.L.; Carbone, A.; et al. Radiogenomics in Clear Cell Renal Cell Carcinoma: Correlations Between Advanced CT Imaging (Texture Analysis) and MicroRNAs Expression. *Technol. Cancer Res. Treat.* **2019**, *18*, 1533033819878458. [CrossRef]
29. Yin, Q.; Hung, S.C.; Rathmell, W.K.; Shen, L.; Wang, L.; Lin, W.; Fielding, J.R.; Khandani, A.H.; Woods, M.E.; Milowsky, M.I.; et al. Integrative radiomics expression predicts molecular subtypes of primary clear cell renal cell carcinoma. *Clin. Radiol.* **2018**, *73*, 782–791. [CrossRef]
30. Cen, D.; Xu, L.; Zhang, S.; Chen, Z.; Huang, Y.; Li, Z.; Liang, B. Renal cell carcinoma: Predicting RUNX3 methylation level and its consequences on survival with CT features. *Eur. Radiol.* **2019**, *29*, 5415–5422. [CrossRef]
31. Huang, Y.; Zeng, H.; Chen, L.; Luo, Y.; Ma, X.; Zhao, Y. Exploration of an Integrative Prognostic Model of Radiogenomics Features With Underlying Gene Expression Patterns in Clear Cell Renal Cell Carcinoma. *Front Oncol.* **2021**, *11*, 640881. [CrossRef] [PubMed]
32. Jamshidi, N.; Jonasch, E.; Zapala, M.; Korn, R.L.; Aganovic, L.; Zhao, H.; Tumkur Sitaram, R.; Tibshirani, R.J.; Banerjee, S.; Brooks, J.D.; et al. The Radiogenomic Risk Score: Construction of a Prognostic Quantitative, Noninvasive Image-based Molecular Assay for Renal Cell Carcinoma. *Radiology* **2015**, *277*, 114–123. [CrossRef] [PubMed]
33. Jamshidi, N.; Jonasch, E.; Zapala, M.; Korn, R.L.; Brooks, J.D.; Ljungberg, B.; Kuo, M.D. The radiogenomic risk score stratifies outcomes in a renal cell cancer phase 2 clinical trial. *Eur. Radiol.* **2016**, *26*, 2798–2807. [CrossRef] [PubMed]
34. Udayakumar, D.; Zhang, Z.; Xi, Y.; Dwivedi, D.K.; Fulkerson, M.; Haldeman, S.; McKenzie, T.; Yousuf, Q.; Joyce, A.; Hajibeigi, A.; et al. Deciphering Intratumoral Molecular Heterogeneity in Clear Cell Renal Cell Carcinoma with a Radiogenomics Platform. *Clin. Cancer Res.* **2021**, *27*, 4794–4806. [CrossRef] [PubMed]
35. Cancer Genome Atlas Research Network. Comprehensive molecular characterization of clear cell renal cell carcinoma. *Nature* **2013**, *499*, 43–49. [CrossRef]
36. Sato, Y.; Yoshizato, T.; Shiraishi, Y.; Maekawa, S.; Okuno, Y.; Kamura, T.; Shimamura, T.; Sato-Otsubo, A.; Nagae, G.; Suzuki, H.; et al. Integrated molecular analysis of clear-cell renal cell carcinoma. *Nat. Genet.* **2013**, *45*, 860–867. [CrossRef]

37. Brauch, H.; Weirich, G.; Brieger, J.; Glavac, D.; Rodl, H.; Eichinger, M.; Feurer, M.; Weidt, E.; Puranakanitstha, C.; Neuhaus, C.; et al. VHL alterations in human clear cell renal cell carcinoma: Association with advanced tumor stage and a novel hot spot mutation. *Cancer Res.* **2000**, *60*, 1942–1948.
38. Maxwell, P.H.; Wiesener, M.S.; Chang, G.W.; Clifford, S.C.; Vaux, E.C.; Cockman, M.E.; Wykoff, C.C.; Pugh, C.W.; Maher, E.R.; Ratcliffe, P.J. The tumour suppressor protein VHL targets hypoxia-inducible factors for oxygen-dependent proteolysis. *Nature* **1999**, *399*, 271–275. [CrossRef]
39. Kim, B.J.; Kim, J.H.; Kim, H.S.; Zang, D.Y. Prognostic and predictive value of VHL gene alteration in renal cell carcinoma: A meta-analysis and review. *Oncotarget* **2017**, *8*, 13979–13985. [CrossRef]
40. Turajlic, S.; Xu, H.; Litchfield, K.; Rowan, A.; Chambers, T.; Lopez, J.I.; Nicol, D.; O'Brien, T.; Larkin, J.; Horswell, S.; et al. Tracking Cancer Evolution Reveals Constrained Routes to Metastases: TRACERx Renal. *Cell* **2018**, *173*, 581–594.e12. [CrossRef]
41. Brugarolas, J. Molecular genetics of clear-cell renal cell carcinoma. *J. Clin. Oncol.* **2014**, *32*, 1968–1976. [CrossRef] [PubMed]
42. Carril-Ajuria, L.; Santos, M.; Roldan-Romero, J.M.; Rodriguez-Antona, C.; De Velasco, G. Prognostic and Predictive Value of PBRM1 in Clear Cell Renal Cell Carcinoma. *Cancers* **2019**, *12*, 16. [CrossRef] [PubMed]
43. Hakimi, A.A.; Chen, Y.B.; Wren, J.; Gonen, M.; Abdel-Wahab, O.; Heguy, A.; Liu, H.; Takeda, S.; Tickoo, S.K.; Reuter, V.E.; et al. Clinical and pathologic impact of select chromatin-modulating tumor suppressors in clear cell renal cell carcinoma. *Eur. Urol.* **2013**, *63*, 848–854. [CrossRef] [PubMed]
44. Kim, S.H.; Park, W.S.; Park, E.Y.; Park, B.; Joo, J.; Joung, J.Y.; Seo, H.K.; Lee, K.H.; Chung, J. The prognostic value of BAP1, PBRM1, pS6, PTEN, TGase2, PD-L1, CA9, PSMA, and Ki-67 tissue markers in localized renal cell carcinoma: A retrospective study of tissue microarrays using immunohistochemistry. *PLoS ONE* **2017**, *12*, e0179610. [CrossRef]
45. Miao, D.; Margolis, C.A.; Gao, W.; Voss, M.H.; Li, W.; Martini, D.J.; Norton, C.; Bosse, D.; Wankowicz, S.M.; Cullen, D.; et al. Genomic correlates of response to immune checkpoint therapies in clear cell renal cell carcinoma. *Science* **2018**, *359*, 801–806. [CrossRef]
46. Joseph, R.W.; Kapur, P.; Serie, D.J.; Parasramka, M.; Ho, T.H.; Cheville, J.C.; Frenkel, E.; Parker, A.S.; Brugarolas, J. Clear Cell Renal Cell Carcinoma Subtypes Identified by BAP1 and PBRM1 Expression. *J. Urol.* **2016**, *195*, 180–187. [CrossRef]
47. Bielecka, Z.F.; Czarnecka, A.M.; Szczylik, C. Genomic Analysis as the First Step toward Personalized Treatment in Renal Cell Carcinoma. *Front Oncol.* **2014**, *4*, 194. [CrossRef]
48. Hakimi, A.A.; Ostrovnaya, I.; Reva, B.; Schultz, N.; Chen, Y.B.; Gonen, M.; Liu, H.; Takeda, S.; Voss, M.H.; Tickoo, S.K.; et al. Adverse outcomes in clear cell renal cell carcinoma with mutations of 3p21 epigenetic regulators BAP1 and SETD2: A report by MSKCC and the KIRC TCGA research network. *Clin. Cancer Res.* **2013**, *19*, 3259–3267. [CrossRef]
49. Pena-Llopis, S.; Vega-Rubin-de-Celis, S.; Liao, A.; Leng, N.; Pavia-Jimenez, A.; Wang, S.; Yamasaki, T.; Zhrebker, L.; Sivanand, S.; Spence, P.; et al. BAP1 loss defines a new class of renal cell carcinoma. *Nat. Genet.* **2012**, *44*, 751–759. [CrossRef]
50. Tennenbaum, D.M.; Manley, B.J.; Zabor, E.; Becerra, M.F.; Carlo, M.I.; Casuscelli, J.; Redzematovic, A.; Khan, N.; Arcila, M.E.; Voss, M.H.; et al. Genomic alterations as predictors of survival among patients within a combined cohort with clear cell renal cell carcinoma undergoing cytoreductive nephrectomy. *Urol. Oncol.* **2017**, *35*, 532.e7–532.e13. [CrossRef]
51. Kumar, V.; Gu, Y.; Basu, S.; Berglund, A.; Eschrich, S.A.; Schabath, M.B.; Forster, K.; Aerts, H.J.; Dekker, A.; Fenstermacher, D.; et al. Radiomics: The process and the challenges. *Magn. Reson. Imaging* **2012**, *30*, 1234–1248. [CrossRef] [PubMed]
52. Gillies, R.J.; Kinahan, P.E.; Hricak, H. Radiomics: Images Are More than Pictures, They Are Data. *Radiology* **2016**, *278*, 563–577. [CrossRef] [PubMed]
53. Wang, Z.; Peng, S.; Guo, L.; Xie, H.; Wang, A.; Shang, Z.; Niu, Y. Prognostic and clinicopathological value of PBRM1 expression in renal cell carcinoma. *Clin. Chim. Acta* **2018**, *486*, 9–17. [CrossRef] [PubMed]
54. Lopez, J.I. Intratumor heterogeneity in clear cell renal cell carcinoma: A review for the practicing pathologist. *APMIS* **2016**, *124*, 153–159. [CrossRef]
55. Lopez, J.I.; Angulo, J.C. Pathological Bases and Clinical Impact of Intratumor Heterogeneity in Clear Cell Renal Cell Carcinoma. *Curr. Urol. Rep.* **2018**, *19*, 3. [CrossRef]
56. Duns, G.; Van den Berg, E.; Van Duivenbode, I.; Osinga, J.; Hollema, H.; Hofstra, R.M.; Kok, K. Histone methyltransferase gene SETD2 is a novel tumor suppressor gene in clear cell renal cell carcinoma. *Cancer Res.* **2010**, *70*, 4287–4291. [CrossRef]
57. Brooks, S.A.; Brannon, A.R.; Parker, J.S.; Fisher, J.C.; Sen, O.; Kattan, M.W.; Hakimi, A.A.; Hsieh, J.J.; Choueiri, T.K.; Tamboli, P.; et al. ClearCode34: A prognostic risk predictor for localized clear cell renal cell carcinoma. *Eur. Urol.* **2014**, *66*, 77–84. [CrossRef]
58. Serie, D.J.; Joseph, R.W.; Cheville, J.C.; Ho, T.H.; Parasramka, M.; Hilton, T.; Thompson, R.H.; Leibovich, B.C.; Parker, A.S.; Eckel-Passow, J.E. Clear Cell Type A and B Molecular Subtypes in Metastatic Clear Cell Renal Cell Carcinoma: Tumor Heterogeneity and Aggressiveness. *Eur. Urol.* **2017**, *71*, 979–985. [CrossRef]
59. Tang, K.; Xu, H. Prognostic value of meta-signature miRNAs in renal cell carcinoma: An integrated miRNA expression profiling analysis. *Sci. Rep.* **2015**, *5*, 10272. [CrossRef]
60. Pourmir, I.; Noel, J.; Simonaggio, A.; Oudard, S.; Vano, Y.A. Update on the most promising biomarkers of response to immune checkpoint inhibitors in clear cell renal cell carcinoma. *World J. Urol.* **2021**, *39*, 1377–1385. [CrossRef]
61. Quail, D.F.; Joyce, J.A. Microenvironmental regulation of tumor progression and metastasis. *Nat. Med.* **2013**, *19*, 1423–1437. [CrossRef] [PubMed]
62. Rappold, P.M.; Silagy, A.W.; Kotecha, R.R.; Hakimi, A.A. Immune checkpoint blockade in renal cell carcinoma. *J. Surg. Oncol.* **2021**, *123*, 739–750. [CrossRef] [PubMed]

63. Rijnders, M.; De Wit, R.; Boormans, J.L.; Lolkema, M.P.J.; Van der Veldt, A.A.M. Systematic Review of Immune Checkpoint Inhibition in Urological Cancers. *Eur. Urol.* **2017**, *72*, 411–423. [CrossRef] [PubMed]
64. Berenguer, R.; Pastor-Juan, M.D.R.; Canales-Vazquez, J.; Castro-Garcia, M.; Villas, M.V.; Mansilla Legorburo, F.; Sabater, S. Radiomics of CT Features May Be Nonreproducible and Redundant: Influence of CT Acquisition Parameters. *Radiology* **2018**, *288*, 407–415. [CrossRef] [PubMed]
65. Zwanenburg, A.; Vallieres, M.; Abdalah, M.A.; Aerts, H.; Andrearczyk, V.; Apte, A.; Ashrafinia, S.; Bakas, S.; Beukinga, R.J.; Boellaard, R.; et al. The Image Biomarker Standardization Initiative: Standardized Quantitative Radiomics for High-Throughput Image-based Phenotyping. *Radiology* **2020**, *295*, 328–338. [CrossRef] [PubMed]

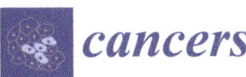

Article

Prognostic Gene Expression-Based Signature in Clear-Cell Renal Cell Carcinoma

Fiorella L. Roldán [1,2,†], Laura Izquierdo [1,2,†], Mercedes Ingelmo-Torres [1,2], Juan José Lozano [3], Raquel Carrasco [1,2], Alexandra Cuñado [1], Oscar Reig [4], Lourdes Mengual [1,2,5,*,‡] and Antonio Alcaraz [1,2,‡]

1. Laboratori i Servei d'Urologia, Hospital Clínic de Barcelona, 08036 Barcelona, Spain; flroldan@clinic.cat (F.L.R.); lizquier@clinic.cat (L.I.); ingelmo@clinic.cat (M.I.-T.); racarrasco@clinic.cat (R.C.); scunado@clinic.cat (A.C.); aalcaraz@clinic.cat (A.A.)
2. Genètica i Tumors Urològics, Institut d'Investigacions Biomèdiques August Pi i Sunyer (IDIBAPS), 08036 Barcelona, Spain
3. Plataforma de Bioinformàtica, Centro de Investigación Biomédica en Red Enfermedades Hepáticas y Digestivas (CIBERehd), Hospital Clínic, 08036 Barcelona, Spain; juanjo.lozano@ciberehd.org
4. Servei d'Oncologia Mèdica, Hospital Clínic de Barcelona, 08036 Barcelona, Spain; oreig@clinic.cat
5. Departament de Biomedicina, Facultat de Medicina i Ciències de la Salut, Universitat de Barcelona (UB), 08036 Barcelona, Spain
* Correspondence: lmengual@clinic.cat; Tel.: +34-93-227-54-00 (ext. 4820)
† These authors contributed equally to this work.
‡ These authors contributed equally to this work.

Simple Summary: In this study, we identified molecular markers for disease progression from ccRCC tissue samples. Using the selected biomarkers and clinical data from the TCGA cohort, we developed a gene expression-based signature which enhances the prognostic prediction of clinicopathological variables and could help to provide personalized disease management.

Abstract: The inaccuracy of the current prognostic algorithms and the potential changes in the therapeutic management of localized ccRCC demands the development of an improved prognostic model for these patients. To this end, we analyzed whole-transcriptome profiling of 26 tissue samples from progressive and non-progressive ccRCCs using Illumina Hi-seq 4000. Differentially expressed genes (DEG) were intersected with the RNA-sequencing data from the TCGA. The overlapping genes were used for further analysis. A total of 132 genes were found to be prognosis-related genes. LASSO regression enabled the development of the best prognostic six-gene panel. Cox regression analyses were performed to identify independent clinical prognostic parameters to construct a combined nomogram which includes the expression of *CERCAM*, *MIA2*, *HS6ST2*, *ONECUT2*, *SOX12*, *TMEM132A*, pT stage, tumor size and ISUP grade. A risk score generated using this model effectively stratified patients at higher risk of disease progression (HR 10.79; $p < 0.001$) and cancer-specific death (HR 19.27; $p < 0.001$). It correlated with the clinicopathological variables, enabling us to discriminate a subset of patients at higher risk of progression within the Stage, Size, Grade and Necrosis score (SSIGN) risk groups, pT and ISUP grade. In summary, a gene expression-based prognostic signature was successfully developed providing a more precise assessment of the individual risk of progression.

Keywords: gene expression; clear-cell renal cell carcinoma; disease progression; prognostic factors; biomarkers; RNA sequencing

1. Introduction

Renal cell carcinoma (RCC) ranks third among the urological cancers with the highest incidence. Over 431,000 new cases and more than 170,000 RCC-related deaths were reported worldwide last year [1]. Clear-cell RCC (ccRCC) is the most common histological subtype and has the worst prognosis among all RCCs [2]. Currently, most of the newly diagnosed ccRCC cases are organ-confined tumors; however, after curative treatment, up to 30–40%

will develop tumor metastases. Unfortunately, metastatic patients have a very poor five-year survival rate, varying between 0–20% [3,4].

According to the European Urological Guidelines, the standard management for all localized ccRCCs receiving surgery is limited to radiographic surveillance. No adjuvant treatment is approved for patients with a higher risk of progression [2]. Moreover, all surveillance recommendations are only based on clinical parameters, even though these have been proven insufficient to accurately predict disease progression, either to select ccRCC patients for adjuvant treatments or guide disease management [5,6].

Gene expression profiling has been used extensively in cancer research and has led to the discovery of new molecular prognostic markers and potential therapeutic targets. Several genetic models have been proposed in ccRCC [7–10]; however, none of those classifiers have been widely accepted nor implemented in routine clinical practice. Biomarker research for ccRCC still faces multiple challenges, mainly due to tumor heterogeneity and lack of validation studies. In addition, the use of high-throughput assays and the identification of a significant number of markers in a relatively small number of patients increase the complexity of data analysis [3]. The currently validated gene signatures comprise a large number of biomarkers, hindering their applicability and reproducibility [8,9]. Therefore, in this study we sought to develop a novel and high-performing gene expression-based signature using data generated from our cohort and The Cancer Genome Atlas (TCGA) cohort, to provide a more accurate assessment of the individual risk of progression for patients with localized ccRCC.

2. Materials and Methods

2.1. Patients, Datasets Sources and Study Design

This study was split into a three-stage approach: an initial molecular profiling, a selection and verification of prognosis-related genes and a signature development phase (Figure 1). The initial molecular profiling phase included a total of 26 localized ccRCCs who underwent partial or radical nephrectomy between 2001 and 2010 in our center (Hospital Clinic of Barcelona, Barcelona, Spain). These 26 cases consisted of 13 progressive and 13 non-progressive patients and met the following criteria: no neoadjuvant or adjuvant treatment, no prior or concomitant malignancies or a history of inherited von Hippel-Lindau disease, all patients had thoracoabdominal CT scan staging within two month before surgery to ensure organ-confined disease. Tumors were considered progressive when local relapse or distant metastasis developed during follow-up. All patients were followed up postoperatively according to the European Urology guidelines. Any progressive patient within two months of surgery was excluded from the study. Non-progressive patients had a minimum follow-up of 10 years to ensure their status as appropriate controls. Tissue samples were obtained under institutional review board-approved protocols (HBC/2016/0333).

The selection of prognosis-related genes and signature development phases was carried out using The Cancer Genome Atlas (TCGA) dataset. Level 3 RNAseq expression data and the corresponding clinical data from TCGA ccRCC samples were obtained from the portal (https://firebrowse.org (accessed on 8 October 2021) [11] (Supplementary Material Table S1). Survival data were obtained from portal (https://www.sciencedirect.com/science/article/pii/S0092867418302290?via%3Dihub#app2 (accessed on 8 October 2021) [12]. After selecting samples matching our selection criteria and excluding patients without survival status or missing clinical data, a total of 356 ccRCC samples from TCGA, 68 progressive and 288 non-progressive, were selected and the gene expression of 20,532 genes was downloaded.

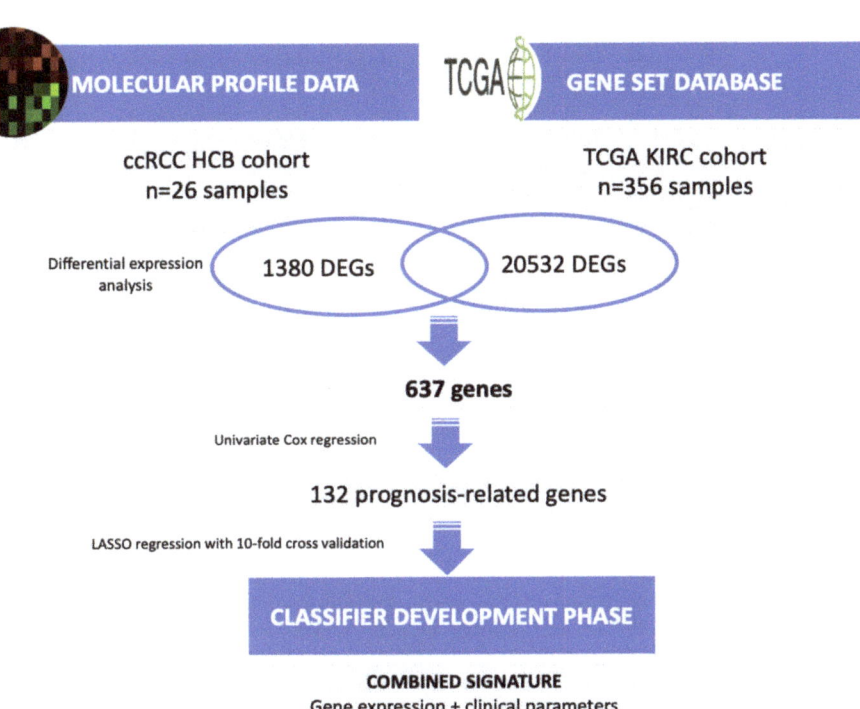

Figure 1. Flowchart of the whole study. Abbreviations: ccRCC, clear-cell renal cell carcinoma; DEGs, differentially expressed genes.

2.2. Tissue Specimens and RNA Isolation

Formalin-fixed paraffin-embedded (FFPE) tissue blocks were reviewed. The tumor area was macro-dissected from slides (total thickness 80 µm) and RNA was isolated from FFPE specimens using the kit RecoverAll™ Total Nucleic Acid Isolation for FFPE (Ambion, Inc. Austin, TX, USA), following manufacturers' instructions. RNA was quantified by spectrophotometric analysis at 260 nm (NanoDrop Technologies, Wilmington, DE, USA) and RNA integrity was assessed using Agilent 2100 Bioanalyzer System.

2.3. Molecular Profiling by RNA Sequencing

Library preparation and sequencing method: Following rRNA removal (Ribo-Zero® rRNA Removal Kit, Illumina), RNA from 26 selected ccRCC samples was processed for library preparation using the TruSeq® RNA Access Library Preparation Kit (Illumina, San Diego, CA, USA) that allows generating libraries starting from degraded RNA. Briefly, cDNA strands were synthetized from input RNA in order to be adaptor-tagged, labeled and amplified. cDNA was then pooled and enriched by a double step of probes hybridization. The enriched targets were captured by streptavidin labeled beads, cleaned up and amplified to obtain the final multiplexed libraries. The libraries were then sequenced on an Illumina HiSeq® 4000 platform (Illumina®).

Read alignment and differential gene expression analysis: Paired-end RNA-Seq FASTQ files were trimmed from a 3′ end to a fixed length based on the Phred quality score (trimmed if score fell below 20, with a minimum read length of 25) [13]. Trimmed RNA-seq reads were aligned to the GRCh38 reference genome with STAR [14] and gene counts were determined using quantMode GeneCounts. Trimmed reads were then aligned using STAR. We used limma-voom transformation and cyclic-loess to normalize the non-biological variability. An assessment of differential expression between groups was evaluated using moderated t-statistics [15].

Significant DEGs between progressive and non-progressive patients were identified based on an adjusted p-value of <0.05 and a fold change (FC) $\geq \pm 2$. The heatmap and statistical analyses were performed using the R statistical package (v3.3.2). Gene set enrichment analysis (GSEA) was performed using GSEA2-2.2.0 software for testing specific gene sets based on Gene Ontology (GO) Biological Processes [16]. The "EnrichmentMap" plug-in of Cytoscape was used to create an enrichment map of the GSEA results, depicting the overlap among pathways, with similar biological processes grouped together as subnetworks [17–19]. A conservative overlap coefficient (0.5) was used to build the enrichment map. The "AutoAnnotate" plug-in identified clusters in an automated manner, visually annotating them with a summary label [20]. RNAseq files and clinical information were deposited in the Gene Expression Omnibus (GEO) with accession number GSE175648.

2.4. Selection and Verification of Prognosis-Related Genes

The DEGs identified in the previous phase were intersected with the TCGA gene expression dataset and overlapping genes were used for further analysis. The raw counts of RNA-sequencing data from the TCGA cohort were normalized using log2-based transformation. This normalized expression was used to build a multigene signature panel. Firstly, we performed univariate Cox regression analysis (considering 637 genes and 3 clinical variables) to identify the potential prognosis-related variables. Then, LASSO (Least Absolute Shrinkage and Selection Operator) regression was applied to construct the gene-based signature for predicting tumor progression in ccRCC using the cvr.glmnet function from ipflasso R package using ten-fold cross-validation and repeated it ten successive runs to increase reliability and robustness [21]. In the machine learning procedure, we fixed the three clinical variables. For all statistical analysis, a p-value < 0.05 was considered significant. All statistical analyses were performed using SPSS 19.0 (Statistical Product and Service Solutions; IBM Corporation, Armonk, NY, USA) and R version 3.4.2 (R Foundation for Statistical Computing, Vienna, Austria).

2.5. Development of a Gene Expression-Based Signature

Based on the expression of each gene discovered and the three clinical variables, each patient's risk score (RS) was calculated according to the risk score model. The risk score model was then used to evaluate the ccRCC prognosis according to the general form RS = exp $\Sigma \beta_i x_i s$, where $i = 1$, k index variables, β_i represents the coefficient for each variable estimated from the Cox regression model, and $x_i s$ the corresponding value for each variable in a given patient. RS was subjected to a Receiver Operating Characteristics (ROC) curve analysis to choose the most appropriate threshold for predicting tumor progression. Thereafter, Kaplan–Meier curves were generated using the selected cut-off point and compared according to the log-rank test.

The endpoints were disease progression, defined as any local relapse or distant metastasis demonstrated by radiological imaging, and cancer-specific survival. We investigated the role of the gene panel alone, clinicopathological variables alone, and a combined model including gene expression and clinicopathological variables as potential predictors of disease progression and cancer-specific survival.

2.6. Pathway Enrichment Analysis

Ingenuity Pathway Analysis (IPA) software was used to identify interactions and networks between the prognostic markers included in our gene signature, possible altered canonical pathways, regulators, diseases and functions based on direct/indirect and experimental targets.

3. Results

3.1. Clinical Features of the Cohort

The clinicopathological characteristics of patients divided by study phase are summarized in Table 1. The median (range) follow-up of the cohort was 45.6 (2.1–135.8) months. During the follow-up period, a total of 68 patients (19.1%) developed tumor progression and a total of 36 patients died of ccRCC. The median time to tumor progression and cancer-related death was 19.9 (2.1–125.5) and 48.5 (2.5–151.2) months, respectively.

Table 1. Demographic and pathological characteristics of enrolled patients.

KERRYPNX	Discovery Phase Hospital Clinic Barcelona (n = 26)	Validation Phase TCGA Cohort (n = 356)
Gender		
Male	18 (69.2)	231 (64.9)
Female	8 (30.8)	125 (35.1)
Age at diagnosis (year)	59 (34–81)	60 (29–90)
Pathological tumor size (cm)	5.5 (1.9–17.5)	5.1 (1.0–25)
ISUP		
ISUP 1	3 (11.5)	4 (1.1)
ISUP 2	12 (46.2)	173 (48.6)
ISUP 3	6 (23.1)	145 (40.7)
ISUP 4	5 (19.2)	34 (9.6)
Tumor stage		
pT1	15 (57.7)	211 (59.3)
pT2	5 (19.2)	41 (11.5)
pT3	5 (19.2)	102 (28.7)
pT4	1 (3.8)	2 (0.6)
N stage		
N0/x	24 (92.3)	346 (97.2)
N1	2 (7.7)	10 (2.8)
Necrosis	10 (38.5)	144 (40.4)
SSIGN score *		
Low risk	12 (46.2)	143 (40.2)
Intermediate risk	8 (30.7)	141 (39.6)
High risk	6 (23.1)	72 (20.2)

* Stage, Size, Grade and Necrosis (SSIGN) score [22].

3.2. Molecular Profiling of ccRCC Samples

Overall, we identified 1380 transcripts that were differentially expressed ($p < 0.05$) between progressive and non-progressive ccRCC samples. Of these, 639 were protein-coding genes; 217 were downregulated and 422 upregulated in progressive compared with non-progressive cases. A heat map based on the most DEGs between the two groups of ccRCC patients is shown in Figure 2A. Gene set enrichment analysis (GSEA) identified several enriched biological processes, such as the dependent toll-like receptor signaling pathway, metabolic process and immune response regulating cell surface receptor signaling pathway (Figure 2B). The full list of GO biological processes is available in Supplementary Materials (Table S2). To aid interpretation of these enriched pathways, we used enrichment maps to create a network-based representation of our results. The most prominent cluster of significantly enriched pathways recapitulated changes in the Catabolism Biological Process and Toll Signaling Pathway (Figure 2C).

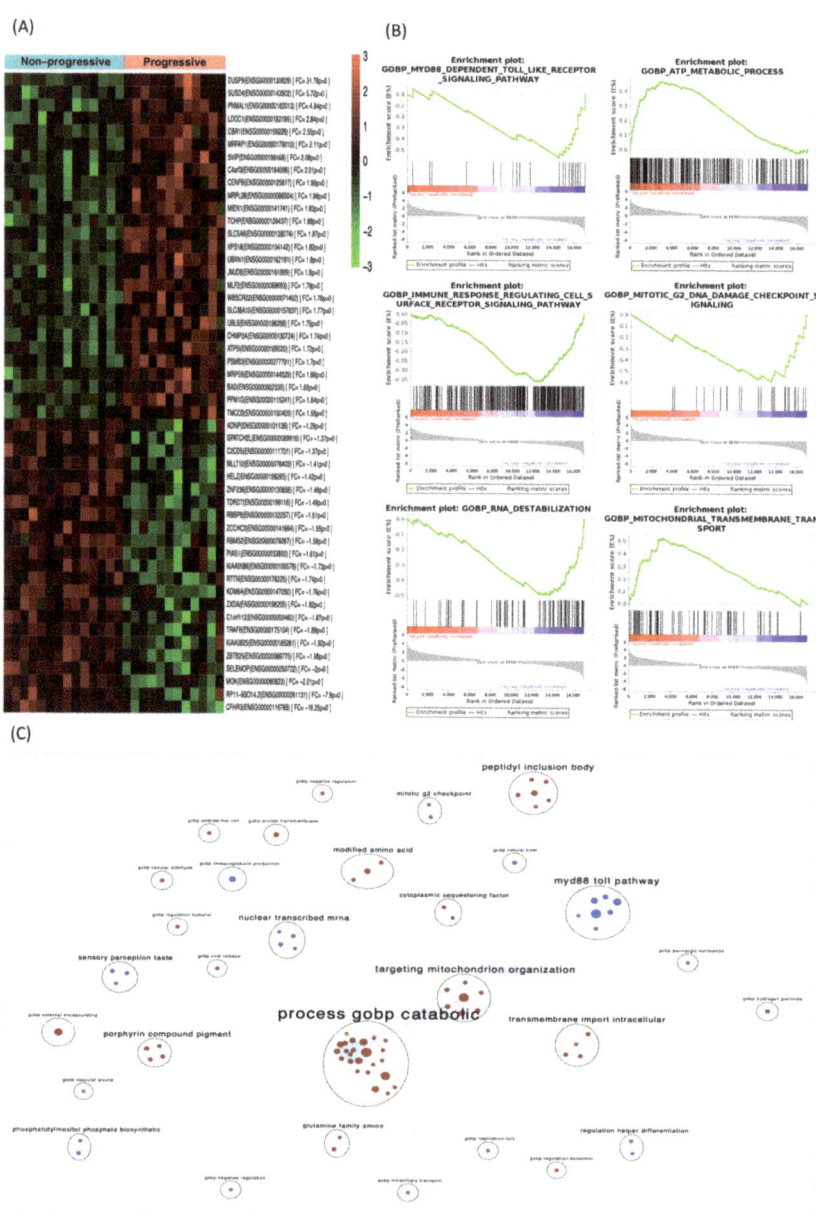

Figure 2. DEGs in the discovery phase and gene-set enrichment analysis. (**A**) Heat map displaying the 50 most DEGs between progressive and non-progressive localized ccRCC patients. Red pixels correspond to upregulated genes, whereas green pixels indicate downregulated genes. (**B**) GSEA shows positive correlation of DEGs in biological processes involved in tumor progression. (**C**) Enrichment map where nodes represent gene sets (pathways) and edges (blue lines) denote overlapping genes between 2 pathways. Node size denotes gene set size. Predicted pathways are grouped as circles, where shades in red correspond to up-regulated gene-sets and shades in light blue correspond to down-regulated gene-sets. Highly redundant gene sets are grouped together as clusters. Abbreviations: DEGs, differentially expressed genes. GSEA, gene set enrichment analysis.

3.3. Identification of Prognosis-Related Genes in an External Data Set

To validate the 639 genes identified as DEGs in the previous study phase, these genes were intersected with the 20,532 genes from the TCGA cohort (Figure 1). As a result, we obtained 637 overlapping genes. Of those, univariate Cox regression analysis identified 132 prognosis-related DEGs and three clinicopathological variables (pT stage, tumor size and ISUP grade).

LASSO regression analysis was used to select the best combination of genes significantly associated with disease progression and to build a six-gene signature. The expressions of five of these genes: CERCAM, HS6ST2, ONECUT2, SOX12 and TMEM132A were upregulated, while MIA2 expression was downregulated in progressive compared with non-progressive cases. According to Ingenuity Pathway Analysis (IPA), these six validated genes were enriched in cancer, organismal injury, abnormalities, cell-to-cell signaling and interactions, cell-mediated immune response, cellular development, cellular growth and proliferation, carbohydrate metabolism, and angiogenesis, among others. Significant IPA canonical pathways are depicted in Supplementary Material Table S3. The network generated shows that there were no direct interactions between the six prognostic genes (Figure S1).

Gene expression values for each selected gene were used for Cox regression analysis. High expression of CERCAM, HS6ST2, ONECUT2, SOX12 and TMEM132A and low expression of MIA2 related to poor outcomes for progression-free survival (Figure S2) and cancer-specific survival (Table 2). Moreover, the clinicopathological variables pT stage, tumor size and ISUP were also found as to be prognostic factors for both survival endpoints.

Table 2. Univariate Cox regression analysis of statistically significant genetic and clinical variables in the validation set (TCGA cohort).

	Progression-Free Survival			Cancer-Specific Survival		
	p	95% CI	HR	p	95% CI	HR
CERCAM	<0.001	1.387–3.807	2.298	<0.001	1.036–1.075	1.055
HS6ST2	<0.001	1.164–3.106	1.902	0.034	1.043–2.866	1.729
MIA2	<0.001	0.222–0.632	0.375	<0.001	0.825–0.935	0.878
ONECUT2	0.015	1.111–2.952	1.811	<0.001	2.443–5.942	3.810
SOX12	0.001	1.354–3.748	2.252	<0.001	1.177–1.488	1.323
TMEM132A	<0.001	1.526–4.288	2.558	<0.001	1.070–1.156	1.112
pT Stage	<0.001	1.775–3.024	2.317	<0.001	2.547–9.940	5.032
Tumor size	<0.001	1.154–1.273	1.212	<0.001	1.125–1.271	1.195
ISUP	<0.001	1.568–3.158	2.225	0.001	1.628–7.845	3.574

3.4. Development of a Prognostic Signature

The risk score (RS) for disease progression was calculated for each patient according to a mathematical algorithm containing the six-gene expression values; pT stage, tumor size and ISUP grade (Supplementary Material Table S4). An ROC analysis of this combined gene expression–clinicopathological model was performed and allowed the selection of a threshold of 0.789 (sensitivity 90% and specificity 60%) and 0.799 (sensitivity 94% and specificity 55%) to categorize patients into high- and low-risk groups for tumor progression and cancer-related death, respectively. The Kaplan–Meier curve of the combined generated gene expression-based model was able to discriminate two groups with significantly different probabilities of tumor progression (hazard ratio (HR) 10.79; 95%, $p < 0.001$) and cancer-specific survival (HR 19.27; 95%, $p < 0.001$) (Figure 3). Notably, the performance of the combined gene expression-based model (Area under the Curve [AUC] 0.824) was higher than that of clinicopathological variables alone (AUC 0.766) or gene expression data alone (AUC 0.753) (Figure S3).

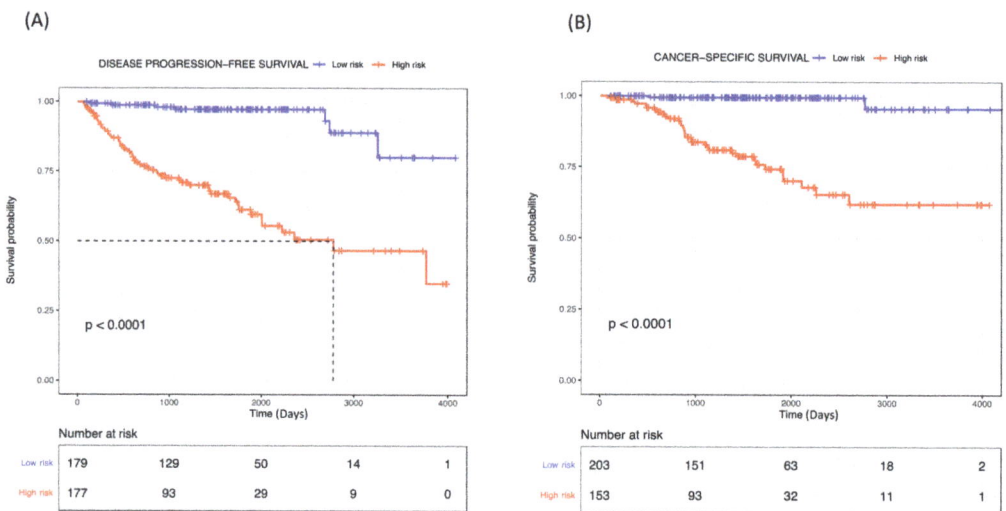

Figure 3. Kaplan–Meier curves of the combined gene expression-based model for (**A**) disease progression-free survival and (**B**) cancer-specific survival for TCGA cohort.

3.5. Correlation Analysis of the RS with Clinical Characteristics for Disease Progression

Given the clinical significance of the RS in ccRCC, we sought to investigate the potential correlation between RS and clinical features. The Mann–Whitney test revealed that higher RSs correlated with a higher risk group within the SSIGN model, higher pT stage and higher ISUP grade (Figure 4). Furthermore, the Kaplan–Meier curve indicated that our established RS was capable of identifying ccRCC patients at the highest risk of progression within the groups stratified by SSIGN, pT stage and ISUP grade (all $p < 0.05$; Figure S4).

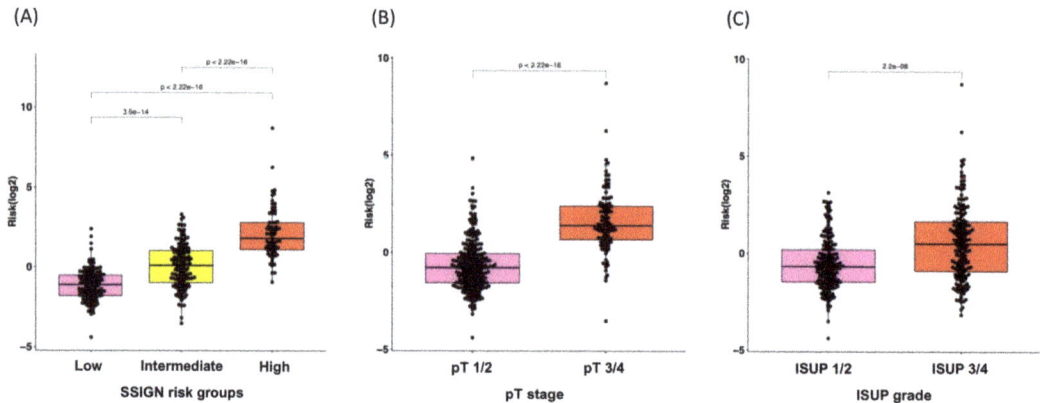

Figure 4. Box plots for the correlation analysis of RS with clinical characteristics for disease progression. (**A**) SSIGN risk groups, (**B**) pT stage and (**C**) ISUP grade.

4. Discussion

Currently, clinicopathological variables are the most valuable tool for predicting disease outcomes in ccRCC. However, due to the highly variable behavior of ccRCC, the prediction of tumor progression is still an important clinical challenge. For decades, surgery has remained the only treatment approved for localized ccRCC [2]. At present, disease management of these patients at high risk of progression is changing and new adjuvant treatments are being considered, opening a door to more personalized medicine in localized renal carcinoma [23,24].

Molecular profiling helps our understanding of the molecular mechanism underlying ccRCC and affords great potential to identify new biomarkers of clinical utility [25,26]. However, intratumor heterogeneity and the methodology for sample processing, readout and expression normalization have been a strong challenge in the development of a robust gene signature. Next-generation sequencing is the most advanced technique for gene expression profiling [27]; here, we used this technology to analyze the entire transcriptome profiling of tissue samples from progressive and non-progressive ccRCC patients. We then established a gene signature for predicting disease progression based on the gene expression and clinical data obtained from the TCGA cohort. We improved the gene selection and accuracy of the model by using LASSO regression analysis; this allowed us to include all DEGs found in the training set and avoid the preselection and validation of only a subset of these DEGs [28].

This study demonstrated that our gene expression-based signature was able to identify localized ccRCC patients with high and low risk of disease progression in the whole cohort and within the SSIGN risk groups. It properly correlated with clinical parameters and was proven to enhance the predictive value of the current clinicopathological variables. Furthermore, it was also predictive of cancer-specific survival. Therefore, our signature may constitute an important step forward in treatment decisions for ccRCC patients.

Remarkably, the developed gene-based panel demonstrated a greater value for prognostic prediction (HR 10.79, $p < 0.001$; AUC = 0.824) compared with similar, previously described models. Dai et al. proposed a four-gene signature with an HR of 3.1, $p < 0.001$, whereas Zhao et al. described a 15-gene model with an AUC of 0.737 [29]. Unfortunately, the different designs and methodologies of several other studies thwart any performance comparisons with their proposed genetic models. Thus, Brook et al. [9] assessed the performance of ClearCode34, which classifies ccRCC into ccA and ccB subtypes, ccB presented tumor relapse more frequently (HR 2.1; $p = 0.001$), whereas Rini et al. [8] generated a 16-gene signature associated with tumor recurrence with an HR per 25-unit increase in score of 3.37 ($p < 0.001$). Likewise, other authors have built molecular signatures aiming to predict overall survival (OS), thus making the classifiers' performance non-comparable [30–32].

Biologically, the genes from our panel are unrelated to each other and many of them have been shown to have either prognostic or biologic relevance in tumor metastasis development. According to previous reports, some of our selected genes were consistent with previously discovered biomarkers; therefore, we have further validated their value for ccRCC progression. Briefly, *CERCAM* (cerebral endothelial cell adhesion molecule) is an adhesion molecule found to be an unfavorable prognostic marker in several tumors [33–35]. Its overexpression promotes cell viability, proliferation and invasion, it is involved in the PI3K/AKT pathway [36] and is part of an immune prognostic signature for colon and rectal cancer [35]. *HS6ST2* (heparan sulfate D-glucosaminyl 6-O-sulfotransferase-2) is a glycolysis-related gene and has also been associated with poor disease outcomes in numerous malignancies [10,37]. Interestingly, our group previously validated this gene as an independent prognosis biomarker in intermediate/high-risk ccRCC and found it to be associated with angiogenesis, epithelia–mesenchymal transition (EMT), and indirectly related to the PD-1, PDL-1 cancer immunotherapy pathway [37–39]. *MIA2* (melanoma inhibitory activity 2) has been found in several malignancies and can act as a tumor suppressor [40] or as a proto-oncogene depending on the receptor-related signaling differences [41]. We found *MIA2* to be downregulated in progressive ccRCC. This is congruent with the human protein atlas findings, where high expression was a favorable prognostic factor in renal cancer [33,42]. *ONECUT2* (One cut domain family member 2) is a transcription factor able to activate oncogenic pathways and lineage-specific genes; hence, it is involved in EMT, angiogenesis, neural differentiation, proliferation, extracellular matrix organization, cell locomotion and migration, among others. Overexpression of *ONECUT2* has been described in several tumors and is related to poor prognosis [43–46]. *SOX12* (Sex-determining region Y-box12) is a transcription factor, its upregulation promotes tumor progression and it is involved in EMT, apoptosis and cell proliferation [47–49]. It functions as an oncogene-regulating Wnt/B-catenin signaling to promote the growth of multiple myeloma cells [50]. As for *TMEM132A*, few studies were found in the literature, so further investigations are required to establish its role in tumor development.

Our study has multiple strengths. The first advantage of our gene expression-based signature is that it contains a low number of genes, making its clinical application easier. Our model did match genes from previous models and some of them exceeded the mere field of ccRCC, highlighting the prognostic power of the selected genes. The fact that they are involved in different carcinogenic mechanisms confers an advantage to our signature compared with others that only target one single pathway [10,51]. The high-throughput technology used to analyze the samples and the statistical methodology makes our gene model a reliable tool for predicting disease progression in ccRCC and adds important prognostic information to the clinicopathological parameters. However, we acknowledge that this study has several limitations. First, the retrospective design and the relatively small sample might have influenced our findings. Second, the definition of CSS in the TCGA cohort should be taken with caution since it was estimated [12]. Finally, despite the good performance of our six-gene model, further validations in larger cohorts are required.

5. Conclusions

A gene expression-based prognostic signature to predict disease progression in ccRCC was successfully developed; it could discriminate two groups with different probabilities of tumor recurrence. In addition, our model was also useful in predicting cancer-specific survival. The combination of genetic and clinical information enhanced the current risk stratification of the localized ccRCC patients. Refining prognostic algorithms could help to improve the disease management and follow-up of ccRCC patients.

Supplementary Materials: The following supporting information can be downloaded at: https://www.mdpi.com/article/10.3390/cancers14153754/s1, Figure S1. Network of gene-gene interactions for the six genes from the gene expression-based signature. Figure S2. Kaplan–Meier curves of each gene of the model evaluating progression free survival (data from the TCGA cohort). Figure S3. ROC curves showing the performance of the gene expression-based signature. The figure depicts that the combined gene expression-based model outperforms clinicopathological variables alone or gene expression data alone. Figure S4. Kaplan–Meier curves of the combined gene expression-based model to evaluate progression-free survival within (A) SSIGN risk groups (low, intermediate and high), (B) pT stage groups (pT1/2 and pT3/4) and (C) ISUP grade groups (ISUP 1/2 and ISUP 3/4) (data from the TCGA cohort). Table S1. Clinical database of TCGA cohort used in this study. Table S2. List of GO biological processes from 1380 differentially expressed transcripts between progressive and non-progressive ccRCC samples. Table S3. Significant IPA canonical pathways from the six genes of the signature. Table S4. Risk Score for disease progression.

Author Contributions: Conceptualization, A.A., L.M., F.L.R. and L.I.; methodology O.R. and F.L.R.; software and validation, F.L.R. and J.J.L.; formal analysis, F.L.R., L.I., L.M. and A.A.; investigation, F.L.R., L.I. and L.M.; resources A.C., M.I.-T. and R.C.; data curation J.J.L. and F.L.R.; writing—original draft preparation, F.L.R. and L.I.; writing—review and editing, all authors contributed to reviewing and editing the writing; visualization, F.L.R. and L.M.; supervision, L.M., L.I. and A.A.; project administration, A.C., M.I.-T. and R.C.; funding acquisition, F.L.R. and A.A. All authors have read and agreed to the published version of the manuscript.

Funding: This work was supported in part by an Emili Letang grant from the Hospital Clínic de Barcelona to FLR/2019.

Institutional Review Board Statement: The study was conducted according to the guidelines of the Declaration of Helsinki and approved by the Institutional Review Board of Hospital clinic of Barcelona (protocol code HBC/2016/0333 and date of approval was 24 January 2019).

Informed Consent Statement: Informed consent was obtained from all subjects involved in the study.

Data Availability Statement: The data presented in this study are available in the article and supplementary material. RNAseq files and clinical information were deposited in the Gene Expression Omnibus (GEO) with accession number GSE175648. Further details can be obtained on request to the corresponding author.

Acknowledgments: We are indebted to the IDIBAPS Biobank for sample and fecha procurement. We thank Azucena Salas and Lluís Revilla for IPA software support. This work was developed at the building Centre de Recerca Biomèdica Cellex, Barcelona. We thank Helena Kruyer the English revision of the manuscript.

Conflicts of Interest: The authors have no conflict of interest to disclose.

References

1. Sung, H.; Ferlay, J.; Siegel, R.L.; Laversanne, M.; Soerjomataram, I.; Jemal, A.; Bray, F. Global Cancer Statistics 2020: GLOBOCAN Estimates of Incidence and Mortality Worldwide for 36 Cancers in 185 Countries. *CA Cancer J. Clin.* **2021**, *71*, 209–249. [CrossRef] [PubMed]
2. Ljungberg, B.; Albiges, L.; Bensalah, K.; Bex, A.; Giles, R.H.; Hora, M.; Kuczyk, M.A.; Lam, T.; Marconi, L.; Canfield, S.; et al. EAU Guidelines. Edn. presented at the EAU Annual Congress Amsterdam 2020. *Eur. Urol.* **2020**, *67*, 913–924. [CrossRef] [PubMed]
3. Klatte, T.; Rossi, S.H.; Stewart, G.D. Prognostic factors and prognostic models for renal cell carcinoma: A literature review. *World J. Urol.* **2018**, *36*, 1943–1952. [CrossRef] [PubMed]
4. Padala, S.A.; Barsouk, A.; Thandra, K.C.; Saginala, K.; Mohammed, A.; Vakiti, A.; Rawla, P.; Barsouk, A. Epidemiology of Renal Cell Carcinoma. *World J. Oncol.* **2020**, *11*, 79. [CrossRef]
5. Motzer, R.J.; Haas, N.B.; Donskov, F.; Gross-Goupil, M.; Varlamov, S.; Kopyltsov, E.; Lee, J.L.; Melichar, B.; Rini, B.I.; Choueiri, T.K.; et al. Randomized phase III trial of adjuvant pazopanib versus placebo after nephrectomy in patients with localized or locally advanced renal cell carcinoma. *J. Clin. Oncol.* **2017**, *35*, 3916–3923. [CrossRef]
6. Haas, N.B.; Manola, J.; Uzzo, R.G.; Flaherty, K.T.; Wood, C.G.; Kane, C.; Jewett, M.; Dutcher, J.P.; Atkins, M.B.; Pins, M.; et al. Adjuvant sunitinib or sorafenib for high-risk, non-metastatic renal-cell carcinoma (ECOG-ACRIN E2805): A double-blind, placebo-controlled, randomised, phase 3 trial. *Lancet* **2016**, *387*, 2008–2016. [CrossRef]
7. Zhao, H.; Cao, Y.; Wang, Y.; Zhang, L.; Chen, C.; Wang, Y.; Lu, X.; Liu, S.; Yan, F. Dynamic prognostic model for kidney renal clear cell carcinoma (KIRC) patients by combining clinical and genetic information. *Sci. Rep.* **2018**, *8*, 17613. [CrossRef]
8. Rini, B.; Goddard, A.; Knezevic, D.; Maddala, T.; Zhou, M.; Aydin, H.; Campbell, S.; Elson, P.; Koscielny, S.; Lopatin, M.; et al. A 16-gene assay to predict recurrence after surgery in localised renal cell carcinoma: Development and validation studies. *Lancet Oncol.* **2015**, *16*, 676–685. [CrossRef]
9. Brooks, S.A.; Brannon, A.R.; Parker, J.S.; Fisher, J.C.; Sen, O.; Kattan, M.W.; Hakimi, A.A.; Hsieh, J.J.; Choueiri, T.K.; Tamboli, P.; et al. ClearCode34: A prognostic risk predictor for localized clear cell renal cell carcinoma. *Eur. Urol.* **2014**, *66*, 77–84. [CrossRef]
10. Xing, Q.; Zeng, T.; Liu, S.; Cheng, H.; Ma, L.; Wang, Y. A novel 10 glycolysis-related genes signature could predict overall survival for clear cell renal cell carcinoma. *BMC Cancer* **2021**, *21*, 381. [CrossRef]
11. FireBrowse. Available online: http://firebrowse.org/ (accessed on 8 October 2021).
12. Liu, J.; Lichtenberg, T.; Hoadley, K.A.; Poisson, L.M.; Lazar, A.J.; Cherniack, A.D.; Kovatich, A.J.; Benz, C.C.; Levine, D.A.; Lee, A.V.; et al. An Integrated TCGA Pan-Cancer Clinical Data Resource to Drive High-Quality Survival Outcome Analytics. *Cell* **2018**, *173*, 400–416.e11. [CrossRef]
13. Babraham Bioinformatics—Trim Galore! Available online: https://www.bioinformatics.babraham.ac.uk/projects/trim_galore/ (accessed on 15 May 2019).
14. Dobin, A.; Davis, C.A.; Schlesinger, F.; Drenkow, J.; Zaleski, C.; Jha, S.; Batut, P.; Chaisson, M.; Gingeras, T.R. STAR: Ultrafast universal RNA-seq aligner. *Bioinformatics* **2013**, *29*, 15–21. [CrossRef]
15. Ritchie, M.E.; Phipson, B.; Wu, D.; Hu, Y.; Law, C.W.; Shi, W.; Smyth, G.K. limma powers differential expression analyses for RNA-sequencing and microarray studies. *Nucleic Acids Res.* **2015**, *43*, e47. [CrossRef]
16. Kanehisa, M.; Goto, S. KEGG: Kyoto Encyclopedia of Genes and Genomes. *Nucleic Acids Res.* **2000**, *28*, 27–30. [CrossRef]
17. Shannon, P.; Markiel, A.; Ozier, O.; Baliga, N.S.; Wang, J.T.; Ramage, D.; Amin, N.; Schwikowski, B.; Ideker, T. Cytoscape: A Software Environment for Integrated Models of Biomolecular Interaction Networks. *Genome Res.* **2003**, *13*, 2498–2504. [CrossRef]
18. Merico, D.; Isserlin, R.; Stueker, O.; Emili, A.; Bader, G.D. Enrichment map: A network-based method for gene-set enrichment visualization and interpretation. *PLoS ONE* **2010**, *5*, e13984. [CrossRef]
19. Reimand, J.; Isserlin, R.; Voisin, V.; Kucera, M.; Tannus-Lopes, C.; Rostamianfar, A.; Wadi, L.; Meyer, M.; Wong, J.; Xu, C.; et al. Pathway enrichment analysis and visualization of omics data using g:Profiler, GSEA, Cytoscape and EnrichmentMap. *Nat. Protoc.* **2019**, *14*, 482–517. [CrossRef]
20. Kucera, M.; Isserlin, R.; Arkhangorodsky, A.; Bader, G.D. AutoAnnotate: A Cytoscape app for summarizing networks with semantic annotations. *F1000Research* **2016**, *5*, 1717. [CrossRef]

21. Boulesteix, A.L.; De Bin, R.; Jiang, X.; Fuchs, M. IPF-LASSO: Integrative L1-Penalized Regression with Penalty Factors for Prediction Based on Multi-Omics Data. *Comput. Math. Methods Med.* **2017**, *2017*, 7691937. [CrossRef]
22. Frank, I.; Blute, M.L.; Cheville, J.C.; Lohse, C.M.; Weaver, A.L.; Zincke, H. An outcome prediction model for patients with clear cell renal cell carcinoma treated with radical nephrectomy based on tumor stage, size, grade and necrosis: The SSIGN score. *J. Urol.* **2002**, *168*, 2395–2400. [CrossRef]
23. Choueiri, T.K.; Tomczak, P.; Park, S.H.; Venugopal, B.; Ferguson, T.; Chang, Y.-H.; Hajek, J.; Symeonides, S.N.; Lee, J.L.; Sarwar, N.; et al. Adjuvant Pembrolizumab after Nephrectomy in Renal-Cell Carcinoma. *N. Engl. J. Med.* **2021**, *385*, 683–694. [CrossRef]
24. Ravaud, A.; Motzer, R.J.; Pandha, H.S.; George, D.J.; Pantuck, A.J.; Patel, A.; Chang, Y.-H.; Escudier, B.; Donskov, F.; Magheli, A.; et al. Adjuvant Sunitinib in High-Risk Renal-Cell Carcinoma after Nephrectomy. *N. Engl. J. Med.* **2016**, *375*, 2246–2254. [CrossRef]
25. Malone, E.R.; Oliva, M.; Sabatini, P.J.B.; Stockley, T.L.; Siu, L.L. Molecular profiling for precision cancer therapies. *Genome Med.* **2020**, *12*, 8. [CrossRef]
26. Dimitrieva, S.; Schlapbach, R.; Rehrauer, H. Prognostic value of cross-omics screening for kidney clear renal cancer survival. *Biol. Direct* **2016**, *11*, 68. [CrossRef]
27. Li, P.; Conley, A.; Zhang, H.; Kim, H.L. Whole-Transcriptome profiling of formalin-fixed, paraffin-embedded renal cell carcinoma by RNA-seq. *BMC Genomics* **2014**, *15*, 1087. [CrossRef]
28. Goeman, J.J. L1 Penalized Estimation in the Cox Proportional Hazards Model. *Biometrical J.* **2010**, *52*, 70–84. [CrossRef]
29. Dai, J.; Lu, Y.; Wang, J.; Yang, L.; Han, Y.; Wang, Y.; Yan, D.; Ruan, Q.; Wang, S. A four-gene signature predicts survival in clear-cell renal-cell carcinoma. *Oncotarget* **2016**, *7*, 82712–82726. [CrossRef]
30. Chen, L.; Luo, Y.; Wang, G.; Qian, K.; Qian, G.; Wu, C.L.; Dan, H.C.; Wang, X.; Xiao, Y. Prognostic value of a gene signature in clear cell renal cell carcinoma. *J. Cell. Physiol.* **2019**, *234*, 10324–10335. [CrossRef]
31. Li, F.; Hu, W.; Zhang, W.; Li, G.; Guo, Y. A 17-Gene Signature Predicted Prognosis in Renal Cell Carcinoma. *Dis. Markers* **2020**, *2020*, 8352809. [CrossRef] [PubMed]
32. Zhang, Z.; Lin, E.; Zhuang, H.; Xie, L.; Feng, X.; Liu, J.; Yu, Y. Construction of a novel gene-based model for prognosis prediction of clear cell renal cell carcinoma. *Cancer Cell Int.* **2020**, *20*, 27. [CrossRef] [PubMed]
33. Uhlen, M.; Zhang, C.; Lee, S.; Sjöstedt, E.; Fagerberg, L.; Bidkhori, G.; Benfeitas, R.; Arif, M.; Liu, Z.; Edfors, F.; et al. A pathology atlas of the human cancer transcriptome. *Science* **2017**, *357*, eaan2507. [CrossRef] [PubMed]
34. Jiang, M.; Wang, H.; Chen, H.; Han, Y. SMARCD3 is a potential prognostic marker and therapeutic target in CAFs. *Aging* **2020**, *12*, 20835–20861. [CrossRef] [PubMed]
35. Wei, R.; Liu, H.; Li, C.; Guan, X.; Zhao, Z.; Ma, C.; Wang, X.; Jiang, Z. Computational identification of 29 colon and rectal cancer-associated signatures and their applications in constructing cancer classification and prognostic models. *Front. Genet.* **2020**, *11*, 740. [CrossRef]
36. Zuo, Y.; Xu, X.; Chen, M.; Qi, L. The oncogenic role of the cerebral endothelial cell adhesion molecule (CERCAM) in bladder cancer cells in vitro and in vivo. *Cancer Med.* **2021**, *10*, 4437–4450. [CrossRef]
37. Roldán, F.L.; Lozano, J.J.; Ingelmo-Torres, M.; Carrasco, R.; Díaz, E.; Ramirez-Backhaus, M.; Rubio, J.; Reig, O.; Alcaraz, A.; Mengual, L.; et al. Clinicopathological and Molecular Prognostic Classifier for Intermediate/High-Risk Clear Cell Renal Cell Carcinoma. *Cancers* **2021**, *13*, 6338. [CrossRef]
38. Lundin, L.; Larsson, H.; Kreuger, J.; Kanda, S.; Lindahl, U.; Salmivirta, M.; Claesson-Welsh, L. Selectively desulfated heparin inhibits fibroblast growth factor-induced mitogenicity and angiogenesis. *J. Biol. Chem.* **2000**, *275*, 24653–24660. [CrossRef]
39. Chen, E.; Stringer, S.E.; Rusch, M.A.; Selleck, S.B.; Ekker, S.C. A unique role for 6-O sulfation modification in zebrafish vascular development. *Dev. Biol.* **2005**, *284*, 364–376. [CrossRef]
40. Hellerbrand, C.; Amann, T.; Schlegel, J.; Wild, P.; Bataille, F.; Spruss, T.; Hartmann, A.; Bosserhoff, A.K. The novel gene MIA2 acts as a tumour suppressor in hepatocellular carcinoma. *Gut* **2008**, *57*, 243–251. [CrossRef]
41. Sasahira, T.; Kirita, T.; Nishiguchi, Y.; Kurihara, M.; Nakashima, C.; Bosserhoff, A.K.; Kuniyasu, H. A comprehensive expression analysis of the MIA gene family in malignancies: MIA gene family members are novel, useful markers of esophageal, lung, and cervical squamous cell carcinoma. *Oncotarget* **2016**, *7*, 31137–31152. [CrossRef]
42. Expression of MIA2 in cancer—Summary—The Human Protein Atlas. Available online: https://www.proteinatlas.org/ENSG00000150527-MIA2/pathology (accessed on 12 May 2022).
43. Ma, Q.; Wu, K.; Li, H.; Li, H.; Zhu, Y.; Hu, G.; Hu, L.; Kong, X. ONECUT2 overexpression promotes RAS-driven lung adenocarcinoma progression. *Sci. Rep.* **2019**, *9*, 20021. [CrossRef]
44. Wu, Y.; Jiang, G.; Zhang, N.; Liu, S.; Lin, X.; Perschon, C.; Zheng, S.L.; Ding, Q.; Wang, X.; Na, R.; et al. HOXA9, PCDH17, POU4F2, and ONECUT2 as a Urinary Biomarker Combination for the Detection of Bladder Cancer in Chinese Patients with Hematuria. *Eur. Urol. Focus* **2020**, *6*, 284–291. [CrossRef] [PubMed]
45. Lu, T.; Wu, B.; Yu, Y.; Zhu, W.; Zhang, S.; Zhang, Y.; Guo, J.; Deng, N. Blockade of ONECUT2 expression in ovarian cancer inhibited tumor cell proliferation, migration, invasion and angiogenesis. *Cancer Sci.* **2018**, *109*, 2221. [CrossRef] [PubMed]
46. Guo, H.; Ci, X.; Ahmed, M.; Hua, J.T.; Soares, F.; Lin, D.; Puca, L.; Vosoughi, A.; Xue, H.; Li, E.; et al. ONECUT2 is a driver of neuroendocrine prostate cancer. *Nat. Commun.* **2019**, *10*, 278. [CrossRef] [PubMed]
47. Wang, L.; Hu, F.; Shen, S.; Xiao, H.; Li, G.; Wang, M.S.; Mei, J. Knockdown of SOX12 expression inhibits the proliferation and metastasis of lung cancer cells. *Am. J. Transl. Res.* **2017**, *9*, 4003.

48. Gu, W.; Wang, B.; Wan, F.; Wu, J.; Lu, X.; Wang, H.; Zhu, Y.; Zhang, H.; Shi, G.; Dai, B.; et al. SOX2 and SOX12 are predictive of prognosis in patients with clear cell renal cell carcinoma. *Oncol. Lett.* **2018**, *15*, 4564–4570. [CrossRef]
49. Huang, W.; Chen, Z.; Shang, X.; Tian, D.; Wang, D.; Wu, K.; Fan, D.; Xia, L. Sox12, a direct target of FoxQ1, promotes hepatocellular carcinoma metastasis through up-regulating Twist1 and FGFBP1. *Hepatology* **2015**, *61*, 1920–1933. [CrossRef]
50. Gao, Y.; Li, L.; Hou, L.; Niu, B.; Ru, X.; Zhang, D. SOX12 promotes the growth of multiple myeloma cells by enhancing Wnt/β-catenin signaling. *Exp. Cell Res.* **2020**, *388*, 111814. [CrossRef]
51. Ghatalia, P.; Gordetsky, J.; Kuo, F.; Dulaimi, E.; Cai, K.Q.; Devarajan, K.; Bae, S.; Naik, G.; Chan, T.A.; Uzzo, R.; et al. Prognostic impact of immune gene expression signature and tumor infiltrating immune cells in localized clear cell renal cell carcinoma. *J. Immunother. Cancer* **2019**, *7*, 139. [CrossRef]

MDPI
St. Alban-Anlage 66
4052 Basel
Switzerland
Tel. +41 61 683 77 34
Fax +41 61 302 89 18
www.mdpi.com

Cancers Editorial Office
E-mail: cancers@mdpi.com
www.mdpi.com/journal/cancers

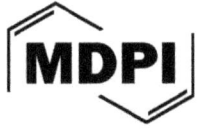

www.ingramcontent.com/pod-product-compliance
Lightning Source LLC
LaVergne TN
LVHW070222100526
838202LV00015B/2076